Colorectal Cancer Liver Metastases

Mauro Monteiro Correia
Michael A. Choti • Flavio G. Rocha
Go Wakabayashi
Editors

Colorectal Cancer Liver Metastases

A Comprehensive Guide to Management

Springer

Editors
Mauro Monteiro Correia
National Cancer Institute
Rio de Janeiro
Brazil

Department of Surgery
UNIVERSIDADE DO GRANDE RIO
Duque de Caxias
Brazil

Flavio G. Rocha
Virginia Mason Medical Center
Seattle, WA
USA

Michael A. Choti
Banner MD Anderson Cancer Center
Phoenix, AZ
USA

Go Wakabayashi
Center for Advanced Treatment
of HBP Diseases
Ageo Central General Hospital
Ageo Shi
Saitama
Japan

ISBN 978-3-030-25485-8 ISBN 978-3-030-25486-5 (eBook)
https://doi.org/10.1007/978-3-030-25486-5

This Springer imprint is published by the registered company Springer Nature Switzerland AG
The registered company address is: Gewerbestrasse 11, 6330 Cham, Switzerland

Preface

This book was originally conceptualized based on our observed need for the practicing clinician to have complete source under one cover that specifically focuses on all aspects of the complex and multidisciplinary management of colorectal liver metastases. Despite an increased emphasis on screening and prevention, colorectal cancer remains one of the most common malignancies worldwide, with an alarming increasing incidence in young patients as well as in many developing countries. Among those diagnosed with this disease, about half will develop metastases, most of which will be involving or confined to the liver. Unlike some other gastrointestinal malignancies where any advanced disease is typically treated with systemic therapies alone, patients with hepatic colorectal metastases are often offered various therapies, including surgical resection, other liver-directed therapies, and combined approaches. In selected cases, long-term survival and even potential for cure may be possible.

Information in this book and the manner in which it is written was designed both for the general clinician or trainee who cares for these cancer patients, as well as for those with specific focus and practice managing patients with liver metastases. We have paid particular attention to providing only the most relevant and up-to-date information necessary for a clinician of different specialties to help manage these patients. More importantly, our goal in this book is to emphasize the importance for an *integrated and multidisciplinary* management approach of this disease.

As one looks thought the table of contents, they will appreciate the complexity and breath of the multidisciplinary approach to patients with hepatic metastases. The book is written by an international team of world-renowned authorities in various specialties, covering topics in their respective areas of expertise. It aims to provide a fully current and referenced text that is succinct as possible, but comprehensive and detailed when necessary. It spans topics ranging from tumor biology, diagnosis, and staging, to advanced aspects of surgical technique. It provides the most updated knowledge in this rapidly advancing field, with specific emphasis on the most complex and multidisciplinary components of care. Debatable topics are discussed by highly regarded authorities, addressing controversies from different perspectives.

We are grateful to our contributors, as well as to our patients who have taught us the importance of much of the subject matter in this book. We believe the result of this comprehensive textbook will serve as an excellent foundation for the understanding of the underlying disease biology, assessment, and patient risk stratification, which are necessary to appropriately select patients for therapy, with the goal of improving survival and quality of life of colorectal cancer patients with liver-only or liver-dominant disease.

Rio de Janeiro, Brazil — Mauro Monteiro Correia
Phoenix, AZ, USA — Michael A. Choti
Seattle, WA, USA — Flavio G. Rocha
Ageo Shi, Saitama, Japan — Go Wakabayashi

Contents

Contributors

Jad Abou Khalil, MD, MSc, FRCSC Department of Surgery, The Ottawa Hospital, Ottawa, ON, Canada

Phillipe Abreu-Reis Brazilian Society of Surgical Oncology, Rio de Janeiro, Brazil

René Adam Centre Hépato-Biliaire, AP-HP Hôpital Paul Brousse, Université Paris Sud, INSERM U935, Villejuif, France

Rehan Ali Department of Radiology, Section of Interventional Radiology, Northwestern Memorial Hospital, Chicago, IL, USA

Marc-Antoine Allard Centre Hépato-Biliaire, AP-HP Hôpital Paul Brousse, Université Paris Sud, INSERM U935, Villejuif, France

Thomas A. Aloia Department of Surgical Oncology, The University of Texas MD Anderson Cancer Center, Houston, TX, USA

Paulo Cezar Galvão do Amaral Department of Gastrointestinal Surgery, San Rafael Hospital, Salvador, Brazil

Blaire Anderson Division of Transplantation Surgery, Department of Surgery at University of Nebraska Medical Center, Omaha, NE, USA

Carlos José Coelho de Andrade Instituto Nacional de Câncer, Americas Centro de Oncologia Integrado, Hospital Pró-Cardíaco, Rio de Janeiro, Brazil

Rodrigo Araújo Department of Abdomino-Pelvic Surgery, Instituto Nacional de Câncer (INCA), Rio de Janeiro, Brazil

André Noronha Arvellos Federal University of Juiz de Fora, Juiz de Fora, Brazil

D. Asano Department of Hepatobiliary and Pancreatic Surgery, Graduate School of Medicine, Tokyo Medical and Dental University, Tokyo, Japan

Mathew M. Augustine Division of Surgical Oncology, Harold C. Simmons Cancer Center, Dallas, TX, USA

Department of Surgery, UT Southwestern Medical Center, Dallas, TX, USA

Bruno Roberto Braga Azevedo Brazilian Society of Surgical Oncology, Rio de Janeiro, Brazil

São Vicente Hospital, São Vicente, Brazil

Hideo Baba Department of Gastroenterological Surgery, Graduate School of Life Sciences, Kumamoto University, Kumamoto, Japan

D. Ban Department of Hepatobiliary and Pancreatic Surgery, Graduate School of Medicine, Tokyo Medical and Dental University, Tokyo, Japan

Toru Beppu Department of Surgery, Yamaga City Medical Center, Yamaga, Japan

Department of Gastroenterological Surgery, Graduate School of Life Sciences, Kumamoto University, Kumamoto, Japan

Giammauro Berardi Center for Advanced Treatment of HBP Diseases, Ageo Central General Hospital, Ageo Shi, Saitama, Japan

Kimberly A. Bertens, MD, MPH, FRCSC Department of Surgery, The Ottawa Hospital, Ottawa, ON, Canada

Marcio Boff Head of Surgical Oncology Mãe de Deus Cancer Center, Mãe de Deus Hospital, Porto Alegre, RS, Brazil

Paulo Henrique Miranda Brandão Department of Abdominal Surgery, Surgical Oncology, A.C. Camargo Cancer Center, São Paulo, Brazil

John Bridgewater University College London Hospital NHS Trust, London, UK

Mariana I. Chavez Division of Surgical Oncology, Medical College of Wisconsin, Milwaukee, WI, USA

Naokazu Chiba Department of Digestive and Transplantation Surgery, Tokyo Medical University Hachioji Medical Center, Tokyo, Japan

Michael A. Choti, MD, MBA Banner MD Anderson Cancer Center, Phoenix, AZ, USA

Jordan M. Cloyd Division of Surgical Oncology, Department of Surgery, The Ohio State University Wexner Medical Center, Columbus, OH, USA

Felipe José Fernández Coimbra Department of Abdominal Surgery, Surgical Oncology, A.C. Camargo Cancer Center, São Paulo, Brazil

Louise C. Connell Memorial Sloan Kettering Cancer Center, New York, NY, USA

Christopher Coon Division of Surgical Oncology, Medical College of Wisconsin, Milwaukee, WI, USA

Mauro Monteiro Correia National Cancer Institute, Rio de Janeiro, Brazil

Department of Surgery, UNIVERSIDADE DO GRANDE RIO, Duque de Caxias, Brazil

Wilson Luiz da Costa Júnior Department of Abdominal Surgery, Surgical Oncology, A.C. Camargo Cancer Center, São Paulo, Brazil

Rinaldo Danesi Hepato-Pancreato-Biliary Surgical Division, Universidade de Blumenau, Santa Catarina Hospital, Blumenau, SC, Brazil

Michael I. D'Angelica Hepatopancreatobiliary Service, Department of Surgery, Memorial Sloan Kettering Cancer Center, New York, NY, USA

Jashodeep Datta Hepatopancreatobiliary Service, Department of Surgery, Memorial Sloan Kettering Cancer Center, New York, NY, USA

The Dewitt Daughtry Family Department of Surgery, Sylvester Comprehensive Cancer Center, University of Miami Miller School of Medicine, Miami, FL, USA

Memorial Sloan Kettering Cancer Center, Weill Cornell Unviersity School of Medicine, Miami, FL, USA

Alessandro Landskron Diniz Department of Abdominal Surgery, Surgical Oncology, A.C. Camargo Cancer Center, São Paulo, Brazil

Svein Dueland Department of Oncology, Oslo University Hospital, Oslo, Norway

Igor Correia de Farias Department of Abdominal Surgery, Surgical Oncology, A.C. Camargo Cancer Center, São Paulo, Brazil

Ryan C. Fields Department of Surgery, Barnes-Jewish Hospital, Washington University School of Medicine, St. Louis, MO, USA

João Paulo Fogacci Hospital dos Servidores do Estado, Rio de Janeiro, Brazil

Yuman Fong City of Hope National Medical Center, Duarte, CA, USA

Ahmed Gabr Department of Radiology, Section of Interventional Radiology, Northwestern Memorial Hospital, Chicago, IL, USA

T. Clark Gamblin Division of Surgical Oncology, Medical College of Wisconsin, Milwaukee, WI, USA

Adriana C. Gamboa Emory University, Atlanta, GA, USA

Roberto de Almeida Gil Department of Medical Oncology, Instituto Nacional de Câncer (INCA), Rio de Janeiro, Brazil

André Luiz de Godoy Department of Abdominal Surgery, Surgical Oncology, A.C. Camargo Cancer Center, São Paulo, Brazil

Laura W. Goff Vanderbilt University Medical Center, Nashville, TN, USA

Rinaldo Gonçalves Department of Abdomino-Pelvic Surgery, Instituto Nacional de Câncer (INCA), Rio de Janeiro, Brazil

Morten Hagness Department of Transplantation Medicine, Oslo University Hospital, Oslo, Norway

Paulo Herman Liver Surgery Unit, Hospital das Clínicas (HC) and Instituto do Câncer do Estado de São Paulo (ICESP), University of São Paulo Medical School, São Paulo, SP, Brazil

Roberto Hernandez-Alejandro University of Rochester, Rochester, NY, USA

Katsunori Imai Department of Gastroenterological Surgery, Graduate School of Life Sciences, Kumamoto University, Kumamoto, Japan

Georgios Karagkounis Department of General Surgery, Cleveland Clinic Foundation, Cleveland, OH, USA

Shigeyuki Kawachi Department of Digestive and Transplantation Surgery, Tokyo Medical University Hachioji Medical Center, Tokyo, Japan

Nancy Kemeny Memorial Sloan Kettering Cancer Center, New York, NY, USA

Sunnie S. Kim The Ruesch Center for the Cure of Gastrointestinal Cancers, Lombardi Comprehensive Cancer Center, Georgetown University Medical Center, Washington, DC, USA

Jaime A. P. Krüger Liver Surgery Unit, Hospital das Clínicas (HC) and Instituto do Câncer do Estado de São Paulo (ICESP), University of São Paulo Medical School, São Paulo, SP, Brazil

Eric C. H. Lai Department of Surgery, Pamela Youde Nethersole Eastern Hospital, Hong Kong, China

Robert Lewandowski Department of Radiology, Section of Interventional Radiology, Northwestern Memorial Hospital, Chicago, IL, USA

Department of Medicine, Division of Hematology and Oncology, Northwestern University, Chicago, IL, USA

Department of surgery, Northwestern University, Chicago, IL, USA

Agnaldo Soares Lima Department of Gastrointestinal Surgery, Hepatopancreatobiliary Unit, Federal University of Minas Gerais, Belo Horizonte, Brazil

Pål-Dag Line Department of Transplantation Medicine, Oslo University Hospital, Oslo, Norway

Institute of Clinical Medicine, University of Oslo, Oslo, Norway

Roberto Heleno Lopes Brazilian Society of Surgical Oncology, Rio de Janeiro, Brazil

University Hospital of the Federal University of Juiz de Fora, Juiz de Fora, Brazil

José Hugo Mendes Luz, MD, EBIR, FCIRSE Head Interventional Radiology Unit, Radiology Department, INCA – Brazilian National Cancer Institute, Rio de Janeiro, Brazil

Shishir K. Maithel Emory University, Atlanta, GA, USA

Ajay V. Maker, MD, FACS Department of Surgery, Division of Surgical Oncology, University of Illinois at Chicago, Chicago, IL, USA

Creticos Cancer Center, Advocate Illinois Masonic Medical Center, Chicago, IL, USA

Rebecca K. Marcus Department of Surgical Oncology, The University of Texas MD Anderson Cancer Center, Houston, TX, USA

Georgios Antonios Margonis Department of Surgery, Johns Hopkins University School of Medicine, Baltimore, MD, USA

John L. Marshall The Ruesch Center for the Cure of Gastrointestinal Cancers, Lombardi Comprehensive Cancer Center, Georgetown University Medical Center, Washington, DC, USA

Guillaume Martel, MD, MSc, FRCSC, FACS Department of Surgery, The Ottawa Hospital, Ottawa, ON, Canada

Ronald Mora Department of Radiology, Section of Interventional Radiology, Northwestern Memorial Hospital, Chicago, IL, USA

Vitor Moutinho AMV Medical Associates, São Paulo, Brazil

Ibrahim Nassour Department of Surgery, UT Southwestern Medical Center, Dallas, TX, USA

Bao Tram Nghiem University of Rochester, Rochester, NY, USA

Marcos Belotto de Oliveira Medical Sciences University—Santa Casa de Misericórdia de São Paulo, São Paulo, Brazil

Medical member of Pancreas MDT of the Santa Casa de Misericórdia de São Paulo, São Paulo, Brazil

Alexandre Ferreira Oliveira Brazilian Society of Surgical Oncology, Rio de Janeiro, Brazil

University Hospital of the Federal University of Juiz de Fora, Juiz de Fora, Brazil

Federal University of Juiz de Fora, Juiz de Fora, Brazil

Timothy M. Pawlik Division of Surgical Oncology, Department of Surgery, The Ohio State University Wexner Medical Center, Columbus, OH, USA

Renata D'Alpino Peixoto Coordinator of Gastrointestinal and Neuroendocrine tumor, Osvaldo Cruz Hospital, São Paulo, Brazil

Ali Pourvaziri Department of Radiology, Massachusetts General Hospital, Harvard Medical School, Boston, MA, USA

Alexandre Prado de Resende Department of Gastrointestinal Surgery, Mater Dei Hospital, Belo Horizonte, Brazil

Ahsun Riaz Department of Radiology, Section of Interventional Radiology, Northwestern Memorial Hospital, Chicago, IL, USA

Heber Salvador de Castro Ribeiro Department of Abdominal Surgery, Surgical Oncology, A.C. Camargo Cancer Center, São Paulo, Brazil

Eliza Dalsasso Ricardo Clinical Oncologist, Osvaldo Cruz Hospital, São Paulo, Brazil

Pablo Duarte Rodrigues Digestive Surgery Division, Universidade Federal de Ciências da Saúde de Porto Alegre, UFCSPA, Centro de Cirurgia Digestiva – CAD, Porto Alegre, RS, Brazil

M. Carmen Rubio Rodriguez Radiation Oncologist, HM Hospitales, Madrid, Spain

Marc T. Roth Vanderbilt University Medical Center, Nashville, TN, USA

Anna Ryan University College London Hospital NHS Trust, London, UK

Dushyant V. Sahani Department of Radiology, Massachusetts General Hospital, Harvard Medical School, Boston, MA, USA

Toru Sano Department of Digestive and Transplantation Surgery, Tokyo Medical University Hachioji Medical Center, Tokyo, Japan

Carlos Eduardo Rodrigues Santos National Cancer Institute, Rio de Janeiro, Brazil

Khalid W. Shaqdan Department of Radiology, Massachusetts General Hospital, Harvard Medical School, Boston, MA, USA

Motohide Shimazu Tama Kyuryo Hospital, Machida, Japan

Raquel Guimarães Domingos da Silva Radiation Oncologist, Instituto Nacional de Câncer, Rio de Janeiro, Brazil

Eve Simoneau Division of Hepatobiliary Surgery and Liver Transplantation, Department of Surgery, University of Montreal, Montreal, Quebec, Canada

Bhavana P. Singh The Ruesch Center for the Cure of Gastrointestinal Cancers, Lombardi Comprehensive Cancer Center, Georgetown University Medical Center, Washington, DC, USA

Mariana Bruno Siqueira D'Or Institute of Research and Education (IDOR), Rio de Janeiro, Brazil

Malcolm H. Squires III Division of Surgical Oncology, Department of Surgery, The Ohio State University Wexner Medical Center, Columbus, OH, USA

Camille Stewart City of Hope National Medical Center, Duarte, CA, USA

M. Tanabe Department of Hepatobiliary and Pancreatic Surgery, Graduate School of Medicine, Tokyo Medical and Dental University, Tokyo, Japan

Chung Ngai Tang Department of Surgery, Pamela Youde Nethersole Eastern Hospital, Hong Kong, China

Uirá Fernandes Teixeira Digestive Surgery Division, Universidade Federal de Ciências da Saúde de Porto Alegre, UFCSPA, Centro de Cirurgia Digestiva – CAD, Porto Alegre, RS, Brazil

Koichi Tomita Department of Digestive and Transplantation Surgery, Tokyo Medical University Hachioji Medical Center, Tokyo, Japan

Orlando Jorge Martins Torres Department of Gastrointestinal Surgery, Hepatopancreatobiliary Unit—Federal University of Maranhão, São Luís, Brazil

Thuy B. Tran, MD Department of Surgery, Division of Surgical Oncology, University of Illinois at Chicago, Chicago, IL, USA

Creticos Cancer Center, Advocate Illinois Masonic Medical Center, Chicago, IL, USA

Ching-Wei D. Tzeng Department of Surgical Oncology, The University of Texas MD Anderson Cancer Center, Houston, TX, USA

Marcus Valadão Department of Abdomino-Pelvic Surgery, Instituto Nacional de Câncer (INCA), Rio de Janeiro, Brazil

Fábio Luiz Waechter Digestive Surgery Division, Universidade Federal de Ciências da Saúde de Porto Alegre, UFCSPA, Centro de Cirurgia Digestiva – CAD, Porto Alegre, RS, Brazil

Go Wakabayashi Center for Advanced Treatment of HBP Diseases, Ageo Central General Hospital, Ageo Shi, Saitama, Japan

Kerollos Nashat Wanis Western University, London, ON, Canada

Benjamin A. Weinberg The Ruesch Center for the Cure of Gastrointestinal Cancers, Lombardi Comprehensive Cancer Center, Georgetown University Medical Center, Washington, DC, USA

Matthew J. Weiss Department of Surgery, Johns Hopkins University School of Medicine, Baltimore, MD, USA

Pancreas Cancer Multidisciplinary Clinic, Liver Cancer Multidisciplinary Clinic, Johns Hopkins University, Baltimore, MD, USA

Yasushi Yoshida Department of Surgery, Yamaga City Medical Center, Yamaga, Japan

Department of Gastroenterological Surgery, Graduate School of Life Sciences, Kumamoto University, Kumamoto, Japan

Surgical Treatment of Colorectal Cancer Liver Metastases (CRLM) - Historical Aspects

1

Carlos Eduardo Rodrigues Santos
and Mauro Monteiro Correia

The history of hepatectomies for metastases relates to the very history of the evolution of liver surgery, and a brief historical review is necessary. This chapter represents our individual view of the evolutionary steps of liver surgery for CRLM biased by our scientific and cultural background. We understand and agree that others might enrich this story with other geographical and historical facts as well as distinct cultural points of view. We have made an effort to include what we understand have been the most relevant milestones and protagonists and we might have failed somewhere in the process. Therefore, we apologize for any data omitted in this chapter, which is not intended to be comprehensive.

The liver was the only organ that summarized the custom of predicting the future among the Babylonians, Etruscans, Greeks, and Romans and was considered the site of the soul, the vital organ, and the central place of the human body [1].

Hepatobiliary surgery, specifically surgery for CRLM, had to await the advent of general anesthesia and antisepsis to evolve, mainly after WW II. But there are some anecdotal reports, such as that of Berta in 1716, when he accomplished a partial hepatectomy in a war open wound. In 1886, Lius described the first elective resection of a hepatic adenoma, followed by the unfortunate death of the patient, and in 1888, Langenbuch in Germany made the first planned partial lobectomy [2]. This patient required reoperation to control bleeding. In 1898, Cantlie described the delimitation of the anatomical division between the two hemilivers, through studies with vascular casts naming it the main lobar fissure. This work was extended by

C. E. R. Santos
National Cancer Institute, Rio de Janeiro, Brazil
e-mail: carloseduardo@cirurgiaonline.com.br

M. M. Correia (✉)
National Cancer Institute, Rio de Janeiro, Brazil

Department of Surgery, UNIVERSIDADE DO GRANDE RIO, Duque de Caxias, Brazil

M. M. Correia et al. (eds.), *Colorectal Cancer Liver Metastases*,
https://doi.org/10.1007/978-3-030-25486-5_1

Hjostsjo and Healy and Schroy, who demonstrated the sectorial lobular divisions, and both paved the way for a few courageous hepatic surgeons [3].

The first surgeon to describe an elective resection of the liver tumor was Tiffany in 1890 [4]. An important step toward a safer liver resection occurred in 1908, when J. Hogarth Pringle, a Scottish surgeon, published an article in the *Annals of Surgery* using the cross-clamping of the liver pedicle for control of hepatic hemorrhage in trauma drawn from his experiences with rabbits. In this initial report, four patients died despite the maneuver [5].

One of the first reports of successful surgery for CRLM was made by Catell in 1940 [6]. In 1948, Raven reported an anatomical lateral left sectorectomy for liver metastasis of colorectal cancer [7]. In 1949, Honjo in Japan performed an anatomical right hepatectomy [8].

For a long time, hepatectomies were considered as exceptions and were mostly performed for biliary disease, until Lortat-Jacob performed the first hepatectomy with vascular control in 1952. Later, the physiologic vascular segmentation of the liver would be described by Couinaud in 1957, in the magnificent book "*Le foie: études anatomiques et chirurgicales. Masson, Paris.*"

In the second half of the twentieth century, important technical advances were introduced, such as anatomic segmentectomies, total hepatic exclusion, and subsegmentectomies [9, 10, 11].

More recently, maneuvers such as Jacques Belghiti's "Liver hanging maneuver" and the use of intra-hepatic Doppler ultrasonography to aid the resection of the venous trunks described by Torzilli have increased the tactical arsenal of surgeons [12, 13].

Hepatectomies for metastasis have remained occasional, since the vast majority of metastases are large or multiple at presentation. The cases usually indicated for resection were initially those of single and indolent metastases in highly selected patients. It was then that some initial publications started to report long-term survivals with the combination of surgery and chemotherapy in the second half of the twentieth century. After the association of 5FU and leucovorin, standardized by the Mayo Clinic, new chemotherapeutic drugs and drug associations with a higher degree of response emerged. The first publication aiming conversion of unresectable metastases was that of Prof. Henri Bismuth, with the article "Resection of Irresectable Metastases" [14]. For the first time, that group obtained an effective response with size reduction of CRLM using the combination of oxaliplatin, 5FU, and leucovorin, in "chronodulation," in about 12% of the patients, which doubled the number of possible resectable patients at that time.

Since then, the association of surgeons with clinical oncologists and radiologists in the process of decision making for multidisciplinary treatment of initially unresectable CRLM has raised the 5-year survival rate from 0% to 38%.

It was also noticed that at least 50% of these patients recurred, and only some could be re-operated. When these surgeries were successful, they led to a survival equivalent to those who had been operated only once. Prof. Rene Adam validated this procedure, and re-hepatectomies and parenchymal-sparing surgery became the standard of care [15].

Chemotherapy continued to evolve, and new drugs appeared with irinotecan and later anti-angiogenic drugs such as anti-VGRF and EGRF antibodies, increasing the tumor response rate to levels never before achieved, sometimes reaching 80% response rates.

Although this response rate has not yet been translated into a long-term survival rate, it has allowed the improvement of new chemotherapeutic treatment protocols. "Conversion chemotherapy," where there is maximum response of chemotherapy, is performed in order to achieve tumor reduction for hepatectomy. The joint analysis of the Hepatobiliary Surgeon and the Clinical Oncologist is fundamental for choosing which patients are eligible for this protocol, whose effective response had a direct impact on survival, as described by Rubbia-Brandt [16]. There is logic that, in parallel, new challenges were emerging as to how best to deal with the damage of chemotherapy in the non-tumor liver, as described by Jean Nicolas Vauthey [17].

Even so, most patients still could not be resected due to the lack of sufficient estimated remnant liver. This was when the observation of the liver behavior of patients with hepatocellular carcinoma involving one-side portal tumor thrombosis showed a contralateral hypertrophy, especially when the surgeon decided to tie this thrombosed side of the portal vein, in order to avoid the tumor thrombus to progress to the portal trunk, as described by Honjo [18]. It was observed that, although there was no direct tumor effect, there was sufficient contralateral hypertrophy to make a hepatectomy possible. Since then, previous portal embolization has been performed with this objective, establishing a functional hepatectomy prior to the now-possible anatomical hepatectomy, as described by Kinoshita [19].

The limits of hepatic hypertrophy were also amplified with the advent of two-time hepatectomy and, more recently, the Associating Liver Partition and Portal Vein Ligation for Staged Hepatectomy - ALLPS, by Schlitt, at Regensburg. Germany, in 2007 [20].

At the same time, methods of local thermal tumor destruction were developed, such as cryoablation (cold) and radioablation (heat), which allowed tumor destruction in those patients who, for technical or clinical reasons, could not be resected and to the use of non-bleeding sections in hepatectomies as proposed by Nagy Habbib [21].

Also, the surgical techniques themselves have been improved, with the use of hepatic parenchymal dissection technologies with less bleeding such as with the use of ultrasonic dissectors or with jet of water, reducing bleeding and allowing the dissection of areas before difficult to access as the vascular pedicles [22].

In hemostasis, there were also advances such as the creation of argon beam coagulators and the invention of new surface hemostatic agents (patch, powder, and glue) and energy equipment such as electrothermal bipolar tissue sealing system and ultrasonic sealer, derived from cable end fusion technology in sailing boats.

Imaging diagnosis also evolved to integrate the surgical field with the use of intraoperative ultrasound, first described by Makuuchi in 1983. Ultrasound makes the liver transparent to the eyes of the surgeon, reducing the risk of intraoperative bleeding and detailing the position of the lesions and their relation with vessels. There is also the added benefit of potentially detecting unsuspected lesions and avoiding unnecessary surgeries, besides allowing guided intraoperative biopsies and treatments [23, 24].

The preoperative imaging tests also evolved greatly with more sensitive CT and magnetic resonance (MR) techniques with specific hepatocellular contrasts, and nuclear medicine was associated with these advances, and positron emission tomography (PET CT) became part of the imaging armamentarium for diagnosis and treatment planning. PET CT impacted the selection of patients, detecting extrahepatic lesions in about 25% of the cases, resulting in a better survival rate in those selected patients [25].

The development of minimally invasive techniques introduced by videolaparoscopy for liver resections, as reported by Gagner in 1992 and, more recently, with robotic liver resections in the twenty-first century, has made possible the diminution of incisions, reduction of postoperative pain, and enhancement of surgical recovery [26, 27, 28].

Besides, Dr. Thomas Aloia, of MD, proposed certain ways to enhance postoperative recovery in conventional open surgeries with the protocol known as enhanced surgery and enhanced recovery, which have been adopted worldwide for liver resections [29].

Even the way of approaching synchronous liver and colorectal lesions evolved to the reverse approach proposed by the late Gilles Mentha, who reversed the paradigm of oncological resections, proposing the resection of the metastatic liver before the primary colorectal, using the rationale that would often be the hepatic metastases that would lead to the patient death, not the primary one, obviously after analyzing the severity of each tumor [30].

Since opportunity has always been the mother of inventions, Pal Dag Line, a Norwegian surgeon, in view of the surplus of organs for liver transplantation in his country, began to transplant patients with unresectable liver disease restricted to the liver, exceeding 60% of survival in 5 years. This experience has revived the curiosity around the world about this indication for liver transplantation [31].

Navigated liver surgery, derived from the neuronavigation, associated or not with the virtual or expanded reality, is in its dawn. This technique has been developed in many different countries and institutes, such as in Strasbourg-France, by Prof. Marescaux's team. The patient's individual anatomy is matched with the reconstructed 3D images, allowing, for example, the location of metastases that have disappeared with chemotherapy (missing metastases) and the navigation of instruments during minimally invasive surgeries.

Presently, the collaboration of Hepatobiliary Surgeons, Clinical Oncologists, Hepatologists, Radiologists and Interventional Radiologists in multidisciplinary meetings have become central in the correct management of patients with CRLM, increasing resectability and survival of many.

The union of all those techniques and approaches had led to what Prof Dong from Beijing calls as "Precision in Liver Surgery," adopting the best way of treatment individualized for each patient [32].

The comprehensive book written by Prof. Leslie H Blumgart entitled "*Hepatobiliary-Pancreatic Surgery*," first released in 1988, was the first occidental of a growing series of international literature on specific hepatobiliary–pancreatic surgery, which have been guiding surgeons for generations [33].

Many other surgeons were instrumental in this evolutionary process, producing scientific publications creating specialized medical societies, such as IHPBA.

IHPBA dates back to 1978 when it was founded as the International Biliary Association (IBA) in San Francisco, California. The new IHPBA was formally inaugurated at its first General Assembly on 31 May 1994 in Boston, Massachusetts, USA. The IHPBA was incorporated as a non-profit organization with the goals of finding effective treatment for the disorders of the liver, pancreas, and biliary tree: to promote understanding, encourage change, study problems, foster friendship in the field of HPB surgery, strive toward the highest ethical standards, and advanced education and career development in the field.

The multiple chapters of IHPBA around countries and continents help spread knowledge about HPB surgery, transforming a disease considered terminal in old days into a treatable one with real hope for cure in some cases.

We are certain that surgery for liver metastases will have a future even brighter than its past.

References

1. Martins ACA, Martins C. History of liver anatomy: Mesopotamian liver clay models. HPB. 2013;115(4):322–3.
2. Lius A. Di un adenoma del fegato. Gazz delle cliniche. 1886;23.
3. Cantlie J. On a new arrangement of the right and left lobes of the liver. J Anat Physiol. 1898;32:4–10.
4. Tiffany L. The removal of a solid tumor from the liver by laparotomy. Maryland Med J. 1890;23:531.
5. Pringle JG. Notes on the arrest of hepatic haemorrhage due to trauma. Ann Surg. 1908;48: 541–9.
6. Cattell RB. Successful removal of liver metastasis from carcinoma of the rectum. Lahey Clinic Bull. 1940;2:7–11.
7. Raven RW. Partial hepatectomy. Br J Surg. 1948;36:397–401.
8. Honjo I, Araki C. Total resection of the right lobe of the liver. J Int Coll Surg. 1955;23:23–8.
9. Bismuth H, et al. Major and minor segmentectomies "reglèes" in liver surgery. World J Surg. 1982;6:10–24.
10. Bismuth H, et al. Major hepatic resection under total vascular exclusion. Ann Surg. 1989;210(1):13–9.
11. Makuuchi M, et al. Ultrasonically guided subsegmentectomy. Surg Gynecol Obstet. 1985;161:346–50.
12. Torzilli G, Procopio F, Viganò L, et al. Vein management in a parenchyma-sparing policy for resecting colorectal liver metastases at the caval confluence. Surgery. 2018;163(2):277–84.
13. Belghiti J, Guevara OA, Noun R, Saldinger PF, Kianmanesh R. Liver hanging maneuver: a safe approach to right hepatectomy without liver mobilization. J Am Coll Surg. 2001;193(1):109–11.
14. Bismuth H, Adam R, Lévi F, et al. Resection of nonresectable liver metastases from colorectal cancer after neoadjuvant chemotherapy. Ann Surg. 1996;224(4):509–20.
15. Adam R, Bismuth H, Castaing D, et al. Repeat hepatectomy for colorectal liver metastases. Ann Surg. 1997;225(1):51–62.
16. Rubbia-Brandt L, Giostra E, Brezault C, et al. Importance of histological tumor response assessment in predicting the outcome in patients with colorectal liver metastases treated with neo-adjuvant chemotherapy followed by liver surgery. Ann Oncol. 2007;18(2):299–04.

17. Kishi Y, Zorzi D, Contreras CM, et al. Extended preoperative chemotherapy does not improve pathologic response and increases postoperative liver insufficiency after hepatic resection for colorectal liver metastases. Ann Surg Oncol. 2010;17(11):2870–6.
18. Honjo I, Suzuki T, Ozawa K, Takasan H, Kitamura O. Ligation of a branch of the portal vein for carcinoma of the liver. Am J Surg. 1975;130(3):296–302.
19. Kinoshita H, Sakai K, Hirohashi K, Igawa S, Yamasaki O, Kubo S. Preoperative portal vein embolization for hepatocellular carcinoma. World J Surg. 1986;10(5):803–8.
20. Schnitzbauer AA, Lang SA, Goessmann H, et al. Right portal vein ligation combined with in situ splitting induces rapid left lateral liver lobe hypertrophy enabling 2-staged extended right hepatic resection in small-for-size settings. Ann Surg. 2012;255:405–14.
21. Weber JC, Navarre G, Jiao LR, Nicholls JP, Jensen SL, Habib NA. New technique for liver resection using heat coagulative necrosis. Ann Surg. 2002;236(5):560–3.
22. Hodgson WJ, DelGuercio LR. Surgical technique, preliminary experience in liver surgery using the ultrasonic scalpel. Surgery. 1984;95(2):230–4.
23. Guimaraes CM, Correia MM, Baldisserotto M, Aires EPQ, Coelho JF. Intraoperative ultrasonography of the liver in patients with abdominal tumors. J Ultrasound Med. 2006;23:1549–55.
24. Makuuchi M, Hasegawa H, Yamazaki S. Intraoperative ultrasonic examination for hepatectomy. Ultrasound Med Biol. 1983;(Suppl 2):493–7.
25. Strasberg SM, Dehdashti F, Siegel BA, Drebin JA, Linehan D. Survival of patients evaluated by FDG-PET before hepatic resection for metastatic colorectal carcinoma: a prospective database study. Ann Surg. 2001;233(3):293–9.
26. Gagner M, Rheault M, Dubuc J. Laparoscopic partial hepatectomy for liver tumor (abstract). Surg Endosc. 1992;6:99.
27. Choi SB, Park JS, Kim JK, et al. Early experiences of robotic-assisted laparoscopic liver resection. Yonsei Med J. 2008;49:632–8.
28. Vasile S, Sgarbură O, Tomulescu V, Popescu I. The robotic-assisted left lateral hepatic segmentectomy: the next step. Chirurgia (Bucur). 2008;103:401–5.
29. Day RW, Cleeland CS, Wang XS, et al. Patient-reported outcomes accurately measure the value of an enhanced recovery program in liver surgery. J Am Coll Surg. 2015;221(6):1023–30.
30. Mentha G, Roth AD, Terraz S, et al. 'Liver first' approach in the treatment of colorectal cancer with synchronous liver metastases. Dig Surg. 2008;25(6):430–5.
31. Hagness M, Foss A, Line PD, et al. Liver transplantation for nonresectable liver metastases from colorectal cancer. Ann Surg. 2013;257(5):800–6.
32. Dong J, Yang S, Zeng J, Cai S, Ji W, Duan W, Zhang A, Ren W, Xu Y, Tan J, Bu X, Zhang N, Wang X, Wang X, Meng X, Jiang K, Gu W, Huang Z. Semin Liver Dis. 2013;33(3):189–203.
33. Belghiti J, Jarnagin WR. Blumgart's surgery of the liver, biliary tract an pancreas. Philadelphia: Elsevier; 2017.

The Biology of Colorectal Liver Metastases

2

Mathew M. Augustine

Introduction

In 2018, colorectal cancer (CRC) was diagnosed in approximately two million people worldwide, accounting for 10% of cancer diagnoses. It is estimated that one million people died from colorectal cancer this past year, accounting for 9% of cancer-related deaths [1, 2]. CRC is the third leading cause of cancer in males and the second leading cause in females. For patients diagnosed with stage 1 and early stage 2 CRC, surgical resection of the primary tumor is considered curative, with a low risk for distant metastatic progression and no systemic chemotherapy requirement. Unfortunately, for approximately 50% of CRC patients, metastatic disease is present at the time of diagnosis or ultimately develops [3]. The consequences of metastasis are significant, as it is the major cause of cancer-related morbidity and death. While systemic cytotoxic and targeted therapies are offered with the hope of eliminating disease progression and metastatic spread, they rarely cure metastasis due to intrinsic or acquired resistance. However, for a very select group of patients with metastatic CRC, surgery offers the only curative option, offering 5-year overall survival rates of 50–60% [4–6].

Despite significant advances in our understanding of CRC tumorigenesis, metastasis remains an investigational and therapeutic challenge. Metastasis is a complex process involving a dynamic interplay of numerous intrinsic and extrinsic factors. For metastasis to succeed, several steps must be successfully executed. Cancer cells undergo genetic and epigenetic alterations that result in their growth and expansion, epithelial–mesenchymal transition (EMT), and invasion of the surrounding tissue including the vasculature of blood vessels or lymphatic channels (intravasation).

M. M. Augustine (✉)
Division of Surgical Oncology, Harold C. Simmons Cancer Center, Dallas, TX, USA

Department of Surgery, UT Southwestern Medical Center, Dallas, TX, USA
e-mail: Mathew.Augustine@UTSouthwestern.edu

M. M. Correia et al. (eds.), *Colorectal Cancer Liver Metastases*,
https://doi.org/10.1007/978-3-030-25486-5_2

Tumor cells that have breached their native environment must survive the hostile conditions of transit through two vascular systems, attach or become lodged in the microvessels of a distant host organ, migrate from the bloodstream into the parenchyma of that organ (extravasation), and survive within the new foreign microenvironment (colonization) [7, 8]. Along this trajectory, cancer cells maintain a dynamic dialogue with cells in their local environment (tumor microenvironment). These multiple layers of biologic complexity involved in the metastatic process underscore why metastasis remains a poorly understood phenomenon. Investigating the biologic factors that underlie metastatic development is crucial in improving both the detection and treatment of CRC liver metastasis.

Metastasis is the terminal step in a multi-step tumorigenic process that takes place over several decades. The average patient age at the time of diagnosis of sporadic colorectal cancer is 65 years. Mathematical estimates reveal that while the timeframe between the development of a large colonic adenoma and invasive adenocarcinoma is close to two decades, progression from advanced carcinoma to the detection of metastasis is less than 2 years, indicating that once invasive carcinoma develops, metastatic dissemination commences quickly thereafter [9]. When considering the proportion of invasive cancers routinely identified, we would expect synchronous metastatic disease to be diagnosed in almost all cases, presenting with innumerable nodules at multiple sites. Clinical experience indicates that this is not the case. Accomplishing all the steps toward metastatic colonization is a very inefficient process, with only a small proportion of cancer cells surviving inhospitable environments and, ultimately, finding the appropriate target organ environment to survive. Once colonized, these cells may lay in a dormant state for years before revealing themselves as macrometastatic nodules.

Colorectal Carcinogenesis

Colorectal cancer tumorigenesis begins within the same anatomic compartment from which intestinal epithelial regeneration occurs. The intestinal epithelium is organized into large numbers of crypt-villus units (of note, the colon has a flat epithelium instead of villi). Residing within the base of the crypts are self-renewing, intestinal stem cells [10, 11]. These cells are exposed to stromal-derived soluble Wnt factors, which engage their cognate stem cell receptor. Activation of Wnt signaling initiates a cascade of events that result in the stabilization and accumulation of nuclear β-catenin, where it associates with DNA-binding proteins that promote transcriptional programs, which maintain the intestinal stem cell phenotype [12]. Wnt signaling is critical in maintaining hierarchical organization along the crypt–villus axis. As these cells undergo proliferation and asymmetric division, a subset of cells remains in the crypt, preserving stem cell properties. A subpopulation of daughter cells migrates out of the crypts, amplifies along the crypt axis (transit-amplifying cells), and differentiates into four intestinal cell types (enterocytes, enteroendocrine cells, goblet cells, and Paneth cells) that function mostly at the epithelial surface where they perform unique functions prior to undergoing cell death.

The successive rounds of DNA replication and cell division imposed on intestinal stem cells expose these cells to acquiring mutational events throughout their lifetime. Environmental and lifestyle factors including diet, gut microbial composition, inflammation, and smoking expedite the mutational rate and compress the timeframe for tumorigenesis. Histological data reveal that most CRCs arise from preexisting benign tumors (adenomas) and follow a succession of mutational events culminating in genomic instability [13, 14]. These mutational events include the activation of key driver oncogenes, inactivation of tumor suppressor genes, and epigenetic modifications. Through these genetic and epigenetic alterations, intestinal stem cells enhance their proliferative advantage, maintain residence within the crypts, and inactivate apoptotic mechanisms. It should come as little surprise that mutations in members of the Wnt pathway are early genetic drivers that initiate CRC development. Adenomatous polyposis coli gene (*APC*), a tumor suppressor that negatively controls β-catenin levels within the cytosol, is the most commonly mutated gene in colon cancer. Truncating mutations in *APC* and epigenetic silencing at the *APC* promoter result in its inactivation and inability to degrade and regulate β-catenin levels. In cases lacking APC alterations, genetic alterations in other members of the Wnt signaling pathway are found including *β-catenin*, *AXIN2*, *SOX9*, *TCF7L1/2*, and R-spondin family members *RSPO2* and *RSPO3* [15, 16]. Overall, the WNT signaling pathway is altered in 93% of all CRC tumors in the TCGA analysis [16]. The genetic alterations that result in aberrant Wnt signaling maintain the intestinal stem cell-like phenotype, make the cells less dependent on stromal Wnt signaling, prevent further differentiation, and preserve the proliferation of cells within the crypts, leading to the outgrowth of adenomatous polyps, the precursor lesion that ultimately develop into colon cancer [10]. The addiction to Wnt signaling is further supported by investigations that revealed how intestinal cells further amplify Wnt signaling through the expression of the soluble factors HGF and PGE2, which are secreted from stromal cells within the initiating tumor microenvironment [17, 18]. Subsequent mutational events resulting in activation of the KRAS/BRAF pathway lead to the development of small adenomas [13]. Acquisition of mutations to *p53*, *PI3KCA*, and loss of signaling through the TGF-β pathway propel adenoma to invasive carcinoma progression. Recently, application of CRISPR-Cas9 genome-editing technology to introduce mutations in these pathways from human intestinal epithelial organoids was employed. Organoids harboring these mutations were capable of growth independent of niche factors and formed tumors in foreign tissues [19–21]. These investigations revealed that mutations in these pathways prove sufficient to support tumor development and survival [19–21]. While DNA sequencing has revealed a wide spectrum of mutational events associated with primary colorectal cancer development [16], paired mutational analysis of primary colorectal and metastatic lesions reveals a few novel mutations in metastatic lesions [9]. This finding supports the concept that metastasis occurs as a late clonal expansion of the primary tumor or that non-genetic factors influence the cellular behavior that promotes metastatic development.

Colon Cancer Stem Cells and the Hierarchical Organization Model

Originally, it was believed that tumors developed along the lines of a "clonal succession model" in which mutational events spawn clonal progeny that expand and mutate, giving rise to successive populations of clones, which undergo further mutational events that result in invasive carcinoma and metastasis. However, over the past decade, a growing body of research supports a "hierarchical organization model" for tumorigenesis that mirrors the normal role of intestinal stem cells in epithelial organization and development. Investigations by several groups revealed that CRC tumors harbor a small sub-population of self-renewing "cancer stem cells" that possess the capacity to give rise to a progressively differentiated population of cells that comprise the original tumor [22–24]. These tumor-initiating cells, identified by unique cell surface marker expression profiles proliferate, generate the full population of cells that comprise the tumor and survive transplantation in foreign tissue microenvironments [22–24]. Cancer stem cells appear to appropriate the genetic programs that exist within normal stem cells. As tumor progression continues, the cancer stem cells exhibit increasing genomic instability and are modified by the tumor microenvironment, giving rise to genetically distinct subclones that propel the development of intratumor heterogeneity (ITH). Through genetic, epigenetic, and microenvironment modifications, ITH fuels the development of subclones that ultimately give rise to metastasis.

CRC Molecular Classification Subtypes and the Role of Stroma

Despite the extensive heterogeneity that marks cancer progression, investigations led by several groups were able to classify CRC into molecular subtypes (CMSs) [25–30]. From these classifications, four consensus molecular subtypes, based on global transcriptional expression analysis, were identified from six independent classification systems [31]: CMS1 (microsatellite instable, hypermutated, *BRAF* mutation, immune), CMS2 (canonical, strong upregulation of WNT and MYC), CMS3 (*KRAS* mutations, metabolic deregulation), and CMS4 (stromal infiltration, TGF-β activation, and angiogenesis). Among the four subtypes, CMS4 displayed elevated expression of mesenchymal genes and was associated with worse relapse-free and overall survival. Initially, this subtype appeared to derive from the population of tumor cells that undergo EMT, exist at the invasion front, and, most likely, contribute to tumor dissemination. However, more recent investigations that applied techniques that separated the potential cellular sources of this gene signature revealed that the CMS4 expression pattern derives from stromal cells, especially cancer-associated fibroblasts (CAFs), and not epithelial tumor cells [32, 33]. The stromal cells associated with this subtype expressed elevated protein levels of CALD1, FAP, IGFBP7, or POSTN (periostin), a signature that predicted shorter disease-free interval. POSTN was previously identified as a differentially expressed gene in metastatic CRC, which promoted CRC metastatic tumor growth in the liver by inhibiting tumor apoptosis and enhancing angiogenesis and endothelial cell survival [34]. POSTN was also shown to antagonize tumor response to anti-VEGFA therapy [35].

Elevated TGF-β expression was a common feature of the CMS4, poor-prognosis subtype [32]. Treatment of colonic fibroblasts with TGF-β increased the expression of CALD1, FAP, IGFBP7, or POSTN [32]. CRC patient-derived organoids, which exhibited biallelic inactivation of *TGFBR2* and *SMAD4*, which expressed elevated levels of TGF-β, were found to be highly metastatic when injected into the spleens of immunodeficient mice. Using a TGF-βR1-specific inhibitor reduced the capacity for these cells to colonize the liver. The lack of TGF-β signaling in the cancer cells supports the role of TGF-β in the tumor microenvironment. A mechanism by which TGF-β exerts its effect was shown when CAFs exposed to TGF-β enhanced secretion of IL-11, which induced STAT3 signaling and increased the efficiency of organ colonization by CRC cells [36]. Conversely, pharmacological inhibition of IL-11 was shown to reduce the invasiveness of gastrointestinal cancers through reduced STAT3 signaling [37]. Pharmacological inhibition of TGF-β signaling resulted in reduced metastasis formation. In addition, expression of IQ motif-containing GTPase-activating protein 1 (IQGAP1) suppressed TGF-β signaling and myofibroblasts associated with human colorectal liver metastases have downregulated expression of IQGAP1 [38]. Loss of the TGF-β signaling member SMAD4 promoted adenoma-to-carcinoma progression and recruitment of CD34+ myeloid cells to the tumor invasion front. These CD34+ myeloid cells expressed the matrix metalloproteinases MMP9 and MMP2, as well as the CC-chemokine receptor 1 (CCR1), which is the cognate receptor for the chemokine CCL15 [39]. A separate study revealed that knockdown of SMAD4, a mediator of TGF-β signal transduction, increased the expression of the chemokine CCL15 and liver metastases that recruit CCR1+ myeloid cells through CCL15 expression result in shorter disease-free survival [40]. These studies reveal that CRC cancer cells acquire genetic alterations to limit the effect of TGF-β, while exposure of mesenchymal cells to TGF-β within the tumor microenvironment supports metastatic colonization.

Endothelial Cells and Angiogenesis

The finding that poor prognosis is correlated with a stromal cellular and molecular signature, along with elevated levels of TGF-β expression, strongly underscores how the dialogue between stroma and cancer cells promotes tumor aggressiveness and metastasis formation. In addition to CAFs, endothelial cells play a critical role in tumor progression and metastasis. As tumors grow and increase metabolism, their requirements for nutrients and oxygen increase. Prior to encroaching on the basement membrane, tumor cells develop the ability to initiate neovascularization, enhancing the opportunity for metastatic dissemination. Tumor-associated angiogenesis, unlike normal angiogenesis, produces abnormal, leaky blood vessels that are associated with metastasis and poor prognosis [41, 42]. CAFs promote angiogenesis by releasing stroma-derived factor 1 (SDF-1), a chemokine that recruits endothelial progenitor cells. Both CAFs and tumor-associated macrophages (TAMs) secrete VEGF (VEGFA/B), an endothelial mitogen that supports endothelial progenitor differentiation and angiogenesis. VEGF is also capable of inducing myofibroblasts to develop into endothelial cells and support tumor neovasculature development. Targeted therapies against the VEGF signaling pathway increase response rates, progression-free survival, and overall survival when combined with cytotoxic chemotherapy in patients with metastatic colorectal cancer [43]. Tumor-derived IL-33, an IL-1 cytokine family member, is elevated in patient tumor tissues and facilitates the recruitment of myeloid cell populations [44]. Increased expression of IL-33 also enhanced tumor angiogenesis by activating endothelial cells. These activities of IL-33 promoted the growth and capacity for liver metastasis, while abrogation of IL-33 in a mouse model of intestinal tumorigenesis suppressed angiogenesis of adenomatous polyps and suppressed mast cell-derived proteases and cytokines [45].

In addition to the role of endothelial cells in facilitating metastasis, these cells are capable of promoting the cancer stem cell phenotype through paracrine signaling [46]. A soluble form of Jagged-1, secreted by endothelial cells and cleaved by the protease ADAM17, activates NOTCH signaling and promotes the development of sphere-forming cells, a phenotype representative of cancer stem cells. NOTCH is implicated in promoting tumor cell intravasation and metastasis [47], and conversely, inhibition of NOTCH signaling prevents colon cancer cell motility and metastasis [48].

Epithelial–Mesenchymal Transition (EMT) and Colorectal Cancer (CRC): Extravasation

Despite clear evidence that stromal cells contribute significantly to CRC development and progression, support exists for the concept of a population of mobile cancer stem cells (MCS) [49] that reside at the tumor–host interface and are derived from stationary cancer stem cells (SCS) that have acquired changes associated with epithelial–mesenchymal transition. These cells shed most of their epithelial phenotype, detach from their cellular interactions, and express genes associated with motility. They are thought to form the "budding region," possess both stem-like and invasive attributes, and appear most likely to contribute to increased metastatic potential and poorer overall prognosis [50, 51]. It should be stated that while the molecular subtype CMS4 is mostly composed of mesenchymal cells, their presence does not disprove the possibility that MCS cells contribute to the mesenchymal gene signature. MCS cells at the invasive front express the highest accumulation of nuclear β-catenin and lose expression of the cell adhesion molecule E-cadherin, a cellular change commonly associated with EMT [52]. Interestingly, just as the levels of cyclin D1 correlated with β-catenin levels, so too was p16INK4a expression, a tumor suppressor important for decelerating G1-S phase cell cycle transition [52]. These areas also exhibited low expression of the proliferation marker Ki-67, revealing a non-proliferative role for β-catenin at the invasive front. Cancer cells at the invasive front, expressing the cancer stem cell marker CD44v6, were sensitive to the presence of Wnt3a and associated with high β-catenin levels, with evidence of the presence of the cancer stem cell phenotype at the interface for metastatic dissemination [53]. Further molecular and histological characterization of MSCs at the budding invasive front has been limited due to the rare and transient nature of this population and the difficulty in separating the genetic signature of these cells from that of the surrounding stromal tissue.

By breaching the basement membrane, exploiting angiogenesis, and branching away from the invasive front, CRCs gain access to the systemic circulation and disseminate. While our understanding of the journey of tumor cells from detachment to metastatic seeding is limited, it is safe to assume that travel from the invasive front into the blood and lymphatic circulation is harsh and fraught with various obstacles. The immediate lack of cellular attachment during travel through the lymphatic and blood circulation may result in anoikis, a form of apoptotic death due to failure of cellular anchorage. While in transit, cancer cells lose contact and communication with the various stromal cells comprising the primary tissue microenvironment that provide a steady supply of soluble factors supporting their growth and expansion. Lastly, sheer forces within the blood vessels may cause injury to metastatic cells in circulation.

Circulating Tumor Cells (CTCs)

The isolation and characterization of circulating tumor cells (CTCs) in patients lend support to the concept that these cells contribute to metastatic colony formation. Several studies report that CTCs predict clinical outcomes in patients with various solid tumors, including colorectal cancer [54–60]. Their isolation from blood before primary tumor detection, after surgical resection, and during disease recurrence, as well as their significance as a prognostic marker for patients with worse outcome, has led to the recommendation of their detection as a tool for determining adjuvant chemotherapy administration. Evidence that both primary and metastatic CTCs harbor cells with the cancer stem cell phenotype raises the question of whether metastatic cells derive from the primary tumor's self-renewing cancer stem cell population. Although not yet established as the main source of CTCs, stem cell markers have been identified on CTCs of patients with colon and metastatic breast cancer, supporting the concept that a subpopulation of SCS or MCS could be the source progenitor population from which CTCs are derived [57, 61]. In a study using a pancreatic cancer cell line, depletion of a unique population of CD133(+) CXCR4(+) cancer stem cells prevented the formation of metastasis [62]. The existence of subpopulations of mobile colorectal cancer stem cells was also demonstrated after identification and enrichment of the cell surface molecule CD26 on metastatic cells. Separation of CD26+ and CD26 subpopulations revealed that while both subsets exhibited tumorigenic potential by cecal implantation, only the CD26+ population was present in the portal vein circulation and capable of establishing liver metastases after direct portal vein injection [63]. A separate study revealed that metastatic CRC stem cells express the aforementioned cancer stem cell surface marker CD44v6, which was required for migration and generation of metastatic tumors [53]. Expression of CD44v6 was positively regulated by multiple soluble factors including Wnt3a, HGF, OPN, and SDF-1 but downregulated in the presence of the differentiation factors BMP2 and 4. CD44v6(−) cells did not give rise to metastatic tumors. In a separate study, three distinct cancer stem cell types were identified in CRC extensively self-renewing long-term tumor-initiating cells (LT-TICs), tumor transient-amplifying cells (T-TACs), and delayed-contributing TICs [64]. Among these populations, only the LT-TICs were capable of metastasis formation. Collectively, these studies indicate that select subpopulations of cells possessing the cancer stem cell phenotype are capable of executing metastatic dissemination.

Extravasation and Metastatic Dormancy

Once CTCs lodge in the blood vessels of tissues, these cells must reprogram themselves to exit the systemic circulation. Extravasation involves a complex interplay between the CTCs and the endothelial cells of the host metastatic organ and requires numerous adaptations to gain access to the metastatic parenchymal tissue. CTCs traverse the endothelium by several mechanisms, physically pushing their way across the endothelial barrier, expanding into a colony that ultimately leads to the formation of gaps between endothelial cells and pericytes or using paracrine signaling to recruit macrophages that allow cancer cells access to the basement membrane [65–68]. CRC cells shed from the primary tumor can reach both the liver and the lungs through blood vessel drainage through the portal and systemic circulation, respectively. In the liver, cells are trapped within the sinusoids and migrate out of the circulation through fenestrations and into the liver parenchyma. This process of migration from the vasculature and through the endothelial layer in different organs can be set by subtle shifts in the activation of downstream molecular pathways. For example, a *KRAS*-mutated colorectal cancer cell line revealed that activation of ERK2 led to liver metastasis, while downregulation of p38 MAPK promoted pulmonary metastasis resulting from increased expression of the cytokine PTHLH, which induced caspase-independent endothelial cell death in the lung endothelial vasculature [69].

To facilitate colonization, changes associated with EMT are reversed as the metastatic tumor nodules recapitulate the histological organization of the primary tumor. Once these micrometastases establish themselves within the parenchymal tissue, cancer cells may transition into a dormant or latent phase, surviving in a state of non-growth. These cells are refractory to conventional chemotherapy or targeted therapy [70]. In colorectal cancer, the dormant period can range for up to 5 years. Dormancy most likely involves one of three phases: cellular dormancy, where cells are maintained in a state of quiescence due to cell intrinsic and/or extrinsic effects; angiogenic dormancy, where tumor nodules are limited in their growth by outstripping their blood supply; and immune-mediated dormancy, where the cytotoxic effects of the immune system control tumor cell growth [70, 71]. What triggers the end of dormancy and the initiation of macrometastatic tumor formation from micrometastases is still unclear. Primary tumors may release suppressive factors that hold micrometastases at bay until resection of the primary tumor unleashes their growth [72, 73]. Determining the intrinsic and extrinsic factors that regulate the transition from dormancy is an important issue for future research and therapeutic discovery.

Immune System

We are only beginning to appreciate the many roles of the immune system in combating tumorigenesis and metastasis, as well as the multitude of ways cancer evades immune detection and clearance. As a recognized hallmark of cancer [74], the immune system is now seen as a critical mediator in sculpting the tumor microenvironment, both in suppressing and in promoting tumor growth. As described above, chemokine signaling can recruit myeloid cells and promote CRC progress and metastasis [39]. Based on the context of the tumor microenvironment, macrophages have the capacity to develop into tumor-associated macrophages (M2), which can secrete VEGF and IL-8, two important angiogenic factors that help ameliorate the effects of hypoxia. In addition, they support invasiveness by secreting matrix metalloproteinases, including MMP9. Macrophages can also perform antitumor effects, involved in the detection and killing of tumor cells. The presence and type of antigen-presenting cells are correlated with outcomes in patients with CRC. The frequency of distant metastases was found to be higher in patients with lower numbers of immature dendritic cells in the tumor stroma and at the invasive margin [75]. However, the presence of myeloid-derived suppressor cells (MDSC) in blood correlated with poor prognosis [76, 77].

It is now well established that the presence of tumor-infiltrating lymphocytes is associated with tumor inhibition and improved prognosis [78–81]. Tumors without signs of early metastatic invasion exhibit increased infiltrates of immune cells and elevated IFN-γ, granulysin, and granzyme B levels [82]. Furthermore, these tumors had increased numbers of CD8+ T cells and displayed markers of migration, activation, and differentiation. Immunologic data, including cell type, density, and location of immune cells within the tumor sample, were found to be better predictors of outcome than classical histological analysis [83]. Patients with tumors harboring high-density CD3(+) T cells had double the 5-year survival of patient with low-density T cell infiltrates. Neoantigen load is also found to be strongly associated with cytolytic activity across numerous tumor types [84]. These neoantigens, absent from the thymus and therefore unable to facilitate deletion of their cognate T-cell receptor, are expressed by cancer cells and exhibit high immunogenicity. A recent longitudinal analysis of clonal evolution, across time and anatomic locations, in two CRC patients, revealed the extraordinary mutational and immunologic diversity that exists between and within tumor nodules and across patients [81]. This study revealed that immune activity is present within metastatic sites and that aneuploidy within metastases was associated with the absence of immunoediting. The absence of immunoediting, low Immunoscore, and higher metastatic burden adversely impacted recurrence-free survival, while the presence of immunoediting, high Immunoscore, and small tumor burden distinguished the lowest risk cohort. Non-immunoedited metastases that harbored immune infiltrates had increased densities of FOXP3+ T cells, increased PD-L1 expression, and significant proximity of T cells to PD-L1+ cells. The presence of PD-L1 expression raises the possibility of targeting this immunophenotype with immune-checkpoint inhibitors. The provision of antibodies directed against PD-1 in MSI-high CRC patients demonstrated that blockade of the PD-1:PD-L1 axis is an effective treatment strategy [85]. These findings illustrate that intratumoral and metastatic heterogeneity are strongly influenced by immunologic pressures.

Conclusion

Colorectal cancer metastasis remains a challenging clinical and laboratory problem. Despite decades of advances in cytotoxic chemotherapy regimens, biologically targeted therapies, radiologic detection, and surgery metastasis continue to be the leading cause of mortality in patients with colorectal cancer. The development of metastasis touches on the foundations of many biologic processes. Metastasis has been described as a sequence of discrete steps. However, within each of these steps are multiple intrinsic and extrinsic factors that drive metastatic progression. As a result, understanding the biology behind the metastatic behavior is complex and requires the development of sophisticated experimental models. Despite these challenges, our understanding of the mechanisms behind metastatic processes has become clearer and our treatment options are expanding into new territories as evidenced by the recognition of the role of the immune system in sculpting clonal and metastatic evolution and the efficacy of immunotherapy in our treatment regimen. Future research should yield new insights into metastatic behavior in colorectal cancer, offering the possibility of newer, more effective therapies in the near future.

References

1. Bray F, Ferlay J, Soerjomataram I, Siegel RL, Torre LA, Jemal A. Global cancer statistics 2018: GLOBOCAN estimates of incidence and mortality worldwide for 36 cancers in 185 countries. CA Cancer J Clin. 2018;68(6):394–424.
2. Torre LA, Bray F, Siegel RL, Ferlay J, Lortet-Tieulent J, Jemal A. Global cancer statistics, 2012. CA Cancer J Clin. 2015;65:87–108.
3. Tzeng C-WD, Aloia TA. Colorectal Liver Metastases. J Gastrointest Surg. 2013;17:195–202.
4. Choti MA, Sitzmann JV, Tiburi MF, et al. Trends in long-term survival following liver resection for hepatic colorectal metastases. Ann Surg. 2002;235:759–66.
5. Brouquet A, Abdalla EK, Kopetz S, et al. High survival rate after two-stage resection of advanced colorectal liver metastases: response-based selection and complete resection define outcome. J Clin Oncol. 2011;29:1083–90.
6. Brouquet A, Mortenson MM, Vauthey JN, et al. Surgical strategies for synchronous colorectal liver metastases in 156 consecutive patients: classic, combined or reverse strategy? J Am Coll Surg. 2010;210:934–41.

7. Fidler IJ. The pathogenesis of cancer metastasis: the 'seed and soil' hypothesis revisited. Nat Rev Cancer. 2003;3:453–8.
8. Chaffer CL, Weinberg RA. A perspective on cancer cell metastasis. Science. 2011;331:1559–64.
9. Jones S, Chen WD, Parmigiani G, et al. Comparative lesion sequencing provides insights into tumor evolution. Proc Natl Acad Sci U S A. 2008;105:4283–8.
10. Barker N, Ridgway RA, van Es JH, et al. Crypt stem cells as the cells-of-origin of intestinal cancer. Nature. 2009;457:608–11.
11. Barker N, van Es JH, Kuipers J, et al. Identification of stem cells in small intestine and colon by marker gene Lgr5. Nature. 2007;449:1003–7.
12. Reya T, Clevers H. Wnt signalling in stem cells and cancer. Nature. 2005;434:843–50.
13. Vogelstein B, Fearon ER, Hamilton SR, et al. Genetic alterations during colorectal-tumor development. N Engl J Med. 1988;319:525–32.
14. Fearon ER, Vogelstein B. A genetic model for colorectal tumorigenesis. Cell. 1990;61:759–67.
15. Seshagiri S, Stawiski EW, Durinck S, et al. Recurrent R-spondin fusions in colon cancer. Nature. 2012;488:660–4.
16. Cancer Genome Atlas Network. Comprehensive molecular characterization of human colon and rectal cancer. Nature. 2012;487:330–7.
17. Vermeulen L, De Sousa EMF, van der Heijden M, et al. Wnt activity defines colon cancer stem cells and is regulated by the microenvironment. Nat Cell Biol. 2010;12:468–76.
18. Li HJ, Reinhardt F, Herschman HR, Weinberg RA. Cancer-stimulated mesenchymal stem cells create a carcinoma stem cell niche via prostaglandin E2 signaling. Cancer Discov. 2012;2:840–55.
19. Drost J, van Jaarsveld RH, Ponsioen B, et al. Sequential cancer mutations in cultured human intestinal stem cells. Nature. 2015;521:43–7.
20. Fujii M, Shimokawa M, Date S, et al. A colorectal tumor organoid library demonstrates progressive loss of niche factor requirements during tumorigenesis. Cell Stem Cell. 2016;18:827–38.
21. Matano M, Date S, Shimokawa M, et al. Modeling colorectal cancer using CRISPR-Cas9-mediated engineering of human intestinal organoids. Nat Med. 2015;21:256–62.
22. Ricci-Vitiani L, Lombardi DG, Pilozzi E, et al. Identification and expansion of human colon-cancer-initiating cells. Nature. 2007;445:111–5.
23. O'Brien CA, Pollett A, Gallinger S, Dick JE. A human colon cancer cell capable of initiating tumour growth in immunodeficient mice. Nature. 2007;445:106–10.
24. Dalerba P, Dylla SJ, Park IK, et al. Phenotypic characterization of human colorectal cancer stem cells. Proc Natl Acad Sci U S A. 2007;104:10158–63.
25. Budinska E, Popovici V, Tejpar S, et al. Gene expression patterns unveil a new level of molecular heterogeneity in colorectal cancer. J Pathol. 2013;231:63–76.
26. Schlicker A, Beran G, Chresta CM, et al. Subtypes of primary colorectal tumors correlate with response to targeted treatment in colorectal cell lines. BMC Med Genet. 2012;5:66.
27. Roepman P, Schlicker A, Tabernero J, et al. Colorectal cancer intrinsic subtypes predict chemotherapy benefit, deficient mismatch repair and epithelial-to-mesenchymal transition. Int J Cancer. 2014;134:552–62.
28. Sadanandam A, Lyssiotis CA, Homicsko K, et al. A colorectal cancer classification system that associates cellular phenotype and responses to therapy. Nat Med. 2013;19:619–25.
29. De Sousa EMF, Wang X, Jansen M, et al. Poor-prognosis colon cancer is defined by a molecularly distinct subtype and develops from serrated precursor lesions. Nat Med. 2013;19:614–8.
30. Marisa L, de Reynies A, Duval A, et al. Gene expression classification of colon cancer into molecular subtypes: characterization, validation, and prognostic value. PLoS Med. 2013;10:e1001453.
31. Guinney J, Dienstmann R, Wang X, et al. The consensus molecular subtypes of colorectal cancer. Nat Med. 2015;21:1350–6.
32. Calon A, Lonardo E, Berenguer-Llergo A, et al. Stromal gene expression defines poor-prognosis subtypes in colorectal cancer. Nat Genet. 2015;47:320–9.
33. Isella C, Terrasi A, Bellomo SE, et al. Stromal contribution to the colorectal cancer transcriptome. Nat Genet. 2015;47:312–9.

34. Bao S, Ouyang G, Bai X, et al. Periostin potently promotes metastatic growth of colon cancer by augmenting cell survival via the Akt/PKB pathway. Cancer Cell. 2004;5:329–39.
35. Keklikoglou I, Kadioglu E, Bissinger S, et al. Periostin limits tumor response to VEGFA inhibition. Cell Rep. 2018;22:2530–40.
36. Calon A, Espinet E, Palomo-Ponce S, et al. Dependency of colorectal cancer on a TGF-beta-driven program in stromal cells for metastasis initiation. Cancer Cell. 2012;22:571–84.
37. Putoczki TL, Thiem S, Loving A, et al. Interleukin-11 is the dominant IL-6 family cytokine during gastrointestinal tumorigenesis and can be targeted therapeutically. Cancer Cell. 2013;24:257–71.
38. Liu C, Billadeau DD, Abdelhakim H, et al. IQGAP1 suppresses TbetaRII-mediated myofibroblastic activation and metastatic growth in liver. J Clin Invest. 2013;123:1138–56.
39. Kitamura T, Kometani K, Hashida H, et al. SMAD4-deficient intestinal tumors recruit CCR1+ myeloid cells that promote invasion. Nat Genet. 2007;39:467–75.
40. Itatani Y, Kawada K, Fujishita T, et al. Loss of SMAD4 from colorectal cancer cells promotes CCL15 expression to recruit CCR1+ myeloid cells and facilitate liver metastasis. Gastroenterology. 2013;145:1064–75. e11
41. Dudley AC. Tumor endothelial cells. Cold Spring Harb Perspect Med. 2012;2:a006536.
42. Yonenaga Y, Mori A, Onodera H, et al. Absence of smooth muscle actin-positive pericyte coverage of tumor vessels correlates with hematogenous metastasis and prognosis of colorectal cancer patients. Oncology. 2005;69:159–66.
43. Hurwitz H, Fehrenbacher L, Novotny W, et al. Bevacizumab plus irinotecan, fluorouracil, and leucovorin for metastatic colorectal cancer. N Engl J Med. 2004;350:2335–42.
44. Zhang Y, Davis C, Shah S, et al. IL-33 promotes growth and liver metastasis of colorectal cancer in mice by remodeling the tumor microenvironment and inducing angiogenesis. Mol Carcinog. 2017;56:272–87.
45. Maywald RL, Doerner SK, Pastorelli L, et al. IL-33 activates tumor stroma to promote intestinal polyposis. Proc Natl Acad Sci U S A. 2015;112:E2487–96.
46. Lu J, Ye X, Fan F, et al. Endothelial cells promote the colorectal cancer stem cell phenotype through a soluble form of Jagged-1. Cancer Cell. 2013;23:171–85.
47. Wieland E, Rodriguez-Vita J, Liebler SS, et al. Endothelial Notch1 activity facilitates metastasis. Cancer Cell. 2017;31:355–67.
48. Sonoshita M, Aoki M, Fuwa H, et al. Suppression of colon cancer metastasis by Aes through inhibition of Notch signaling. Cancer Cell. 2011;19:125–37.
49. Brabletz T, Jung A, Spaderna S, Hlubek F, Kirchner T. Opinion: migrating cancer stem cells – an integrated concept of malignant tumour progression. Nat Rev Cancer. 2005;5:744–9.
50. Ueno H, Price AB, Wilkinson KH, Jass JR, Mochizuki H, Talbot IC. A new prognostic staging system for rectal cancer. Ann Surg. 2004;240:832–9.
51. Ueno H, Murphy J, Jass JR, Mochizuki H, Talbot IC. Tumour 'budding' as an index to estimate the potential of aggressiveness in rectal cancer. Histopathology. 2002;40:127–32.
52. Jung A, Schrauder M, Oswald U, et al. The invasion front of human colorectal adenocarcinomas shows co-localization of nuclear beta-catenin, cyclin D1, and p16INK4A and is a region of low proliferation. Am J Pathol. 2001;159:1613–7.
53. Todaro M, Gaggianesi M, Catalano V, et al. CD44v6 is a marker of constitutive and reprogrammed cancer stem cells driving colon cancer metastasis. Cell Stem Cell. 2014;14:342–56.
54. Engell HC. Cancer cells in the circulating blood; a clinical study on the occurrence of cancer cells in the peripheral blood and in venous blood draining the tumour area at operation. Ugeskr Laeger. 1955;117:822–3.
55. Peach G, Kim C, Zacharakis E, Purkayastha S, Ziprin P. Prognostic significance of circulating tumour cells following surgical resection of colorectal cancers: a systematic review. Br J Cancer. 2010;102:1327–34.
56. Iinuma H, Okinaga K, Egami H, et al. Usefulness and clinical significance of quantitative real-time RT-PCR to detect isolated tumor cells in the peripheral blood and tumor drainage blood of patients with colorectal cancer. Int J Oncol. 2006;28:297–306.

57. Iinuma H, Watanabe T, Mimori K, et al. Clinical significance of circulating tumor cells, including cancer stem-like cells, in peripheral blood for recurrence and prognosis in patients with Dukes' stage B and C colorectal cancer. J Clin Oncol. 2011;29:1547–55.
58. Cristofanilli M, Budd GT, Ellis MJ, et al. Circulating tumor cells, disease progression, and survival in metastatic breast cancer. N Engl J Med. 2004;351:781–91.
59. Cohen SJ, Punt CJ, Iannotti N, et al. Relationship of circulating tumor cells to tumor response, progression-free survival, and overall survival in patients with metastatic colorectal cancer. J Clin Oncol. 2008;26:3213–21.
60. Rahbari NN, Aigner M, Thorlund K, et al. Meta-analysis shows that detection of circulating tumor cells indicates poor prognosis in patients with colorectal cancer. Gastroenterology. 2010;138:1714–26.
61. Aktas B, Tewes M, Fehm T, Hauch S, Kimmig R, Kasimir-Bauer S. Stem cell and epithelial-mesenchymal transition markers are frequently overexpressed in circulating tumor cells of metastatic breast cancer patients. Breast Cancer Res. 2009;11:R46.
62. Hermann PC, Huber SL, Herrler T, et al. Distinct populations of cancer stem cells determine tumor growth and metastatic activity in human pancreatic cancer. Cell Stem Cell. 2007;1:313–23.
63. Pang R, Law WL, Chu AC, et al. A subpopulation of CD26+ cancer stem cells with metastatic capacity in human colorectal cancer. Cell Stem Cell. 2010;6:603–15.
64. Dieter SM, Ball CR, Hoffmann CM, et al. Distinct types of tumor-initiating cells form human colon cancer tumors and metastases. Cell Stem Cell. 2011;9:357–65.
65. Chambers AF, Groom AC, MacDonald IC. Dissemination and growth of cancer cells in metastatic sites. Nat Rev Cancer. 2002;2:563–72.
66. Luzzi KJ, MacDonald IC, Schmidt EE, et al. Multistep nature of metastatic inefficiency: dormancy of solitary cells after successful extravasation and limited survival of early micrometastases. Am J Pathol. 1998;153:865–73.
67. Al-Mehdi AB, Tozawa K, Fisher AB, Shientag L, Lee A, Muschel RJ. Intravascular origin of metastasis from the proliferation of endothelium-attached tumor cells: a new model for metastasis. Nat Med. 2000;6:100–2.
68. Nguyen DX, Bos PD, Massague J. Metastasis: from dissemination to organ-specific colonization. Nat Rev Cancer. 2009;9:274–84.
69. Urosevic J, Garcia-Albeniz X, Planet E, et al. Colon cancer cells colonize the lung from established liver metastases through p38 MAPK signalling and PTHLH. Nat Cell Biol. 2014;16:685–94.
70. Sosa MS, Bragado P, Aguirre-Ghiso JA. Mechanisms of disseminated cancer cell dormancy: an awakening field. Nat Rev Cancer. 2014;14:611–22.
71. Aguirre-Ghiso JA. Models, mechanisms and clinical evidence for cancer dormancy. Nat Rev Cancer. 2007;7:834–46.
72. Folkman J. Role of angiogenesis in tumor growth and metastasis. Semin Oncol. 2002;29:15–8.
73. Demicheli R, Retsky MW, Hrushesky WJ, Baum M, Gukas ID. The effects of surgery on tumor growth: a century of investigations. Ann Oncol. 2008;19:1821–8.
74. Hanahan D, Weinberg RA. Hallmarks of cancer: the next generation. Cell. 2011;144:646–74.
75. Gulubova MV, Ananiev JR, Vlaykova TI, Yovchev Y, Tsoneva V, Manolova IM. Role of dendritic cells in progression and clinical outcome of colon cancer. Int J Color Dis. 2012;27:159–69.
76. Solito S, Falisi E, Diaz-Montero CM, et al. A human promyelocytic-like population is responsible for the immune suppression mediated by myeloid-derived suppressor cells. Blood. 2011;118:2254–65.
77. Sun HL, Zhou X, Xue YF, et al. Increased frequency and clinical significance of myeloid-derived suppressor cells in human colorectal carcinoma. World J Gastroenterol. 2012;18:3303–9.
78. Baier PK, Wimmenauer S, Hirsch T, et al. Analysis of the T cell receptor variability of tumor-infiltrating lymphocytes in colorectal carcinomas. Tumour Biol. 1998;19:205–12.
79. Naito Y, Saito K, Shiiba K, et al. CD8+ T cells infiltrated within cancer cell nests as a prognostic factor in human colorectal cancer. Cancer Res. 1998;58:3491–4.

80. Diederichsen AC, Hjelmborg J, Christensen PB, Zeuthen J, Fenger C. Prognostic value of the CD4+/CD8+ ratio of tumour infiltrating lymphocytes in colorectal cancer and HLA-DR expression on tumour cells. Cancer Immunol Immunother. 2003;52:423–8.
81. Angelova M, Mlecnik B, Vasaturo A, et al. Evolution of metastases in space and time under immune selection. Cell. 2018;175:751–65 e16.
82. Pages F, Berger A, Camus M, et al. Effector memory T cells, early metastasis, and survival in colorectal cancer. N Engl J Med. 2005;353:2654–66.
83. Galon J, Costes A, Sanchez-Cabo F, et al. Type, density, and location of immune cells within human colorectal tumors predict clinical outcome. Science. 2006;313:1960–4.
84. Rooney MS, Shukla SA, Wu CJ, Getz G, Hacohen N. Molecular and genetic properties of tumors associated with local immune cytolytic activity. Cell. 2015;160:48–61.
85. Le DT, Uram JN, Wang H, et al. PD-1 blockade in tumors with mismatch-repair deficiency. N Engl J Med. 2015;372:2509–20.

Molecular Biomarkers for the Management of Colorectal Cancer Liver Metastases

3

Malcolm H. Squires III, Jordan M. Cloyd, and Timothy M. Pawlik

Introduction

As the efficacy of systemic therapies for metastatic colorectal cancer improves and the number of patients with colorectal liver metastases (CRLM) eligible for curative-intent resection increases, the need for careful patient selection and individualized prognostication has become increasingly important. Historically, traditional clinicopathologic features such as the number and size of liver metastases, primary tumor stage and nodal status, the presence of extrahepatic disease, disease-free interval, and serum carcinoembryonic antigen (CEA) level have been used as biomarkers to extrapolate prognostic data and guide patient selection for treatment decisions regarding CRLM [1, 2]. These prognostic biomarkers have been used to predict important oncologic endpoints such as progression-free survival (PFS), recurrence-free survival (RFS), or overall survival (OS) [3]. As many of these clinical variables have demonstrated inconsistent correlations with oncologic outcomes, however, more recently, there has been increasing interest in the prognostic capabilities of molecular and genetic biomarkers. In fact, a rapidly expanding understanding of the molecular mechanisms underlying the tumor biology of CRLM has provided new opportunities to identify potential molecular biomarkers with predictive and prognostic utility. In this chapter, we explore the molecular underpinnings and clinical utility of emerging biomarkers for CRLM, including KRAS, BRAF, and PIK3CA, among others.

M. H. Squires III · J. M. Cloyd · T. M. Pawlik (✉)
Division of Surgical Oncology, Department of Surgery, The Ohio State University Wexner Medical Center, Columbus, OH, USA
e-mail: Malcolm.Squires@osumc.edu; Jordan.Cloyd@osumc.edu; Tim.Pawlik@osumc.edu

M. M. Correia et al. (eds.), *Colorectal Cancer Liver Metastases*,
https://doi.org/10.1007/978-3-030-25486-5_3

KRAS

KRAS is a member of the RAS family of proto-oncogenes and functions as a membrane-bound GTP-binding protein downstream of the epidermal growth factor receptor (EGFR). Activation of KRAS in turn leads to the activation of the mitogen activated protein kinase (MAPK) cascade, promoting cell growth and proliferation (Fig. 3.1):

RAS → RAF → MEK → ERK. Mutations in KRAS lead to constitutive activation of this pathway and render tumors largely unresponsive to treatment with anti-EGFR antibody therapies [4].

KRAS mutations have been observed in 30–50% of patients with CRLM and are among the best-characterized prognostic biomarkers in metastatic colorectal cancer (CRC) [4–6]. In CRC, concordance of KRAS mutation status between the primary

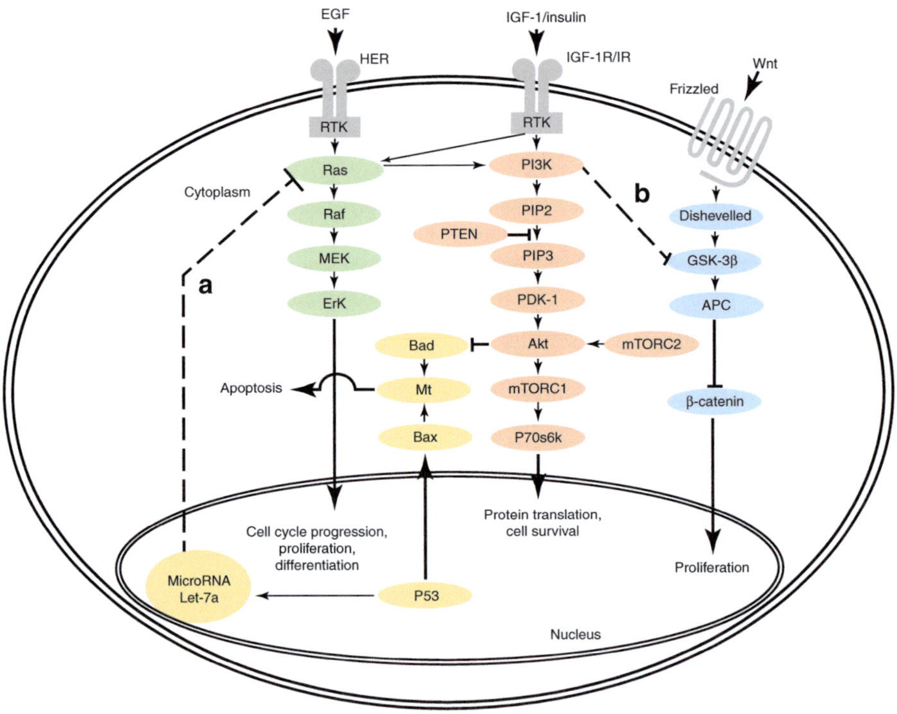

Fig. 3.1 Signaling pathways involved in the proliferation and progression of colorectal cancer. (Reprinted with permission from Yamashita et al. [23]). Abbreviations: EGF epidermal growth factor, HER human epidermal growth factor receptor, RTK receptor tyrosine kinase, MEK mitogen-activated protein kinase, ErK extracellular signal-regulated kinase, Mt mitochondria, IGF-1 insulin-like growth factor 1, IGF-1R/IR IGF-1 receptor/insulin receptor, PIP2 phosphatidyl inositol 4,5-bisphosphate, PTEN phosphatase and tensin homolog, PIP3 phosphatidyl inositol (3,4,5)-triphosphate, PDK-1 phosphoinositide-dependent protein kinase 1, mTORC1/2 mammalian target of rapamycin complex 1/2, P70s6k P70s6 kinase, APC adenomatous polyposis coli, Let-7a lethal 7a, PI3k phosphoinositide 3-kinase, GSK-3β glycogen synthase kinase-3β. (**a**) TP53 inhibits activated RAS through lethal (Let) 7a. When TP53 is mutated, Let-7a is not able to regulate activated RAS. (**b**) Dysregulated phosphoinositide 3-kinase (PI3K) inhibits glycogen synthase kinase (GSK)3β, leading to accumulation of β-catenin

tumor and liver metastasis is as high as 96% in one large series; thus, KRAS testing can be performed on either the primary tumor or metastatic lesions [7]. Generally, KRAS mutant status is associated with worse prognosis, more aggressive disease, and increased risk of disease recurrence after resection of CRLM compared to patients with KRAS wild-type (wt) tumors. For example, a recent meta-analysis of 1800 patients demonstrated that mutant KRAS status was an independent negative prognostic factor associated with significantly decreased OS (HR = 2.24) and RFS (HR = 1.89) after resection of CRLM [4].

In a large, single-institution study of patients treated with neoadjuvant chemotherapy followed by curative-intent hepatectomy, mutant RAS status (KRAS or NRAS) was associated with worse prognosis and a specific pattern of recurrence following resection of CRLM [5]. Specifically, mutant RAS status was associated with significantly decreased 3-year OS (52% vs. 81%) and 3-year RFS (16% vs. 34%) after resection of CRLM compared to patients with wtRAS tumors. In addition, RAS mutation was associated with significantly increased risk of disease recurrence in the lungs at 3-year post-CRLM resection (65% vs. 41%) but not intrahepatic recurrence. Kemeny et al. similarly reported that mutant KRAS status was independently associated with significantly decreased RFS (HR 1.9; $p = 0.01$) after CRLM resection compared to wtKRAS tumors and was associated with increased risk of distant bone ($p = 0.01$), brain ($p = 0.05$), and lung metastases ($p < 0.01$) but not intrahepatic recurrence [8]. In contrast, in a single-institution series of 334 patients undergoing hepatic resection for CRLM, Margonis et al. found that while KRAS status was not associated with RFS or site of recurrence, mutant KRAS status was associated with decreased survival among all patients and particularly among the subset of patients who developed recurrent disease after CRLM resection (HR 2.02; $p = 0.002$) [9].

Other studies have failed to show a prognostic association with KRAS status or have suggested a more nuanced relationship with outcomes for patients with CRLM. Primary tumor location, for example, may influence the prognostic impact of KRAS mutation status on patients with CRLM [10]. Recent studies suggest that the negative prognostic impact of mutant KRAS status among patients undergoing hepatic resection of CRLM was only present for left-sided primary colon cancers, whereas no association of RFS or OS with KRAS mutation status was observed for patients with right-sided primary tumors [11, 12].

The prognostic impact of KRAS mutations may also vary according to specific point mutations and codons with the KRAS gene locus. Previous analyses have identified worse RFS among patients with stage I–IV CRC who have G12V or G12S point mutations on codon 12 of the KRAS locus [13, 14]. In addition, a study by Imamura et al. of 1075 patients with CRC demonstrated that KRAS codon 12 mutations, particularly the G12V point mutation, were associated with significantly worse survival compared to wtKRAS, whereas KRAS codon 13 mutations had no association with prognosis [15]. Subsequent analyses of specific KRAS mutations among patients who underwent resection of CRLM have similarly shown that the G12V (HR 1.78; $p = 0.05$) and G12S (HR 3.33; $p = 0.02$) point mutations were associated with significantly worse OS compared to wtKRAS tumors [16]. In patients with recurrent CRLMs, the negative prognostic impact of G12V, G12C, and G12S mutations was even greater.

Given the negative prognostic impact of RAS mutations on survival, the management of patients with RAS-mutant CRLM remains controversial. As previously mentioned, patients with KRAS mutant CRLM are not responsive to systemic EGFR antibody therapy, and no agents directly targeting KRAS are available. Vascular endothelial growth factor (VEGF) inhibitors may, however, still provide benefit and elicit tumor response in patients with KRAS mutant tumors [17]. Development of MEK inhibitors and additional targeting of the RAS-RAF-ERK signaling cascade may offer future treatment options [18, 19]. RAS mutations are also known to impact the response to traditional systemic chemotherapy as well. For example, among patients treated with neoadjuvant chemotherapy prior to undergoing resection of CRLM, RAS mutant status has been associated with significantly decreased rates of radiographic (11% vs. 33%, $p = 0.006$) and major pathologic response (37% vs. 59%; $p = 0.015$), in addition to decreased RFS and OS [20].

Several studies have shown an increased risk of microscopically positive (R1) resection margins (11.4% vs. 5.4%, $p = 0.007$) and narrower width of negative margins for R0 resections (4 mm vs. 7 mm, $p = 0.03$) among patients undergoing resection of RAS mutant CRLM versus wtRAS tumors [21]. Similarly, mutant RAS status has been associated with earlier and more frequent local disease recurrence/progression following percutaneous ablation of CRLM compared to patients with wtRAS tumors, even if greater ablation margins are attempted [22, 23]. These clinical findings have led some groups to advocate wider resection or ablation margins for the treatment of mutant RAS CRLM in order to overcome the more infiltrative growth pattern of KRAS-mutant tumors. Nevertheless, whether such aggressive measures translate into improved outcomes has not yet been demonstrated [21, 23, 24]. Other data suggest that margin clearance for patients with mutant KRAS CRLM resection may in fact have little impact on negative survival outcomes, as any distance of negative margin width failed to show any improvement in OS compared to R1 resections [25]. The more invasive cellular behavior of RAS mutant tumors perhaps may be driving the adverse outcomes observed for these patients rather than potentially modifiable surgical variables [26]. While nonanatomic liver resections with 1–10 mm margin distance for CRLM have been deemed the standard of care, an intriguing recent analysis further clouded the issue of resection extent. Retrospective analysis of a cohort of patients with KRAS mutant CRLM found that more extensive anatomical resections were associated with significantly improved 5-year DFS versus traditional nonanatomic resections (46.4% vs. 14.4%; $p < 0.001$) [27]. No such difference in DFS was observed among patients with wtKRAS CRLM treated with anatomical versus nonanatomic hepatic resections. Additional prospective investigations of the interaction between margin width and RAS mutation status for patients with CRLM are clearly needed.

Despite the growing evidence that RAS mutation status affects the prognosis of patients undergoing resection and/or ablation of CRLM, there is likely insufficient research to demonstrate that it should be routinely used to select patients for or against surgical resection. Instead, RAS mutation status remains an important prognostic biomarker for patients undergoing multidisciplinary evaluation of CRLM. In fact, a recent work has led to the development of a modified clinical risk score that incorporates RAS status, along with the risk factors of primary colorectal tumor lymph node status and CRLM lesion diameter > 5 cm into a validated prognostic tool for predicting patient survival after CRLM resection [28]. Based on this risk score, the presence of extra-hepatic disease or a short disease-free interval may be relative contraindications to resection of CRLM in patients with KRAS mutant disease, given the comparatively worse outcomes observed in patients with wtRAS tumors.

BRAF

The BRAF kinase functions downstream of KRAS within the MAPK signaling cascade (Fig. 3.1). Among patients with microsatellite stable sporadic colorectal primary tumors, the incidence of BRAF mutations is 5–10%, whereas among tumors with microsatellite instability, the reported incidence is as high as 40–60% [29]. The overall rate of BRAF mutations observed in patients with resected CRLM is rare, at only 2–4% [30]. This is likely the case because BRAF mutations appear to be associated with less likelihood of resectable metastatic disease and, among patients who do undergo resection of CRLM, worse overall outcomes. Unlike KRAS mutations, however, patients with BRAF mutations retain more systemic therapy options, as BRAF mutations do not appear to confer resistance to anti-EGFR therapies [17, 31].

Multiple studies have demonstrated that the presence of BRAF mutation is associated with significantly worse RFS and OS among patients undergoing resection of CRLM, with some studies suggesting that BRAF mutations may be a stronger adverse prognostic marker than RAS mutations [29, 32–35]. In a series of patients with resected CRLM, mutant BRAF status was an independent adverse risk factor associated with decreased 5-year OS (HR 5.18; $p = 0.002$) on multivariate analysis, while KRAS status failed to demonstrate prognostic significance within this cohort [33]. In a pooled analysis of 845 patients with wtKRAS CRLM from the CRYSTAL and OPUS randomized clinical trials assessing the benefit of cetuximab added to cytotoxic chemotherapy, mutant BRAF tumors were associated with significantly decreased OS compared to wtBRAF tumors, regardless of treatment arm [31]. While the addition of the anti-EGFR antibody cetuximab was associated with improved survival versus traditional chemotherapy alone in both mutant BRAF and wtBRAF patients, patients with BRAF mutant tumors demonstrated significantly worse OS ($p < 0.01$) than their wild-type counterparts [31]. Interestingly, the prognostic impact of BRAF mutant status among patients with resectable CRLM may vary over time, according to a recent multi-institutional retrospective analysis of conditional overall survival [36]. Within the first year after resection of CRLM, mutant BRAF status has a profound impact on prognosis but does not maintain its prognostic significance beyond 12 months post-hepatectomy; clinicopathologic variables such as resection margin status and presence of extrahepatic disease drive prognosis after the first year [36].

In a recent single-institution, 10-year series of 709 patients with CRLM, *BRAF* mutations were overall more commonly observed among patients treated with chemotherapy alone ($n = 313$) than among those who underwent surgical resection ($n = 396$), (8.9% vs. 3.5%, $p < 0.001$) [23]. In particular, the V600E mutation of *BRAF* was significantly more common among patients with CRLM treated with chemotherapy alone versus those with resectable disease (89% [25/28 patients] vs. 43% [6/14 patients], $p = 0.001$), reflecting the adverse prognostic association with the V600E *BRAF* mutation [23]. By contrast, *BRAF* mutations other than codon 600, while significantly less common, appear to be associated with a more favorable prognosis among patients with CRLM. In a multi-institutional retrospective analysis of 9600 patients with metastatic CRC, non-V600 BRAF mutations were identified in 208 patients (2.2% of the entire cohort), encompassing 22% of all BRAF mutations observed [37]. Non-V600 BRAF mutations were associated with fewer right-sided primary colon cancers and fewer high-grade tumors, both known to be adverse prognostic factors. Patients with non-V600E BRAF mutations demonstrated significantly improved median OS compared to patients with V600 mutations and even patients with wild-type BRAF (60.7 vs. 11.4 vs. 43.0 months, $p < 0.001$). Unfortunately, insufficient evidence is available to evaluate the prognostic impact of non-V600E BRAF mutations on the outcomes following resection of CRLM. Current guidelines recommend evaluation of BRAF mutational status for all patients with CRLM, given its implications as a potential prognostic biomarker and as a predictive marker for guiding chemotherapy options [38].

TP53

The tumor suppressor gene TP53 encodes a transcription factor that regulates DNA repair, apoptosis, and a host of other cellular functions, and loss-of-function mutations in TP53 are widely implicated in cancer development [39]. As such, TP53 mutations are widely present and have been reported in 50–66% of patients with CRLM [40–43]. To date, studies have reported widely conflicting results regarding the prognostic impact of TP53 mutations on survival outcomes after CRLM resection, with some series reporting a positive association on OS, while others have reported no association or even a negative prognostic association [40–45].

The discrepancy in previously published studies may be a result of more complicated molecular pathways in which synchronous, synergistic mutations are required to exhibit a worse biological phenotype. For example, recent evidence has elucidated the role of concomitant somatic double mutations in TP53 and RAS among patients undergoing resection of CRLM. A recent single-institution series reported by Chun et al. found double TP53-RAS mutations in 31% of patients with CRLM [46]. While isolated mutations in RAS or TP53 were not associated with worse prognosis, the presence of a RAS/TP53 double mutation remained an independent risk factor for decreased OS (HR 2.62, $p = 0.002$) on multivariate analysis.

PIK3CA

The proto-oncogene PIK3CA encodes the catalytic subunit of the phosphoinositide-3 kinase (PI3K), which controls the activation of the PI3K/Akt/mTOR signaling cascade involved in cell survival and proliferation [47]. Mutations in PIK3CA have been associated with the transition from adenoma to invasive colorectal cancer [48] and are reportedly present in 7–28% of patients with CRLM [5, 49–52].

The prognostic effect of isolated PIK3CA mutations on survival outcomes of patients with CRLM remains somewhat unclear, as some studies have shown an association with decreased RFS and OS, while others have found no prognostic association [53–55]. Additionally, PIK3CA mutations frequently occur in the context of concurrent KRAS and/or BRAF mutations, which appear to have a greater impact on prognosis [55, 56]. Mutations in PIK3CA are also associated with relative resistance to systemic chemotherapy, including resistance to anti-EGFR therapy even in the absence of KRAS mutations [55, 57, 58]. Different mutations within the PIK3CA locus may have variable prognostic impact, as one large retrospective cohort analysis found exon 9 mutations in PIK3CA had no effect on outcomes, while exon 20 mutations were associated with significantly worse response rates, PFS, and OS compared to patients with wild-type exon 20 [55]. Mutations in both the PIK3CA and the adenomatous polyposis coli (APC) genes appear to interact synergistically, leading to dramatically increased tumor growth and invasiveness [59]. The presence of concurrent somatic mutations in PIK3CA and APC in patients with CRLM was an independent adverse prognostic factor associated with decreased response to neoadjuvant chemotherapy (OR 2.91; $p = 0.002$) and significantly decreased OS (HR 3.09; $p < 0.001$) compared to patients without the double mutation [52].

APC

Inherited or somatic loss-of-function mutations in the APC tumor suppressor gene are one of the earliest steps in colorectal cancer tumorigenesis, leading to beta-catenin dysregulation and overactivity of the Wnt signaling pathway [47]. As a result, APC mutations are extremely common, observed at a frequency of 42–73% in patients with CRLM [60–62]. The influence of isolated APC mutations on patients with CRLM remains unclear, with some studies reporting a negative prognostic association, while others found no relationship with recurrence or survival outcomes [53, 63]. While the prognostic role of isolated APC mutations on outcomes after CRLM resection is poorly understood, increasing evidence suggests that APC may affect tumor biology by interacting synergistically with other mutations such as PIK3CA, as described above [64].

SMAD4

Drosophila protein, mothers against decapentaplegic homolog 4 (SMAD4), is an important mediator in the transforming growth factor (TGF)-β signaling pathway and is known to have an essential role in colorectal cancer progression. Sporadic *SMAD4* gene mutations occur in approximately 2–20% of patients with colorectal cancer [65]. Recent evidence has found that SMAD4 mutations are associated with a significantly worse overall survival following resection of CRLM, even after controlling for KRAS mutation status [66].

Microsatellite Instability

The mismatch repair (MMR) system comprises multiple proteins including MLH1, MSH2, MSH6, and PMS2, which function to recognize and repair insertions and deletions within microsatellites, repetitive units within the DNA sequence. Deficiencies within the MMR system, whether from sporadic or germline mutations, result in a state of microsatellite instability (MSI) that predisposes to mutation accumulation and tumorigenesis [67]. Sporadic MMR mutations among colorectal cancers (10–20% of primary tumors) most commonly result from MLH1 promoter hypermethylation and are more common than germline mutations in MMR genes associated with Lynch syndrome or hereditary nonpolyposis colorectal cancer (HNPCC) syndrome, which account for 1–5% of primary colorectal cancers [67, 68].

High microsatellite instability (MSI-H) is defined as the absence of expression of any one of the MMR proteins, based on immunohistochemical analysis, or instability in >30% of microsatellite markers within a tumor [69]. MSI-H tumors are commonly associated with poor tumor differentiation, mucinous histology, and a high concentration of tumor-infiltrating lymphocytes, and typically arise in the right colon [70]. Microsatellite instability is actually less common in more advanced stages of colorectal cancer, with rates of MSI-H reported as approximately 20% for stage II colorectal cancers, 12% for stage III, and only 4% for stage IV cancers [67, 69]. While stage II and III MSI-H colorectal cancers are associated with decreased risk of distant metastases and improved outcomes compared to microsatellite stable (MSS) tumors, this does not appear to hold true for stage IV MSI-H cancers [69, 71]. Given the rarity of MSI-H status among patients with CRLM (2.5–4%), the prognostic impact of microsatellite instability within this patient population has been difficult to determine, with several studies failing to demonstrate any association of MSI-H status in CRLM with progression-free survival (PFS), RFS, or OS [72–74]. Other studies, however, have shown significantly worse outcomes associated with MSI-H CRLM compared to MSS tumors [32, 67, 68]. This discrepancy may be due to the frequency of concurrent BRAF mutations in sporadic MMR-deficient tumors, with its known disproportionate adverse prognostic impact.

MSI status may influence the selection of systemic therapies for patients with CRLM. For example, although stage II and III MSI-H colorectal cancers are often chemoresistant to traditional 5-fluorouracil (5-FU)-based retrospective studies suggest that 5-FU maintains efficacy for treatment of CRLM with MSI-H status [68, 69]. In addition, immunotherapy targeting the programmed death-1 (PD-1) receptor or its ligand (PD-L1) has shown exciting promise in patients with MSI-H metastatic colorectal cancer. The landmark phase II study by Le et al. in 2015 demonstrated a remarkable 90% disease control rate with the anti-PD1 antibody pembrolizumab among patients with MSI-H metastatic colorectal cancer who had progressed on prior lines of systemic chemotherapy [75]. Numerous ongoing studies are investigating the role of checkpoint inhibitors for the subset of patients with CRLM and MSI.

Circulating Tumor Cells

The presence of detectable circulating tumor cells (CTCs) in the peripheral blood of patients with CRLM may hold promise as a novel prognostic biomarker [76]. A study by Koch et al. was among the first to demonstrate that detection of CTCs at the time of R0 hepatic resection for CRLM was independently associated with significantly decreased median DFS, versus patients without CTCs (13 vs. 25 months; $p = 0.03$) [77]. A subsequent meta-analysis in 2013 including 12 studies of patients with metastatic colorectal cancer, including patients with resectable CRLM, similarly demonstrated that the presence of CTCs was associated with significantly worse PFS (HR 2.07; $p = 0.0001$) and OS (HR 2.47; $p = 0.01$) compared to that in patients without detectable CTCs [78]. Analysis of CTC levels at specific time points in patients with CRLM may also be a measurable indicator of response to systemic therapy and serve as a complementary tool to traditional measurement of radiographic response using Response Evaluation Criteria in Solid Tumors (RECIST) criteria [79]. The use of CTCs as a potential biomarker for patients with CRLM remains under active clinical investigation.

Conclusion

Prognostic biomarkers for patients with CRLM have traditionally consisted of clinicopathologic variables such as tumor size and focality, primary colon cancer nodal status, disease-free interval, and serum CEA level. Many of these variables have in turn been incorporated into prognostic nomograms or risk scores to better stratify the recurrence and survival of individual patients undergoing resection of CRLM. Evolving insights into the molecular pathways underlying the development and metastasis of colorectal cancer have led to a growing appreciation for the prognostic importance of mutations in KRAS, BRAF, and MMR genes, among others. In addition to their prognostic importance, specific mutations, such as KRAS status, may influence the selection of systemic therapies, the sequencing of treatments, or the planned resection/ablation margin of CRLM. As our understanding of the molecular and genetic determinants of the outcomes of metastatic colorectal cancer continues to expand, the importance of these molecular biomarkers in the personalized management of CRLM will only continue to increase.

References

1. Fong Y, Fortner J, Sun RL, Brennan MF, Blumgart LH. Clinical score for predicting recurrence after hepatic resection for metastatic colorectal cancer: analysis of 1001 consecutive cases. Ann Surg. 1999;230(3):309–18; discussion 318–21.
2. Maithel SK, Gonen M, Ito H, Dematteo RP, Allen PJ, Fong Y, et al. Improving the clinical risk score: an analysis of molecular biomarkers in the era of modern chemotherapy for resectable hepatic colorectal cancer metastases. Surgery. 2012;151(2):162–70.
3. Oldenhuis CN, Oosting SF, Gietema JA, de Vries EG. Prognostic versus predictive value of biomarkers in oncology. Eur J Cancer. 2008;44(7):946–53.
4. Brudvik KW, Kopetz SE, Li L, Conrad C, Aloia TA, Vauthey JN. Meta-analysis of KRAS mutations and survival after resection of colorectal liver metastases. Br J Surg. 2015;102(10):1175–83.
5. Vauthey JN, Zimmitti G, Kopetz SE, Shindoh J, Chen SS, Andreou A, et al. RAS mutation status predicts survival and patterns of recurrence in patients undergoing hepatectomy for colorectal liver metastases. Ann Surg. 2013;258(4):619–26; discussion 626–7.
6. Yaeger R, Cowell E, Chou JF, Gewirtz AN, Borsu L, Vakiani E, et al. RAS mutations affect pattern of metastatic spread and increase propensity for brain metastasis in colorectal cancer. Cancer. 2015;121(8):1195–203.
7. Knijn N, Mekenkamp LJ, Klomp M, Vink-Borger ME, Tol J, Teerenstra S, et al. KRAS mutation analysis: a comparison between primary tumours and matched liver metastases in 305 colorectal cancer patients. Br J Cancer. 2011;104(6):1020–6.
8. Kemeny NE, Chou JF, Capanu M, Gewirtz AN, Cercek A, Kingham TP, et al. KRAS mutation influences recurrence patterns in patients undergoing hepatic resection of colorectal metastases. Cancer. 2014;120(24):3965–71.
9. Margonis GA, Spolverato G, Kim Y, Karagkounis G, Choti MA, Pawlik TM. Effect of KRAS mutation on long-term outcomes of patients undergoing hepatic resection for colorectal liver metastases. Ann Surg Oncol. 2015;22(13):4158–65.
10. Barbon C, Margonis GA, Andreatos N, Rezaee N, Sasaki K, Buettner S, et al. Colorectal liver metastases: does the future of precision medicine lie in genetic testing? J Gastrointest Surg. 2018;22(7):1286–96.
11. Sasaki K, Andreatos N, Margonis GA, He J, Weiss M, Johnston F, et al. The prognostic implications of primary colorectal tumor location on recurrence and overall survival in patients undergoing resection for colorectal liver metastasis. J Surg Oncol. 2016;114(7):803–9.
12. Sasaki K, Margonis GA, Wilson A, Kim Y, Buettner S, Andreatos N, et al. Prognostic implication of KRAS status after hepatectomy for colorectal liver metastases varies according to primary colorectal tumor location. Ann Surg Oncol. 2016;23(11):3736–43.
13. Andreyev HJ, Norman AR, Cunningham D, Oates J, Dix BR, Iacopetta BJ, et al. Kirsten ras mutations in patients with colorectal cancer: the 'RASCAL II' study. Br J Cancer. 2001;85(5):692–6.
14. Andreyev HJ, Norman AR, Cunningham D, Oates JR, Clarke PA. Kirsten ras mutations in patients with colorectal cancer: the multicenter 'RASCAL' study. J Natl Cancer Inst. 1998;90(9):675–84.
15. Imamura Y, Morikawa T, Liao X, Lochhead P, Kuchiba A, Yamauchi M, et al. Specific mutations in KRAS codons 12 and 13, and patient prognosis in 1075 BRAF wild-type colorectal cancers. Clin Cancer Res. 2012;18(17):4753–63.
16. Margonis GA, Kim Y, Spolverato G, Ejaz A, Gupta R, Cosgrove D, et al. Association between specific mutations in KRAS codon 12 and colorectal liver metastasis. JAMA Surg. 2015;150(8):722–9.
17. Hurwitz HI, Yi J, Ince W, Novotny WF, Rosen O. The clinical benefit of bevacizumab in metastatic colorectal cancer is independent of K-ras mutation status: analysis of a phase III study of bevacizumab with chemotherapy in previously untreated metastatic colorectal cancer. Oncologist. 2009;14(1):22–8.

18. Cheng Y, Tian H. Current development status of MEK inhibitors. Molecules. 2017;22(10):1551.
19. Samatar AA, Poulikakos PI. Targeting RAS-ERK signalling in cancer: promises and challenges. Nat Rev Drug Discov. 2014;13(12):928–42.
20. Zimmitti G, Shindoh J, Mise Y, Kopetz S, Loyer EM, Andreou A, et al. RAS mutations predict radiologic and pathologic response in patients treated with chemotherapy before resection of colorectal liver metastases. Ann Surg Oncol. 2015;22(3):834–42.
21. Brudvik KW, Mise Y, Chung MH, Chun YS, Kopetz SE, Passot G, et al. RAS mutation predicts positive resection margins and narrower resection margins in patients undergoing resection of colorectal liver metastases. Ann Surg Oncol. 2016;23(8):2635–43.
22. Odisio BC, Yamashita S, Huang SY, Harmoush S, Kopetz SE, Ahrar K, et al. Local tumour progression after percutaneous ablation of colorectal liver metastases according to RAS mutation status. Br J Surg. 2017;104(6):760–8.
23. Yamashita S, Chun YS, Kopetz SE, Vauthey JN. Biomarkers in colorectal liver metastases. Br J Surg. 2018;105(6):618–27.
24. Brudvik KW, Vauthey JN. Surgery: KRAS mutations and hepatic recurrence after treatment of colorectal liver metastases. Nat Rev Gastroenterol Hepatol. 2017;14(11):638–9.
25. Margonis GA, Sasaki K, Andreatos N, Kim Y, Merath K, Wagner D, et al. KRAS mutation status dictates optimal surgical margin width in patients undergoing resection of colorectal liver metastases. Ann Surg Oncol. 2017;24(1):264–71.
26. Serova M, Astorgues-Xerri L, Bieche I, Albert S, Vidaud M, Benhadji KA, et al. Epithelial-to-mesenchymal transition and oncogenic Ras expression in resistance to the protein kinase Cbeta inhibitor enzastaurin in colon cancer cells. Mol Cancer Ther. 2010;9(5):1308–17.
27. Margonis GA, Buettner S, Andreatos N, Sasaki K, Ijzermans JNM, van Vugt JLA, et al. Anatomical resections improve disease-free survival in patients with KRAS-mutated colorectal liver metastases. Ann Surg. 2017;266(4):641–9.
28. Brudvik KW, Jones RP, Giuliante F, Shindoh J, Passot G, Chung MH, et al. RAS mutation clinical risk score to predict survival after resection of colorectal liver metastases. Ann Surg. 2019;269(1):120–6.
29. Tie J, Desai J. Targeting BRAF mutant metastatic colorectal cancer: clinical implications and emerging therapeutic strategies. Target Oncol. 2015;10(2):179–88.
30. Passiglia F, Bronte G, Bazan V, Galvano A, Vincenzi B, Russo A. Can KRAS and BRAF mutations limit the benefit of liver resection in metastatic colorectal cancer patients? A systematic review and meta-analysis. Crit Rev Oncol Hematol. 2016;99:150–7.
31. Bokemeyer C, Van Cutsem E, Rougier P, Ciardiello F, Heeger S, Schlichting M, et al. Addition of cetuximab to chemotherapy as first-line treatment for KRAS wild-type metastatic colorectal cancer: pooled analysis of the CRYSTAL and OPUS randomised clinical trials. Eur J Cancer. 2012;48(10):1466–75.
32. Tran B, Kopetz S, Tie J, Gibbs P, Jiang ZQ, Lieu CH, et al. Impact of BRAF mutation and microsatellite instability on the pattern of metastatic spread and prognosis in metastatic colorectal cancer. Cancer. 2011;117(20):4623–32.
33. Teng HW, Huang YC, Lin JK, Chen WS, Lin TC, Jiang JK, et al. BRAF mutation is a prognostic biomarker for colorectal liver metastasectomy. J Surg Oncol. 2012;106(2):123–9.
34. Karagkounis G, Torbenson MS, Daniel HD, Azad NS, Diaz LA Jr, Donehower RC, et al. Incidence and prognostic impact of KRAS and BRAF mutation in patients undergoing liver surgery for colorectal metastases. Cancer. 2013;119(23):4137–44.
35. Schirripa M, Bergamo F, Cremolini C, Casagrande M, Lonardi S, Aprile G, et al. BRAF and RAS mutations as prognostic factors in metastatic colorectal cancer patients undergoing liver resection. Br J Cancer. 2015;112(12):1921–8.
36. Margonis GA, Buettner S, Andreatos N, Wagner D, Sasaki K, Barbon C, et al. Prognostic factors change over time after hepatectomy for colorectal liver metastases: a multi-institutional, international analysis of 1099 patients. Ann Surg. 2019;269(6):1129–37.
37. Jones JC, Renfro LA, Al-Shamsi HO, Schrock AB, Rankin A, Zhang BY, et al. (Non-V600) BRAF mutations define a clinically distinct molecular subtype of metastatic colorectal cancer. J Clin Oncol. 2017;35(23):2624–30.

38. Benson AB 3rd, Venook AP, Bekaii-Saab T, Chan E, Chen YJ, Cooper HS, et al. Colon cancer, version 3.2014. J Natl Compr Cancer Netw. 2014;12(7):1028–59.
39. Vogelstein B, Lane D, Levine AJ. Surfing the p53 network. Nature. 2000;408(6810):307–10.
40. Ivanecz A, Kavalar R, Palfy M, Pivec V, Sremec M, Horvat M, et al. Can we improve the clinical risk score? The prognostic value of p53, Ki-67 and thymidylate synthase in patients undergoing radical resection of colorectal liver metastases. HPB (Oxford). 2014;16(3):235–42.
41. Nitti D, Belluco C, Montesco MC, Bertorelle R, Da Pian PP, Fassina A, et al. Nuclear p53 protein expression in resected hepatic metastases from colorectal cancer: an independent prognostic factor of survival. Eur J Cancer. 1998;34(6):851–5.
42. Pilat N, Grunberger T, Langle F, Mittlbock M, Perisanidis B, Kappel S, et al. Assessing the TP53 marker type in patients treated with or without neoadjuvant chemotherapy for resectable colorectal liver metastases: a p53 Research Group study. Eur J Surg Oncol. 2015;41(5):683–9.
43. Yang Y, Forslund A, Remotti H, Lonnroth C, Andersson M, Brevinge H, et al. P53 mutations in primary tumors and subsequent liver metastases are related to survival in patients with colorectal carcinoma who undergo liver resection. Cancer. 2001;91(4):727–36.
44. Popat S, Chen Z, Zhao D, Pan H, Hearle N, Chandler I, et al. A prospective, blinded analysis of thymidylate synthase and p53 expression as prognostic markers in the adjuvant treatment of colorectal cancer. Ann Oncol. 2006;17(12):1810–7.
45. Belluco C, Guillem JG, Kemeny N, Huang Y, Klimstra D, Berger MF, et al. p53 nuclear protein overexpression in colorectal cancer: a dominant predictor of survival in patients with advanced hepatic metastases. J Clin Oncol. 1996;14(10):2696–701.
46. Chun YS, Passot G, Yamashita S, Nusrat M, Katsonis P, Loree JM, et al. Deleterious effect of RAS and evolutionary high-risk TP53 double mutation in colorectal liver metastases. Ann Surg. 2019;269(5):917–23.
47. Cancer Genome Atlas N. Comprehensive molecular characterization of human colon and rectal cancer. Nature. 2012;487(7407):330–7.
48. Samuels Y, Diaz LA Jr, Schmidt-Kittler O, Cummins JM, Delong L, Cheong I, et al. Mutant PIK3CA promotes cell growth and invasion of human cancer cells. Cancer Cell. 2005;7(6):561–73.
49. Holdhoff M, Schmidt K, Diehl F, Aggrawal N, Angenendt P, Romans K, et al. Detection of tumor DNA at the margins of colorectal cancer liver metastasis. Clin Cancer Res. 2011;17(11):3551–7.
50. Loes IM, Immervoll H, Sorbye H, Angelsen JH, Horn A, Knappskog S, et al. Impact of KRAS, BRAF, PIK3CA, TP53 status and intraindividual mutation heterogeneity on outcome after liver resection for colorectal cancer metastases. Int J Cancer. 2016;139(3):647–56.
51. Bruin SC, He Y, Mikolajewska-Hanclich I, Liefers GJ, Klijn C, Vincent A, et al. Molecular alterations associated with liver metastases development in colorectal cancer patients. Br J Cancer. 2011;105(2):281–7.
52. Yamashita S, Chun YS, Kopetz SE, Maru D, Conrad C, Aloia TA, et al. APC and PIK3CA mutational cooperativity predicts pathologic response and survival in patients undergoing resection for colorectal liver metastases. 2017 Apr 4. PMID: 28379870. [Epub ahead of print].
53. Dallol A, Buhmeida A, Al-Ahwal MS, Al-Maghrabi J, Bajouh O, Al-Khayyat S, et al. Clinical significance of frequent somatic mutations detected by high-throughput targeted sequencing in archived colorectal cancer samples. J Transl Med. 2016;14(1):118.
54. Ogino S, Nosho K, Kirkner GJ, Shima K, Irahara N, Kure S, et al. PIK3CA mutation is associated with poor prognosis among patients with curatively resected colon cancer. J Clin Oncol. 2009;27(9):1477–84.
55. De Roock W, Claes B, Bernasconi D, De Schutter J, Biesmans B, Fountzilas G, et al. Effects of KRAS, BRAF, NRAS, and PIK3CA mutations on the efficacy of cetuximab plus chemotherapy in chemotherapy-refractory metastatic colorectal cancer: a retrospective consortium analysis. Lancet Oncol. 2010;11(8):753–62.
56. Souglakos J, Philips J, Wang R, Marwah S, Silver M, Tzardi M, et al. Prognostic and predictive value of common mutations for treatment response and survival in patients with metastatic colorectal cancer. Br J Cancer. 2009;101(3):465–72.

57. Yang ZY, Wu XY, Huang YF, Di MY, Zheng DY, Chen JZ, et al. Promising biomarkers for predicting the outcomes of patients with KRAS wild-type metastatic colorectal cancer treated with anti-epidermal growth factor receptor monoclonal antibodies: a systematic review with meta-analysis. Int J Cancer. 2013;133(8):1914–25.
58. Sartore-Bianchi A, Martini M, Molinari F, Veronese S, Nichelatti M, Artale S, et al. PIK3CA mutations in colorectal cancer are associated with clinical resistance to EGFR-targeted monoclonal antibodies. Cancer Res. 2009;69(5):1851–7.
59. Deming DA, Leystra AA, Nettekoven L, Sievers C, Miller D, Middlebrooks M, et al. PIK3CA and APC mutations are synergistic in the development of intestinal cancers. Oncogene. 2014;33(17):2245–54.
60. Chen J, Rocken C, Lofton-Day C, Schulz HU, Muller O, Kutzner N, et al. Molecular analysis of APC promoter methylation and protein expression in colorectal cancer metastasis. Carcinogenesis. 2005;26(1):37–43.
61. Lim B, Mun J, Kim JH, Kim CW, Roh SA, Cho DH, et al. Genome-wide mutation profiles of colorectal tumors and associated liver metastases at the exome and transcriptome levels. Oncotarget. 2015;6(26):22179–90.
62. Lee SY, Haq F, Kim D, Jun C, Jo HJ, Ahn SM, et al. Comparative genomic analysis of primary and synchronous metastatic colorectal cancers. PLoS One. 2014;9(3):e90459.
63. Schell MJ, Yang M, Teer JK, Lo FY, Madan A, Coppola D, et al. A multigene mutation classification of 468 colorectal cancers reveals a prognostic role for APC. Nat Commun. 2016;7:11743.
64. McMurray HR, Sampson ER, Compitello G, Kinsey C, Newman L, Smith B, et al. Synergistic response to oncogenic mutations defines gene class critical to cancer phenotype. Nature. 2008;453(7198):1112–6.
65. Fleming NI, Jorissen RN, Mouradov D, Christie M, Sakthianandeswaren A, Palmieri M, et al. SMAD2, SMAD3 and SMAD4 mutations in colorectal cancer. Cancer Res. 2013;73(2):725–35.
66. Mizuno T, Cloyd JM, Vicente D, Omichi K, Chun YS, Kopetz SE, et al. SMAD4 gene mutation predicts poor prognosis in patients undergoing resection for colorectal liver metastases. Eur J Surg Oncol. 2018;44(5):684–92.
67. Koopman M, Kortman GA, Mekenkamp L, Ligtenberg MJ, Hoogerbrugge N, Antonini NF, et al. Deficient mismatch repair system in patients with sporadic advanced colorectal cancer. Br J Cancer. 2009;100(2):266–73.
68. Goldstein J, Tran B, Ensor J, Gibbs P, Wong HL, Wong SF, et al. Multicenter retrospective analysis of metastatic colorectal cancer (CRC) with high-level microsatellite instability (MSI-H). Ann Oncol. 2014;25(5):1032–8.
69. Vilar E, Tabernero J. Molecular dissection of microsatellite instable colorectal cancer. Cancer Discov. 2013;3(5):502–11.
70. Popat S, Hubner R, Houlston RS. Systematic review of microsatellite instability and colorectal cancer prognosis. J Clin Oncol. 2005;23(3):609–18.
71. Sinicrope FA, Foster NR, Thibodeau SN, Marsoni S, Monges G, Labianca R, et al. DNA mismatch repair status and colon cancer recurrence and survival in clinical trials of 5-fluorouracil-based adjuvant therapy. J Natl Cancer Inst. 2011;103(11):863–75.
72. Muller CI, Schulmann K, Reinacher-Schick A, Andre N, Arnold D, Tannapfel A, et al. Predictive and prognostic value of microsatellite instability in patients with advanced colorectal cancer treated with a fluoropyrimidine and oxaliplatin containing first-line chemotherapy. A report of the AIO Colorectal Study Group. Int J Color Dis. 2008;23(11):1033–9.
73. Haddad R, Ogilvie RT, Croitoru M, Muniz V, Gryfe R, Pollet A, et al. Microsatellite instability as a prognostic factor in resected colorectal cancer liver metastases. Ann Surg Oncol. 2004;11(11):977–82.
74. Kochhar R, Halling KC, McDonnell S, Schaid DJ, French AJ, O'Connell MJ, et al. Allelic imbalance and microsatellite instability in resected Duke's D colorectal cancer. Diagn Mol Pathol. 1997;6(2):78–84.
75. Le DT, Uram JN, Wang H, Bartlett BR, Kemberling H, Eyring AD, et al. PD-1 blockade in tumors with mismatch-repair deficiency. N Engl J Med. 2015;372(26):2509–20.

76. Ronnekleiv-Kelly SM, Burkhart RA, Pawlik TM. Molecular markers of prognosis and therapeutic targets in metastatic colorectal cancer. Surg Oncol. 2016;25(3):190–9.
77. Koch M, Kienle P, Hinz U, Antolovic D, Schmidt J, Herfarth C, et al. Detection of hematogenous tumor cell dissemination predicts tumor relapse in patients undergoing surgical resection of colorectal liver metastases. Ann Surg. 2005;241(2):199–205.
78. Groot Koerkamp B, Rahbari NN, Buchler MW, Koch M, Weitz J. Circulating tumor cells and prognosis of patients with resectable colorectal liver metastases or widespread metastatic colorectal cancer: a meta-analysis. Ann Surg Oncol. 2013;20(7):2156–65.
79. Barbazan J, Muinelo-Romay L, Vieito M, Candamio S, Diaz-Lopez A, Cano A, et al. A multimarker panel for circulating tumor cells detection predicts patient outcome and therapy response in metastatic colorectal cancer. Int J Cancer. 2014;135(11):2633–43.

Diagnosis of Colorectal Liver Metastases

4

Roberto Heleno Lopes, Bruno Roberto Braga Azevedo, André Noronha Arvellos, Phillipe Abreu-Reis, and Alexandre Ferreira Oliveira

Worldwide incidence of colorectal cancer (CRC) is estimated at 1,200,000 new cases and 609,000 deaths each year [1]. According to the US Centers for Disease Control and Prevention (CDC), there will be 141,000 new cases and 51,000 deaths from CRC in the country, in 2018 [2, 3].

In Brazil, CRC represents the third leading cause of cancer among men (17,380 new cases, 7.8% of all cancer diagnosis each year) and the second among women (18,980 new cases, 8.6%) [4].

R. H. Lopes
Brazilian Society of Surgical Oncology, Rio de Janeiro, Brazil

University Hospital of the Federal University of Juiz de Fora, Juiz de Fora, Brazil

B. R. B. Azevedo
Brazilian Society of Surgical Oncology, Rio de Janeiro, Brazil

São Vicente Hospital, São Vicente, Brazil

A. N. Arvellos
Federal University of Juiz de Fora, Juiz de Fora, Brazil

P. Abreu-Reis
Brazilian Society of Surgical Oncology, Rio de Janeiro, Brazil

A. F. Oliveira (✉)
Brazilian Society of Surgical Oncology, Rio de Janeiro, Brazil

University Hospital of the Federal University of Juiz de Fora, Juiz de Fora, Brazil

Federal University of Juiz de Fora, Juiz de Fora, Brazil

M. M. Correia et al. (eds.), *Colorectal Cancer Liver Metastases*,
https://doi.org/10.1007/978-3-030-25486-5_4

Definition

In approximately 50–60% of colorectal cancer patients, the disease progresses with distant metastases. The liver is the most common site for disease progression and accounts for up to 80% of cases [5–11]. Isolated liver metastases occur in 20–50% of the advanced stage disease [12, 13].

Metastases are more frequently observed after locoregional primary treatment of colorectal cancer [14], during the follow-up period. In 15–34% of the cases, the diagnosis of metastatic disease is synchronous, meaning detection within 6 months from primary diagnosis [10–17].

Follow-Up After Treatment of the Primary Tumor

Disease progression commonly occurs within 2.5–5 years of the subclinical phase, in which clinical and laboratory changes are absent [18–20].

Patients with treated initial stage disease should be followed up with clinical examination, CT imaging studies (including chest and abdomen), and laboratory samples (serum CEA) every 3–6 months for 2 years, and every 6 months from the third to the fifth year and, annually, after the fifth year. In addition, colonoscopy should be performed 1 year after the resection of the primary [21, 22].

CEA describes a set of glycoproteins highly related to cell adhesion, being present only at very low levels in healthy adults. In colorectal cancer patients, serum CEA levels may be elevated, which means that it can be used as a tumor marker. This marker may be elevated in 80% of patients with hepatic metastases [23].

Clinical Diagnosis

Some symptoms may be present at the time of recurrence, including fever, thromboembolism, abdominal pain, weight loss, progressive liver failure with nausea, jaundice, and encephalopathy, hepatomegaly, and ascites [24, 25].

Laboratory Diagnosis

In specific laboratory results may occur, including mild elevation of serum bilirubin, alkaline phosphatase (AF), and gamma-glutamyltransferase (GGT) may occur [26, 27].

After surgery for complete resection of localized CRC, approximately half of the CEA elevations are false positives. Variation levels range from 5 to 15 ng/mL. Virtually all cases with results greater than 35 ng/mL are true positives. According to meta-analyses and systematic reviews, considering the cut-off value of 10 ng/mL, the sensitivity and specificity of CEA are respectively 68% and

97%. Other markers may show nonspecific elevations, such as CA 19.9, CA 72.4 [28–30].

Biological Diagnosis

Serum evaluation techniques of mutated genetic clones have been used as potential markers of tumor activity. In this context, the technique of liquid biopsy has been demonstrated. Circulating tumor cells and circulating tumor DNA may become useful at initial evaluation, as a personalized approach. Follow-up could be performed by testing circulating serum genetic tumor load [31].

Main limitations for a personalized approach are related to costs and potential unmeasurable benefits at the moment.

Although circulating tumor cells often correlate with a poor prognosis of CRC metastasis, its application in clinical practice has not yet been proven. Likewise, the usefulness of circulating tumor DNA to guide treatment is still under investigation [32–34].

Imaging Diagnosis

Better detection rates of hepatic metastases are achieved with imaging studies at the time a CRC is diagnosed or during follow-up. Imaging is the initial step, regardless of treatment status or clinical and laboratory results [35–37].

Methods

Ultrasonography

Conventional ultrasonography is not currently recommended as the sole liver exams for colorectal tumor patients because of their inferior performance compared to the other methods [38, 39].

However, many teams alternate liver ultrasound (US) and computerized tomography (CT) for disease detection in order to reduce patient exposure to radiation resulting from repeated CT scans [40].

Contrasted Ultrasonography

The introduction of ultrasound with venous contrast can change this trend by allowing the identification of more hepatic metastases than conventional ultrasound, also emphasizing the specificity for characterization of focal liver lesions.

Recent works have shown similar results to contrast computed tomography, already being adopted in some treatment centers as an alternative method to CT, with the main gain of non-radiation exposure [38].

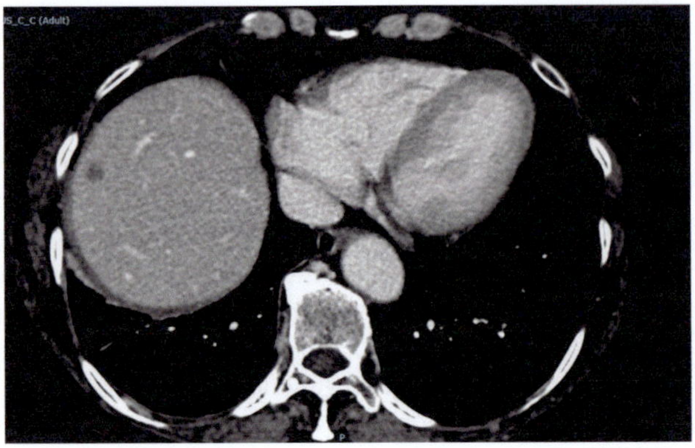

Fig. 4.1 Usual hypodense aspect of colon tumor liver metastasis in post-contrast venous phase on computed tomography image

Its main limitation is the sensitivity for lesions smaller than 1.0 cm, adding to the limitations inherent in the method such as obesity, intestinal gas interposition, and operator experience.

Computed Tomography

The advantages of computed tomography include its fast imaging acquisition, relatively low cost, and the probability of detecting extra-hepatic metastases in addition to liver lesions at the same time, such as pulmonary and lymph nodes (Fig. 4.1).

The portal venous phase persists as the ideal time to detect hepatic metastasis on CT. The thickness of acquisition is important for visualization of the smaller hepatic lesions, from 2.5 to 3.7 mm with better results and sensitivity greater than 5 mm.

However, when using thinner cuts, no improvement in the detection of hepatic lesions was observed, the ideal thickness being 2–3 mm [41].

The main drawbacks of the method are exposure to radiation and the difficulty to characterize injuries smaller than 1.0 cm.

Positron Emission Computed Tomography (PET-CT)

Due to the high metabolic activity of normal hepatic tissue, positron emission computed tomography (PET-CT) may not be useful in assessing intrahepatic lesions, notably small lesions (Fig. 4.2), although the method can identify radiologically extra-hepatic hidden disease, and this is its greatest applicability, changing the treatment plan in up to 24% of cases [42–45] (Fig. 4.3).

However, the value of this test for staging has been questioned, since its results do not seem to change as often the surgical management as initially reported [46].

The primary limitations of PET-CT include its low sensitivity for detection of lesions lower than 1.0 cm and lesions with high mucin content, and a decrease in sensitivity for the detection of lesions of patients submitted to neoadjuvant chemotherapy. The sensitivity post chemo is 60–70%, compared to 90% of patients without previous chemotherapy.

The combination of PET with magnetic resonance imaging (PET-MRI) is preferable to PET with computed tomography due to lower radiation exposure and better tissue magnetic resonance imaging contrast.

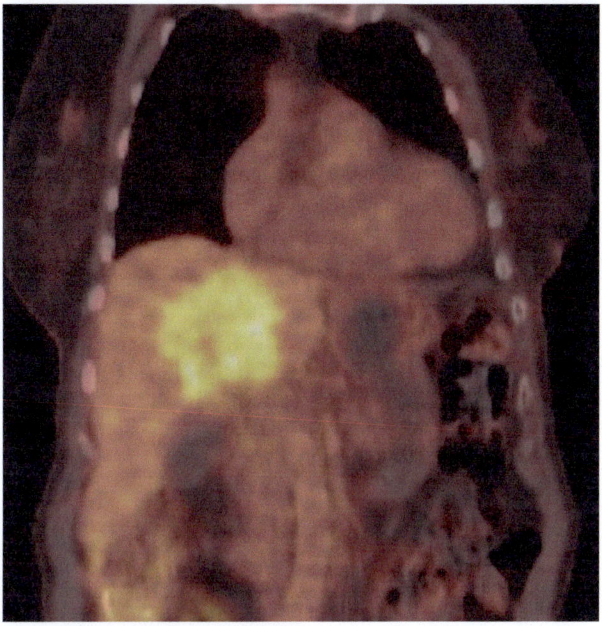

Fig. 4.2 Liver metastasis of colon with high metabolic activity observed on PET-CT exam

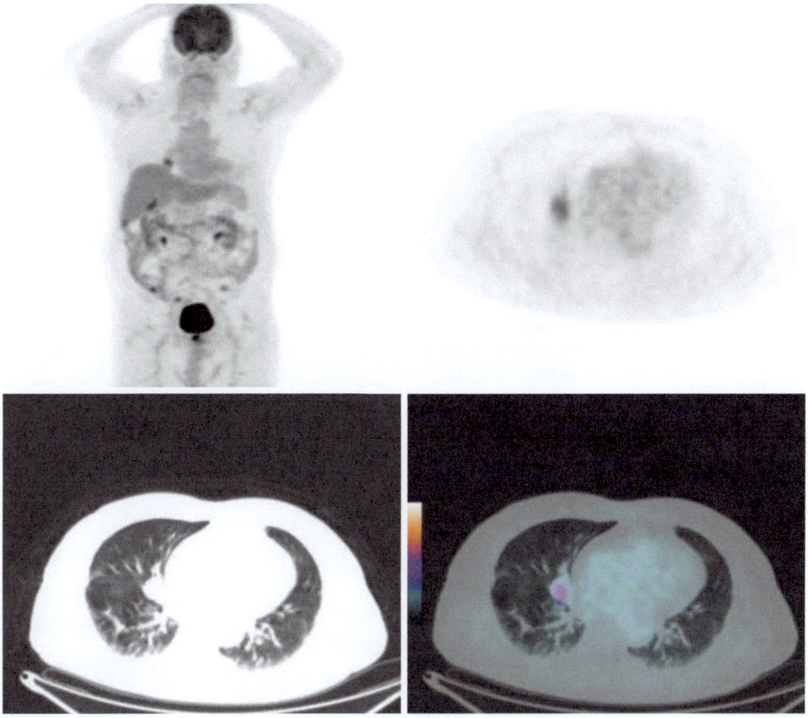

Fig. 4.3 Pulmonary nodule characterized in PET-CT as a secondary lesion, showing the usefulness of the method in extrahepatic staging

The MRI scan added to PET is complementary to the diagnosis of colorectal liver metastasis, since it has a better sensitivity and specificity in PET deficiencies, which are the detection and characterization of the small hepatic lesion and evaluation of the lesion post-chemo.

Magnetic Resonance Imaging

Based on meta-analyses, magnetic resonance imaging is the most sensitive imaging modality of the liver in patients with colorectal cancer metastasis (Figs. 4.4 and 4.5), particularly for lesions smaller than 1.0 cm (sensitivity 88.2% and mean specificity 92.5%) [47].

Nevertheless, a large number of institutions still use computed tomography as the primary imaging modality, reserving magnetic resonance imaging for situations where the CT scan was not able to characterize the lesions observed and for those

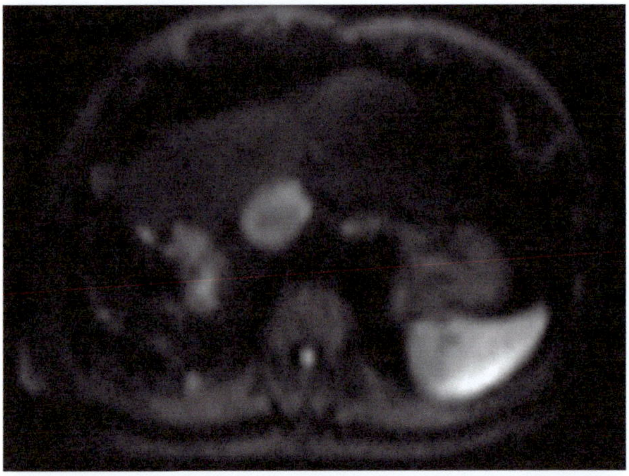

Fig. 4.4 Magnetic resonance imaging in the diffusion sequence showing lesions on the surgical margin of previous resection and another secondary lesion in the transition of segments I and IVa

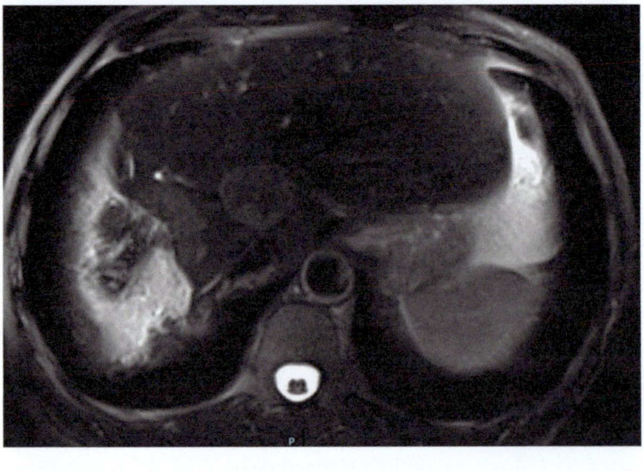

Fig. 4.5 The same patient as in the previous figure shows the lower repercussion of the hepatic lesions in the T2-weighted sequence of the MRI

patients who are candidates for surgical resection where the most accurate detection of the number of lesions is required.

Computed tomography as the primary method of routine liver evaluation is due to the greater familiarity of the method by surgeons than magnetic resonance imaging or PET, as well as its greater availability. Computed tomography shows a high performance in the detection of lesions, especially due to the greater experience of radiologists with the method [48].

In fact, the addition to the diagnosis of magnetic resonance imaging for hepatic metastases in patients newly diagnosed with colorectal carcinoma is low on negative computed tomography, but there is a low superiority in the presence of small lesions that cannot be characterized by tomography [49].

Magnetic Resonance with Specific Hepatobiliary Contrast

Specific hepatobiliary contrast has a similar extra-cellular effect to the usual gadolinium in the arterial, venous-portal, and late phases and should always be performed for the complete study, allowing a better characterization of the lesions, increasing the specificity of the examination.

Magnetic resonance imaging with the use of specific hepatocellular contrast, such as gadoxetic acid, has shown a greater sensitivity of around 92–98%

than conventional magnetic resonance with extracellular contrast agents [50–52].

It is a useful technique to evaluate the hepatic lesions identified and not definitively characterized in the preoperative tomography of newly diagnosed colorectal cancer patients [53].

There is also superiority in the evaluation of small lesions identified in localized diffusion sequences adjacent to the vessels due to their low signal in the hepatobiliary phase, often obscured in the conventional resonance in the post-contrast phases by the high vascular signal [54].

Although magnetic resonance imaging with specific hepatobiliary contrast shows higher isolated cost between imaging modalities, with the exception of PET, it presents final savings, since it prevents the need for other methods and unnecessary surgical procedures by allowing more precise staging [55]. Magnetic resonance imaging with gadoxic acid can be considered the first-line method in the evaluation of colorectal hepatic metastases, especially in patients who are candidates for surgery.

Intraoperative Ultrasound

Intraoperative ultrasound is the most sensitive imaging method for the detection of focal liver lesions, with a specific chapter dedicated to this description.

Typical Presentation of Hepatic Colorectal Metastases

Metastatic hepatic lesions of colorectal origin show a varied appearance, but the typical presentation in the computed tomography has the same hypodense feature of the normal hepatic parenchyma in the non-contrast phase, due to the absence of glycogen inside the lesions and of the relative increase in water content in the extracellular spaces commonly observed in malignant neoplasias.

In the presence of hepatic steatosis, however, the metastatic lesions may be isodense or hyperdense due to the low attenuation of the hepatic tissue by the presence of fat [56].

Heterogeneity is the pattern of appearance of metastatic liver lesions on CT scan due to the varied presence and proportion of mucin, fibrosis, and calcification [57].

About 11% of colorectal metastases may present at the initial evaluation with calcifications, better characterized in the non-contrast phase [41].

The presence of peripheral annular enhancement during the arterial phase corresponds to changes in non-tumor inflammatory pattern and perilesional vascular proliferation [56].

Metastatic hepatic lesions may also present centripetal filling in subsequent post-contrast phases, requiring differentiation with hepatic hemangiomas that usually show discontinuous peripheral enhancement and complete filling, and the density of the latter's enhancement areas similar to the aorta in the same acquisition phase [58].

In MRI, colorectal liver metastases are typically poorly defined with a moderately hypointense sign in relation to the adjacent liver parenchyma in the T1 sequences and hyperintense in the T2 sequences, may often present absence of filling in the central region suggesting necrosis. Hepatobiliary contrast enhancers both peripheral enhancement and target appearance with hyperintense center and hypointense periphery have been described for metastases in the hepatobiliary phase, although the most common usual pattern is homogeneous hypointense aspect [55].

Imaging tests are essential to differentiate metastases from benign lesions, in a way that each of these display a typical presentation. It is usually possible to exclude cysts, granulomatous calcifications, hemangiomas, focal nodular hyperplasias, adenomas with fat content, focal steatosis, and perfusion changes from the diagnosis of liver metastases.

Particular Situations

Small Hepatic Lesions

Small hepatic lesions are defined as lesions smaller than 15 mm, and the likelihood of benign lesions is high even in patients with known hepatic neoplasms [59].

A specific study evaluating hepatic lesions smaller than 10 mm in diameter in patients with several primary neoplasms found 14% of malignancy in patients with colorectal carcinoma [60].

Comparisons with previous imaging studies are the most useful tactics in the evaluation of these cases, since stability greater than 12 months suggests benignity, while the appearance of new lesions increases the suspicion for malignancy.

Magnetic resonance imaging is the next method in the evaluation of the small hepatic lesion detected in the initial CT study when its immediate characterization is necessary. The close monitoring of the small indeterminate lesions in imaging studies is fundamental.

According to the guidelines of the American College of Radiology (2017), injuries smaller than 1.0 cm and injuries unable to be characterized by imaging in patients with a higher risk, such as patients with colorectal tumors, should be followed up by magnetic resonance imaging in 3–6 months [61].

Neoadjuvant Chemotherapy Imaging Workup

The possibility of steatosis and steatohepatitis associated with chemotherapy is highlighted, as it occurs after the use of irinotecan and oxaliplatin. Another situation that may lead to confusion in the post-chemotherapy evaluation is the occurrence of hepatic peliosis associated with some drugs such as oxaliplatin, and it should not be confused as the appearance of a new lesion in the course of chemotherapy. Magnetic resonance imaging is a method of preference in the evaluation of patients with colorectal metastasis treated with neoadjuvant chemotherapy with sensitivity of around 85.7%, mainly because it does not have a great impact on the quality of their images in the presence of steatosis [62].

Specifically, hepatobiliary contrast resonance has been shown to be superior to CT in steatosis contexts and most notably in the presence of metastases smaller than 1 cm [63].

Computed tomography is the best alternative method to MRI, since PET shows a worse performance among these three modalities in the persence of reduction of the size of the metastatic lesions, reduction of the metabolic activity of tumor cells, and presence of necrosis. Computed tomography has a lower sensitivity due to low attenuation of the liver parenchyma and less prominence of the liver in the presence of chemotherapy-induced steatosis, resulting in the reduction of the parenchymal contrast [62].

The identification of new hypoattenuating or hyperattenuating lesions on post-treatment CT scans may represent lesions that have been overlooked in pretreatment examinations due to isodensity and are now observed due to the steatosis, mimicking progression of disease in the period of chemotherapy.

Final Recommendation

Computed tomography should be the initial assessment method at the time of diagnosis of the primary lesion and during the follow-up of the patient treated without liver injury as recommended by the guidelines the European Consensus on the European Society of Oncology Medicine, the Brazilian consensus of multidisciplinary treatment of colorectal liver metastasis, and by the National Comprehensive Cancer Network (NCCN) [63–66].

As a recent alternative, ultrasound with venous contrast seems to show similar results to those of CT and has already been adopted in some treatment centers.

Conventional magnetic resonance or hepatobiliary contrast is the method reserved for better characterization of undetermined lesion on CT, notably of the small lesion, in the context of steatosis, presurgical hepatic evaluation, and post-chemotherapy evaluation.

Specific hepatobiliary contrast resonance is also indicated in the preoperative period by allowing better surgery programming by detecting the highest number of liver lesions.

PET in the hepatic evaluation, with CT or MRI, has a role in post-surgical patients or post-radioablation when CT and MRI cannot differentiate the presence of residual or recurrent lesion (Figs. 4.6 and 4.7).

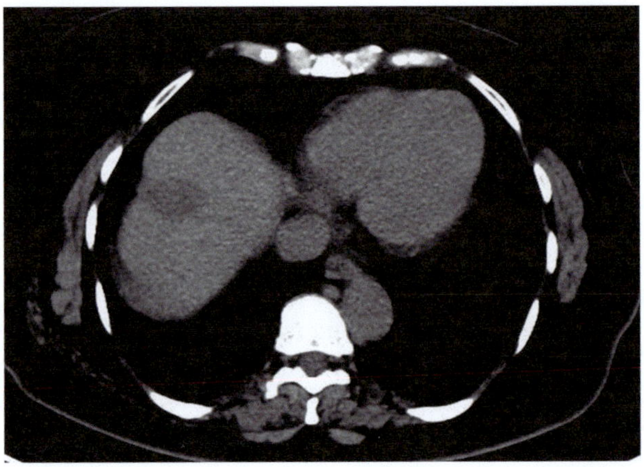

Fig. 4.6 Follow-up examination after local resection of liver metastasis showing non-specific hypodense focal change on CT

Fig. 4.7 PET image of the previous patient without signs of radiotracer uptake denoting area of post-surgical alteration without residual or recurrent lesion

The accomplishment of the step-by-step examinations in the image evaluation of the liver related to the therapeutic possibilities and patient's treatment is the most rational and appropriate use of imaging methods.

References

1. Siegel RL, Miller KD, Jemal A. Cancer statistics, 2016. CA Cancer J Clin. 2016;66(1):7–30.
2. Cheng L, Eng C, Nieman LZ, Kapadia AS, Du XL. Trends in colorectal cancer incidence by anatomic site and disease stage in the United States from 1976 to 2005. Am J Clin Oncol. 2011;34(6):573–80.
3. Henley SJ, Singh SD, King J, Wilson R, O'Neil ME, Ryerson AB, et al. Invasive cancer incidence and survival–United States, 2011. MMWR Morb Mortal Wkly Rep. 2015;64(9):237–42.
4. INCA – Instituto Nacional de Câncer – Estimativa 2018 [Internet]. [cited 2018 Apr 23]. Available from: http://www.inca.gov.br/estimativa/2018/.
5. Abdalla EK, Adam R, Bilchik AJ, Jaeck D, Vauthey JN, Mahvi D. Improving resectability of hepatic colorectal metastases: expert consensus statement. Ann Surg Oncol. 2006;13(10):1271–80.
6. Fong Y, Cohen AM, Fortner JG, Enker WE, Turnbull AD, Coit DG, et al. Liver resection for colorectal metastases. J Clin Oncol. 1997;15(3):938–46. 6. Sheth KR, Clary BM. Management of hepatic metastases from colorrectal cancer. Clin Colon Rectal Surg. 2005;18(3):215–23.
7. Pozzo C, Basso M, Cassano A, Quirino M, Schinzari G, Trigila N, et al. Neoadjuvant treatment of unresectable liver disease with irinotecan and 5-fluorouracil plus folinic acid in colorrectal cancer patients. Ann Oncol. 2004;15:933–9.
8. Manfredi S, Lepage C, Hatem C, Coatmeur O, Faivre J, Bouvier AM. Epidemiology and management of liver metastases from colorectal cancer. Ann Surg. 2006;244(2):254–9.
9. Welch JP, Donaldson GA. The clinical correlation of an autopsy study of recurrent colorectal cancer. Ann Surg. 1979;189(4):496–502.
10. Mantke R, Schmidt U, WolffS KR, Lippert H. Incidence of synchronous liver metastases in patients with colorectal cancer in relationship to clinico-pathologic characteristics. Results of a German prospective multicenter observational study. Eur J Surg Oncol. 2012;38(3):259–65.
11. Lupinacci RM, Coelho FF, Perini MV, Lobo EJ, Ferreira FG, Szutan LA, et al. Current management of liver metastases from colorectal cancer: recommendations of the São Paulo Liver Club. Rev Col Bras Cir. 2013;40(3):251–60.
12. Ghiringhelli F, Hennequin A, Drouillard A, Lepage C, Faivre J, Bouvier AM. Epidemiology and prognosis of synchronous and metachronous colon cancer metastases: a French population-based study. Dig Liver Dis. 2014;46(9):854–8.
13. Pugh S, Fuller A, Rose P, Perera-Salazar R, Mellor J, George S, et al. What is the true incidence of metachronous colorectal liver metástases? Evidence from the UK FACS (follow-up after colorectal surgery) trial. Gut (Medical Abstracts). 2012;61(Suppl 2):A24.
14. Paschos KA, Majeed AW, Bird NC. Natural history of hepatic metastases from colorectal cancer--pathobiological pathways with clinical significance. World J Gastroenterol. 2014;20(14):3719–37.
15. Sugarbaker PH. Colorectal cancer: prevention and management of metastatic disease. Biomed Res Int. 2014;2014:782890.
16. Haddad JD, You DM. Colorectal cancer screening and race in an equal access medical system. J Community Health. 2016;41(1):78–81.
17. Haddad AJ, Bani Hani M, Pawlik TM, Cunningham SC. Colorectal liver metastases. Int J Surg Oncol. 2011;2011:285840.
18. Sargent D, Sobrero A, Grothey A, et al. Evidence for cure by adjuvant therapy in colon cancer: observations based on individual patient data from 20,898 patients on 18 randomized trials. J Clin Oncol. 2009;27:872–7. Available at: http://www.ncbi.nlm.nih.gov/pubmed/19124803.

19. Seo SI, Lim SB, Yoon YS, et al. Comparison of recurrence patterns between </=5 years and >5 years after curative operations in colorectal cancer patients. J Surg Oncol. 2013;108:9–13. Available at: http://www.ncbi.nlm.nih.gov/pubmed/23754582.
20. Smith JJ, D'Angelica MI. Surgical management of hepatic metastases of colorectal cancer. Hematol Oncol Clin North Am. 2015;29(1):61–84.
21. Lepage C, Phelip JM, Cany L, et al. Effect of 5 years of imaging and CEA follow-up to detect recurrence of colorectal cancer: the FFCD PRODIGE 13 randomised phase III trial. Dig Liver Dis. 2015;47:529–31. Available at: http://www.ncbi.nlm.nih.gov/pubmed/25933809.
22. Kahi CJ, Boland CR, Dominitz JA, et al. Colonoscopy surveillance after colorectal cancer resection: recommendations of the US Multi- Society Task Force on Colorectal Cancer. Gastroenterology. 2016;150:758–768 e711. Available at: https://www.ncbi.nlm.nih.gov/pubmed/26892199.
23. Rosati G, Ambrosini G, Barni S, et al. A randomized trial of intensive versus minimal surveillance of patients with resected Dukes B2-C colorectal carcinoma. Ann Oncol. 2016;27:274–80. Available at: https://www.ncbi.nlm.nih.gov/pubmed/26578734.
24. Rex DK, Kahi CJ, Levin B, Smith RA, Bond JH, Brooks D, Burt RW, Byers T, Fletcher RH, Hyman N, Johnson D, Kirk L, Lieberman DA, Levin TR, O'Brien MJ, Simmang C, Thorson AG, Winawer SJ. Guidelines for colonoscopy surveillance after cancer resection: a consensus update by the American Cancer Society and the US Multi-Society Task Force on Colorectal Cancer. Gastroenterology. 2006;130(6):1865–71.
25. Pedruzzi PAG, Hoeldtke E, Tomasich FDS, Dias LAN, Kato M. Metástase hepática – Estudo de 115 casos. Rev Soc Bras Cancerol. 2003;24(4):06–12.
26. Slesser AA, Khan F, Chau I, Khan AZ, Mudan S, Tekkis PP, Brown G, Rao S. The effect of a primary tumour resection on the progression of synchronous colorectal liver metastases: an exploratory study. Eur J Surg Oncol [Internet]. Elsevier Ltd. 2015;41(4):484–92. Available from: http://www.ncbi.nlm.nih.gov/pubmed/25638603.
27. Bendell JC, Bekaii-Saab TS, Cohn AL, Hurwitz HI, Kozloff M, Tezcan H, et al. Treatment patterns and clinical outcomes in patients with metastatic colorectal cancer initially treated with FOLFOX-bevacizumab or FOLFIRI-bevacizumab: results from ARIES, a bevacizumab observational cohort study. Oncologist [Internet]. 2012;17(12):1486–95. Available from: http://www.pubmedcentral.nih.gov/articlerender.fcgi?artid=3528380&tool=pmcentrez&rendertype=abstract.
28. Litvka A, Cercek A, Segal N, et al. False-positive elevations of carcinoembryonic antigen in patients with a history of resected colorectal cancer. J Natl Compr Canc Netw. 2014;12:907–13. Available at: http://www.ncbi.nlm.nih.gov/pubmed/24925201.
29. Nicholson BD, Shinkins B, Pathiraja I, et al. Blood CEA levels for detecting recurrent colorectal cancer. Cochrane Database Syst Rev. 2015:CD011134. Available at: http://www.ncbi.nlm.nih.gov/pubmed/26661580.
30. Nicholson BD, Shinkins B, Mant D. Blood measurement of carcinoembryonic antigen level for detecting recurrence of colorectal cancer. JAMA. 2016;316:1310–1. Available at: https://www.ncbi.nlm.nih.gov/pubmed/27673308.
31. Cohen SJ, Punt CJ, Iannotti N, et al. Relationship of circulating tumor cells to tumor response, progression-free survival, and overall survival in patients with metastatic colorectal cancer. J Clin Oncol. 2008;26:3213–21.
32. Diaz LA Jr, Bardelli A. Liquid biopsies: genotyping circulating tumor DNA. J Clin Oncol. 2014;32:579–86.
33. Siravegna G, Bardelli A. Genotyping cell-free tumor DNA in the blood to detect residual disease and drug resistance. Genome Biol. 2014;15:449.
34. Montagut C, Dalmases A, Bellosillo B, et al. Identification of a mutation in the extracellular domain of the Epidermal Growth Factor Receptor conferring cetuximab resistance in colorectal cancer. Nat Med. 2012;18:221–3.
35. Meyerhardt JA, Mangu PB, Flynn PJ, et al. Follow-up care, surveillance protocol, and secondary prevention measures for survivors of colorectal cancer: American society of clinical

oncology clinical practice guideline endorsement. J Clin Oncol. 2013;31:4465–70. Available at: http://www.ncbi.nlm.nih.gov/pubmed/24220554.
36. Follow-up care, surveillance protocol, and secondary prevention measures for survivors of colorectal cancer. Cancer Care Ontario. 2016. Available at: https://www.cancercare.on.ca/common/pages/UserFile.aspx?fileId=124839. Accessed 15 Aug 2016.
37. Steele SR, Chang GJ, Hendren S, et al. Practice guideline for the surveillance of patients after curative treatment of colon and rectal cancer. Dis Colon Rectum. 2015;58:713–25. Available at: http://www.ncbi.nlm.nih.gov/pubmed/26163950
38. Floriani I, Torri V, Rulli E, et al. Performance of imaging modalities in diagnosis of liver metastases from colorectal cancer: a systematic review and meta-analysis. J Magn Reson Imaging. 2010;31:19–31.
39. Reiter MJ, Hannemann NP, Schwope RB, Lisanti CJ, Learn PA. Role of imaging for patients with colorectal hepatic metastases: what the radiologist needs to know. Abdom Imaging. 2015;40(8):3029–42.
40. Bartolotta TV, Taibbi A, Midiri M, et al. Characterisationof focal liverlesionsundeterminedatgrey-scale US: contrast-enhanced US versus 64-row MDCT and MRI withliver-specificcontrastagent. Radiol Med. 2010;115:714–31.
41. Weg N, Scheer MR, Gabor MP. Liver lesions: improved detection with dual-detector-array CT and routine 2.5 mm thin collimation. Radiology. 1998;209:417–26.
42. Adams RB, Aloia TA, Loyer E, et al. Selection for hepatic resection of colorectal liver metastases: expert consensus statement. HPB. 2013;15:91–103.
43. Frankel TL, D'Angelica MI. Hepatic resection for colorectal metastases. J Surg Oncol. 2014;109:2–7.
44. Wiering B, Krabbe PF, Jager GJ, Oyen WJ, Ruers TJ. The impact of fluorine-18-deoxyglucose-positron emission tomography in the management of colorectal liver metastases. Cancer. 2005;104:2658–70.
45. Zhuang H, Sinha P, Pourdehnad M, et al. The role of positron emission tomography with fluorine-18-deoxyglucose in identifying colorectal cancer metastases to liver. Nucl Med Commun. 2000;21:793–8.
46. Moulton CA, Gu CS, Law CH, et al. Effect of PET before liver resection on surgical management for colorectal adenocarcinoma metastases: a randomized clinical trial. JAMA. 2004;311:1863–9.
47. Niekel MC, Bipat S, Stoker J. Diagnostic imaging of colorectal liver metastases with CT, MR imaging, FDG PET, and/or FDG PET/CT: a meta-analysis of prospective studies including patients who have not previously undergone treatment. Radiology. 2010;257:674–84.
48. Scharitzer M, Ba-Ssalamah A, Ringl H, et al. Preoperative evaluation of colorectal liver metastases: comparison between gadoxetic acid-enhanced 3.0-T MRI and contrast-enhanced MDCT with histopathological correlation. Eur Radiol. 2013;23:2187–96.
49. Han K, Park SH, Kim KW, et al. Use of liver magnetic resonance imaging after standard staging abdominopelvic computed tomography to evaluate newly diagnosed colorectal cancer patients. Ann Surg. 2015;261:480–6.
50. Patel S, Cheek S, Osman H, Jeyarajah DH. MRI with gadoxetate disodium for colorectal liver metastasis: is it the new "imaging modality of choice"? J Gastrointest Surg. 2014;18:2130–5.
51. Zech CJ, Korpraphong P, Huppertz A, et al. Randomized multicentre trial of gadoxetic acid-enhanced MRI vs. Conventional MRI or CT in the staging of colorectal cancer liver metastases. Br J Surg. 2014;101:613–21.
52. Kim HJ, Lee SS, Byun JH, et al. Incremental valueofliver MR imaging in patientswithpotentiallycurablecolorectalhepaticmetastasisdetectedat CT: a prospective comparison of diffusion weighted imaging, gadoxetic acid-enhanced MR imaging, and a combination of both MR techniques. Radiology. 2015;274:712–22.
53. Cho JY, Lee YJ, Han HS, et al. Role of gadoxetic acid enhanced magnetic resonance imaging in the preoperative evaluation of small hepatic lesions in patients with colorectal cancer. World J Surg. 2015;39:1161–6.

54. Donati OF, Fischer MA, Chuck N, et al. Accuracy and confidence of Gd-EOB-DTPA enhanced MRI and diffusion weighted imaging alone and in combination for the diagnosis of liver metastases. Eur J Radiol. 2013;82:822–8.
55. Lafaro KJ, Roumanis P, Demirjian A, Lall C, Imagawa DK. Gd-EOB-DTPA-enhanced MRI for detection of liver metastases from colorectal cancer: a surgeon's perspective! Int J Hepatol. 2013;2013:572307.
56. Kanematsu M, Kondo H, Goshima S, et al. Imaging liver metastases: review and update. Eur J Radiol. 2006;58:217–28.
57. Boonsirikamchai P, Asran MA, Maru DM, et al. CT findings of response and recurrence, independent of change in tumor size, in colorectal liver metastasis treated with bevacizumab. Am J Roentgenol. 2011;197:W1060–6.
58. Sica GT, Ji H, Ros PR. CT and MR imaging of hepatic metastases. Am J Roentgenol. 2000;174:691–8.
59. Jones EC, Chezmar JL, Nelson RC, Bernardino ME. The frequency and significance of small (<15 mm) hepatic lesions detected by CT. AJR Am J Roentgenol. 1992;158:535–9.
60. Schwartz LH, Gandras EJ, Colangelo SM, Ercolani MC, Panicek DM. Prevalence and importance of small hepatic lesions found at CT in patients with cancer. Radiology. 1999;210:71–4.
61. Gore RM, Pickhardt PJ, Mortele KJ, Fishman EK, Horowitz JM, Fimmel CJ, Talamonti MS, Berland LL, Pandharipande PV. Management of incidental liver lesions on CT: a white paper of the ACR Incidental Findings Committee. J Am Coll Radiol. 2017;14(11):1429–37.
62. van Kessel CS, Buckens CF, van den Bosch MA, et al. Preoperative imaging of colorectal liver metastases after neoadjuvant chemotherapy: a meta-analysis. Ann Surg Oncol. 2012;19:2805–13.
63. Kulemann V, Schima W, Tamandl D, et al. Preoperative detection of colorectal liver metastases in fatty liver: MDCT or MRI? Eur J Radiol. 2011;79:e1–6.
64. Van Cutsem E, Cervantes A, Adam R, et al. ESMO consensus guidelines for the management of patients with metastatic colorectal cancer. Ann Oncol. 2016;27(8):1386–422.
65. Coimbra FJF, Ribeiro HSC, Marques MC. I Consenso brasileiro de tratamento multidisciplinar de metástase hepática colorretais. Módulo 1: Avaliação pré-tratamento. ABCD Arq Bras Cir Dig. 2015;28(4):222–30.
66. Benson AB 3rd, Venook AP, Al-Hawary MM, et al. NCCN guidelines insights: colon cancer, version 2.2018. J Natl Compr Canc Netw. 2018;16(4):359–69.

Role of Imaging in the Management of Patients with Potentially Resectable CRLM

5

Khalid W. Shaqdan, Ali Pourvaziri, and Dushyant V. Sahani

Introduction

Assessment of CRLM resection has rapidly changed over the years, as more lesions are deemed operable due to the expanding criteria for resectability [1]. Liver resection with curative intent necessitates addressing or removing all detectable disease sites. Preoperative imaging is essential to determine the location and extent of CRLM, proximity of lesions to vascular structures, predicting future liver remnant and identifying extrahepatic disease [2]. Moreover, full imaging assessment such as with MRI is important prior to chemotherapy, as treatment can change the appearance of metastatic lesions and affect hepatic parenchyma reducing sensitivity of CT and/or PET for CRLM evaluation [3]. In this chapter, we discuss the integral role of current imaging techniques in the management of patients with potentially resectable CRLM.

Role of Imaging in Detection of CRLM

Ultrasound

Conventional ultrasound (US) is widely used for the assessment of CRLM due to its low cost, absence of radiation exposure, and wide availability. US provides a pooled sensitivity of 63% and specificity of 97.6% for CRLM detection [4]. However, it is the addition of contrast-enhanced US (CEUS) with agents that has dramatically

K. W. Shaqdan (✉) · A. Pourvaziri · D. V. Sahani
Department of Radiology, Massachusetts General Hospital, Harvard Medical School, Boston, MA, USA
e-mail: kshaqdan@mgh.harvard.edu; apourvaziri@mgh.harvard.edu; dsahani@mgh.harvard.edu

M. M. Correia et al. (eds.), *Colorectal Cancer Liver Metastases*,
https://doi.org/10.1007/978-3-030-25486-5_5

increased the sensitivity for CRLM detection up to 80–90%, which is comparable to that by computed tomography [5, 6]. US contrast agents consist of tiny microbubbles that carry a strong safety profile and can be used in patients with impaired renal function [7]. In patients who have contraindications to iodinated contrast material, CEUS is a viable alternative and superior to non-contrast-enhanced CT in the characterization of focal liver pathology [8].

On US, CRLM often appear as hypoechoic lesions and less commonly may have similar or higher echogenicity relative to normal hepatic parenchyma [9]. CRLM, which are not visualized during preoperative imaging assessment, may be detected with the use of real-time ultrasound intraoperatively [10]. Intraoperative US (IOUS) also facilitates localization of deep-seated, nonpalpable lesions while mapping major hepatic veins, providing real-time guidance during surgery [10]. Patients with multiple CRLM benefit greatly from IOUS due to its high specificity (94–98%) and detection rate of tumors missed on prior imaging [11]. Additionally, contrast-enhanced IOUS may identify small tumor residuals, which is important to ensure microscopically margin-negative resection [12].

While some limitations regarding lesion characterization can be overcome with CEUS, accurate diagnosis is highly examiner dependent and requires experienced operator training [13]. Evaluation of multiple lesions simultaneously is also challenging with CEUS [14]. Neoadjuvant chemotherapy (NAC) can significantly alter liver echotexture (lesion and parenchyma) interfering with sensitivity and specificity of US [14]. Other challenges include limited spatial resolution of transcutaneous probes, assessing patients with obese habitus, high-lying diaphragm, and uncooperative patients [13].

Computed Tomography (CT)

Multidetector CT (MDCT) is the preferred modality for CLRM assessment in the USA due to its ability to image the liver and potential sites of extrahepatic metastases (e.g., chest, nodes, and peritoneum) in one examination [15]. MDCT is also widely available, reliable, and able to accommodate patients with body habitus limitations (e.g., obesity). Improved resolution and faster scanning speed with MDCT has enabled imaging of the entire abdomen and pelvis during a single breath hold, effectively eliminating respiratory motion artifacts [16]. Acquisition of thin slices allows for reconstruction of high-quality images in different planes and rendering reformatted images are now integral to any CT protocol [17]. The use of iodinated contrast media (ICM) to adequately detect and characterize CRLM has been advocated and is recommended by the current national comprehensive cancer network (NCCN) guidelines [18]. A recent meta-analysis reported 82% sensitivity and 73.5% specificity for CRLM detection using contrast-enhanced CT (CECT) [19] (Table 5.1). Oral contrast media is desirable but not mandatory, as it helps with better evaluation of extrahepatic pathologies, such as eliminating false-positive peritoneal metastases.

Table 5.1 Diagnostic performance of CECT, EOB-MRI, and PET-CT for CRLM detection

Modality	Diagnostic performance	
CT	Sensitivity	82% (74.0–88.1)
	Specificity	73.5% (53.7–86.9)
EOB-MRI	Sensitivity	93.1% (88.4–96.0)
	Specificity	87.3% (77.5–93.2)
PET-CT	Sensitivity	74.1% (62.1–83.3)
	Specificity	93.9% (83.9–97.8)

Reported 95% confidence interval for mean sensitivity and specificity in a meta-analysis between 2004 and 2016 [19].
This table compares the diagnostic performance of MDCT, gadoxetate disodium-enhanced MRI, and FDG PET-CT for diagnosing CRLM. The meta-analysis found that MRI was significantly more sensitive than CT ($p < 0.001$) and PET-CT ($p < 0.001$). PET-CT had the highest specificity, but not statistically significant compared to MRI ($p = 0.59$). MRI and PET-CT had significantly higher specificity than CT ($P = 0.01$ and $P < 0.001$). EOB = Gadoxetate disodium (Gd-EOB-DTPA, Eovist in the USA)

Dynamic contrast-enhanced CT (CECT) involves multi-phase acquisition including true non-contrast, arterial, portal-venous and delayed phase. CRLM are typically hypovascular lesions and appear hypoattenuating compared to normal liver tissue with heterogeneous enhancement on portal venous phase [17]. Since CRLM are hypovascular, arterial phase is typically used for presurgical planning [20]. On delayed images, CRLM can show wash-out contrary to benign pathologies (e.g., hemangiomas) [17]. Newer generation dual-energy CT scanners (DECT), which are becoming mainstream, have further bolstered the role of CT with novel post-processing techniques that improve lesion conspicuity by enhancing the liver-to-lesion contrast [21, 22] (Fig. 5.1).

Limitations of CT include low sensitivity for detecting small lesions (<10 mm) and identifying CRLM in patients receiving NAC (Tables 5.1 and 5.2) [19, 23]. NAC significantly decreases the sensitivity of CRLM detection as treated lesions shrink in size [3]. Furthermore, NAC may also cause liver steatosis which reduces hepatic parenchymal attenuation leading to diminished lesion to liver contrast [24]. Patients with a history of iodinated contrast media allergies or impaired renal function are not ideal candidates for CECT [25]. In addition, ionizing radiation exposure for oncologic patients who often require repeated imaging can be of concern. These limitations can be addressed to some extent with DECT scanners, which can minimize radiation exposure by eliminating the need for true non-contrast images and allow for reduced contrast media dose while maintaining high image quality [26–28]. Moreover, DECT applications are empowering CT with better diagnostic capabilities for small lesion detection and characterization [29, 30].

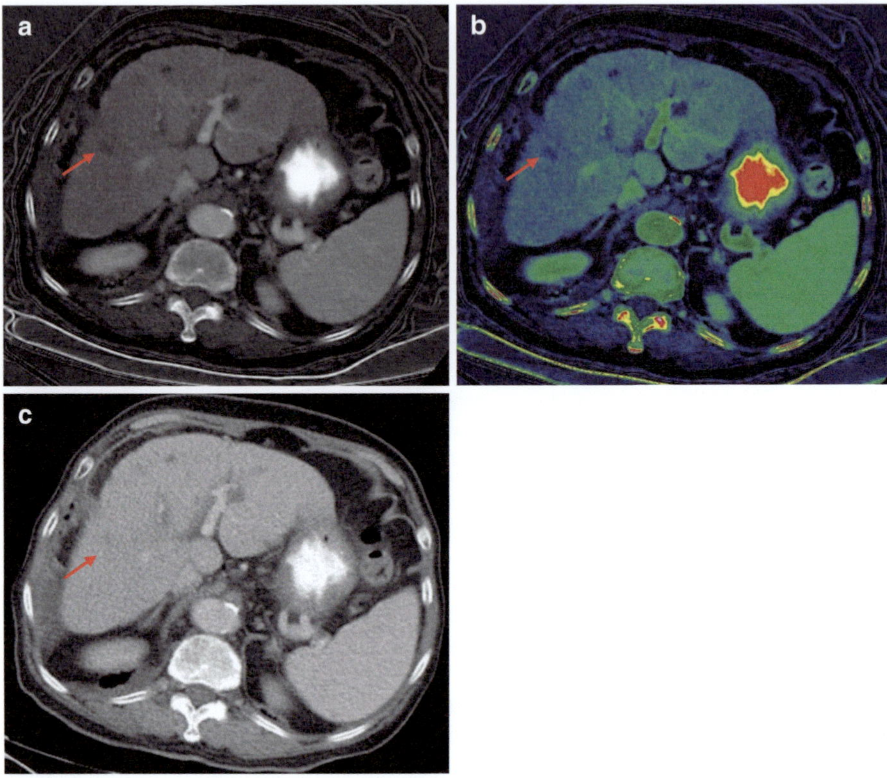

Fig. 5.1 Dual-Energy CT to improve lesion conspicuity. An 85-year-old male with multiple CRLM. Post-contrast axial reconstructions of material density-iodine in gray scale (**a**) and color-overlay (**b**) show better conspicuity of a hepatic lesion (arrows), which is hard to visualize on conventional single-energy CT image (**c**)

Table 5.2 Diagnostic performance of CECT and CEMRI for CRLM detection according to size

		Lesion size	
Modality	Diagnostic performance	<10 mm	≥10 mm
CECT	Sensitivity PL	47.3% (40–55)	86.7% (78–93)
CE-MRI	Sensitivity PL	60.2%, $p < 0.006$ (54–66)	89% (82–94)

Reported 95% confidence interval for mean sensitivity on a per lesion basis in a meta-analysis between 1990 and 2010 [23]. *PL* per-lesion

This table compares the diagnostic performance of contrast enhanced CT (CECT) and contrast-enhanced MRI (CE-MRI) for diagnosing CRLM based on lesion size. For lesions less than 10 mm, MRI had significantly higher sensitivity than CT ($p = 0.006$). There was no statistical significance between CT and MRI for lesions of size 10 mm or more ($p = 0.617$)

Magnetic Resonance Imaging (MRI)

MRI is the modality of choice for evaluating CRLM and has proven to be highly effective for hepatic parenchymal assessment. Compared to CT, MR images offer superb soft tissue contrast, which improves diagnoses of intrahepatic lesions due to greater liver-to-lesion contrast difference (Fig. 5.2) [17]. MRI also excels in detecting small lesions (<10 mm) and identifying CRLM in patients undergoing NAC or have hepatic steatosis (Tables 5.2 and 5.3) [19, 23, 31]. Dynamic contrast-enhanced MRI (CE-MRI) with hepatobiliary agents and diffusion-weighted imaging (DWI) has further improved CRLM detection and characterization of indeterminate lesions, especially for small lesions [32–35]. Gadoxetate disodium (Gd-EOB-DTPA, Eovist in the USA) is the most commonly used hepatobiliary agent with MRI for CRLM detection with a pooled sensitivity of 93.1% (Table 5.3) [19].

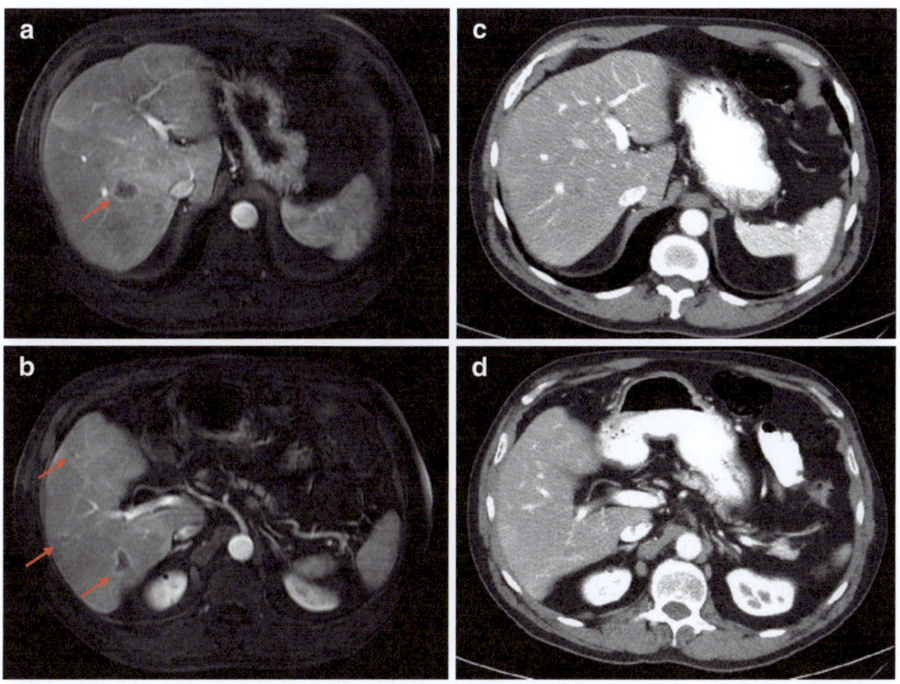

Fig. 5.2 Value of MRI for detection of metastasis in background of fatty liver. A 58-year-old male with CRLM and diffuse hepatic steatosis. Post-contrast T1-weighted axial MR images (**a**, **b**) reveal peripherally enhancing hypointense lesions (arrows) that are not discernible on post-contrast axial CT (**c**, **d**) images due to uniformly low attenuation of background liver parenchyma suggesting diffuse hepatic steatosis

Table 5.3 Diagnostic performance of CECT, EOB-MRI, and PET-CT for CRLM detection according to chemotherapy status

		Chemotherapy status	
Modality	Diagnostic performance	Without NAC	With NAC or mixed
CECT	Sensitivity	88%	78%, $p < 0.001$
		(80–96)	(69–87)
	Specificity	76%	72%
		(50–100)	(49–94)
EOB-MRI	Sensitivity	96%	89%, $p < 0.001$
		(93–99)	(82–95)
	Specificity	88%	86%
		(78–98)	(74–97)
PET-CT	Sensitivity	79%	72%
		(63–95)	(58–85)
	Specificity	92%	95%
		(79–100)	(88–100)

Reported 95% confidence interval for mean sensitivity and specificity in a meta-analysis between 2004 and 2016 [19].
This table compares the diagnostic performance of MDCT, gadoxetate disodium-enhanced MRI, and FDG PET-CT for diagnosing CRLM based on neoadjuvant chemotherapy (NAC) status. The meta-analysis found that neoadjuvant chemotherapy significantly decreased the sensitivity for CT (78% vs. 88%) and MRI (89% vs. 96%), although it did not significantly decrease the sensitivity for PET-CT ($P = 0.19$)

MRI sequences for CRLM assessment usually include a combination of T1-weighted (T1W), T2-weighted (T2W), and diffusion-weighted images (DWI) [36]. CRLM typically appear hypointense in precontrast T1W images and hyperintense in T2W images [36]. On dynamic CE-MRI, CRLM appear mostly hypointense, similar to CECT [36]. Eovist allows for further assessment of intrahepatic lesions with hepatobiliary (HB) phase (20 minutes after contrast injection) [37]. On HB phase, normal hepatocytes appear hyperintense due to eovist uptake, whereas CRLM do not retain contrast remaining hypointense and appear more conspicuous [37]. On DWI, CRLM become hyperintense compared to the normal liver due to diffusion restriction [38]. However, some benign lesions may also appear hyperintense (T2 shine-through effect) on DWI and can be differentiated from CRLM by the use of apparent diffusion coefficients (the "ADC" map) [35] (Fig. 5.3).

Limitations of MRI include contraindications such as imaging patients with metal implants and claustrophobia. Increased patient compliance such as longer breath holds and lying still for a lengthy period is required to avoid motion-related imaging artifacts, which can adversely affect diagnostic image quality [36]. Additionally, DWI have inherent limitations due to low spatial resolution and poor signal-to-noise ratio [39]. However, technological advancements in MRI scanners with more dedicated software can address some of these limitations to improve image quality [39].

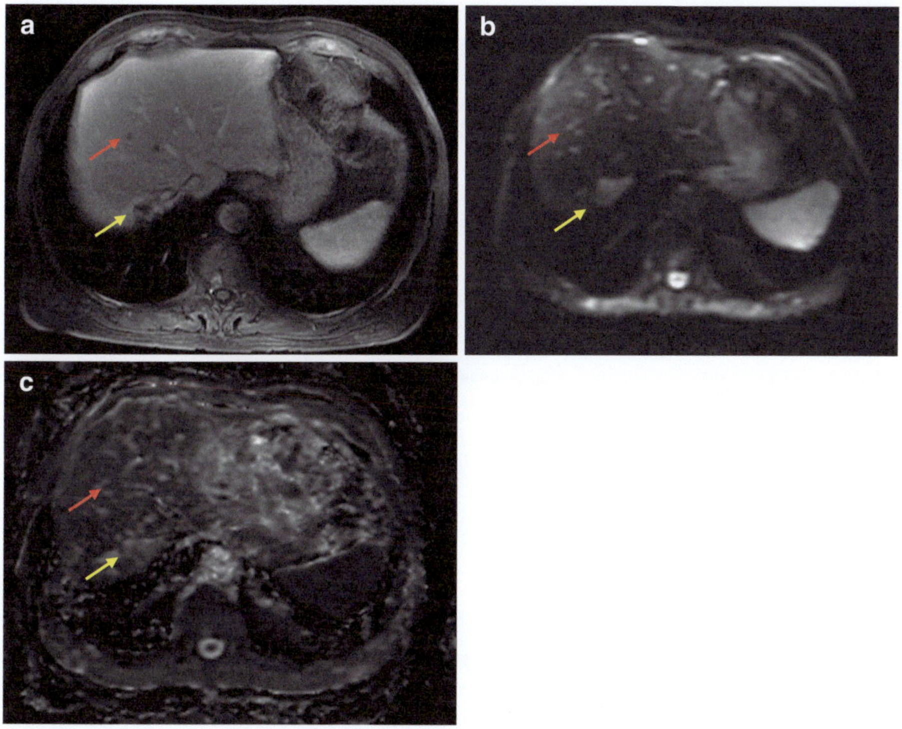

Fig. 5.3 Advantage of DWI for distinguishing benign vs. malignant lesions. A 45-year-old female with CRLM. Post-contrast axial T1 weighted (**a**) reveal tiny hypoenhancing lesions (red arrow) in segment VIII and a larger nodular peripherally enhancing lesion in segment VII (yellow arrow). All lesions appear hyperintense on DWI (**b**). Corresponding ADC map (**c**) shows segment VIII lesions as hypointense suggestive of restricted diffusion that indicates metastasis, whereas the segment VII lesion remains hyperintense suggestive of T2 shine through indicating benign etiology

Positron Emission Tomography (PET)

PET with 18-fluoride deoxyglucose (FDG) analogue is a whole-body imaging technique providing molecular and metabolic information for CRC evaluation [40]. The main advantage of PET imaging is the superior detection of extrahepatic metastases, which can eliminate unnecessary surgical intervention (Table 5.4) [40–43]. FDG-PET has also demonstrated great value in clarifying equivocal findings for the presence of metastases on CT or MRI [40–43]. On FDG-PET, diagnosis of metastases is based on focal FDG uptake exceeding the uptake of the surrounding tissue (Fig. 5.4) [44]. Currently, FDG-PET is routinely

Table 5.4 Advantages and disadvantages of CT, MRI and PET imaging for CRLM assessment

Modality	Advantages	Disadvantages
CT	Quick, reliable method for initial screening and detection of CRLM High-quality images can be generated for vascular assessment when planning for resection	Small lesion detectability and characterization (<10 mm) Poor lesion conspicuity in hepatic steatosis Low sensitivity for detecting CRLM in patients receiving NAC Radiation exposure concern
MRI	Detecting small lesions (<10 mm) Superior lesion conspicuity higher tissue contrast and availability of hepatocyte contrast agents	DWI and ADC maps have inherent image quality limitations Patient-related factors (claustrophobia, uncooperative, metallic prosthesis)
PET	Detecting extrahepatic metastases and disease recurrence Determining management if conventional imaging is equivocal for the presence of metastatic disease	Small lesion detectability and characterization (<10 mm) Hypermetabolic processes may lead to false-positive FDG uptake. Patients receiving NAC within 4 weeks of their PET scan may have high false-negative results

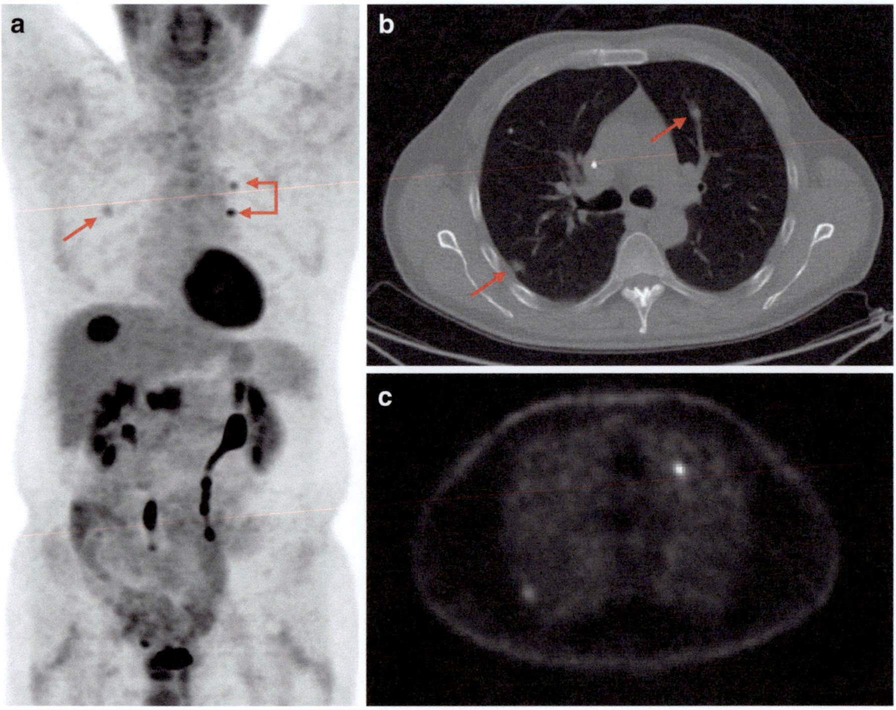

Fig. 5.4 Role of PET-CT. A 46-year-old male with CRLM. PET (**a**) shows moderate FDG uptake by lung nodules in the left upper lobe and one in the right lower lobe, which is suggestive of extra-hepatic metastases (arrows). Axial CT scan (**b**) and its corresponding FDG-PET (**c**) showing the pulmonary nodules

performed with CT (PET-CT) to improve localization of lesions and detection of CRLM [44, 45]. Through the detection of additional liver CRLM and/or extrahepatic disease, PET-CT was shown to change planned surgical management in 24% of patients [46]. FDG-PET with MRI (PET-MRI) is a relatively newer technique that has shown great potential in CRLM detection [47, 48]. In a recent comparative study, PET-MRI had significantly higher sensitivity and diagnostic accuracy (92.2% and 96.1%, respectively) than PET-CT (67.8% and 82.4%, respectively) [49]. This is likely due to the inherent advantages of MRI in differentiating tissue contrast and lesion detection. However, literature data regarding diagnostic performance are limited, as PET-MRI is available only in a few highly specialized centers.

Limitations with PET imaging include reduced sensitivity for small lesion detection and assessing lesions in patients receiving NAC [50, 51]. The physiologic hepatic parenchymal uptake of FDG along with the inherent low resolution of PET can limit the sensitivity for small lesion detection [51]. Additionally, patients receiving NAC within 4 weeks of their PET scan may have high false-negative results due to reduction in lesion size and tumor metabolic activity [50]. Hypermetabolic processes such as chronic infection or inflammation may also lead to false-positive FDG uptake [52]. Studies have reported that 5–8% of CRC patients are falsely upstaged by PET-CT preoperatively [53]. Patient compliance factor such as respiratory motion is an additional challenge when performing PET-CT [54].

Role of Imaging in Surgical Planning for CRLM

Vascular Assessment

The localization of CRLM relative to vascular structures is important to determine feasibility and planning of hepatic resection. A preoperative vascular "road map" can identify anomalous or aberrant hepatic vascular supply to avoid inadvertent injury to the liver (Fig. 5.5). In addition, knowledge of the vascular map aids in determining the best hepatectomy plane. CT angiography (CTA) is preferred over MR angiography, especially for complex hepatic resection due to rapid acquisition, less susceptibility to motion artifacts, and thin collimation [55]. High-quality multiplanar reconstruction (MPR) and three-dimensional images can be obtained with CT to display the liver vascular anatomy in any desired plane [55]. The proximity of liver lesions to the hepatic vasculature can then be illustrated to decide the best surgical approach [56].

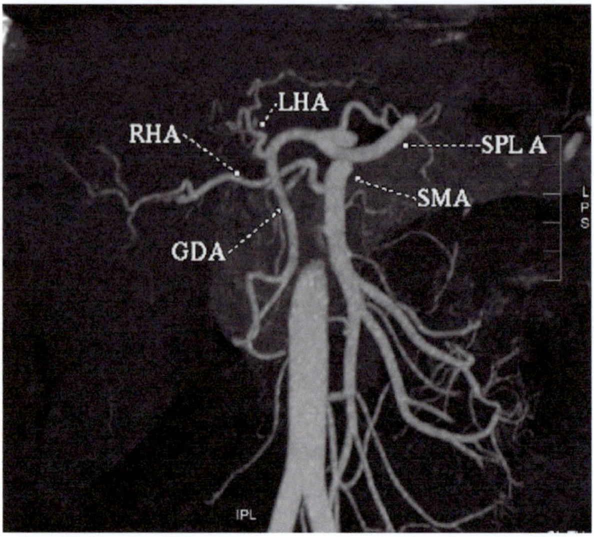

Fig. 5.5 Image post processing for Vascular Mapping. A 36-year-old male with CRLM. Coronal reformatted CT angiography in maximum intensity projection (MIP) reconstruction shows replaced right hepatic artery (RHA) arising from the superior mesenteric artery (SMA). *LHA* left hepatic artery, *SPL A* splenic artery, *GDA* gastroduodenal artery

Liver Volumetry

A crucial factor for planning surgical resection is predicting the future liver remnant (FLR) volume to avoid risk of hepatic insufficiency and subsequent mortality [57]. Preoperative estimation of the FLR is used to determine whether the functional reserve is enough to meet metabolic demands of the liver after surgery [57]. Three-dimensional reconstruction images can be used to generate precise volume measurements of the liver lobes [57, 58]. Approximately 25–30% and 40% of the preoperative liver volume should be preserved for those with normal and abnormal parenchyma (e.g., steatosis, fibrosis), respectively [59]. When FLR is deemed inadequate and CRLM is unresectable, portal vein embolization (PVE) can be performed. PVE induces hypertrophy in the remaining liver to maximize the remnant liver volume and increase resectability rate with high clinical success (Fig. 5.6) [60]. A recent meta-analysis showed that 96.1% of patients who undergo PVE develop sufficient liver lobe hypertrophy [60]. CT performed 1 month following embolization can then estimate any increase in FLR [61]. Any remaining CRLM lesions in the non-resected lobe can be treated with other methods such as radiofrequency ablation (Fig. 5.7) [62]. An area of high density or signal intensity on non-contrast CT and thin regular peripheral rim enhancement are expected after ablative therapy. Complete non-enhancement of the ablated lesions is considered evidence of full tumor necrosis at subsequent follow-up.

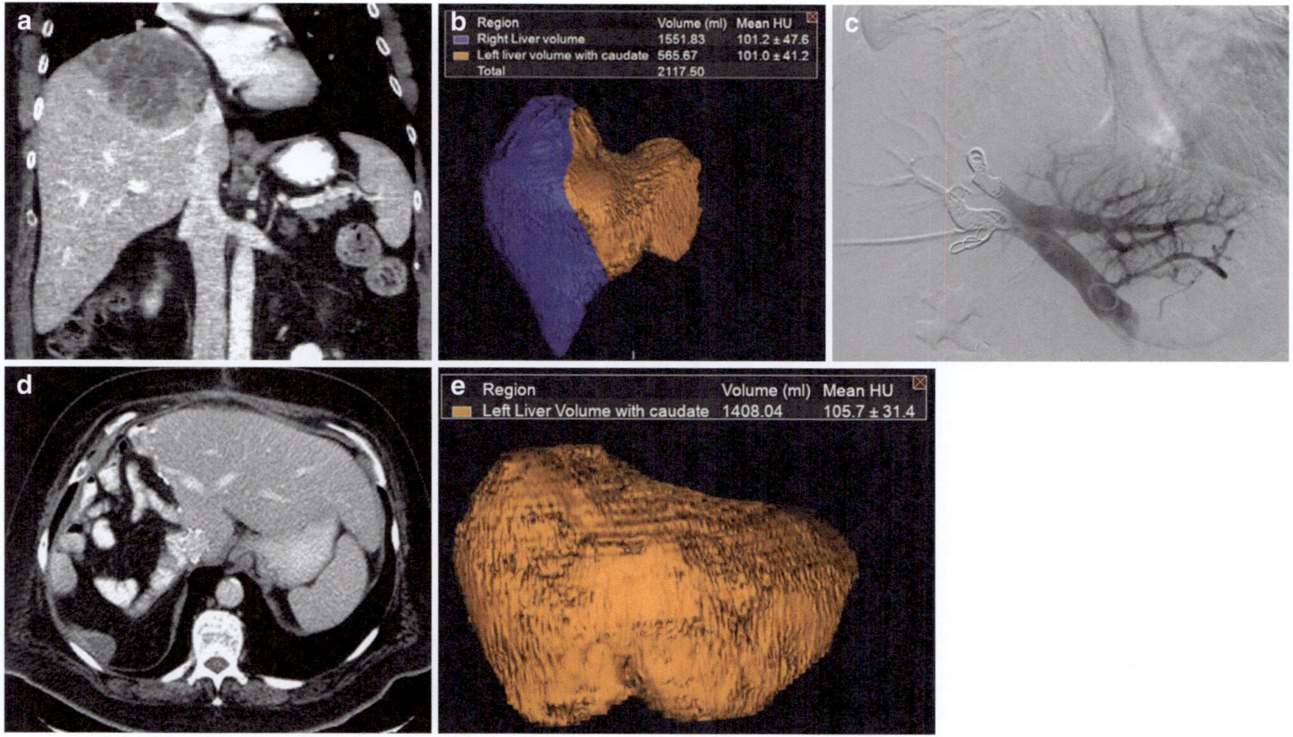

Fig. 5.6 CT volumetric analysis of the liver. A 56-year-old female with liver metastases who underwent portal vein embolization prior to right hepatectomy. CECT axial (**a**) image and corresponding 3D volumetric analysis (**b**) shows the pre-embolization volume of the right lobe (volume = 1552 cm) and left lobe with caudate (volume = 566 cm). Digital subtraction angiography image (**c**) demonstrates successful embolization of the anterior and posterior branches of right portal vein with particles and coils. (**c**) Axial CT (**d**) and three-dimensional volume-rendered CT image (**e**) obtained 3 months after embolization and resection reveal left hepatic lobe hypertrophy (volume = 1408 cm^3). Note: Blue = right hepatic lobe; Gold = left hepatic lobe with caudate

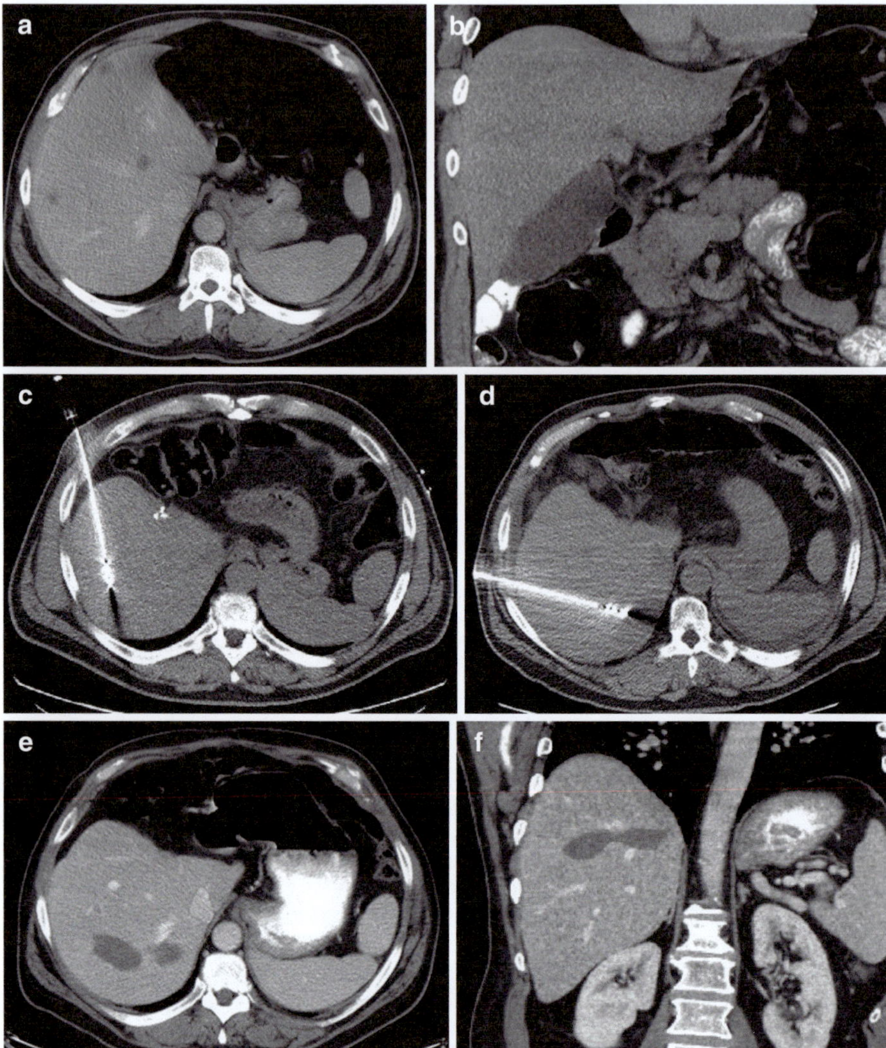

Fig. 5.7 Imaging of ablation zone. A 56-year-old male status pre and post left hepatectomy for CRLM. Post-contrast CT in axial (**a**) and coronal (**b**) planes show multiple liver metastases in both lobes of the liver. Left hepatectomy was performed and right lobe lesions in segment VII were treated with radio-frequency ablation (**c**, **d**). Follow-up CT, after 3 months, (**e**, **f**) shows two non-enhancing hypodense regions suggestive of normal post ablation zone changes with no evidence of residual tumor

Conclusion

Imaging studies play a crucial role in the detection and characterization of CRLM to identify potential surgical candidates. The role of ultrasound has improved with the addition of microbubble contrast agents and remains a valuable tool for intraoperative decision-making. MDCT is most commonly used for initial CRLM detection and staging. MRI is the modality of choice for CRLM assessment, particularly for characterizing and detecting small lesions. MRI is also superior to CT and PET for hepatic evaluation in patients receiving NAC or have underlying hepatic steatosis. High-quality 3D images can be reconstructed from CT or MRI for vascular assessment and FLR estimation to guide the surgical approach. PET has proven essential prior to surgery for its superior extrahepatic disease detection. While each modality has its advantages for patient assessment, a multi-modal imaging approach is required to maximize safety and efficacy of CRLM resection.

Acknowledgments The authors would like to thank Anushri Parakh, MD, for her feedback during the editing process of the manuscript and assistance with the liver volumetry application.

Disclosures Grant support was received from GE Healthcare and the Advisory Board of Allena Pharma; royalties are received from Elsevier Publishing for textbook on Abdomen Imaging.

References

1. House MG. Safely expanding the criteria for resectability of hepatic colorectal metastases. Ann Surg. 2011;253:1080–1.
2. Legou F, Chiaradia M, Baranes L, et al. Imaging strategies before beginning treatment of colorectal liver metastases. Diagn Interv Imaging. 2014;95(5):505–12.
3. Robinson PJ. The effects of cancer chemotherapy on liver imaging. Eur Radiol. 2009;19(7):1752–62.
4. Florani I, Torri V, Rulli E, et al. Performance of imaging modalities in diagnosis of liver metastases from colorectal cancer: a systematic review and meta-analysis. J Magn Reson Imaging. 2010;31:19–31.
5. Larsen LP, Rosenkilde M, Christensen H, et al. Can contrast-enhanced ultrasonography replace multidetector-computed tomography in the detection of liver metastases from colorectal cancer? Eur J Radiol. 2009;69:308–13.
6. Cantisani V, Ricci P, Erturk M, et al. Detection of hepatic metastases from colorectal cancer: prospective evaluation of gray scale US versus SonoVue® low mechanical index real time-enhanced US as compared with multidetector-CT or Gd-BOPTA-MRI. Ultraschall Med. 2010;31:500–5.
7. Piscaglia F, Bolondi L, Italian Society for Ultrasound in M, Biology Study Group on Ultrasound Contrast A. The safety of Sonovue in abdominal applications: retrospective analysis of 23188 investigations. Ultrasound Med Biol. 2006;32:1369–75.

8. Sawhney S, Wilson SR. Can ultrasound with contrast enhancement replace nonenhanced computed tomography scans in patients with contraindication to computed tomography contrast agents? Ultrasound Q. 2017;33(2):125–32.
9. D'Onofrio M, Crosara S, De Robertis R, et al. Contrast-enhanced ultrasound of focal liver lesions. AJR Am J Roentgenol. 2015;205(1):W56–66.
10. Lucchese AM, Kalil AN, Schwengber A, Suwa E, Rolim de Moura GG. Usefulness of intraoperative ultrasonography in liver resections due to colon cancer metastasis. Int J Surg. 2015;20:140–4.
11. Ellebæk SB, Fristrup CW, Mortensen MB, et al. Intraoperative ultrasound as a screening modality for the detection of liver metastases during resection of primary colorectal cancer-a systematic review. Ultrasound Int Open. 2017;3(2):E60–8.
12. Ruzzenente A, Conci S, Iacono C, et al. Usefulness of contrast-enhanced intraoperative ultrasonography (CE-IOUS) in patients with colorectal liver metastases after preoperative chemotherapy. J Gastrointest Surg. 2013;17:281–7.
13. Claudon M, Dietrich CF, Choi BI, et al. Guidelines and good clinical practice recommendations for contrast enhanced ultrasound (CEUS) in the liver–update 2012: a WFUMB-EFSUMB initiative in cooperation with representatives of AFSUMB, AIUM, ASUM, FLAUS and ICUS. Ultraschall Med. 2013;34(1):11–29.
14. Dietrich CF, Ignee A, Greis C, et al. Artifacts and pitfalls in contrast-enhanced ultrasound of the liver. Ultraschall Med. 2014;35:108–25.
15. Kaur H, Hindman NM, Al-Refaie WB, et al. ACR appropriateness criteria® suspected liver metastases. J Am Coll Radiol. 2017;14:S314–25.
16. Ong KO, Leen E. Radiological staging of colorectal liver metastases. Surg Oncol. 2007;16(1):7–14.
17. Tirumani S, Kim KW, Nishino M, Howard SA, Krajewski KM, Jagannathan JP. Update on the role of imaging in management of metastatic colorectal cancer. Radiographics. 2014;34:1908–28.
18. National Comprehensive Cancer Network. NCCN clinical practice guidelines in oncology. Colon Cancer (version 1. 2017). Accessed 30 Apr 2018. Available from: http://www.nccn.org.
19. Choi SH, Kim SY, Park SH, et al. Diagnostic performance of CT, gadoxetate disodium-enhanced MRI, and PET/CT for the diagnosis of colorectal liver metastasis: systematic review and meta-analysis. J Magn Reson Imaging. 2018;47(5):1237–50.
20. Wicherts DA, de Haas RJ, van Kessel CS, et al. Incremental value of arterial and equilibrium phase compared to hepatic venous phase CT in the preoperative staging of colorectal liver metastases: an evaluation with different reference standards. Eur J Radiol. 2011;77:305–11.
21. Agrawal MD, Pinho DF, Kulkarni NM, Hahn PF, Guimaraes AR, Sahani DV. Oncologic applications of dual-energy CT in the abdomen. Radiographics. 2014;34(3):589–612.
22. Leng S, Yu L, Fletcher JG, McCollough CH. Maximizing iodine contrast-to-noise ratios in abdominal CT imaging through use of energy domain noise reduction and virtual monoenergetic dual-energy CT. Radiology. 2015;276(2):562–70.
23. Niekel MC, Bipat S, Stoker J. Diagnostic imaging of colorectal liver metastases with CT, MR imaging, FDG PET, and/or FDG PET/CT: a meta-analysis of prospective studies including patients who have not previously undergone treatment. Radiology. 2010;257(3):674–84.
24. Pawlik TM, Olino K, Gleisner AL, Torbenson M, Schulick R, Choti MA. Preoperative chemotherapy for colorectal liver metastases: impact on hepatic histology and postoperative outcome. J Gastrointest Surg. 2007;11(7):860–8.
25. Nicola R, Shaqdan KW, Aran S, Mansouri M, Abujudeh HH. Contrast-induced nephropathy: identifying the risks, choosing the right agent, and reviewing effective prevention and management methods. Curr Probl Diagn Radiol. 2015;44(6):501–4.
26. Chung YE, You JS, Lee HJ, et al. Possible contrast media reduction with low keV monoenergetic images in the detection of focal liver lesions: a dual-energy CT animal study. PLoS One. 2015;10(7):e0133170.
27. Zhang LJ, Peng J, Wu SY, et al. Liver virtual non-enhanced CT with dual-source, dual-energy CT: a preliminary study. Eur Radiol. 2010;20:2257–64.

28. De Cecco CN, Buffa V, Fedeli S, et al. Dual energy CT (DECT) of the liver: conventional versus virtual unenhanced images. Eur Radiol. 2010;20(12):2870–5.
29. Robinson E, Babb J, Chandarana H, et al. Dual source dual energy MDCT: comparison of 80 kVp and weighted average 120 kVp data for conspicuity of hypo-vascular liver metastases. Investig Radiol. 2010;45(7):413–8.
30. Yamada Y, Jinzaki M, Tanami Y, Abe T, Kuribayashi S. Virtual monochromatic spectral imaging for the evaluation of hypovascular hepatic metastases: the optimal monochromatic level with fast kilovoltage switching dual-energy computed tomography. Investig Radiol. 2012;47(5):292–8.
31. Kulemann V, Schima W, Tamandl D, et al. Preoperative detection of colorectal liver metastases in fatty liver: MDCT or MRI? Eur J Radiol. 2011;79(2):e1–6.
32. Vilgrain V, Esvan M, Ronot M, Caumont-Prim A, Aube C, Chatellier G. A meta-analysis of diffusion-weighted and gadoxetic acid-enhanced MR imaging for the detection of liver metastases. Eur Radiol. 2016;26(12):4595–615.
33. Zech CJ, Korpraphong P, Huppertz A, et al. Randomized multicentre trial of gadoxetic acid-enhanced MRI versus conventional MRI or CT in the staging of colorectal cancer liver metastases. Br J Surg. 2014;101(6):613–21.
34. Kim HJ, Lee SS, Byun JH, et al. Incremental value of liver MR imaging in patients with potentially curable colorectal hepatic metastasis detected at CT: a prospective comparison of diffusion-weighted imaging, gadoxetic acid-enhanced MR imaging, and a combination of both MR techniques. Radiology. 2015;274(3):712–22.
35. Colagrande S, Castellani A, Nardi C, Lorini C, Calistri L, Filippone A. The role of diffusion-weighted imaging in the detection of hepatic metastases from colorectal cancer: a comparison with unenhanced and Gd-EOB-DTPA enhanced MRI. Eur J Radiol. 2016;85:1027–34.
36. Siegelman ES, Chauhan A. MR characterization of focal liver lesions: pearls and pitfalls. Magn Reson Imaging Clin N Am. 2014;22:295–313.
37. Owen JW, Fowler KJ, Doyle MB, Saad NE, Linehan DC, Chapman WC. Colorectal liver metastases: disappearing lesions in the era of Eovist hepatobiliary magnetic resonance imaging. HPB (Oxford). 2016;18:296–303.
38. Hardie AD, Egbert RE, Rissing MS. Improved differentiation between hepatic hemangioma and metastases on diffusion-weighted MRI by measurement of standard deviation of apparent diffusion coefficient. Clin Imaging. 2015;39:654–8.
39. Shenoy-Bhangle A, Baliyan V, Kordbacheh H, Guimaraes AR, Kambadakone A. Diffusion weighted magnetic resonance imaging of liver: principles, clinical applications and recent updates. World J Hepatol. 2017;9(26):1081–91.
40. Papathanassiou D, Bruna-Muraille C, Liehn JC, et al. Positron emission tomography in oncology: present and future of PET and PET/CT. Crit Rev Oncol Hematol. 2008;72:239–54.
41. Maas M, Rutten IJ, Nelemans PJ, Lambregts DM, Cappendijk VC, Beets GL, Beets-Tan RG. What is the most accurate whole-body imaging modality for assessment of local and distant recurrent disease in colorectal cancer? A meta-analysis : imaging for recurrent colorectal cancer. Eur J Nucl Med Mol Imaging. 2011;38:1560–71.
42. Cantwell CP, Setty BN, Holalkere N, et al. Liver lesion detection and characterization in patients with colorectal cancer: a comparison of low radiation dose non-enhanced PET/CT, contrast-enhanced PET/CT, and liver MRI. J Comput Assist Tomogr. 2008;32:738–44.
43. Wiering B, Adang EM, van der Sijp JR, et al. Added value of positron emission tomography imaging in the surgical treatment of colorectal liver metastases. Nucl Med Comm. 2010;31:938–44.
44. Agarwal A, Marcus C, Xiao J, et al. FDG PET/CT in the management of colorectal and anal cancers. AJR Am J Roentgenol. 2014;203:1109–19.
45. Pelosi E, Messa C, Sironi S, et al. Value of integrated PET/CT for lesion localization in cancer patients: a comparative study. J Comput Assist Tomogr. 2005;29(4):554–9.
46. Maffione AM, Lopci E, Bluemel C, Giammarile F, Herrmann K, Rubello D. Diagnostic accuracy and impact on management of 18F-FDG PET and PET/CT in colorectal liver metastasis: a meta-analysis and systematic review. Eur J Nucl Med Mol Imaging. 2015;42:152–63.

47. Lee DH, Lee JM, Hur BY, Joo I, Yi NJ, Suh KS, et al. Colorectal cancer liver metastases: diagnostic performance and prognostic value of PET/MR imaging. Radiology. 2016;280:782–92.
48. Lee DH, Lee JM. Whole-body PET/MRI for colorectal cancer staging: is it the way forward? J Magn Reson Imaging. 2017;45(1):25–35.
49. Beiderwellen K, Geraldo L, Ruhlmann V, et al. Accuracy of [18F]FDG PET/MRI for the detection of liver metastases. PLoS One. 2015;10:e0137285.
50. Kong G, Jackson C, Koh DM, et al. The use of 18F-FDG PET/CT in colorectal liver metastases–comparison with CT and liver MRI. Eur J Nucl Med Mol Imaging. 2008;35:1323–9.
51. Adie S, Yip C, Chu F, Morris DL. Resection of liver metastases from colorectal cancer: does preoperative chemotherapy affect the accuracy of PET in preoperative planning? ANZ J Surg. 2009;79:358–61.
52. Zhu A, Lee D, Shim H. Metabolic positron emission tomography imaging in cancer detection and therapy response. Semin Oncol. 2011;38:55–69.
53. Ruers TJ, Wiering B, Joost R, et al. Improved selection of patients for hepatic surgery of colorectal liver metastases with 18F-FDG PET: a randomized study. J Nucl Med. 2009;50:1036–41.
54. Fayad H, Schmidt H, Wuerslin C, et al. Reconstruction-incorporated respiratory motion correction in clinical simultaneous PET/MR imaging for oncology applications. J Nucl Med. 2015;56:884–9.
55. Sahani D, Mehta A, Blake M, Prasad S, Harris G, Saini S. Preoperative hepatic vascular evaluation with CT and MR angiography: implications for surgery. Radiographics. 2004;24:1367–80.
56. Catalano OA, Singh AH, Uppot RN, et al. Vascular and biliary variants in the liver: implications for liver surgery. Radiographics. 2008;28:359–78.
57. Karlo C, Reiner CS, Stolzmann P, et al. CT- and MRI-based volumetry of resected liver specimen: comparison to intraoperative volume and weight measurements and calculation of conversion factors. Eur J Radiol. 2010;75(1):e107–11.
58. D'Onofrio M, De Robertis R, Demozzi E, Crosara S, Canestrini S, Pozzi Mucelli R. Liver volumetry: is imaging reliable? Personal experience and review of the literature. World J Radiol. 2014;6:62–71.
59. Ferrero A, Vigano L, Polastri R, Muratore A, Eminefendic H, Regge D, Capussotti L. Postoperative liver dysfunction and future remnant liver: where is the limit? Results of a prospective study. World J Surg. 2007;31:1643–51.
60. van Lienden KP, van den Esschert JW, de Graaf W, Bipat S, Lameris JS, van Gulik TM, et al. Portal vein embolization before liver resection: a systematic review. Cardiovasc Intervent Radiol. 2013;36(1):25–34.
61. Ulla M, Ardiles V, Levy-Yeyati E, Alvarez FA, Spina JC, Garcia-Mónaco RD, De Santibañes E. New surgical strategy to induce liver hypertrophy: role of MDCT-volumetry to monitor and predict liver growth. Hepato-Gastroenterology. 2013;60:337–42.
62. Evrard S, Rivoire M, Arnaud J-P, et al. Unresectable colorectal cancer liver metastases treated by intraoperative radiofrequency ablation with or without resection. Br J Surg. 2012;99:558–65.

Staging Classifications of Colorectal Liver Metastases

6

Toru Beppu, Go Wakabayashi, Katsunori Imai, Yasushi Yoshida, and Hideo Baba

Introduction

Various factors have been proposed to estimate the recurrence or long-term prognosis of patients with colorectal liver metastases (CRLM) undergoing liver resection [1–20]. On the basis of such investigations, several staging and classification systems, and nomograms have been developed [1–12, 20–31]. Surgical techniques, as well as the perioperative management of liver resection, have markedly progressed, and modern chemotherapeutic agents including molecular targeted drugs have been formulated. Because of these innovations, the outcomes of resected CRLM have drastically improved [32–34]. Additionally, some useful biomarkers and molecular markers have recently been introduced.

In this chapter, along with the summary of the history of classification systems, we focus on the classification systems for CRLM and their role in the era of modern multidisciplinary treatment.

T. Beppu (✉) · Y. Yoshida
Department of Surgery, Yamaga City Medical Center, Yamaga, Japan

Department of Gastroenterological Surgery, Graduate School of Life Sciences, Kumamoto University, Kumamoto, Japan
e-mail: tbeppu@yamaga-mc.jp

G. Wakabayashi
Center for Advanced Treatment of HBP Diseases, Ageo Central General Hospital, Ageo Shi, Saitama, Japan

K. Imai · H. Baba
Department of Gastroenterological Surgery, Graduate School of Life Sciences, Kumamoto University, Kumamoto, Japan

M. M. Correia et al. (eds.), *Colorectal Cancer Liver Metastases*,
https://doi.org/10.1007/978-3-030-25486-5_6

Prognostic Factors for CRLM Patients Undergoing Liver Resection

Numerous studies have reportedly identified predictive markers for the recurrence and long-term prognosis of CRLM. Prognostic factors and their classification methods or cutoff values are summarized (Table 6.1) [20, 1–12, 26–31]. Various

Table 6.1 Prognostic factors assessed for in CRLM patients undergoing liver resection

Variables	Classification method, cut-off value
CRLM factor	
Tumor number	1–2, 3–4, 4–5, 6–7, 7–8
Largest tumor diameter (cm)	5, 8
Timing of CRLM	Synchronous/metachronous
Bilobar distribution	Yes/no
Liver invasion	30%
Hepatoduodenal node metastasis	Yes/no
Short doubling time of CRLM	Yes/no
Disease progression during first-line chemotherapy	Yes/no
Patients' factor	
Age	60, 70
Disease-free interval (months)	12, 24, 30
CEA (ng/ml)	5, 10, 50, 60, 100, 200
CA19-9 (U/ml)	37, 100
ALT level	≥55 U/L
Alkaline phosphatase level	>125 U/L
Albumin level	<3.6 g/dL
Inflammatory response (CRP >10 mg/L or Neut/Lym >5:1)	Yes/No
Extra-hepatic metastasis	Yes/No, resectable/non-, lung metastasis/others, metastatic sites
Surgical factor	
Nonanatomical resection	Yes/No
Lobectomy or more	Yes/No
Bilateral resection	Yes/No
Surgical margin	Positive/negative, 5 mm, 10 mm
Blood loss at operation	1000 ml
Surgical treatment	Yes/no
Primary site factor	
Duke's stage	A or B/C
Lymph node metastasis	Yes/No, N1 (1–3)/N2 (≥4)
Location	Colon/rectum, right colon/others
Tumor differentiation	Poor or mucinous/others, poor/others
Serosal invasion	Yes/No
Lymphatic or venous invasion	Yes/No
Marked tumor budding	Yes/No
Biomarker	
(K-)RAS, BRAF	Wild/mutant
Integration score	
MSKCC-CRS	CRS ≤2/CRS >2

Abbreviations: *CRLM* colorectal liver metastases, *CEA* carcinoembryonic antigen, *CA19-9* carbohydrate antigen 19-9, *CRS* clinical risk score, *ALT* alanine aminotransferase, *CRP* C-reactive protein, *Neut* neutrophil, *Lym* lymphocyte, *MSKCC-CRS* Memorial Sloan-Kettering Cancer Center-Clinical Risk Score prognostic variables were elucidated, including patient characteristics, presence of primary colorectal tumor, CRLM, biomarkers, and perioperative findings. Among them, four factors were most frequently included: number and maximum size of CRLM, regional lymph node metastasis of primary tumor, and preoperative carcinoembryonic antigen (CEA) level. The most cited prognostic factor was the number of CRLM. Differing cutoff values of tumor number have been proposed; in this study, cutoff values of 1–2, 3–4, and 4–5 were frequently utilized. Project Committee of the Liver of the Japanese Society of Hepato-Biliary-Pancreatic Surgery (JSHBPS) analyzed 727 patients who had undergone CRLM resections and clearly demonstrated that 4–5 was the most reliable cutoff value [hazard ratio (HR), 2.35], followed by 1–2 (HR, 1.81) and 3–4 (HR, 2.14) [29]. The maximum size of the CRLM was indicated as a prognostic factor in approximately half of the papers. We had previously reported that the often used maximum size of 5 cm had less impact compared with the number of CRLM (≥4) in the Beppu nomogram by JSHBPS [35]. Two-thirds of the papers referred to lymph node metastasis as an independent prognostic factor and indicated that it had a strong impact, especially in patients with N2 or N3 status, according to the American Joint Committee on Cancer (AJCC) Cancer Staging System [22]. In half of the papers, a preoperative high CEA level was a significant poor prognostic factor. Various cutoff values were used ranging from 5 to 200 ng/mL; unfortunately, the most suitable cutoff of CEA level is unclear at the present time.

Staging System for CRLM

TNM Cancer Staging System for Colon and Rectum Cancer

In the Tumor–Node–Metastasis (TNM) cancer staging system for colorectal carcinomas of the Union for International Cancer Control (UICC) and the AJCC, M factor has been simply divided into M0 (distant metastasis negative) and M1 (positive). In 2010, the seventh TNM cancer staging system introduced a subdivision of M1 [21]. Focusing on CRLM, liver-only CRLM was classified as M1a (Stage IVA) and multiple-site distant metastases including CRLM as M1b (Stage IVB). These sub-classifications did not indicate the site of the distant metastasis merger with the CRLM.

In 2017, the eighth TNM cancer staging system of the UICC and the AJCC introduced a novel subdivision of M1 in the TNM classification [22]. Focusing on CRLM, liver-only CRLM, metastasis to multiple sites or organs including CRLM without peritoneal metastasis, and CRLM with peritoneal metastasis were classified into M1a, M1b, and M1c, respectively. Peritoneal metastasis was distinguished from other distant metastases based on poor prognosis. Stage classification was decided as follows: Stage IVA (Any T, Any N, M1a), Stage IVB (Any T, Any N, M1b), and Stage IVC (Any T, Any N, M1c).

Japanese Staging System for CRLM

The Study Group for Liver Metastasis project by the Japanese Society for Cancer of the Colon and Rectum (JSCCR) [23] developed a new classification limited to CRLM. The H-factor category consisted of H1, four or less metastases with the largest diameter of ≤5 cm; H2, lesions other than H1 and H3; and H3, five or more metastases with the largest diameter of >5 cm. Thereafter, the comprehensive Japanese classification system for CRLM was created on the basis of H-factor category, nodal status of the primary site, and extrahepatic metastases (EM) [24, 25]. The N-factor category consisted of N0, no regional lymph node metastasis; N1, 1–3 regional lymph node metastasis; and N2, metastasis in four or more regional lymph nodes. The EM-factor category consisted of M0, no distant metastasis; and M1, distant metastasis. This classification included Stage A, H1 and N0/1; Stage B, H2 and N0/1, or H1 and N2; and Stage C, H2 and N2, H3 with any N, or EM with any H/N. This classification system has been successfully validated using independent patients undergoing the latest chemotherapy and Stage C was further recommended to divide into C-I, HT3 and N0/1, HT2 and N2, or HT1 and EM1; and Stage C-II, HT3 and N2, or HT2/3 and EM1 [36]. In the latest guidelines of JSCCR, M factor was divided into M0, distant metastasis negative; M1a, distant metastasis in one organ; and M1b, distant metastasis in two or more organs. The entire number of metastatic sites should be noted [24].

Risk Scoring Systems for CRLM Patients Undergoing Liver Resection

Many prognostic scoring systems have been proposed to stratify patients into risk categories (Table 6.2) [1–11]. The timing of the classification system is very important (especially before or after the beginning of modern chemotherapy). Further more, the utility of a prognostic model or scoring system requires internal and external validation before general use [37].

The first large-scale prognostic Nordlinger score [1] for CRLM patients undergoing liver resection was reported. There were five preoperative and one postoperative factor. Giving one point to each factor, the population was divided into three risk groups with different 2-year survival rates: 79%, 60%, and 43% in patients with 0–2, 3–4, and 5–7 points, respectively.

The Memorial Sloan-Kettering Cancer Center–Clinical Risk Score (MSKCC-CRS) [2] was developed in CRLM patients who underwent liver resection and has been the most widely used scoring system worldwide. MSKCC-CRS consists of five preoperative clinical factors. The coefficient for each factor in the multivariate analysis was similar; therefore, weighting of each factor was not performed. Six risk groups were stratified by the sum of the individual prognostic factors, and a survival curve was well separated in each group; 3- and 5-year survival was 72% and 60%, 66% and 44%, 51% and 40%, 42% and 20%, 38% and 25%, and 27% and 14% in sores 0–5, respectively. In the clinical setting, CRLM patients were sometimes divided into two groups: low risk, CRS ≤2; and high risk, CRS >2 [38]. Recently,

Table 6.2 Risk scoring systems for CRLM patients undergoing liver resection

Scoring system (ref)	Pt number	Pt's recruitment year	Criteria	Score
Nordlinger score [1]	1568	1968–1990	Age ≥60 years	Low risk: 0–2
			Largest CRLM >5 cm	Intermediate risk: 3–4
			CRLM number ≥4	High risk: 5–7
			Disease-free interval from primary tumor to liver metastasis <2 years	
			Serosal invasion of primary tumor	
			Lymphatic spread of primary tumor	
			Surgical margin <10 mm	
MSKCC-CRS [2]	1001	1985–1998	Largest CRLM >5 cm	Low risk: 0–2
			CRLM number ≥2	High risk: 3–5
			Node positive primary	
			Disease-free interval from primary to metastases <12 months	
			Preoperative CEA level >200 ng/ml	
Iwatsuki score [3]	305	1981–1996	Exclusion of patients with positive margins or extra-hepatic tumor	Grade 1, no risk factors Grade 2, one risk factor
			Largest CRLM >8 cm	Grade 3, two risk factors
			CRLM number ≥3	Grade 4, three risk factors
			Time to hepatic recurrence ≤30 months	Grade 5, four risk factors
			Bilobar tumor	Grade 6, positive margin or extrahepatic metastasis
Nagashima grading [4]	81	1981–1997	Largest CRLM >5 cm	A (0 ≤ Y ≤ 1)
			CRLM number ≥2	B (1 < Y ≤ 3)
			Serosal invasion of primary tumor	C (3 < Y)
			Node positive primary	
			Resectable extrahepatic metastases	
Schindl Prognostic Score [5]	337	1988–2002	Dukes stage C	Good (score, 0–10)
			CRLM number ≥4	Moderate (score, 11–25)
			Increased alkaline phosphatase level (normal range, 40–125 U/L)	Poor (score, >25)
			Increased CEA level (normal range, <5 μg/L)	
			Decreased albumin level (normal range, 3.6–4.7 g/dl)	

(continued)

Table 6.2 (continued)

Scoring system (ref)	Pt number	Pt's recruitment year	Criteria	Score
Minagawa Staging System [6]	369	1980–2002	CRLM number ≥2	Stages I–IV
			Preoperative CEA level >50 ng/ml	
			Node positive primary ≥4	
			Hepatic lymph node metastasis positive	
Malik Prognostic Score [7]	687	1993–2006	Inflammatory response to tumor (IRT)	Preoperative prognostic score 0–2
			C-reactive protein (>10 mg/L)	
			Neutrophil/lymphocyte ratio of >5:1	
			CRLM number ≥8	
Basingstoke Predictive Index (BPI) [8]	929	1987–2005	Largest CRLM >5 cm	0–30 points
			CRLM number ≥4	
			Preoperative CEA level >60 ng/ml	
			Poor differentiation of primary tumor	
			Node positive for primary tumor	
			Extrahepatic metastasis	
Konopke Clinical Score [9]	265	1993–2006	CRLM ≥4	Low risk, zero factor Intermediate risk, one factor
			Preoperative CEA level >200 ng/ml	High risk, two factors
Dexiang Scoring System [10]	1613	2000–2010	Synchronous CRLM	Low-risk group (0–2 points)
			Largest CRLM ≥5 cm	High-risk group (3–5 points)
			CRLM number ≥4	
			Poor differentiation of primary tumor	
			No surgical treatment of CRLM	
Tumor Burden Score [11]	604	2000–2015	Maximum size of CRLM	
			CRLM number	
Minagawa Staging System [6]	369	1980–2002	CRLM number ≥2	Stages I–IV
			Preoperative CEA level >50 ng/ml	
			Node positive primary ≥4	
			Hepatic lymph node metastasis positive	
Malik Prognostic Score [7]	700	1993–2006	Inflammatory response to tumor (IRT)	Preoperative prognostic score 0–2
			C-reactive protein (>10 mg/L)	
			Neutrophil/lymphocyte ratio of >5:1	
			CRLM number ≥8	

Table 6.2 (continued)

Scoring system (ref)	Pt number	Pt's recruitment year	Criteria	Score
Basingstoke Predictive Index [8]	929	1987–2005	Largest CRLM >5 cm	Basingstoke Predictive Index (BPI)
			CRLM number ≥4	0–30 points
			Preoperative CEA level >60 ng/ml	
			Poor differentiation of primary tumor	
			Node positive for primary tumor	
			Extrahepatic metastasis	
Konopke Clinical Score [9]	265	1993–2006	CRLM ≥4	Low risk, zero prognostic factors
			Preoperative CEA level >200 ng/ml	Intermediate risk, one factor
Dexiang Scoring System [10]	1613	2000–2010	Synchronous CRLM	Low-risk group (0–2 points)
			Largest CRLM ≥5 cm	High-risk group (3–5 points)
			CRLM number ≥4	
			Poor differentiation of primary tumor	
			No surgical treatment of CRLM	
Tumor Burden Score [11]	604	2000–2015	Maximum size of CRLM	
			CRLM number	

Abbreviations: *CRLM* colorectal liver metastases, *MSKCC-CRS* Memorial Sloan-Kettering Cancer Center–Clinical Risk Score, *CEA* carcinoembryonic antigen

adjuvant chemotherapy was found to be effective only in the high-risk group; therefore, the clinical study of neoadjuvant therapy (NAC) followed by hepatic resection (CHARISMA study) limited to high-risk CRS patients had already started [39]. Rat sarcoma viral oncogene homolog (RAS) mutations are found in 15–35% of patients with resectable CRLM and have been associated with poor overall and recurrence-free survival after hepatic resection [40–42]. RAS mutation status on the traditional CRS was determined to predict survival after resection of CRLM. Modifying the traditional MSKCC-CRS by replacing the disease-free interval (DFI), the number of metastases, and CEA level with RAS mutation status produced a modified MSKCC-CRS that outperformed the traditional one [43].

The Iwatsuki score [3] was developed on the basis of CRLM patients who underwent primary liver resections. First, patients with positive margins or extrahepatic tumors were excluded because their prognoses were consistently very poor. The second analysis demonstrated independent four poor prognostic factors. Risk scores for tumor recurrence of the culled cohort were calculated and were divided into six groups. Estimated 5-year overall survival rates were well separated in patients with grades 1–6: 48.3%, 36.6%, 19.9%, 11.9%, 0%, and 0%, respectively ($p < 0.0001$).

The Nagashima Grading System [4] was developed for patients with CRLM after liver resection. Total score: $Y = 0.8057 \times$ serosal invasion (+) of primary, $1 + 0.8375 \times n$ (+) of primary, $1 + 0.8609 \times$ multiple, $1 + 1.4532 \times$ diameter >5 cm, $1 + 1.3957 \times$ extrahepatic metastases (+), 1. Cancer-related survival curves were well separated; 5-year survival rates were 85%, 56%, and 0%, in Grades A, B, and C, respectively. This grading system was well validated in the other cohort (72 patients between 1981 and 2001).

The Schindl Prognostic Score [5] was developed and validated. First, a mathematical equation was formulated that included all significant variables and coefficients from the final regression model. Prognostic Score = [(4 × Duke code) + (6 × Metcode 3) + (6 × lnAlkphos) + (2 × lnCEA) − Albumin] + 22, rounded to the nearest whole number, where the Duke code indicates Dukes' stage A/B (score, 0) or C (score, 1); Metcode 3, one to three metastases (score, 0) or more than three metastases (score, 1); in alkphos, natural logarithmic function of the serum alkaline phosphatase level; in CEA, natural logarithmic function of the serum CEA level; and in albumin, the serum albumin level. Patients were separated into three categories on the basis of their individual scores. The median survival time (MST) was significantly different in the three groups of overall patients: 35.7 months for good, 23.5 months for moderate, and 10.6 months for poor prognosis. Similar results were obtained in the validation of the cohort containing all patients.

The Minagawa Staging System [6] is a simplified staging system to predict the prognosis of CRLM patients undergoing liver resection. The validation cohort consisted of 229 unrelated patients with CRLM from 1991 to 2003. Patients with hepatic lymph node metastasis were assigned to stage IV, and the remaining patients were divided according to the number of factors: none, stage I; one, stage II; two or three, stage III. In the original cohort, MST in stages I, II, III, and IV were 7.2, 3.5, 2.0, and 1.3 years, respectively, and in the validation cohort were 9.6, 4.1, 2.8, and 1.6 years, respectively. This staging system was highly predictive of the long-term outcome in both cohorts ($P < 0.001$).

The Malik Prognostic Score [7] was used to assess clinicopathological data of patients underwent liver resection for CRLM. The most interesting point of this paper was the focus on an inflammatory response to tumor (IRT), which was noted in 24.5% of patients. A preoperative prognostic score was classified: 0, less than eight metastases and absence of IRT; one, eight, or more metastases or IRT; and two, eight, or more metastases and IRT. Patients with a score of 0 had a significantly better 5-year overall survival of 49% compared with 34% for those with a score of 1 ($P < 0.001$). Those patients with a score of 2 had a poor prognosis, with none of the patients being 5-years from resection (MST: 21.3 months, $P < 0.005$). Unfortunately, MSKCC-CRS showed no predictive value for overall survival (OS) in this cohort.

The Basingstoke Predictive Index (BPI) [8] identified the relationship between preoperative and postoperative factors related to disease-specific survival (DSS) after liver resection for CRLM. Values were derived from the beta-coefficients of the survival analysis and multiplied by a factor of 10. The BPI calculated was shown in Table 6.3. Five-year DSS was 66%, 51%, 35%, 21%, 12%, 5%, and 2% for points of 0, 5, 10, 15, 20, 25, and 30 for the preoperative score, respectively.

The Konopke Clinical Score [9] was developed for CRLM patients undergoing liver resection. The presence of CRLM ≥4 and a CEA level ≥ 200 ng/mL were

Table 6.3 The "Basingstoke Predictive Index" (BPI) predicting cancer-specific survival after primary liver resection for CRLM

Risk factors	Preoperative score	Postoperative score
Primary tumor LN status		
Negative	0	0
Positive	2	2
Primary tumor differentiation		
Well	0	0
Moderate	3	2
Poor	5	4
CEA level at hepatectomy		
<6 ng/mL	0	0
6–60 ng/mL	2	1
>60 ng/mL	3	3
No. hepatic metastases		
1–3	0	—
>3	4	—
Largest tumor diameter		
<5 cm	0	0
5–10 cm	2	2
>10 cm	8	7
Hepatic resection margin		
Negative	—	0
Positive	—	11
Extrahepatic metastatic disease		
No	0	0
Yes	7	4

Reproduced with permission from Rees et al. [8]

independent prognostic factors. The MSTs for low, intermediate, and high risk were 94.0, 40.0, and 33.0 months, respectively. Compared with the low-risk group, patients with intermediate risk and high risk demonstrated an increased HR of 1.91-fold ($P = 0.007$) and 3.10-fold for OS ($P = 0.001$), respectively. Furthermore, the prognostic value of the risk stratification could be confirmed even in a subgroup of 43 patients undergoing liver resection following NAC.

The Dexiang Scoring System [10] was created for all CRLM patients (including unresectable cases). There were 530 patients undergoing liver surgery, including upfront surgery ($n = 345$), NAC ($n = 121$), and conversion therapy ($n = 64$). Six independent predictors of poor survival ($P < 0.001$) were identified. After giving one point to each factor, all patients were divided into low-risk group (0–2 points) and high-risk group (3–5 points), with a 5-year survival of 47% and 7%, respectively ($P < 0.001$).

Recently, a unique prognostic model named "Tumor Burden Score (TBS)" [11] was developed by Sasaki K, et al. Patients undergoing liver resection of CRLM were assessed in the era of new chemotherapy. The TBS was created with reference to the "Metro-ticket" prognostic tool for patients with hepatocellular carcinoma [44]. The TBS also utilized a continuum of tumor size and number, indicating a paradigm shift from a dichotomous to continuous prognostic stratification. It was defined as the distance from the origin on a Cartesian plane that incorporated two variables: maximum tumor size (x-axis) and number of liver lesions (y-axis). The Pythagorean theorem was then used to calculate the distance of any given point from the origin of the plane (0, 0) whereby [TBS^2 (maximum tumor diameter)^2 + (tumor number)^2]

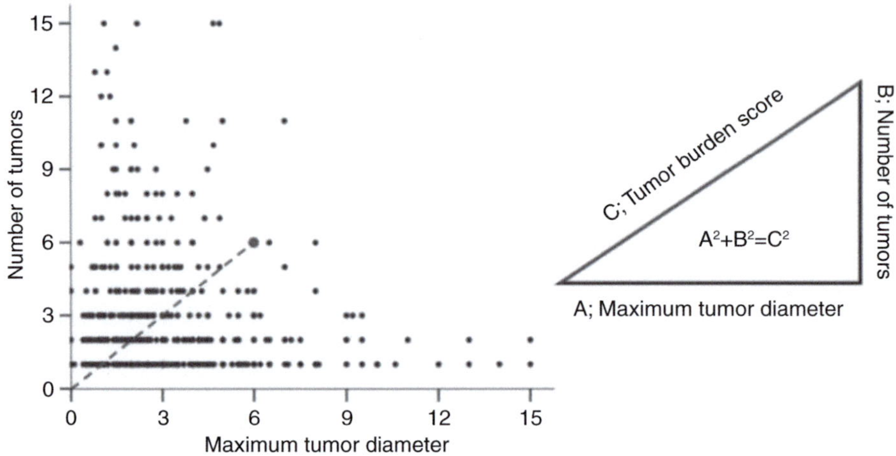

Fig. 6.1 Tumor burden score (TBS). (Reproduced with permission from Sasaki et al. [11])

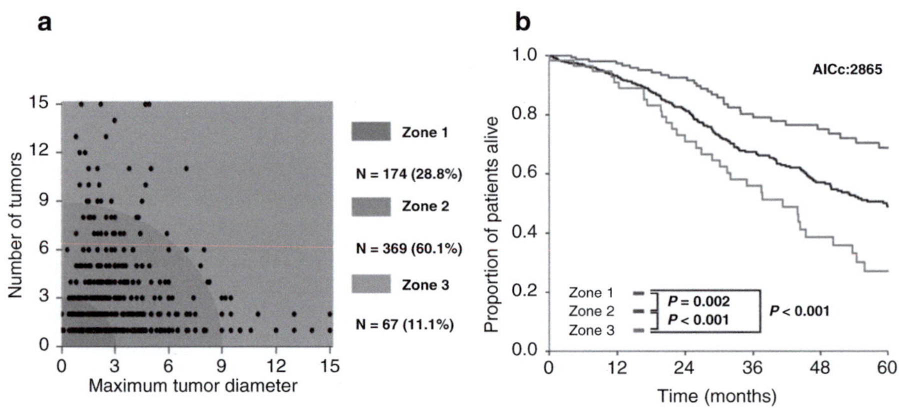

Fig. 6.2 Distribution of patients according to tumor burden score (TBS) and their overall survival. (**a**) Distribution of patients according to the TBS model in the Johns Hopkins' cohort. (**b**) Overall survival stratified by TBS (Zones 1, 2, and 3). (Reproduced with permission from Sasaki et al. [11])

(Fig. 6.1). The cutoff values of TBS were selected to divide the cohort into three groups: lowest 25% of TBS (zone 1), medium TBS between the 25th and 90th percentiles (zone 2), and the highest 10% of TBS (zone 3), respectively. The optimal cutoff points for the TBS model were set at 3 (28.8%, lowest 25%) and 9 (88.9%, highest 10%) according to the cumulative percentage of TBS distribution. The TBS increased, overall survival gradually deteriorated (5-year OS: 68.9% for zone 1, 49.4% for zone 2, and 25.5% for zone 3; $P < 0.05$) (Fig. 6.2). The "Metro-ticket" TBS model has excellent prognostic discriminatory power that has been externally validated by the other Japanese and Italian cohort.

Validation Study of Risk Scoring Systems for CRLM Patients Treated with Liver Resection

Patients' selection and/or treatment period can influence the impact of a risk scoring system. It should be clearly described when CRLM patients in the validation group were treated and contents of the chemotherapeutic regimen should be detailed.

Zakaria S, et al. [12] set out to create a new Mayo scoring system and to validate previous risk scoring systems. A total of 662 consecutive CRLM patients undergoing liver resection from 1960 to 1995 were assessed. Perioperative blood transfusion and positive hepatoduodenal nodes were the major determinants of survival and recurrence. CRLM diameter >8 cm and interval to CRLM <30 months were also prognostic factors for survival. The Mayo prognostic model had the highest concordance probability for DSS; scoring system of Mayo (0.61), Nordlinger (0.55), Fong (0.56), and Iwatsuki (0.53) [1–3].

Reissfelder C et al. [13] conducted validation of five scoring systems using 281 patients underwent liver resection for CRLM from 2002 to 2008. Over 60% of all patients received modern chemotherapy and approximately 30% of patients received molecular targeted therapy with bevacizumab and/or cetuximab. As for the Nordlinger score [1], MSKCC-CRS [2], Iwatsuki score [3], Basingstoke index [8], and Mayo scoring system [12], only the MSKCC-CRS ($P = 0.006$) and the Iwatsuki score ($P = 0.01$) provided a statistically significant stratification of patients with regard to OS. In the modern chemotherapy era, the MSKCC-CRS and the Iwatsuki score also had predictive value and was particularly evident for patients in high-risk categories.

Merkel S et al. [14] analyzed 282 consecutive CRLM patients undergoing 303 liver resections between 1995 and 2006. For the MSKCC-CRS [2], patients were divided into three groups: low risk, no risk factors; intermediate risk, one to two risk factors; and high risk, three to five risk factors. For the Nordlinger score [1], patients were divided into three groups. For the TNM classification [22], patients were divided into three categories: M2a, M2b, and M2c. Only MSKCC-CRS was a reliable preoperative prognostic tool for selecting patients for surgical resection of CRLM. Survival between the intermediate- and high-risk groups differed significantly (5-year survival: 42.8% vs. 29.1%; $P < 0.03$).

Nathan H et al. [15] investigated 949 CRLM patients from an international multi-institutional database who underwent liver resection between 1982 and 2008. Conditional survival estimates were calculated as $CS = S_{(x+5)}/S(x)$. All of the prognostic scoring systems had fair-to-moderate prognostic discriminatory ability and a low concordance index (MSKCC-CRS [2]: 0.57, Nordlinger's score [1]: 0.56, MSKCC-nomogram [26]: 0.58). The inadequate performance of the prognostic scoring systems was explained by the fact that as postoperative survival increased from 0 to 5 years, the 5-year observed conditional survival improved markedly for patients who were initially predicted to have poor survival at the time of surgery.

Previous prognostic scoring systems were validated by CRLM patients treated with liver resection following NAC using modern chemotherapeutic agents between 2000 and 2008 [16]. Unfortunately, the contents of the NAC were unclear. Patients were divided into two groups: 193 patients who did not receive NAC (no-NAC group), and 159 patients who received NAC (NAC group). In the no-NAC group, all scoring systems had a statistically significant predictive value. In the NAC group, only the Nordlinger score had a predictive value before the administration of NAC and all scoring systems had a predictive value again, except for the Konopke score [9] after the administration of NAC. Three traditional scoring systems are not a reliable prognostic tool when used in CRLM patients before treatment with NAC. However, scoring systems assessed after the administration of NAC are useful predicting prognosis.

Barkhatov [17] validated the MSKCC-CRS [2], preoperative and postoperative BPI [8], Nordlinger's score [1], and Iwatsuki's score [3] in CRLM 406 patients treated with laparoscopic liver resection from 1998 to 2015. NAC was conducted on one-third of the patients. Four scoring systems divided patients into risk groups with significant difference in survival between the groups. However, predicted 5-year survival rates were lower (13–30% than the actual 5-year survival in these scoring systems). These scoring systems can be used to predict survival for CRLM patients undergoing laparoscopic liver resection in the era of multidisciplinary treatment after adjusting for survival rates.

The HPB CONCEPT Team [18] re-evaluated the utility of previous CRS in the modern chemotherapy era. Between 2008 and 2012, 740 CRLM patients undergoing liver resection were enrolled. Details of the chemotherapy were not described. The original MSKCC-CRS [2] was a significant ($P < 0.001$) predictor of both OS (5-year OS: 0; 75%, 1; 71%, 2; 57%, 3; 57%, 4; 46%) and RFS (5-year RFS: 0; 39%, 1; 33%, 2; 21%, 3; 21%, and 4; 8%). The presence of extrahepatic hepatic disease decreased RFS (HR of 1.32), and the use of intraoperative portal pedicle clamping increased RFS (HR of 0.78).

Dupré et al. [19] developed a unique validation study focusing on CRLM patients with liver-limited recurrence who were treated with curative liver resection. From 2010 to 2015, 375 CRLM patients received primary liver resection. Among them, 73 patients developed liver-limited recurrence that was treated with curative intent. One-third of the patients received preoperative chemotherapy. The predictive value of six scores (Fong [2], Sofocleous [46], Nagashima [4], Nordlinger [1], Konopke [9], and the Basingstoke index [8]) was assessed in this dataset. Sofocleous et al. [46] proposed using a modified Fong's score for percutaneous radiofrequency ablation, excluding CEA level and modifying the cutoff level for the maximal size of the CRLM (3 cm instead of 5 cm). [45] Only Nagashima's score showed a significant difference in OS between patients from the low-risk group and those from the intermediate- and high-risk groups (40.8 vs. 30.5 months, $P = 0.039$). For PFS, only Fong's score showed a statistically significant stratification (6.6 vs. 4.7 months, $P = 0.027$). Previous scoring systems had limited value in stratifying CRLM patients undergoing repeated liver resection.

New Aspects of the Prognostic Score System

KRAS and BRAF mutations have been reported as prognostic biomarkers for CRLM patients. A recent meta-analysis of seven eligible trials (1403 patients) clearly showed that KRAS and BRAF mutations predicted a significantly worse OS with HRs of 1.86 and 3.90, respectively, in patients who underwent liver resection of CRLM [41].

In the study population of resected 309 CRLM patients, BRAF mutant and RAS mutant patients were 12 (4%) and 160 (52%), respectively. At multivariate analyses, patients with the BRAF mutant had a higher risk of recurrence in comparison with all wild (HR: 2.31, $P = 0.029$) and to patients with the RAS mutant (HR: 2.06, $P = 0.044$). Similar tendencies were confirmed in terms of OS, but such effect was vanished after multivariate analyses [42]. The RAS mutation rate was significantly higher in patients with right-sided tumors ($P < 0.007$). The site of the primary tumor had no significant impact on the long-term survival in patients with CRLM undergoing radical surgery. The multivariate analysis showed that the RAS mutant is an independent factor influencing OS only in patients with left-sided primary tumors [46]. mtKRAS was an independent predictor of worse OS, and the effect was more pronounced among patients who experienced a recurrence after the resection of CRLM [47].

The survival impact of primary lymph node status, circulating tumor cells (CTCs), and disseminated tumor cells (DTCs) in the bone marrow were assessed in patients with resectable CRLM [48]. CTCs were detected in 5.3% of patients in the N0 group. In multivariate analysis, positivity CTC, not DTC, was significantly associated with poor OS [HR: 2.31 (1.00–4.28), $P = 0.05$]. Assessment of CTC in addition to nodal status may contribute to the improvement of clarity as far as a classification of patients into high- and low-risk groups.

Nomogram to Predict Prognosis of Resected CRLM

Kattan et al. [26] first developed a MSKCC-nomogram for predicting the 96-month DSS of CRLM patients between 1986 and 1999. The nomogram consisted of ten factors: gender, age, primary cancer site (colon vs. rectum), DFI (months), preoperative CEA level, number and the largest size of CRLM, bilateral resection, extensive resection (lobectomy or more), and nodal status of the primary cancer (Fig. 6.3). A concordance index was 0.612. Reddy et al. [27] investigated the effect of preoperative chemotherapy on the accuracy of a MSKCC-nomogram. An external cohort of 203 patients who underwent resection of CRLM between 1996 and 2006 was used. Estimated 3-, 5-, and 8-year DSS were 56%, 41%, and 32%, respectively (similar to nomogram predicted probabilities for DSS). The concordance index for the nomogram (0.602) was higher than that for the MSKCC-CRS

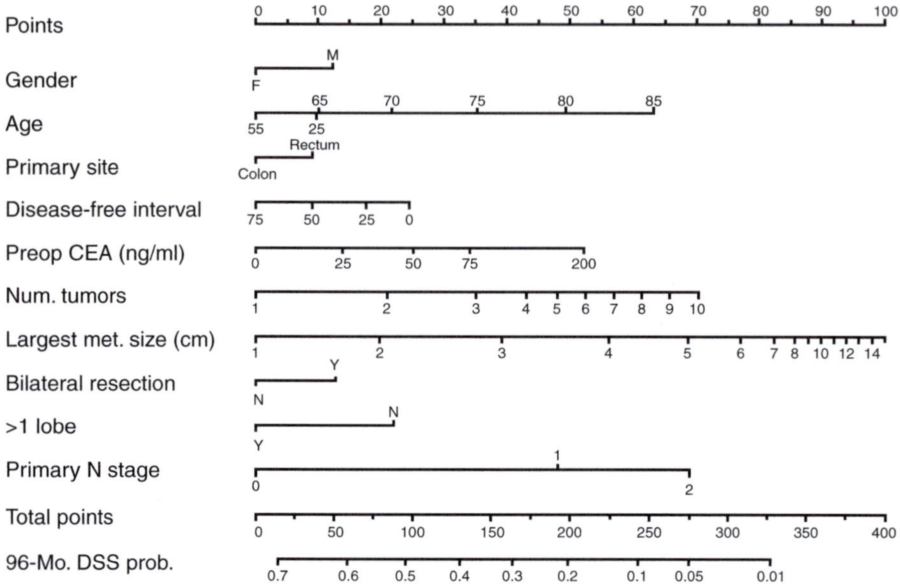

Fig. 6.3 MSKCC-nomogram. (Reproduced with permission from Kattan et al. [26])

(0.533). DSS was longer for patients ($n = 50$) treated with at least 6 months of perioperative irinotecan or oxaliplatin compared with all other patients (median 66 vs. 40 months, $P = 0.06$). The actual DSS was greater than nomogram predicted DSS for treated patients and less than nomogram predicted DSS for all other patients. The prediction ability of the nomogram may reflect the therapeutic effect of perioperative chemotherapy.

The nomogram established by Kanemitsu et al. [28] included 578 CRLM patients undergoing hepatic resection between 1990 and 1998. Pre- and post-treatment prognostic nomograms were developed. The preoperative nomogram included the five prognostic factors: primary histology, number of metastatic lymph nodes in primary lesion, number of CRLM, extrahepatic disease, and pre-hepatectomy CEA level. The concordance index of the nomogram was 0.66. Unfortunately, the preoperative nomogram estimated death after liver resection as a maximum of 3 years; therefore, the preoperative nomogram does not provide a true probability of cure after surgery.

The Beppu nomogram was created to predict disease-free survival (DFS) for CRLM patients undergoing upfront liver resection [35]. Patients were enrolled between 2000 and 2004 at the 11 institutions from all over Japan. The nomogram consisted of only six preoperative factors: synchronous metastases for 3 points, primary LN positive for 3 points, two to four tumors for 4 points and five or more tumors for 9 points, largest tumor diameter >5 cm for 2 points, extrahepatic metastasis at hepatectomy for 4 points, and preoperative Carbohydrate antigen 19-9 (CA19-9) level >100 U/mL for 4 points (Table 6.4). Figure 6.4 shows that drawing a straight line from the total points of the "preoperative score" to the DFS axis can demonstrate the patient's probability of DFS at 3 and 5 years. The concordance index of the nomogram was 0.66. The nomogram can be easily used in clinics or at the patients' bedsides and is a very useful tool for determining the likelihood of early recurrence and the necessity of perioperative chemotherapy. Patients with over 10 points may be good candidates for perioperative chemotherapy because their DFS is shorter than that for 1 year (Fig. 6.5). This nomogram was validated using 234 CRLM patients who underwent liver resection in the new chemotherapy era between 2005 and 2010 [30]. The c-index of the patients who received preoperative chemotherapy was inferior to that of the patients who did not (0.56 and 0.61, respectively). Only in patients without preoperative chemotherapy, DFS among the quintiles clustered by the nomogram score indicated significant differences ($P < 0.0001$). Surprisingly, in patients with no risk factors determined by the nomogram, NAC followed by liver resection provided significantly lower DFS than upfront liver resection (DFS at 3-year: 42.9% vs. 80.0%, $P = 0.03$).

Table 6.4 The "preoperative score" predicting disease-free survival after hepatic resection for CRLM

Risk factors	Preoperative score
Timing of liver metastases	
Metachronous	0
Synchronous	3
Primary tumor LN status	
Negative	0
Positive	3
Number of tumors	
1	0
2–4	4
5<	9
Largest tumor diameter	
≤5 cm	0
>5 cm	2
Extrahepatic metastatic disease (at hepatectomy)	
No	0
Yes	4
CA19-9 level (before hepatectomy)	
≤100	0
>100	4

Reproduced with permission from Beppu et al. [35]

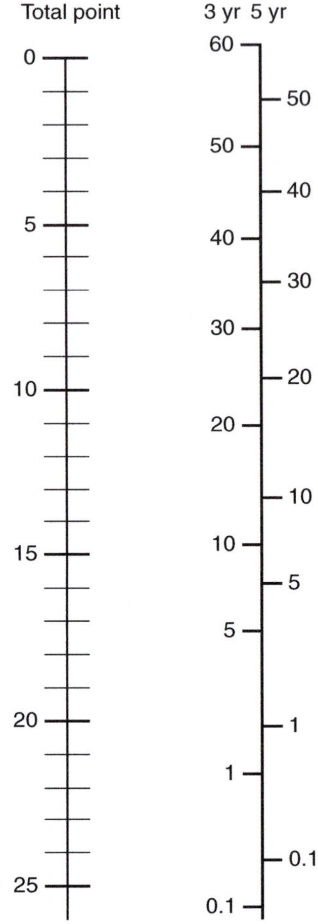

Fig. 6.4 A nomogram to predict disease-free survival after liver resection for CRLM. (Reproduced with permission from Beppu et al. [35])

Recently, a unique nomogram has been developed by Imai et al. [31] to predict survival after liver resection for initially unresectable CRLM. Between 1990 and 2012, 444 (38.2%) patients were identified as undergoing hepatectomy for initially unresectable CRLM. The following five factors were independent prognostic indicators: node-positive primary, 5; more than six CRLM at hepatectomy, 7; CA 19–9 level at hepatectomy above 37 U/mL, 10; disease progression during first-line chemotherapy, 9; and presence of extrahepatic disease, 4 (Fig. 6.6a). Unlike previous nomograms for upfront hepatectomy, disease progression during

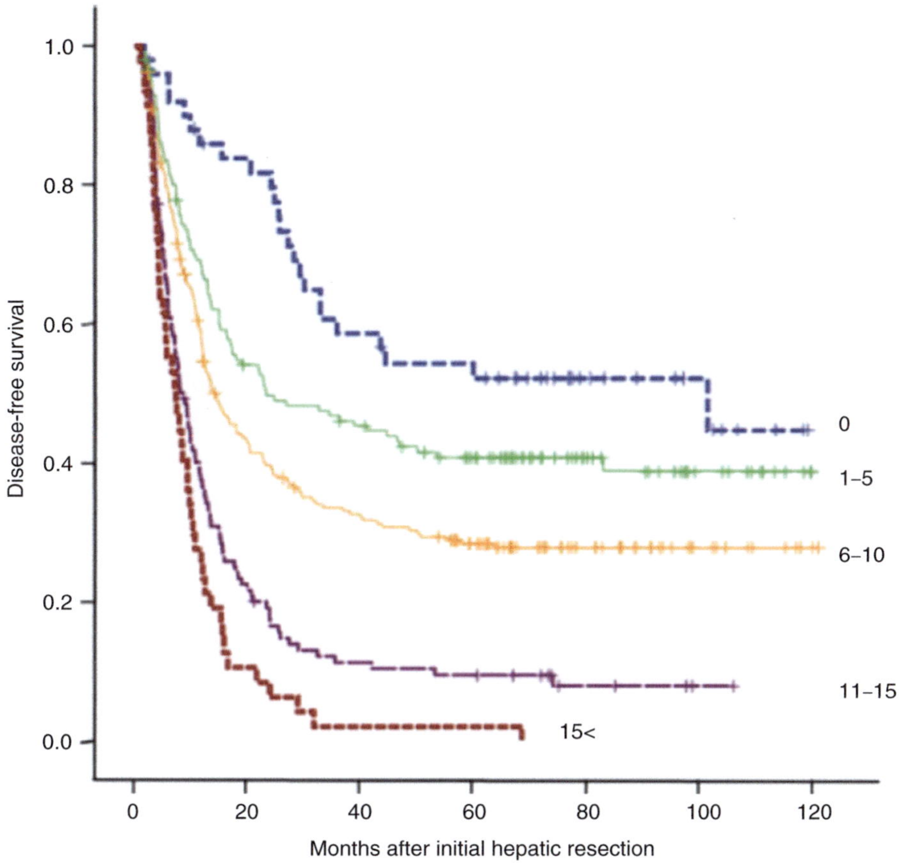

Fig. 6.5 Disease-free survival after liver resection of five groups, each with a five-point increase in "preoperative score." Estimated median DFS time was calculated as follows: >8.4 years for patients with 0 points, 1.9 years for 5 points, 1.0 year for 10 points; rates were lower than 0.6 years for patients with more than 10 points. (Reproduced with permission from Beppu et al. [35])

first-line chemotherapy was selected. The model achieved relatively good discrimination and calibration, with a concordance index of 0.66. The OS rate of patients with a score greater than 16 was significantly worse than that of patients with a score of 16 or less (5-year survival rate: 4% vs. 46.3%, respectively; $P < 0.001$) (Fig. 6.6b).

Factor	Score
Primary tumour N category	
N0	0
N1–2	5
Tumour no. at hepatectomy	
≤6	0
>6	7
CA19-91evel at hepatectomy (units/ml)	
≤37	0
>37	10
Response to first-line chemotherapy	
Response/stabilization	0
Progression	9
Concomitant extrahepatic disease	
No	0
Yes	4

a Prognostic factor scores

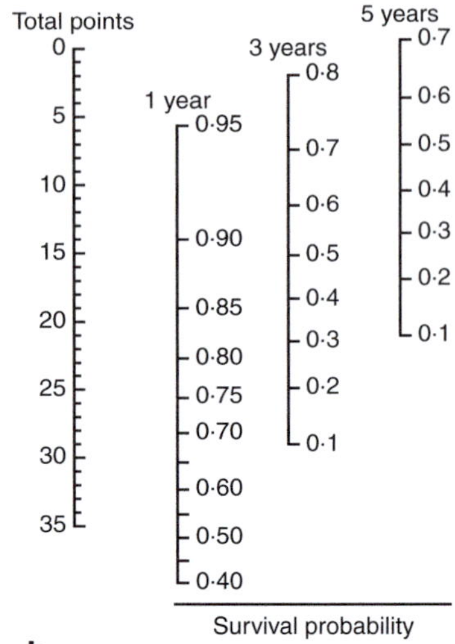

b Nomogram to predict survival after hepatectomy

Fig. 6.6 A nomogram to predict survival after liver resection in patients with initially unresectable colorectal liver metastases. A nomogram can predict 1-, 3-, and 5-year survival probabilities. The sum of the scores for each variable (**a**) was plotted on the total point axis, and the estimated probabilities of survival at 1, 3, and 5 years (**b**) were obtained by drawing a line horizontally from the plotted total point axis straight to the survival axis. (Reproduced with permission from Imai et al. [31])

Conclusion

Due to state-of-the-art chemotherapy and improved surgical techniques for liver resection, the appropriate staging classification for CRLM has been changing. A multicenter prospective study limited to CRLM patients is necessary. A new staging classification limited to CRLM patients in for the era of multidisciplinary treatment will be required.

References

1. Nordlinger B, Guiguet M, Vaillant JC, et al. Surgical resection of colorectal carcinoma metastases to the liver. A prognostic scoring system to improve case selection, based on 1568 patients. Association Francaise de Chirurgie. Cancer. 1996;77:1254–62.
2. Fong Y, Fortner J, Sun RL, et al. Clinical score for predicting recurrence after hepatic resection for metastatic colorectal cancer: analysis of 1001 consecutive cases. Ann Surg. 1999;230:309–18.
3. Iwatsuki S, Dvorchik I, Madariaga JR, et al. Hepatic resection for metastatic colorectal adenocarcinoma: a proposal of a prognostic scoring system. J Am Coll Surg. 1999;189:291–9.
4. Nagashima I, Takada T, Matsuda K, et al. A new scoring system to classify patients with colorectal liver metastases: proposal of criteria to select candidates for hepatic resection. J Hepato-Biliary-Pancreat Surg. 2004;11:79–83.

5. Schindl M, Wigmore SJ, Currie EJ, et al. Prognostic scoring in colorectal cancer liver metastases: development and validation. Arch Surg. 2005;140:183–9.
6. Minagawa M, Yamamoto J, Kosuge T, et al. Simplified staging system for predicting the prognosis of patients with resectable liver metastasis: development and validation. Arch Surg. 2007;142:269–27.
7. Malik HZ, Prasad KR, Halazun KJ, et al. Preoperative prognostic score for predicting survival after hepatic resection for colorectal liver metastases. Ann Surg. 2007;246:806–14.
8. Rees M, Tekkis PP, Welsh FK, et al. Evaluation of long-term survival after hepatic resection for metastatic colorectal cancer: a multifactorial model of 929 patients. Ann Surg. 2008;247:125–35.
9. Konopke R, Kersting S, Distler M, et al. Prognostic factors and evaluation of a clinical score for predicting survival after resection of colorectal liver metastases. Liver Int. 2009;29:89–102.
10. Dexiang Z, Li R, Ye W, et al. Outcome of patients with colorectal liver metastasis: analysis of 1,613 consecutive cases. Ann Surg Oncol. 2012;19:2860–8.
11. Sasaki K, Morioka D, Conci S, et al. The tumor burden score: a new "metro-ticket" prognostic tool for colorectal liver metastases based on tumor size and number of tumors. Ann Surg. 2018;267(1):132–41.
12. Zakaria S, Donohue JH, Que FG, et al. Hepatic resection for colorectal metastases: value for risk scoring systems? Ann Surg. 2007;246:183–91.
13. Reissfelder C, Rahbari NN, Koch M, et al. Validation of prognostic scoring systems for patients undergoing resection of colorectal cancer liver metastases. Ann Surg Oncol. 2009;16(12):3279–88.
14. Merkel S, Bialecki D, Meyer T, et al. Comparison of clinical risk scores predicting prognosis after resection of colorectal liver metastases. J Surg Oncol. 2009;100(5):349–57.
15. Nathan H, de Jong MC, Pulitano C, et al. Conditional survival after surgical resection of colorectal liver metastasis: an international multi-institutional analysis of 949 patients. J Am Coll Surg. 2010;210(5):755–64.
16. Ayez N, Lalmahomed ZS, van der Pool AE, et al. Is the clinical risk score for patients with colorectal liver metastases still useable in the era of effective neoadjuvant chemotherapy? Ann Surg Oncol. 2011;18(10):2757–63.
17. Barkhatov L, Fretland ÅA, Kazaryan AM, et al. Validation of clinical risk scores for laparoscopic liver resections of colorectal liver metastases: a 10-year observed follow-up study. J Surg Oncol. 2016;114(6):757–63.
18. Beamish P, Lemke M, Li J, Dixon E, et al. HPB CONCEPT team. Validation of clinical risk score for colorectal liver metastases resected in a contemporary multicenter cohort. HPB (Oxford). 2017;19(8):675–81.
19. Dupré A, Rehman A, Jones RP, et al. Validation of clinical prognostic scores for patients treated with curative-intent for recurrent colorectal liver metastases. J Surg Oncol. 2018;117:1330. https://doi.org/10.1002/jso.24959. [Epub ahead of print].
20. Matias M, Casa-Nova M, Faria M, et al. Prognostic factors after liver resection for colorectal liver metastasis. Acta Medica Port. 2015;28(3):357–69.
21. Edge SB, Compton CC. The American joint committee on cancer: the 7th edition of the AJCC cancer staging manual and the future of TNM. Ann Surg Oncol. 2010;17(6):1471–4.
22. AJCC Cancer staging manual. 8th ed. New York: Springer. p. 2017.
23. Kato T, Yasui K, Hirai T, et al. Therapeutic results for hepatic metastasis of colorectal cancer with special reference to effectiveness of hepatectomy: analysis of prognostic factors for 763 cases recorded at 18 institutions. Dis Colon Rectum. 2003;46(10 suppl):S22–31.
24. Japanese Society for Cancer of the Colon and Rectum. Rectum and Anus. 8th ed. Tokyo: Kanehara & CO., LTD; 2013.
25. Yamaguchi T, Mori T, Takahashi K, et al. A new classification system for liver metastases from colorectal cancer in Japanese multicenter analysis. Hepato-Gastroenterology. 2008;55:173–8.
26. Kattan MW, Gonen M, Jarnagin WR, et al. A nomogram for predicting disease-specific survival after hepatic resection for metastatic colorectal cancer. Ann Surg. 2008;247:282–7.

27. Reddy SK, Kattan MW, Yu C, et al. Evaluation of peri-operative chemotherapy using a prognostic nomogram for survival after resection of colorectal liver metastases. HPB (Oxford). 2009;11(7):592–9.
28. Kanemitsu Y, Kato T. Prognostic models for predicting death after hepatectomy in individuals with hepatic metastases from colorectal cancer. World J Surg. 2008;32:1097–107.
29. Beppu T, Sakamoto Y, Hasegawa K, et al. Optimal cut-off value for the number of colorectal liver metastases: a project study for hepatic surgery of the Japanese Society of Hepato-Biliary-Pancreatic Surgery. J Hepatobiliary Pancreat Sci. 2014;21(3):169–75.
30. Okuno M, Hatano E, Seo S, et al. Indication for neoadjuvant chemotherapy in patients with colorectal liver metastases based on a nomogram that predicts disease-free survival. J Hepatobiliary Pancreat Sci. 2014;21(12):881–8.
31. Imai K, Allard MA, Castro Benitez C, et al. Nomogram for prediction of prognosis in patients with initially unresectable colorectal liver metastases. Br J Surg. 2016;103(5):590–9.
32. Adam R, De Gramont A, Figueras J, EGOSLIM (Expert Group on OncoSurgery management of Liver Metastases) Group, et al. The oncosurgery approach to managing liver metastases from colorectal cancer: a multidisciplinary international consensus. Oncologist. 2012;17(10):1225–39.
33. Khoo E, O'Neill S, Brown E, et al. Systematic review of systemic adjuvant, neoadjuvant and perioperative chemotherapy for resectable colorectal-liver metastases. HPB (Oxford). 2016;18(6):485–93.
34. Jones RP, Poston GJ. Resection of liver metastases in colorectal cancer in the era of expanding systemic therapy. Annu Rev Med. 2017;68:183–96.
35. Beppu T, Sakamoto Y, Hasegawa K, et al. A nomogram predicting disease-free survival in patients with colorectal liver metastases treated with hepatic resection: multicenter data collection as a project study for hepatic surgery of the Japanese Society of Hepato-Biliary-Pancreatic Surgery. J Hepatobiliary Pancreat Sci. 2012;19(1):72–84.
36. Shinto E, Takahashi K, Yamaguchi T, Study Group for Liver Metastasis projected by the Japanese Society for Cancer of the Colon and Rectum (JSCCR), et al. Validation and modification of the Japanese classification system for liver metastases from colorectal cancer: a multi-institutional study. Ann Surg Oncol. 2015;22(12):3888–95.
37. Altman DG, Royston P. What do we mean by validating a prognostic model? Stat Med. 2000;19:453–73.
38. Rahbari NN, Reissfelder C, Schulze-Bergkamen H, et al. Adjuvant therapy after resection of colorectal liver metastases: the predictive value of the MSKCC clinical risk score in the era of modern chemotherapy. BMC Cancer. 2014;14:174.
39. Ayez N, van der Stok EP, de Wilt H, et al. Neo-adjuvant chemotherapy followed by surgery versus surgery alone in high-risk patients with resectable colorectal liver metastases: the CHARISMA randomized multicenter clinical trial. BMC Cancer. 2015;15:180. https://doi.org/10.1186/s12885-015-1199-8.
40. Vauthey JN, Zimmitti G, Kopetz SE, et al. RAS mutation status predicts survival and patterns of recurrence in patients undergoing hepatectomy for colorectal liver metastases. Ann Surg. 2013;258:619–26.
41. Passiglia F, Bronte G, Bazan V, et al. Can KRAS and BRAF mutations limit the benefit of liver resection in metastatic colorectal cancer patients? A systematic review and meta-analysis. Crit Rev Oncol Hematol. 2016;99:150.
42. Schirripa M, Bergamo F, Cremolini C, et al. BRAF and RAS mutations as prognostic factors in metastatic colorectal cancer patients undergoing liver resection. Br J Cancer. 2015;112(12):1921–8.
43. Brudvik KW, Jones RP, Giuliante F, et al. RAS mutation clinical risk score to predict survival after resection of colorectal liver metastases. Ann Surg. 2019;269(1):120–6.
44. Mazzaferro V, Llovet JM, Miceli R, et al. Predicting survival after liver transplantation in patients with hepatocellular carcinoma beyond the Milan criteria: a retrospective, exploratory analysis. Lancet Oncol. 2009;10:35–43.

45. Sofocleous CT, Petre EN, Gonen M, et al. CT-guided radiofrequency ablation as a salvage treatment of colorectal cancer hepatic metastases developing after hepatectomy. J Vasc Interv Radiol. 2011;22:755–61.
46. Wang K, Xu D, Yan XL, et al. The impact of primary tumour location in patients undergoing hepatic resection for colorectal liver metastasis. Eur J Surg Oncol. 2018. pii: S0748-7983(18)30884-9;44:771.
47. Margonis GA, Spolverato G, Kim Y, et al. Effect of KRAS mutation on long-term outcomes of patients undergoing hepatic resection for colorectal liver metastases. Ann Surg Oncol. 2015;22(13):4158–65.
48. Seeberg LT, Brunborg C, Waage A, et al. Survival impact of primary tumor lymph node status and circulating tumor cells in patients with colorectal liver metastases. Ann Surg Oncol. 2017;24(8):2113–21.

Prognostic Factors of Colorectal Cancer Liver Metastasis

7

Felipe José Fernández Coimbra, Paulo Henrique Miranda Brandão, Alessandro Landskron Diniz, Heber Salvador de Castro Ribeiro, Wilson Luiz da Costa Júnior, André Luiz de Godoy, and Igor Correia de Farias

Introduction

Approximately 1,200,000 cases of colorectal cancer occur annually throughout the world. It is one of the most common tumors and the third leading cause of cancer-related death in both sexes. Half of these patients will develop liver metastases in 2 years, and 25% will present it synchronously, being the most common site of dissemination and cause of death in two-thirds of colorectal tumors [1, 2].

The likelihood of cure consists of R0 resection of metastatic liver disease, which can transform 5-year survival from 11% in nonsurgical patients to 38–58%, with progressively better results with the evolution of multimodal treatment [3–6]. However, this patient group is quite heterogeneous presenting variable prognoses and different therapeutic proposals depending on the characteristics of the patient, the characteristics of the primary and metastatic tumor, and the presence and volume of extrahepatic disease [7].

Since the first publications that demonstrated the benefit of hepatic resection in metastatic disease, the studies turned to the investigation of prognostic factors for the best selection of patients who would benefit from surgical resection and exclusion from those who should be directed to exclusive palliative treatment. Predictive models were developed that helped to categorize risk and selection of treatments, the most important being those published in the late 1990s by Fong et al. and Nordlinger et al. [8, 9].

These studies are based on data collection from the 1980s in which several known prognostic factors were not yet studied, such as genetic tumor characteristics and the influence of multimodal treatment. In 2015, Schreckenbach et al.

F. J. F. Coimbra (✉) · P. H. M. Brandão · A. L. Diniz · H. S. de Castro Ribeiro
W. L. da Costa Júnior · A. L. de Godoy · I. C. de Farias
Department of Abdominal Surgery, Surgical Oncology, A.C. Camargo Cancer Center, São Paulo, Brazil

M. M. Correia et al. (eds.), *Colorectal Cancer Liver Metastases*,
https://doi.org/10.1007/978-3-030-25486-5_7

retrospectively applied the risk scores of Fong et al. and Nordlinger et al. in patients undergoing neoadjuvant chemotherapy and identified that these scores lost their validity in this context [10]. Considering the evolution of systemic treatment and local treatment (portal vein embolization, two-stage hepatectomy, chemoembolization, and radioablation), other articles question the validity of these risk scores in the current scenario [7, 11].

In this chapter, we will evaluate the prognostic characteristics of colorectal liver metastases, considering the constant evolution in research on biological and genetic tumor factors, multimodal treatment, and systemic therapy in addition to the classically studied factors related to staging, disease volume, and surgical characteristics. Didactically, we will divide the factors into those related to the patient, related to the primary tumor, related to the liver disease, and related to the extrahepatic metastatic disease.

Factors Related to the Patient

Considering that a good performance status is indispensable for the complete therapeutic follow-up involving at least systemic treatment and major surgery, it can be inferred that patients with better clinical conditions would have higher rates of treatment with curative intent and better prognoses. This assumption is confirmed by studies that correlate, in multivariate analysis, the clinical condition and comorbidities with a worse overall survival, although they have no association with less disease-free time [1, 12].

In the same sense, *age* also manifested as a prognostic factor. Margonis et al. found in multivariate analysis that age above 65 years is an independent prognostic factor for overall survival. Using the 60-year cut, Liu et al. found only a prognostic association in overall survival of 1–3 and 5 years in univariate analysis, losing the effect in multivariate analysis [13, 14].

Age is also a controversial factor, since many consider the chronological age isolated, without evaluation of functional conditions and fragility. Certainly, it should not be considered an isolated prognostic factor but rather as an item in the preoperative decision, which implies a possible decrease in clinical reserves and recovery capacity in the case of more severe complications, but not an exclusion factor per se only.

Intra- and postoperative complications are related not only to surgical size (change size for extension) and tumor characteristics but also to the clinical conditions of the patients. In a study conducted in a Brazilian cancer center, Salvador et al. evaluated the postoperative complications, estimated by the Clavien-Dindo classification [15] and their prognostic impact. Patients with mild complications (Clavien-Dindo grade 1 and 2) had overall 5-year survival of 70.1% versus 50.2% in patients with more severe complications (Clavien-Dindo 3 and 4). The same trend was found in multivariate analysis with a hazard ratio of 2.7 in patients with complications of degrees 3 and 4. However, no negative association of these patients with disease-free survival was found. As interpreted by other studies, this finding seems to demonstrate that postoperative complications result in a worse outcome due to systemic/immunological changes rather than to tumor progression itself [5, 16]. Another fact classically related to a worse operative outcome is blood transfusion, being associated with a higher postoperative mortality rate at 90 days and a higher incidence of postoperative liver failure [17].

Factors Related to Primary Tumor

It is known that the staging and biological characteristics of the primary colorectal tumor, even when resected, have an influence on the prognosis of patients who develop metastatic disease. However, the impact of this influence is variable and some characteristics have greater impact than others.

T staging of the primary tumor is questionable as a prognostic factor in colorectal tumors with hepatic metastasis. Most studies do not find an unfavorable overall survival outcome in patients who underwent resection of hepatic metastases with more advanced T staging [13, 14], despite evidence of shorter disease-free survival for T3–T4 patients [5, 6].

The *lymph node status* of the primary tumor is a commonly described prognostic factor in patients with colorectal liver metastases. In a systematic review of prognostic factors in patients undergoing hepatectomy, Spelt et al. described lymph node positivity as one of the most cited prognostic factors [7]. Creasy et al., analyzing factors that predict cure in patients undergoing hepatectomy at 10 years of follow-up at Memorial Sloan Kettering Cancer Center, also found lymph node negativity of the primary tumor as a relevant factor [18]. In the same sense, Liu et al., studying patients not candidates for surgery, also found a worse survival overall survival at 1, 3, and 5 years associated with positive lymph node status [14].

The *degree of histological differentiation* of the primary tumor is another factor commonly related to the prognosis in these patients [13, 14]. However, Acciuffi et al., analyzing for 22 years patients with single liver metastases submitted to adequate surgical resection, found that histological differentiation loses prognostic impact and can show that even in unfavorable histologies, adequate resection with low volume of disease seems to overcome the factors of lower impact [12].

The *elevated tumor marker* (CEA and CA 19-9) at the time of surgery is considered a well-established prognostic factor. Margonis et al. analyzed the prognostic significance of CEA over the years and found that it remains a significant prognostic factor [13]. In a study developed at the A.C. Camargo Cancer Center, CEA remained a prognostic factor in both overall and disease-free survival [5]. In addition, the value of postoperative CEA >15 also showed an independent recurrence factor in patients submitted to hepatic resection [19].

The *genetic characteristics* of colorectal tumors have been addressed in several studies. Key molecules involved in the Epidermal Growth Factor Receptor (EGFR) cascade appear to be important in the response to systemic therapy and present as important prognostic factors. Mutations in the *KRAS*, *BRAF*, *MEK*, *PI3K*, and *PTEN* genes are identified at varying frequencies in these tumors and are of diverse prognostic importance.

The mutation most frequently found in colorectal metastases is KRAS, ranging from 25% to 52%. Analyzing patients with resectable liver disease, the KRAS mutation is a negative prognostic factor in both overall survival and disease-free survival, decreasing the overall survival expectancy of 70 months in wild-type KRAS to 19–50.9 months in mutated patients. In the scenario of unresectable liver disease, the KRAS mutation is also associated with poorer overall survival and disease-free survival [13, 20].

The BRAF mutation ranges from 0 to 9.1% in patients with resectable liver disease. This prevalence reaches higher rates in unresectable patients, since most of these patients present with advanced disease at diagnosis. When analyzed together, mutated BRAF patients (V600E and non-V600E) presented with worse prognosis for both overall survival and disease-free survival. However, analyzed separately, the BRAF V600E mutation is associated with a significantly worse prognosis and greater risk of recurrence and is even the most important prognostic factor in some cohorts. Conversely, the non-V600E mutation loses its prognostic value when analyzed separately. Interestingly, when analyzing these results temporally, the BRAF mutation presents an important prognostic factor in the first year after hepatic resection, decreasing its importance after this period [13, 21].

Other studies corroborate the prognostic significance of the KRAS mutation. Vauthey et al. showed that mutated KRAS patients undergoing chemotherapy followed by liver resection had worse overall survival and disease-free survival and less time for pulmonary recurrence. The same group, analyzing 524 patients submitted to hepatic resection with curative intent, identified three main factors associated with a worse prognosis in mutated KRAS patients (positive lymph nodes, more than seven cycles of preoperative chemotherapy and tumor >3 cm). Overall survival decreased from 72 months in wild-type KRAS to 21.5 months in mutated KRAS patients with the three risk factors, prompting the authors to discourage hepatectomy in this high-risk setting [22, 23].

Mutations of TP53 and PI3K are found in a high proportion of these patients, and in isolation, do not appear to have a prognostic influence in cases of resectable colorectal metastases. Alternatively, in unresectable patients, the mutation of p53 is associated with a shorter overall survival and less response to therapies with fluorinated pyrimidines. For a subgroup of patients with mutation in PI3K who underwent radioembolization, there is greater local disease-free survival, demonstrating possible radiosensitivity in this subgroup [20].

As for the *laterality of the primary tumor*, tumors of the right colon (from the cecum to the first two-thirds of the transverse colon) have an embryological origin distinct from the so-called left colon tumors, resulting in distinct clinical and molecular characteristics. Recent randomized trials have shown that in patients with metastatic unresectable tumors, primary right colon lesions have been shown to have a worse prognosis, resulting in worse overall survival and progression-free survival, and objective response to chemotherapy [24, 25]. Some tumor genetic characteristics that are more common in right colon tumors are known to be associated with a worse response to chemotherapy: BRAF mutation, MSI-H, and ERCC1 expression, explaining at least partially the worst outcomes of patients undergoing palliative chemotherapy.

After these results, some studies have sought to clarify whether the location of the primary tumor in metastatic patients undergoing hepatectomy also has a prognostic effect. Theoretically, the importance of systemic treatment in these cases is comparatively smaller, minimizing the differences between the genetic characteristics of the two groups. Several studies have found that the location of the primary tumor has no prognostic influence on the group undergoing hepatectomy in colorectal liver metastases [26, 27].

Factors Related to Liver Tumor

Several factors associated with metastatic liver disease are associated with prognosis in patients with colorectal tumors. Some of these factors may be intuitively associated with a worse prognosis, such as number and size of hepatic nodules, disease-free interval, and resection margins. However, these factors have different importance in several scenarios.

Several *histological features* of colorectal metastases were analyzed and discussed as prognostic factors. Vascular, lymphatic perineural and bile duct invasion, and presence of fibrotic capsule are some of the factors studied. Among these factors,, *intrahepatic lymphatic invasion* is associated with lower overall survival (41.9 versus 61 months), especially when associated with vascular invasion (28.1 versus 62.2 months) [28].

The *number of hepatic nodules* is described as a prognostic factor in several studies, independently of other factors such as surgical margins and resectability. However, the established cutoff point is variable, ranging from two to seven nodules. In the same line, the size of the largest nodule, bilobar disease, and multiple involved segments are also negative prognostic factors for overall survival and recurrence [5, 7, 14, 16, 28].

From the anatomical point of view, some studies have sought to associate *tumor location* as a prognostic factor. In resectable patients, central metastases are associated with earlier recurrence and lower overall survival, independent of other factors. However, it is worth noting that these data are quite controversial [16].

The *interval between primary and metastatic disease* is known to be a prognostic factor described in most studies. However, the time interval for metastatic disease is the subject of controversy. There is discrepancy about the cutoff point to delimit synchronic or metachronous disease, with 6 months being the most commonly used [29]. However, the definition of synchronic and metachronous disease does not seem to have as much prognostic influence in most of the studies, demonstrating that between the 6 or 12 month cutoff points there may be no such relevant difference [5, 7, 29]. For many, the interval for 12-month metastatic disease appears to be a more realistic cutoff point from a prognostic point of view [5, 28].

Complete surgical resection (R0) is historically a decisive factor in curing patients undergoing liver resection. Several studies have demonstrated the importance of obtaining negative margins for a greater chance of cure and disease-free survival [5, 7, 13, 14]. In temporal analysis, the R0 surgical margin assumes a positive prognostic factor of progressively greater impact with the passage of time, being the most important factor from the second year of follow-up after liver resection [13]. An important counterpoint refers to recent studies that found similar cure rates among patients undergoing resection of R1 and R0 (18% versus 23%) in the era of modern chemotherapy regimens, demonstrating a possible path of paradigm shift [30, 31]. In the same sense, in specific subgroups, the surgical margin seems to lose prognostic importance. In patients with mutated KRAS, R0 vs. R1 liver resection does not give a better prognosis, as margins larger than 1–4 mm do not seem to benefit these patients [20]. However, in these patients, anatomical resections seem to confer better disease-free survival at 5 years, but results are not found in other subgroups [32].

Conclusion

Patients with colorectal liver metastases present a therapeutic challenge for the various specialties involved in their treatment. Over time, treatment options have been broadened and lead to better rates of cure and disease-free survival. In this same line, much progress has been made on the prognostic factors involved. These patients are known to have a very distinct molecular and genetic spectrum, and the advances of the studies in these subgroups of patients are bringing more personalized prognostic information, individualizing these patients according to their genetic and molecular characteristics.

References

1. Siberhumer GR, Paty PB, Denton B, et al. Long-termoncologic outcomes for simultaneous resection of synchronous metastatic liver and primary colorectal cancer. Surgery. 2016;160(1):67–73.
2. Coimbra FJ, Ribeiro HS, Marques MC, et al. First brazilian consensus on multimodal treatment of colorectal liver metastases. Module 1: pre-treatment evaluation. Arq Bras Cir Dig. 2015;28(4):222–30.
3. Ihnát P, Vávra P, Zonca P. Treatment strategies for colorectal carinoma with synchronoues liver metastases: which way to go? World J Gastroenterol. 2015;21(22):7014–21.
4. Rees M, Elias D, Coimbra FJF, et al. Selection for hepatic resection: expert consensus conference. HPB. 2013;15(2):104–5.
5. Ribeiro HSC, Stevanato-Filho PR, Costa WL Jr, et al. Prognostic factors for survival in patients with colorectal liver metastases: experience of a single Brazilian center. Arq Gastroenterol. 2012;49(4):266–72.
6. Coimbra FJ, Pires TC, Costa Junior WL, et al. Advances in surgical treatment of colorectal liver metastases. Rev Assoc Med Bras. 2011;57(2):220–7.
7. Spelt L, Andersson B, Nilsson J, et al. Prognostic models for outcome following iver resection for colorectal cancer metastases: a systematic review. EJSO. 2011;38(2012):16–24.
8. Fong Y, Fortner J, Sun RL, et al. Clinical score for predicting recurrence after hepatic resection for metastatic colorectal cancer: analysis of 1001 consecutie cases. Ann Surg. 1999;230(3):309–21.
9. Nordilinger B, Guiguet M, Vailant JC, et al. Surgical ressection for colorectal carcinoma metastases to the liver: a prognostic score system to improve case selection, based in 1568 patients. Cancer. 1996;77(7):1254–62.

10. Schreckenbach T, Malkomes P, Bechstein W, et al. The clinical relevance of the Fong and Nordlinger scores in the era pf effective neoadjuvant chemotherapy for colorectal liver metastases. Surg Today. 2015;45:1527–34.
11. Adam R, Avisar E, Ariche A, et al. Five year survival following hepatic resection after neoadjuvant therapy for nonresectable colorectal liver metastases. Ann Surg Oncol. 2001;8:347–53.
12. Acciuffi S, Meyer F, Bauschke A, et al. Analysis of factors after resection of solitary liver metastasis in colorectal cancer: a 22-year bicentre study. J Cancer Res and Clin Oncol. 2018;144:593–9.
13. Margonis GA, Buettner S, Andreatos N, et al. Prognostic factors change over time after hepatectomy for colorectal liver metastases. Ann Surg. 2018;20(20):1–9.
14. Liu Q, Hao L, Lou Z, et al. Survival time and prognostic factors of patients with initial noncurative colorectal liver metastases. Medicine. 2017;96(51):1–5.
15. Dindo D, Demartines N, Clavien PA. Classification of surgical complications: a new proposal with evaluation in a cohort of 6336 patients and results of a survey. Ann Surg. 2004;240(2):205–13.
16. Kuo IM, Huang SF, Chiang JM, et al. Clinical features and prognosis in hepatectomy for colorectal cancer with centrally located liver metastasis. World J Surg Oncol. 2015;13(92):1–12.
17. Ribeiro HSC, Costa WL Jr, Diniz AL, et al. Extended preoperative chemotherapy, extent of liver resection and blood transfusion are predictive factors of liver failure following resection of colorectal liver metastasis. Eur J Surg Oncol. 2013;39(4):380–5.
18. Creasy JM, Sadot E, Koerkamp BS, et al. Actual 10-year survival after hepatic resection of colorectal liver metastases: what factors preclude cure? Surgery. 2018;163:1238–44.
19. Araujo RLC, Gonen M, Allen P, et al. Positive postoperative CEA is a strong predictor of recurrence for patients after resection for colorectal liver metastases. Ann Surg Oncol. 2015;22(9):3087–93.
20. Tsilimigras DI, Stathopoulos IN, Bagante F, et al. Clinical significance and prognostic relevance of KRAS, BRAF, PI3K and TP53 genetic mutation analysis for resectable and unresectable colorectal liver metastases: a systematic review of the current evidence. Surg Oncol. 2018;27:280–8.
21. Margonis GA, Buettner S, Andreatos N, et al. Association of BRAF mutations with survival and recurrence in surgically treated patients with metastatic colorectal liver cancer. JAMA Surg. 2018;153(7):E1–8.
22. Vauthey JN, Zimmitti G, Kopetz SE, et al. RAS mutation status predicts survival and patterns of recurrence in patients undergoing hepatectomy for colorectal liver metastases. Ann Surg. 2013;258(4):619–26.
23. Passot G, Denbo JW, Yamashita S, et al. Is hepatectomy justified for patients with RAS mutant colorectal liver metastases? An analysis of 524 patients undergoing curative liver resection. Surgery. 2017;161(2):332–40.
24. Modest DP, Stintzing S, Weikersthal LF, et al. Primary tumor location and efficacy of second-line therapy after initial treatment with FOLFIRI in combination with cetuximab or bevacizumab in patients with metastatic colorectal cancer. J Clin Oncol. 2017;35:3525.
25. Venook AP, Ou FS, Lenz HJ, et al. Primary tumor location as an independent prognostic maker from molecular features for overall survival in patients with metastatic colorectal câncer: analysis of CALGB/SWOG 80405 (Alliance). J Clin Oncol. 2017;35:3503.
26. Marques MC, Ribeiro HS, Costa WL Jr, et al. Is primary sidedness a prognostic factor in patients with resected colon câncer liver metastases (CLM)? J Surg Oncol. 2018;117(5):858–63.
27. Wang K, Xu D, Yan XL, et al. The impact of primary tumor location in patients undergoing hepatic resection for colorectal liver metástasis. Eur J Surg Oncol. 2018;44:771–7.
28. Ridder JAM, Knijn N, Wiering B, et al. Lymphatic invasion is an independent adverse prognostic factor in patients with colorectal liver metastasis. Ann Surg Oncol. 2015;22: 638–45.
29. Coimbra FJF, Ribeiro HSC, Torres OJM. I Brazilian consensus for multimodal treatment of colorectal liver metastases. Arq Bras Cir Dig. 2015;28(4):221.

30. Hosokawa I, Allard MA, Gelli M, et al. Long-term survival benefit and potential for cure after R1 resection for colorectal liver metastases. Ann Surg Oncol. 2016;23(6):1897–905.
31. Adam R, Delvart V, Pascal G, et al. Rescue surgery for unresectable colorectal liver metastases downstaged by chemotherapy: a model to predict long-term survival. Ann Surg. 2004;240:644–57.
32. Margonis GA, Buettner S, Andreatos N, et al. Anatomical resections improve disease-free survival in patients with KRAS-mutated colorectal liver metastases. Ann Surg. 2017;266(4):641–9.

Clinical Scoring Systems for Colorectal Cancer Liver Metastases

8

Camille Stewart and Yuman Fong

Introduction

Clinical scoring systems are frequently used for predicting outcomes in medicine. These scoring systems take into account that patient outcomes such as morbidity and mortality are seldom based on a single variable and generally are multi-factorial in nature. While physicians may have working knowledge of positive or negative influences on the outcomes, understanding the most important variables and assessing the weight of these variables in patients can be difficult. For the surgeon, challenges arise when determining who should be offered an operation and also when providing information regarding prognosis, especially when patients are perceived to possess both favorable and poor prognostic features. Beyond risk stratification, clinical scoring systems importantly facilitate communication between physicians and assist in patient selection for participation in clinical research. As such, clinical scoring systems have proved very useful for the evaluation of a wide variety of patients.

Commonly used systems include the Apgar score [1], the Glasgow coma scale [2], the Injury Severity Score [3], and the Acute Physiology and Chronic Health Evaluation (APACHE) scoring system [4]. Within surgery, scoring systems have been developed for a number of high-risk operations, including cardiac surgery [5], liver transplantation [6], and cytoreductive surgery with heated intraperitoneal chemotherapy [7]. As surgeons continue to push the limits of their technical ability, the question "can an operation be done?" shifts to "should an operation be done?". Further questions are raised regarding who are the best patient candidates for trials of new methodologies and innovative therapies. Patients with colorectal cancer liver metastases openly lend themselves to this type of stratification, since a percentage

C. Stewart · Y. Fong (✉)
City of Hope National Medical Center, Duarte, CA, USA
e-mail: cstewart@coh.org; yfong@coh.org

M. M. Correia et al. (eds.), *Colorectal Cancer Liver Metastases*,
https://doi.org/10.1007/978-3-030-25486-5_8

of these patients will be cured with surgery, whereas a percentage will likely incur little or no benefit. A number of manuscripts have been published over the last two decades to facilitate the evaluation and care of these patients.

During this time frame, however, the standard of care has evolved, and now frequently includes neoadjuvant chemotherapy. This change in care has increased the number of surgical candidates and overall survival of these patients, requiring validation of previous scoring systems. Here we review 17 scoring systems for patients with colorectal liver metastases that are summarized in Tables 8.1, 8.2, 8.3, and 8.4. The discussion is divided into early scoring systems, prior to the widespread use of neoadjuvant chemotherapy, and contemporary systems that include patients treated after the year 2000, when modern neoadjuvant chemotherapy started being given more frequently. We then discuss comparison studies and conclude with how to best apply scoring systems to practice in the present day.

Table 8.1 Colorectal liver metastases scoring systems by institution and patient characteristics

Study (first author, publication date)	Years included in the study	N used to develop score	Patient group specifics	Neoadjuvant chemotherapy (%)	Institution	Locations of external validation
Sasaki et al. [36]	2000–2015	604	CRLM treated surgically, excluded combination ablations	65	Johns Hopkins, Baltimore, Maryland	Yokohama City University, Japan; University of Verona, Italy
Brudvik et al. [34]	2005–2013	564	CRLM treated surgically, known RAS status, CEA level	87	MD Anderson Cancer Center, Houston, Texas	Oslo University Hospital, Norway; Aintree University Hospital, Liverpool, UK; Gemelli Medical School, Rome, Italy; University of Tokyo, Japan
Wang et al. [35]	2006–2016	300	Neoadjuvant chemotherapy, CRLM treated surgically	100	Peking University Cancer Hospital, China	N/A

Table 8.1 (continued)

Study (first author, publication date)	Years included in the study	N used to develop score	Patient group specifics	Neoadjuvant chemotherapy (%)	Institution	Locations of external validation
Imai et al. [24]	1990–2012	439	Initially unresectable, neoadjuvant chemotherapy, CRLM treated surgically	100	Hôpital Universitaire Paul Brousse, Villejuif, France	N/A
Rees et al. [21]	1987–2005	929	CRLM treated surgically	21	North Hampshire Hospital, Basingstoke, UK	N/A
Lee et al. [10]	1994–2005	138	CRLM treated surgically, only synchronous resections	0	Samsung Medical Center, Seoul, South Korea	N/A
Konopke et al. [20]	1993–2006	201	CRLM treated surgically	21	University of Technology, Dresden, Germany	N/A
Malik et al. [19]	1993–2006	687	CRLM treated surgically	10	St. James's University Hospital, Leeds, UK	N/A
Schindl et al. [18]	1988–2002	150	CRLM treated surgically, no extra-hepatic disease	NR	Royal Infirmary of Edinburgh, Scotland	University of Vienna, Italy
Zakaria et al. [14]	1960–1995	662	CRLM treated surgically, excluded combination ablations	NR	Mayo Clinic, Rochester, Minnesota	N/A
Adam et al. [23]	1988–1999	138	Initially unresectable, neoadjuvant chemotherapy, CRLM treated surgically	100	Hôpital Universitaire Paul Brousse, Villejuif, France	N/A
Nagashima et al. [41]	1997–2001	83	CRLM treated surgically	NR	Tokyo University Hospital, Japan	Teikyo University Hospital, Tokyo, Japan

(continued)

Table 8.1 (continued)

Study (first author, publication date)	Years included in the study	N used to develop score	Patient group specifics	Neoadjuvant chemotherapy (%)	Institution	Locations of external validation
Lise et al. [13]	1977–1997	135	CRLM treated surgically	NR	University of Padova, Italy	N/A
Ueno et al. [12]	1985–1996	85	CRLM treated surgically	NR	National Defense Medical College, Saitama, Japan	N/A
Fong et al. [9]	1985–1998	1001	CRLM treated surgically	NR	Memorial Sloan-Kettering Cancer Center, New York, New York	N/A
Iwatsuki et al. [11]	1981–1996	306	CRLM treated surgically	NR	University of Pittsburgh Medical Center, Pennsylvania	N/A
Nordlinger et al. [8]	1968–1990	1568	CRLM treated surgically	NR	85 institutions within the Association Française de Chirurgie	N/A

Notes: *CRLM* colorectal liver metastases, *N/A* not applicable, *NR* not reported. Number of patients represents those who underwent surgery for colorectal metastases, except as noted under patient specifics

Early Scoring Systems

Nordlinger et al. derived one of the earliest scoring systems in 1996, using a French multi-institutional database including 1568 patients from 1968 to 1990. In this study, 95% of the patients included were treated after 1980 [8]. The authors observed a 2.3% perioperative mortality rate, and a 28% 5-year overall survival after liver resection. In addition, the authors used regression analysis and identified features significantly associated with disease-free survival and overall survival. They selected seven clinical criteria, each getting one point, given that each factor had a relative risk between 1.0 and 2.0 (Fig. 8.1a), which were dependent on age, stage of the primary tumor, disease-free interval, size and number of the liver metastases, and margin status.

These patients were divided into low risk (scores 0–2), intermediate risk (scores 3–4), and high risk (scores 5–7). Two-year (instead of 5-year) survival rates were

Table 8.2 Colorectal liver metastasis scoring systems by publication and reported metrics

Study (first author, publication date)	Mortality (%)	Five-year OS (%)	Low group 5-year OS (%)	High group 5-year OS (%)	High group median survival (months)	Follow-up (months)
Sasaki et al. [36]	NR	50	69	26	NR	30.3
Brudvik et al. [34]	NR	NR (median OS 51.8 months)	NR	NR	NR	NR
Wang et al. [35]	0.0	46	64	14	NR	45
Imai et al. [24]	1.1	40	58	4	NR	42.1
Rees et al. [21]	1.5	36	64	2	8.5	26.4
Lee et al. [10]	0.0	43	46	11	23.5	47.2
Konopke et al. [20]	0.5	43	57	0	38	31
Malik et al. [19]	3.1	45	49	0	21.3	34
Schindl et al. [18]	NR	36	63	0	21.9	16.4
Zakaria et al. [14]	3.0	37	55	20	NR	36
Adam et al. [23]	0.7	33	59	0	NR	48.7
Nagashima et al. [41]	2.4	49	85	0	NR	36.3
Lise et al. [13]	2.2	29	72	0	NR	22
Ueno et al. [12]	3.4	28	55	0	14	52
Fong et al. [9]	2.8	37	60	0	22	32
Iwatsuki et al. [11]	1.0	32	48	0	NR	32
Nordlinger et al. [8]	2.3	28	NR	NR	NR	19

Notes: Number of patients and reported metrics are for patients who underwent surgery for colorectal metastases, except as noted under patient specifics. Low group refers to patients in each scoring system who score the lowest/have the fewest risk factors, and high group refers to patients who score the highest/have the most risk factors for recurrence/death. *CRLM* colorectal liver metastases, *N/A* not applicable, *NR* not reported, *OS* overall survival

reported and were significantly higher in the low-risk (79%) versus the intermediate- (60%), and high-risk groups (43%) (Fig. 8.1b). Of note, CEA was not available for all patients in this study – when it was included in the model, age and size of largest tumor dropped out, and an alternative scoring system was proposed using CEA >5 μg/L or > 30 μg/L worth one or two additional points, to again make a total of seven possible points.

Fong et al. created a frequently cited scoring system in 1999, utilizing data of 1001 patients treated from 1985 to 1999 at the Memorial Sloan-Kettering Cancer Center [9]. In this study, there was a 2.8% perioperative mortality rate, and the 5-year survival after liver resection was 37%. The authors performed regression analyses to identify features that correlated with disease-free and overall survival,

Table 8.3 Colorectal liver metastases scoring systems by common prognostic factors

Study (first author, publication date)	Number of variables	Preoperative labs	Tumor size	Nodal status	Number of liver tumors	Disease-free interval
Sasaki et al. [36]	2	NR	Max. diameter (cm)	NR	Number of tumors	NR
Brudvik et al. [34]	3	NR	>5 cm	Positive	NR	NR
Wang et al. [35]	7	CEA >200 ng/ml	>5 cm	Positive	>1	<12 months
Imai et al. [24]	5	CA 19–9 >37 units/ml	NR	Positive	>6	NR
Rees et al. [21]	7	CEA >6 or > 60 ng/mL	>5 or >10 cm	Positive	>3	NR
Lee et al. [10]	4	CEA >5 ng/ml	NR	>4 positive	>1	NR
Konopke et al. [20]	3	CEA >200 ng/ml	NR	NR	>3	Synchronous
Malik et al. [19]	2	CRP >10 mg/L or Neutrophil:Lymphocyte ratio >5:1	NR	NR	>7	NR
Schindl et al. [18]	4	CEA >5 μg/ml Albumin <3.6 Alk phos[a] >125 U/L	NR	Positive	>3	NR
Zakaria et al.	2	NR	NR	Positive hepatoduodenal lymph node	NR	NR
Adam et al. [23]	4	CA 19–9 >100 UI/L	>10 cm	NR	>2	NR
Nagashima et al. [41]	5	NR	>5 cm	Positive	>1	NR
Lise et al. [13]	5	ALT >55 U/L	NR	Positive	>1	NR
Ueno et al. [12]	5	"Elevated" CEA	NR	Positive lymph nodes distal from tumor	>2	<12 months
Fong et al. [9]	5	CEA >200 ng/ml	>5 cm	Positive	>1	<12 months
Iwatsuki et al. [11]	4	NR	>8 cm	NR	>2	<30 months
Nordlinger et al. [8]	8	CEA >5 or >30 ug/L	>5 cm	Positive	>3	<24 months

Notes: *CEA* carcinoembryonic antigen, *CA* cancer antigen, *CRP* C-reactive protein, *ALT* alanine aminotransferase, *Alk phos* alkaline phosphatase, *NR* not reported

Table 8.4 Additional prognostic factors considered in scoring systems for colorectal liver metastases prognosis

Study (First author, publication date)	"Unique" considerations for scoring system development
Brudvik et al. [34]	KRAS/NRAS mutation
Wang et al. [35]	Progressive or stable disease per RECIST KRAS mutation
Imai et al. [24]	Presence of extra-hepatic metastases Progressive disease on first-line chemo per RECIST
Rees et al. [21]	Presence of extra-hepatic metastases Margin status: positive Moderate or poorly differentiated primary tumor features
Lee et al. [10]	Margin status of <5 mm
Zakaria et al. [14]	Positive hepatoduodenal lymph node Transfusion − 7 to +14 days relative to surgery
Adam et al. [23]	Rectal cancer primary
Nagashima et al. [41]	Presence of extra-hepatic metastases T-stage of primary disease with evidence of serosal invasion
Lise et al. [13]	>30% tumor invasion of liver Nonanatomic resection
Ueno et al. [12]	Moderate or severe primary tumor budding
Iwatsuki et al. [11]	Presence of bilobar tumors
Nordlinger et al. [8]	Margin status of <1 cm T-stage of primary disease with evidence of serosal invasion; Patient age > 60 years

Notes: *RECIST* Response Evaluation Criteria in Solid Tumors

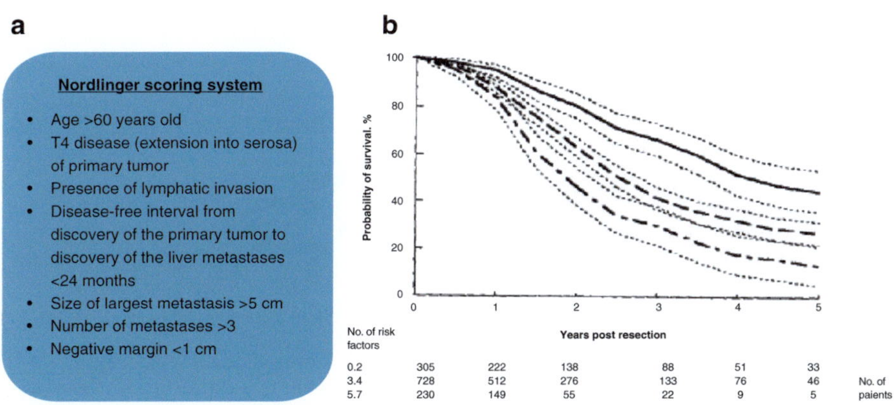

Fig. 8.1 Nordlinger et al. 1996 Clinical Scoring System. Scoring system variables (**a**) and overall survival curve demonstrating stratification between groups (**b**) in Nordlinger et al. 1996. (Reproduced with permission from Nordlinger et al. [8])

resulting in the selection of five clinical criteria, each getting one point (Fig. 8.2a): positive colorectal lymph nodes, disease-free interval < 12 months, number and size of liver tumors, and preoperative CEA level. When this scoring system was applied, the 5-year survival correlation coefficient was $r^2 = 0.92$; patients with 0 points had a 5-year survival of 60%, compared to 14% for patients with 5/5 points (Fig. 8.2b). This score was superior to prediction based on a number of tumors alone and was considered more practical than the Nordlinger score by the authors, since all criteria could generally be known prior to surgery (excluding patients with planned synchronous resections).

Of note, Lee et al. (2008) created a scoring system based on 138 patients who had synchronous liver and colorectal resections from 1994 to 2005 [10]. Risk factors included in their scoring system, however, were similar to those identified in Fong et al. (1999) [9], including nodal status, number of liver tumors, preoperative CEA, and margin status and thus could not be easily applied preoperatively. Iwatsuki et al. (1999), Ueno et al. (2000), Lise et al. (2001), and Zakaria et al. (2007) also published scoring systems during this early time frame [11–14]. Additional risk factors for mortality in their scoring systems included >30% tumor invasion of the liver (relative risk 9.21) [13], bilobar tumors (relative risk 1.25) [11], serum alanine aminotransferase >55 U/L (relative risk 3.56) [13], hepatoduodenal lymph node positivity (hazard ratio 2.8) [14], and need for perioperative blood transfusion (hazard ratio 1.5) [14].

The treatment and prognosis of colorectal cancer liver metastases were significantly altered by the approval of multiple chemotherapeutic regimens in the early 2000s. Irinotecan was approved in April 2000 as first-line therapy for patients with metastatic colorectal cancer in conjunction with fluorouracil and leucovorin [15]. Oxaliplatin was then approved in August 2002 for use also in combination with

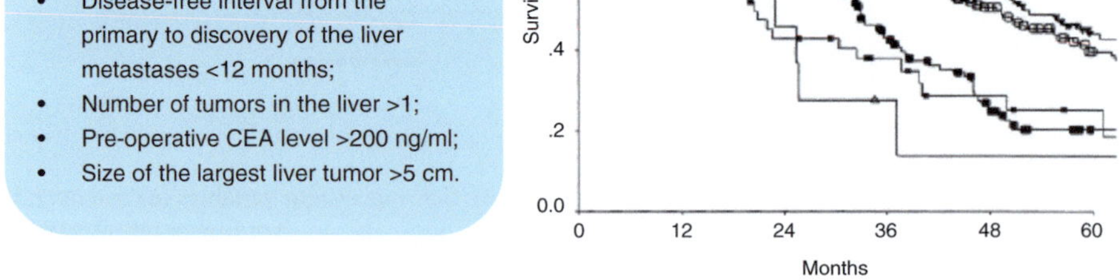

Fig. 8.2 Fong et al. 1999 Clinical Scoring System. Scoring system variables (**a**) and overall survival curve demonstrating stratification between groups (**b**) in Fong et al. 1999. (Reproduced with permission from Fong et al. [9])

fluorouracil and leucovorin for patients with metastatic colorectal cancer whose disease has recurred or progressed during or within 6 months of completion of first-line therapy [16]. These combination treatments doubled the median overall survival for metastatic colorectal cancer from 10 to 20 months [17].

A number of clinical scoring systems that straddled the time periods of infrequent and frequent use of neoadjuvant chemotherapy have been published (see Table 8.1, years included in the study) and thus may be more difficult to interpret. Schindl et al. (2005) reported that both neoadjuvant and adjuvant therapy were not used routinely in their cohort [18]. Malik et al. (2007) reported that neoadjuvant therapy was used in 10.3% of their cohort and that it did not alter the prognosis of patients who were high scoring [19]. Interestingly, the authors of this study hypothesized that preoperative inflammatory markers were clinically important and criticized previous scoring systems for requiring pathologic information not available at the time of clinical decision-making. In multivariate analysis, they showed that disease-free and overall survival were significantly associated with serum C-reactive protein >10 mg/L or a serum neutrophil-to-lymphocyte ratio > 5:1. They also showed no difference in survival between patients in the highest scoring group who had a liver resection and patients who were deemed inoperable because of advanced disease discovered after laparotomy. Konopke et al. (2008) reported that neoadjuvant therapy was used in 21% of patients in their cohort but that these patients were not well stratified using the scoring system proposed [20]. Those who were high scoring, however, lived longer than patients who did not receive neoadjuvant therapy. Rees et al. reported that 21% of patients received chemotherapy as a "downsizing strategy" but reported that its use was not associated with outcome [21].

House et al. (2010) examined the same group of patients from the original Fong et al. (1999) scoring system, and updated patients through 2004. Patients were compared before and after 1999, when neoadjuvant therapy had shifted at this institution [22]. Patients in the latter group were more likely to be treated with neoadjuvant chemotherapy, adjuvant chemotherapy, and adjuvant hepatic artery infusion pump, when compared to the earlier group. The 5-year overall survival was improved in patients treated in the later years (1999–2004) compared to those treated earlier (43% vs. 35%). They found that low-risk patients accounted for the difference in survival, whereas higher risk patients (clinical risk >2 points) had similar survival between time periods. The authors concluded that improved patient selection in combination with better chemotherapy was the likely reason for the difference in survival. This study did not address how many patients, however, were converted from unresectable to resectable status based on neoadjuvant treatment.

Two scoring systems that included patients from this early era focused exclusively on those initially deemed unresectable, both out of the same institution, Hôpital Universitaire Paul Brousse, in Villejuif, France. Adam et al. 2004, defined unresectability as <30% expected liver remnant, or concomitant extra-hepatic disease [23]. Of 1104 patients identified from 1988 to 1999, 138 (13%) went on to surgery and 58% who had FOLFOX as first-line therapy. Points were assigned for rectal primary disease, CA 19–9 > 100 IU/L, and maximum liver tumor diameter > 10 cm. Patients with three and four points had 0–6% 3-year survival. Imai et al.

2016 updated this cohort to include 439 patients treated from 1990 to 2012 [24]. Inoperability included <30% expected liver remnant, but additionally considered <40% in patients who had received more than eight cycles of chemotherapy. This is because the effect of neoadjuvant chemotherapy on liver parenchyma was better understood at that time [25]. Chemotherapy regimens used in Imai et al. (2016), however, were not reported. Scoring in this manuscript included node-positive primary disease, number of liver tumors, CA 19-9, concomitant extra-hepatic disease, and radiologic response to first-line chemotherapy based on Response Evaluation Criteria in Solid Tumors (RECIST) criteria [26].

Contemporary Scoring Systems

In 2008, Nordlinger et al. published a randomized controlled trial on the perioperative administration of FOLFOX to patients with potentially resectable colorectal liver metastases, and showed that progression-free survival was increased by 9.2% in patients who later underwent resection [27]. The follow-up to this study in 2013 showed a non-significant trend toward an increase in disease-specific survival in the treatment arm but no difference in overall survival [28]. Randomized controlled trials also demonstrated an increased number of patients with colorectal liver metastases who become surgical candidates after treatment with FOLFOXIRI regimens [29, 30]. As such, chemotherapy is now often given prior to surgical resection of colorectal liver metastases. RAS mutational status and epidermal growth factor receptor inhibitors are further relevant factors in the twenty-first century. Initially, inoperable patients with wild-type KRAS colorectal cancers and who were treated with cetuximab more frequently converted to surgical candidates in a number of randomized studies [31–33]. These advancements in treatment have prognostic implications and raise questions about the validity of previous colorectal liver metastasis scoring systems.

Three scoring systems have been published based on patient populations treated after the year 2000 [34–36]. Brudvik et al. (2017) examined 564 patients who had surgical treatment of colorectal liver metastases from 2005 to 2013, of whom 87% were treated with neoadjuvant chemotherapy [34]. They tested two different scoring systems – a traditional system that included nodal status, disease-free interval, number of liver tumors, size of the largest liver tumor, and CEA level, and a modified system that included nodal status, size of largest liver tumor, and RAS mutational status of the liver tumor. The modified scoring system was a better discriminator of recurrence-free survival and overall survival than the traditional scoring system for this cohort and four international validation cohorts. The number of viable tumor cells in the pathologic specimen was evaluated, which did not improve the discrimination of the score, but preoperative response to chemotherapy by imaging was not addressed. They also specifically examined the KRAS and NRAS status of the liver metastases postoperatively but commented that there is generally a high concordance of RAS mutational status between the primary tumor and liver metastases. Other limitations of this scoring system are that recurrence-free and overall survival rates were not reported by year and score, and that the median follow-up time for the cohort was also not reported.

Wang et al. (2017) published a scoring system based on 300 patients who all had been treated with neoadjuvant chemotherapy from 2006 to 2016 [35]. The final value, called a tumor biology score, was calculated with positive KRAS mutational status, Fong score >2, and poor radiologic response to neoadjuvant chemotherapy (progressive or stable disease according to RECIST criteria) [26], with each risk factor counting as a point. The tumor biology score correlated with survival: patients with 0 points had 64% 5-year survival, whereas patients with three points had 14% 5-year survival.

Sasaki et al. (2018) published a scoring system that included 604 patients treated from 2000 to 2015, 65% of whom were treated with neoadjuvant chemotherapy [36]. Points were calculated based on tumor size and number of tumors in a Cartesian schema to create a tumor burden score (tumor burden score^2 = (maximum tumor diameter)^2 + (number of liver lesions)^2). Patients were then stratified into the lowest 25% (score <3.0), the intermediate 25–90% percentile (score 3.0–8.9), and the top 10% (≥9.0). Tumor burden score correlated with survival: scores <3.0 had 69% 5-year survival, and scores >9.0 had 26% 5-year survival. Scoring was validated using two other international cohorts, and maintained discrimination between patient groups who were treated with neoadjuvant chemotherapy and those who were not.

Validation and Comparison of Existing Scoring Systems

A number of the above studies compared their own scoring system to others, including Malik et al. (2007), Wang et al. (2017), and Sasaki et al. (2018) [19, 35, 36]. Universally, each study found that their own scoring system was superior for their own cohort. Wang et al. (2017), examining patients treated with neoadjuvant chemotherapy, compared their score to nine others for prognostic predictive power, including the Fong et al., Iwatsuki et al., Konopke et al., Nagashima et al., Nordlinger et al., Sasaki et al., Rees et al., and Brudvik et al. scores, and found that only the Fong et al., Brudvik et al., and Wang et al. scores had significant predictive power in their patient population [35].

Zakaria et al. (2007) compared predictive capacity of Fong et al., Nordlinger et al., and Iwatsuki et al. scoring systems and found that the Fong et al. score was the best for predicting survival and recurrence in their cohort [14]. Concordance probability estimates were performed for the three previous scoring systems and their own and found that all models were "only marginally better than chance alone" in predicting disease-specific survival and recurrence, thus concluding that the broad application of risk scoring systems had limited clinical value. They proposed that it be used to provide prognostic information postoperatively and to determine the value of adjuvant therapies.

Ayez et al. (2011) examined 352 patients treated from 2000 to 2008 [37], who were divided based on neoadjuvant chemotherapy administration, and then compared based on four different scoring systems: Fong et al., Konopke et al., Nagashima et al., and Nordlinger et al. Those who received neoadjuvant treatment had scores calculated before and after chemotherapy. Significant differences between scoring groups were detected for disease-free and overall survival in patients who did not receive neoadjuvant therapy. Differences were generally lost when scoring the neoadjuvant chemotherapy group before chemotherapy but then were generally recovered when scoring after neoadjuvant chemotherapy. Patients whose scores dropped after chemotherapy had the same outcome as patients who started with a lower score and did not receive chemotherapy. Remarkably, patients whose Nagashima scores dropped after chemotherapy had a better outcome than those with the same score who did not get chemotherapy.

A meta-analysis by Kanas et al. in 2012 critically evaluated 54 studies that examined survival of patients with colorectal liver metastases status post-liver resection and at least 24 months of median follow-up [38]. They found that the lowest meta-relative risk feature for survival was for liver tumors >3 cm (overall meta-relative risk of 1.52 (1.28–1.80) and the highest was for patients with a positive resection margin (overall meta-relative risk of 2.02 (1.65–2.48); it also found significant negative associations with high CEA level, high tumor grade, and multiple liver tumors.

Should I Use a Scoring System? If So, Which One? When Should I Use a Scoring System?

The above studies highlight a number of important factors related to patients with colorectal liver metastases. Features including extra-hepatic metastases, presence of positive lymph nodes, multiple liver tumors, and larger liver tumors generally have a negative prognostic value. They were the most frequently included features in the 17 scoring systems reviewed (Table 8.3) and thus can likely be used to estimate prognosis for patients at any institution. These studies also demonstrate that there is a group of surgically treated patients that have similar outcomes as those who do not have surgery; this is beyond the 1one in 100 patients who do not survive the perioperative period. Patients with colorectal liver metastases who are not resected have a 0% 5-year survival rate and median survival time of 13.3–21.4 [18, 39, 40].

Those who can be converted to curative resection on average experience better survival; however, patients who attain the highest values in these scoring systems also have median survivals that range from 14 to 22 months. Ueno et al. (2000) and Lise et al. (2001) specifically addressed this group. Ueno et al. (2000) reported that patients with a recurrence within 6 months had a median survival of 13 months, and that scoring highly was associated with this outcome [12]. Lise et al. (2001) reported that 92% of patients who had an early recurrence were identified in their highest scoring group [13]. Therefore, scoring systems that identify a group with 0% 5-year survival and <24 months median survival are of the greatest value in determining surgical candidacy. As chemotherapy and interventional radiology treatments continue to improve, this group of patients may enjoy the same survival as that of marginal candidates who get surgery but without the associated postoperative discomforts. These patients are also the best for consideration into clinical trials. Colorectal liver metastasis scoring systems further emphasize a group of patients who experience significant longevity and can potentially be cured. Patients who score the lowest have 48–85% 5-year survival depending on the system used. One might consider foregoing the modest improvement in recurrence-free survival afforded by neoadjuvant chemotherapy for patients without risk factors who are clearly resectable upfront.

The above rationale suggests that scoring systems should be used to assist in decision-making for the upper and bottom tiers of patients with respect to expected survival. While imperfect, they serve as an additional data point to drive discussion within a multi-disciplinary environment. The question of which scoring system to use should be answered based on some additional factors. Scoring systems tended to perform best in the institution where they were created. If no such scoring system exists within your own institution, it is worth considering the country where a scoring system was created or if it was validated using an external dataset that may be similar to your patient population. Scoring systems have been created based on patients in the United States, the United Kingdom, France, Italy, South Korea, Japan, and China and have been validated in Norway. The number of patients used to create a scoring system and the average follow-up should also be considered since validity is presumably increased with greater patient numbers and longer follow-up. Study cohorts reviewed here ranged from 83 to 1568 patients, and median follow-up ranged from 16.4 to 52 months. These metrics are presented for comparison in Table 8.2.

One should exercise caution using a scoring system without all of the data points needed to derive a score (Tables 8.3 and 8.4, Fig. 8.3). Scoring systems that require information only available postoperatively are best used for prognostic information, and are not well suited to be used in preoperative decision-making (Fig. 8.3). Preoperative decision-making can be to include or exclude patients for surgery, to estimate the extent of imaging, or even to decide whether a patient should have a different surgical procedure such as staging laparoscopy. If a synchronous

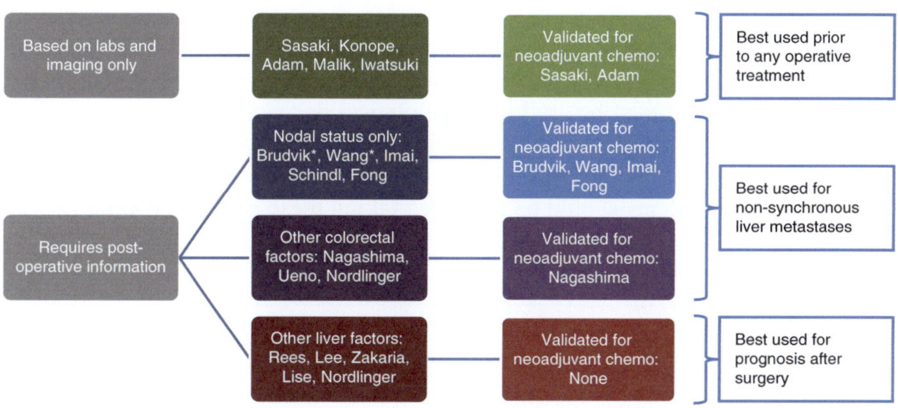

Fig. 8.3 Colorectal Liver Metastasis Scoring Systems. Schematic of colorectal liver metastasis scoring systems based on time frame of treatment and treatment with neoadjuvant chemotherapy. (Note: *Requires biopsy for mutational status)

colorectal and hepatic resection is being considered, a scoring system that requires nodal status may not be accurate if calculated preoperatively. Many institutions consider extra-hepatic disease or anticipated positive margin as contraindications to surgery. Scoring systems that are predicated on these factors, such as Imai et al., Rees et al., Nagashima et al., Lee et al., and Nordlinger et al. may be less useful if these patients are already clinically excluded from surgery in your practice. Lastly, for patients who are receiving neoadjuvant chemotherapy, scoring systems appear to have the best prognostic value when applied after this treatment.

Many scoring systems created prior to the widespread use of neoadjuvant chemotherapy are less effective in predicting outcomes of patients before treatment has been initiated. Scoring systems created based on patients treated in the neoadjuvant setting generally use data from patients after chemotherapy. Scoring systems validated for use in patients treated with neoadjuvant chemotherapy are presented in Fig. 8.3. Reviewing the Figures and Tables in this chapter can assist in identification of the best scoring system to use for your patient, which will improve predictive accuracy. The preoperative scoring system most used worldwide remains the Fong score because it incorporates criteria available for any patient. Thus, Fong plus, meaning Fong score plus response to chemotherapy, is practical and is still the system against which most newly proposed scoring systems are compared.

Conclusion

A number of clinical scoring systems exist for colorectal liver metastases that may assist in clinical decision-making and provide prognostic information. Limitations of these scoring systems include that they were all devised in a retrospective fashion and without a power analysis. Many include patients from a wide range of time periods while the standard of care was in evolution. They also frequently require information for calculation that is only available postoperatively. Clinical scoring systems are useful, however, as an additional data point when appropriately applied, to help predict which patients will have the best and poorest long-term outcomes. This information can then be used to guide clinical decision-making and facilitate patient discussions. In the future, as medical and interventional radiologic treatments advance for this population, older scoring systems will need to be validated, and new scoring systems should be evaluated taking these additional variables into account.

References

1. Apgar V. A proposal for a new method of evaluation of the newborn infant. Curr Res Anesth Analg. 1953;32(4):260–7. PubMed PMID: 13083014. Epub 1953/07/01. eng.
2. Teasdale G, Jennett B. Assessment of coma and impaired consciousness. A practical scale. Lancet (London, England). 1974;2(7872):81–4. PubMed PMID: 4136544. Epub 1974/07/13. eng.

3. Baker SP, O'Neill B, Haddon W Jr, Long WB. The injury severity score: a method for describing patients with multiple injuries and evaluating emergency care. J Trauma. 1974;14(3):187–96. PubMed PMID: 4814394. Epub 1974/03/01. eng.
4. Vincent JL, Moreno R. Clinical review: scoring systems in the critically ill. Crit Care (London, England). 2010;14(2):207. PubMed PMID: 20392287. Pubmed Central PMCID: PMC2887099. Epub 2010/04/16. eng.
5. Geissler HJ, Holzl P, Marohl S, Kuhn-Regnier F, Mehlhorn U, Sudkamp M, et al. Risk stratification in heart surgery: comparison of six score systems. Eur J Cardio-Thorac Surg. 2000;17(4):400–6. PubMed PMID: 10773562. Epub 2000/04/25. eng.
6. Botta F, Giannini E, Romagnoli P, Fasoli A, Malfatti F, Chiarbonello B, et al. MELD scoring system is useful for predicting prognosis in patients with liver cirrhosis and is correlated with residual liver function: a European study. Gut. 2003;52(1):134–9. PubMed PMID: 12477775. Pubmed Central PMCID: PMC1773509. Epub 2002/12/13. eng
7. Harmon RL, Sugarbaker PH. Prognostic indicators in peritoneal carcinomatosis from gastrointestinal cancer. Int Semin Surg Oncol: ISSO. 2005;2(1):3. PubMed PMID: 15701175. Pubmed Central PMCID: PMC549516. Epub 2005/02/11. eng.
8. Nordlinger B, Guiguet M, Vaillant JC, Balladur P, Boudjema K, Bachellier P, et al. Surgical resection of colorectal carcinoma metastases to the liver. A prognostic scoring system to improve case selection, based on 1568 patients. Association Francaise de Chirurgie. Cancer. 1996;77(7):1254–62. PubMed PMID: 8608500. Epub 1996/04/01. eng.
9. Fong Y, Fortner J, Sun RL, Brennan MF, Blumgart LH. Clinical score for predicting recurrence after hepatic resection for metastatic colorectal cancer: analysis of 1001 consecutive cases. Ann Surg. 1999;230(3):309–18; discussion 18–21. PubMed PMID: 10493478. Pubmed Central PMCID: PMC1420876. Epub 1999/09/24. eng.
10. Lee WS, Kim MJ, Yun SH, Chun HK, Lee WY, Kim SJ, et al. Risk factor stratification after simultaneous liver and colorectal resection for synchronous colorectal metastasis. Langenbeck's Arch Surg. 2008;393(1):13–9. PubMed PMID: 17909846. Epub 2007/10/03. eng.
11. Iwatsuki S, Dvorchik I, Madariaga JR, Marsh JW, Dodson F, Bonham AC, et al. Hepatic resection for metastatic colorectal adenocarcinoma: a proposal of a prognostic scoring system. J Am Coll Surg. 1999;189(3):291–9. PubMed PMID: 10472930. Pubmed Central PMCID: PMC2967754. Epub 1999/09/03. eng.
12. Ueno H, Mochizuki H, Hatsuse K, Hase K, Yamamoto T. Indicators for treatment strategies of colorectal liver metastases. Ann Surg. 2000;231(1):59–66. PubMed PMID: 10636103. Pubmed Central PMCID: PMC1420966. Epub 2000/01/15. eng.
13. Lise M, Bacchetti S, Da Pian P, Nitti D, Pilati P. Patterns of recurrence after resection of colorectal liver metastases: prediction by models of outcome analysis. World J Surg. 2001;25(5):638–44. PubMed PMID: 11369992. Epub 2001/05/23. eng.
14. Zakaria S, Donohue JH, Que FG, Farnell MB, Schleck CD, Ilstrup DM, et al. Hepatic resection for colorectal metastases: value for risk scoring systems? Ann Surg. 2007;246(2):183–91. PubMed PMID: 17667495. Pubmed Central PMCID: PMC1933577. Epub 2007/08/02. eng.
15. Medscape. FDA grants marketing approval to irinotecan for first-line treatment of metastatic colorectal cancer2000. Available from: https://www.medscape.com/viewarticle/411816.
16. Ibrahim A, Hirschfeld S, Cohen MH, Griebel DJ, Williams GA, Pazdur R. FDA drug approval summaries: oxaliplatin. Oncologist. 2004;9(1):8–12. PubMed PMID: 14755010. Epub 2004/02/03. eng.
17. Kelly H, Goldberg RM. Systemic therapy for metastatic colorectal cancer: current options, current evidence. J Clin Oncol. 2005;23(20):4553–60. PubMed PMID: 16002847. Epub 2005/07/09. eng.
18. Schindl M, Wigmore SJ, Currie EJ, Laengle F, Garden OJ. Prognostic scoring in colorectal cancer liver metastases: development and validation. Arch Surg (Chicago, Ill : 1960). 2005;140(2):183–9. PubMed PMID: 15724001. Epub 2005/02/23. eng.

19. Malik HZ, Prasad KR, Halazun KJ, Aldoori A, Al-Mukhtar A, Gomez D, et al. Preoperative prognostic score for predicting survival after hepatic resection for colorectal liver metastases. Ann Surg. 2007;246(5):806–14. PubMed PMID: 17968173. Epub 2007/10/31. eng.
20. Konopke R, Kersting S, Distler M, Dietrich J, Gastmeier J, Heller A, et al. Prognostic factors and evaluation of a clinical score for predicting survival after resection of colorectal liver metastases. Liver int. 2009;29(1):89–102. PubMed PMID: 18673436. Epub 2008/08/05. eng.
21. Rees M, Tekkis PP, Welsh FK, O'Rourke T, John TG. Evaluation of long-term survival after hepatic resection for metastatic colorectal cancer: a multifactorial model of 929 patients. Ann Surg. 2008;247(1):125–35. PubMed PMID: 18156932. Epub 2007/12/25. eng.
22. House MG, Ito H, Gonen M, Fong Y, Allen PJ, DeMatteo RP, et al. Survival after hepatic resection for metastatic colorectal cancer: trends in outcomes for 1,600 patients during two decades at a single institution. J Am Coll Surg. 2010;210(5):744–52. 52-5. PubMed PMID: 20421043. Epub 2010/04/28. eng.
23. Adam R, Delvart V, Pascal G, Valeanu A, Castaing D, Azoulay D, et al. Rescue surgery for unresectable colorectal liver metastases downstaged by chemotherapy: a model to predict long-term survival. Ann Surg. 2004;240(4):644–57; discussion 57-8. PubMed PMID: 15383792. Pubmed Central PMCID: PMC1356466. Epub 2004/09/24. eng.
24. Imai K, Allard MA, Castro Benitez C, Vibert E, Sa Cunha A, Cherqui D, et al. Nomogram for prediction of prognosis in patients with initially unresectable colorectal liver metastases. Br J Surg. 2016;103(5):590–9. PubMed PMID: 26780341. Epub 2016/01/19. eng.
25. Rubbia-Brandt L, Audard V, Sartoretti P, Roth AD, Brezault C, Le Charpentier M, et al. Severe hepatic sinusoidal obstruction associated with oxaliplatin-based chemotherapy in patients with metastatic colorectal cancer. Ann Oncol. 2004;15(3):460–6. PubMed PMID: 14998849. Epub 2004/03/05. eng.
26. Eisenhauer EA, Therasse P, Bogaerts J, Schwartz LH, Sargent D, Ford R, et al. New response evaluation criteria in solid tumours: revised RECIST guideline (version 1.1). Eur J Cancer (Oxford, England : 1990). 2009;45(2):228–47. PubMed PMID: 19097774. Epub 2008/12/23. eng.
27. Nordlinger B, Sorbye H, Glimelius B, Poston GJ, Schlag PM, Rougier P, et al. Perioperative chemotherapy with FOLFOX4 and surgery versus surgery alone for resectable liver metastases from colorectal cancer (EORTC Intergroup trial 40983): a randomised controlled trial. Lancet (London, England). 2008;371(9617):1007–16. PubMed PMID: 18358928. Pubmed Central PMCID: PMC2277487. Epub 2008/03/25. eng.
28. Nordlinger B, Sorbye H, Glimelius B, Poston GJ, Schlag PM, Rougier P, et al. Perioperative FOLFOX4 chemotherapy and surgery versus surgery alone for resectable liver metastases from colorectal cancer (EORTC 40983): long-term results of a randomised, controlled, phase 3 trial. Lancet Oncol. 2013;14(12):1208–15. PubMed PMID: 24120480. Epub 2013/10/15. eng.
29. Falcone A, Ricci S, Brunetti I, Pfanner E, Allegrini G, Barbara C, et al. Phase III trial of infusional fluorouracil, leucovorin, oxaliplatin, and irinotecan (FOLFOXIRI) compared with infusional fluorouracil, leucovorin, and irinotecan (FOLFIRI) as first-line treatment for metastatic colorectal cancer: the Gruppo Oncologico Nord Ovest. J Clin Oncol. 2007;25(13):1670–6. PubMed PMID: 17470860. Epub 2007/05/02. eng.
30. Masi G, Vasile E, Loupakis F, Cupini S, Fornaro L, Baldi G, et al. Randomized trial of two induction chemotherapy regimens in metastatic colorectal cancer: an updated analysis. J Natl Cancer Inst. 2011;103(1):21–30. PubMed PMID: 21123833. Epub 2010/12/03. eng.
31. Van Cutsem E, Kohne CH, Hitre E, Zaluski J, Chang Chien CR, Makhson A, et al. Cetuximab and chemotherapy as initial treatment for metastatic colorectal cancer. N Engl J Med. 2009;360(14):1408–17. PubMed PMID: 19339720. Epub 2009/04/03. eng.
32. Bokemeyer C, Bondarenko I, Hartmann JT, de Braud F, Schuch G, Zubel A, et al. Efficacy according to biomarker status of cetuximab plus FOLFOX-4 as first-line treatment for metastatic colorectal cancer: the OPUS study. Ann Oncol. 2011;22(7):1535–46. PubMed PMID: 21228335. Epub 2011/01/14. eng

33. Ye LC, Liu TS, Ren L, Wei Y, Zhu DX, Zai SY, et al. Randomized controlled trial of cetuximab plus chemotherapy for patients with KRAS wild-type unresectable colorectal liver-limited metastases. J Clin Oncol. 2013;31(16):1931–8. PubMed PMID: 23569301. Epub 2013/04/10. eng
34. Brudvik KW, Jones RP, Giuliante F, Shindoh J, Passot G, Chung MH, et al. RAS mutation clinical risk score to predict survival after resection of colorectal liver metastases. Ann Surg. 2019;269(1):120–6. PubMed PMID: 28549012. Epub 2017/05/27. eng.
35. Wang K, Liu W, Yan XL, Li J, Xing BC. Long-term postoperative survival prediction in patients with colorectal liver metastasis. Oncotarget. 2017;8(45):79927–34. Pubmed Central PMCID: PMC5668107. Epub 2017/11/08. eng.
36. Sasaki K, Morioka D, Conci S, Margonis GA, Sawada Y, Ruzzenente A, et al. The tumor burden score: a new "metro-ticket" prognostic tool for colorectal liver metastases based on tumor size and number of tumors. Ann Surg. 2018;267(1):132–41. Epub 2016/10/21. eng.
37. Ayez N, Lalmahomed ZS, van der Pool AE, Vergouwe Y, van Montfort K, de Jonge J, et al. Is the clinical risk score for patients with colorectal liver metastases still useable in the era of effective neoadjuvant chemotherapy? Ann Surg Oncol. 2011;18(10):2757–63. Pubmed Central PMCID: PMC3171666. Epub 2011/06/04. eng.
38. Kanas GP, Taylor A, Primrose JN, Langeberg WJ, Kelsh MA, Mowat FS, et al. Survival after liver resection in metastatic colorectal cancer: review and meta-analysis of prognostic factors. Clin Epidemiol. 2012;4:283–301. Pubmed Central PMCID: PMC3496330. Epub 2012/11/16. eng.
39. Giacchetti S, Itzhaki M, Gruia G, Adam R, Zidani R, Kunstlinger F, et al. Long-term survival of patients with unresectable colorectal cancer liver metastases following infusional chemotherapy with 5-fluorouracil, leucovorin, oxaliplatin and surgery. Ann Oncol. 1999;10(6):663–9. Epub 1999/08/12. eng.
40. Beppu T, Miyamoto Y, Sakamoto Y, Imai K, Nitta H, Hayashi H, et al. Chemotherapy and targeted therapy for patients with initially unresectable colorectal liver metastases, focusing on conversion hepatectomy and long-term survival. Ann Surg Oncol. 2014;21(Suppl 3):S405–13. Epub 2014/02/27. eng.
41. Nagashima I, Takada T, Matsuda K, Adachi M, Nagawa H, Muto T, et al. A new scoring system to classify patients with colorectal liver metastases: proposal of criteria to select candidates for hepatic resection. J Hepato-Biliary-Pancreat Surg. 2004;11(2):79–83. PubMed PMID: 15127268. Epub 2004/05/06. eng.

What Is the Impact of Positive Margins in the Liver?

9

Ibrahim Nassour and Michael A. Choti

Introduction

Many patients with colorectal cancer will develop metastatic disease, with the majority being in the liver. Unfortunately, even with extended criteria, most of the patients with colorectal cancer liver metastasis (CRLM) are unresectable, with only approximately 25% potentially resectable. Liver resection is one of the only therapies associated with long-term survival, with 5-year survival rates reported as 50–60% [1, 2]. With the advances of surgical techniques and newer chemotherapy regimens, a larger number of patients are potentially eligible for resection, including some patients who were deemed unresectable in the past. Yet, even with this approach, the aim remains to remove all the evident macroscopic metastatic disease while preserving sufficient functional hepatic tissue. While long-term survival can be achieved, prognosis can vary. Several clinicopathological factors have been found to be independent predictors of survival, including the number and size of the metastases, preoperative CEA, disease-free interval, primary nodal status, and histologic grade [3–5]. Resection margin status and width have also been historically an important prognostic factor. Yet, more recent studies have challenged the oncologic impact of close or microscopically positive (R1) resection. This is particularly important to understand, as this is one factor which is potentially under the control of the surgeon. In this chapter, we will discuss what is the impact of positive margin and the optimal width after hepatectomy for CRLM.

I. Nassour
Department of Surgery, UT Southwestern Medical Center, Dallas, TX, USA
e-mail: IBRAHIM.NASSOUR@phhs.org

M. A. Choti (✉)
Banner MD Anderson Cancer Center, Phoenix, AZ, USA
e-mail: Michael.Choti@bannerhealth.com

M. M. Correia et al. (eds.), *Colorectal Cancer Liver Metastases*,
https://doi.org/10.1007/978-3-030-25486-5_9

Defining a Negative Margin

One of the challenges in examining the literature on this topic is the varying definition of resection margin in CRLM, particularly when defining a "positive" or R1 resection. Specifically, some have defined R1 as an actual histologically involved microscopic (inked) margin, while others have defined R1 as a margin width of <1 mm [6]. A recent study demonstrated that patients with involved or ≤1 mm margin have similar inferior overall survival as that of patients with a margin width >1 mm, suggesting that a uniform definition of R1 as a margin width <1 mm should be employed [6]. However, studies reporting the impact of margin status on outcomes have varied or often not made this distinction.

Importance of R0 Resection

A critical principle of oncologic surgery is to remove all diseases with negative margins. Indeed, the prognostic impact of a microscopically positive resection margin has been clearly demonstrated in other malignancies, including breast, pancreas, and rectal cancer. While it is clear that incomplete removal of CRLM, resecting with gross residual disease (R2) is associated with worse outcome, strong evidence for improved outcomes following R1 resection of CRLM remains more obscure. In part, this may be because long-term prognosis can often be dominated by other oncologic prognostic factors, independent of margin. Patients who have positive margins often have more extensive disease and therefore worse disease biology [7, 8].

In a meta-analysis of 18 retrospective studies, patients who underwent R1 resection were shown to have worse 5-year overall survival compared to those who underwent R0 resection (Pooled HR: 1.60; 95% CI: 1.46–1.75) [9]. In contrast, De Haas et al. argued that an anticipated R1 resection should not be a contraindication for surgery in the current era of effective chemotherapy [7]. In a study comparing 202 R1 resections to 234 R0 resections, the 5-year survival was not different between groups after median follow-up of 40 months (R0 61% vs. R1 57%, $P = 0.27$). The intrahepatic recurrences were higher in the R1 group (28%) than in the R0 group (17%, $P = 0.004$).

Recent reports from experienced hepatobiliary centers reported the incidence of R1 resection to range from 10% to 30% and often over 50% in patients with bilateral or initially unresectable disease, reflecting the increasing aggressiveness in the surgical management of CRLM [10–20]. Some have argued that not all R1 resection cases behave the same. Vigano et al. showed that patients with positive parenchymal margin have higher local recurrence and worse survival than those who underwent R0 resection, while patients who had R1 resection with detachment of CRLM from major intrahepatic vessels had equivalent outcomes to R0 resection [14].

The reasons why margin status may be less important in liver surgery compared to other cancer surgery may also be due to some technical factors associated with hepatectomy. The use of crush techniques or aspirating dissectors may achieve a wider margin that is seen by the pathologist in the specimen. During the resection process, some disruption or cracking of the specimen liver may result in positive ink on the resection surface, which could overcall a microscopically positive margin. In addition, the remnant liver resection surface is often treated with energy devices such as bipolar coagulation or argon beam, likely achieving an additional "ablation margin" of 2–5 mm of hepatic tissue not appreciated on the pathologic specimen. Unlike other cancer resections, attempting to perform frozen section intraoperatively and re-resecting an R1 margin to convert it to R0 has not been advocated, as it does not confer survival advantage [21]. Likewise, the recommendation for any postoperative adjuvant local therapy such as radiation is not indicated following an R1 resection for CRLM.

Is the Width of Surgical Margin Important?

Beyond the attainment of a negative margin, traditionally, the width of the negative margin has been advocated by some as an important surgical principle when resecting CRLM. In the past, many hepatic surgeons adopted the "1 cm rule" as a goal for optimal resection and even a contraindication for surgery if not achievable. More recently, this criterion has been rejected by some. Provided all macroscopic diseases are resected with a negative microscopic margin, most agree that this is sufficient and associated with a comparably favorable outcome. As for R1 vs. R0 controversy, challenges with definitions, measurement criteria, and pathologic variability can impact on determining the prognostic impact of margin width on the outcome.

In a meta-analysis of 34 studies, a wider resection margin (>1 cm vs. <1 cm) was shown to be associated with improved overall survival at 3 years (pooled RR = 0.86; 95% CI: 0.79–0.95), 5 years (pooled RR = 0.91; 95% CI: 0.85–0.97), and 10 years (pooled RR = 0.94; 95% CI: 0.88–1.00) [22]. Similarly, in a large single-institution retrospective report of 1019 patients, Are et al. showed that patients with a margin width <1–10 mm and >10 mm had a median survival of 42 and 55 months, respectively [23]. Survival increased incrementally with increasing width of the margin with a plateau at 25 mm and two inflection points: one at 0 mm and another one at 10 mm. After adjusting for type of resection, number and size of tumors, transfusion, and nodal disease, margin width >10 mm was found to be an independent predictor of survival. In this study, they concluded that while achieving a 1 cm margin is preferable, this does not negate offering surgery for patients who potentially will a narrower margin, as this group still has a favorable long-term outcome. Others who have addressed this question have failed to demonstrate an effect of margin width on survival. In one multicenter study of 557 patients, no difference in recurrence or survival was found based on the margin width [8]. Of note, in this study, local recurrence at the margin was low, ranging from 2–5% for patients with a negative margin. In another study, Hamady et al. found in an analysis of 2715 patients who underwent resection of CRLM in two major hepatobiliary centers a margin beyond 1 mm did not offer a survival advantage, advocating for 1 mm margin as an acceptable standard of care [24].

As with the achievement of an R0 resection margin, a wider margin of 1 cm should likely be the goal for the metastasectomy, when it can be done without increased morbidity. This aim may be useful because by striving for a wider margin, the probability of complete resection without tumor disruption may be greater. However, what is clear is that concern of or failure to offer curative-intent resection should be tempered based on more recent evidence and current trends. As such, surgeons have moved away from the 1-cm rule as the standard of care to the negative margin rule (≥1 mm) [25].

Conclusion

Among factors associated with prognosis following resection of CRLM, the surgical margin remains a persistent point of controversy, particularly because it is one factor that theoretically is in control of the surgeon. Yet, as outlined in this chapter, the emphasis on the importance of margin status as a predictor of outcome has clearly diminished in recent years. Moreover, evidence suggests that the width of the surgical margin likely has limited significance in predicting survival in patients undergoing resection. Even the value of achieving an R0 resection is not consistently substantiated in the modern literature. Rather than dogmatically adhering to "1-cm rule" or even the "R0 rule," the surgeon should assess resectability based on the goal for curative-intent resection of CRLM – complete and safe removal of all macroscopic disease.

References

1. Siegel RL, Ward EM, Jemal A. Trends in colorectal cancer incidence rates in the United States by tumor location and stage, 1992–2008. Cancer Epidemiol Biomark Prev. 2012;21:411–6. https://doi.org/10.1158/1055-9965.EPI-11-1020.
2. Nassour I, Polanco PM. Minimally invasive liver surgery for hepatic colorectal metastases. Curr Colorectal Cancer Rep. 2016;12:1–10. https://doi.org/10.1007/s11888-016-0316-7.
3. Scheele J, Stangl R, Altendorf-Hofmann A, Gall FP. Indicators of prognosis after hepatic resection for colorectal secondaries. Surgery. 1991;110:13–29.
4. Hughes KS, Rosenstein RB, Songhorabodi S, et al. Resection of the liver for colorectal carcinoma metastases. A multi-institutional study of long-term survivors. Dis Colon Rectum. 1988;31:1–4. https://doi.org/10.1007/BF02552560.
5. Fong Y, Fortner J, Sun RL, et al. Clinical score for predicting recurrence after hepatic resection for metastatic colorectal cancer: analysis of 1001 consecutive cases. Ann Surg. 1999;230:309–18. – discussion 318–21.
6. Wang J, Margonis GA, Amini N, et al. The prognostic value of varying definitions of positive resection margin in patients with colorectal cancer liver metastases. J Gastrointest Surg. 2018;22:1350–7. https://doi.org/10.1007/s11605-018-3748-3.
7. de Haas RJ, Wicherts DA, Flores E, et al. R1 resection by necessity for colorectal liver metastases: is it still a contraindication to surgery? Ann Surg. 2008;248(4):626–37. https://doi.org/10.1097/SLA.0b013e31818a07f1.
8. Pawlik TM, Scoggins CR, Zorzi D, et al. Effect of surgical margin status on survival and site of recurrence after hepatic resection for colorectal metastases. Ann Surg. 2005;241:715–22–discussion 722–4. https://doi.org/10.1097/01.sla.0000160703.75808.7d.

9. Liu W, Sun Y, Zhang L, Xing B-C. Negative surgical margin improved long-term survival of colorectal cancer liver metastases after hepatic resection: a systematic review and meta-analysis. Int J Color Dis. 2015;30:1365–73. https://doi.org/10.1007/s00384-015-2323-6.
10. Van Dam RM, Lodewick TM, van den Broek MAJ, et al. Outcomes of extended versus limited indications for patients undergoing a liver resection for colorectal cancer liver metastases. HPB (Oxford). 2014;16:550–9. https://doi.org/10.1111/hpb.12181.
11. Viganò L, Capussotti L, Majno P, et al. Liver resection in patients with eight or more colorectal liver metastases. Br J Surg. 2015;102:92–101. https://doi.org/10.1002/bjs.9680.
12. Andreou A, Aloia TA, Brouquet A, et al. Margin status remains an important determinant of survival after surgical resection of colorectal liver metastases in the era of modern chemotherapy. Ann Surg. 2013;257:1079–88. https://doi.org/10.1097/SLA.0b013e318283a4d1.
13. Sadot E, Groot Koerkamp B, Leal JN, et al. Resection margin and survival in 2368 patients undergoing hepatic resection for metastatic colorectal cancer: surgical technique or biologic surrogate? Ann Surg. 2015;262:476–85– discussion 483–5. https://doi.org/10.1097/SLA.0000000000001427.
14. Viganò L, Procopio F, Cimino MM, et al. Is tumor detachment from vascular structures equivalent to R0 resection in surgery for colorectal liver metastases? An observational cohort. Ann Surg Oncol. 2016;23:1352–60. https://doi.org/10.1245/s10434-015-5009-y.
15. Eveno C, Karoui M, Gayat E, et al. Liver resection for colorectal liver metastases with perioperative chemotherapy: oncological results of R1 resections. HPB (Oxford). 2013;15:359–64. https://doi.org/10.1111/j.1477-2574.2012.00581.x.
16. Kornprat P, Jarnagin WR, Gonen M, et al. Outcome after hepatectomy for multiple (four or more) colorectal metastases in the era of effective chemotherapy. Ann Surg Oncol. 2007;14:1151–60. https://doi.org/10.1245/s10434-006-9068-y.
17. Malik HZ, Hamady ZZR, Adair R, et al. Prognostic influence of multiple hepatic metastases from colorectal cancer. Eur J Surg Oncol. 2007;33:468–73. https://doi.org/10.1016/j.ejso.2006.09.030.
18. Tanaka K, Shimada H, Ueda M, et al. Role of hepatectomy in treating multiple bilobar colorectal cancer metastases. Surgery. 2008;143:259–70. https://doi.org/10.1016/j.surg.2007.08.015.
19. Adam R, Delvart V, Pascal G, et al. Rescue surgery for unresectable colorectal liver metastases downstaged by chemotherapy: a model to predict long-term survival. Ann Surg. 2004;240(4):644–58.
20. Yamashita S, Hasegawa K, Takahashi M, et al. One-stage hepatectomy following portal vein embolization for colorectal liver metastasis. World J Surg. 2013;37:622–8. https://doi.org/10.1007/s00268-012-1861-0.
21. Margonis GA, Spolverato G, Kim Y, et al. Intraoperative surgical margin re-resection for colorectal liver metastasis: is it worth the effort? J Gastrointest Surg. 2015;19:699–707. https://doi.org/10.1007/s11605-014-2710-2.
22. Margonis GA, Sergentanis TN, Ntanasis-Stathopoulos I, et al. Impact of surgical margin width on recurrence and overall survival following R0 hepatic resection of colorectal metastases: a systematic review and meta-analysis. Ann Surg. 2018;267:1047–55. https://doi.org/10.1097/SLA.0000000000002552.
23. Are C, Gonen M, Zazzali K, et al. The impact of margins on outcome after hepatic resection for colorectal metastasis. Ann Surg. 2007;246:295–300. https://doi.org/10.1097/SLA.0b013e31811ea962.
24. Hamady ZZR, Lodge JPA, Welsh FK, et al. One-millimeter cancer-free margin is curative for colorectal liver metastases: a propensity score case-match approach. Ann Surg. 2014;259:543–8. https://doi.org/10.1097/SLA.0b013e3182902b6e.
25. Viganò L, Costa G, Cimino MM, et al. R1 resection for colorectal liver metastases: a survey questioning surgeons about its incidence, clinical impact, and management. J Gastrointest Surg. 2018;22:1752–63. https://doi.org/10.1007/s11605-018-3820-z.

Multidisciplinary Team (MDT) and the Management of Colorectal Cancer Liver Metastases

10

Mauro Monteiro Correia

Introduction

Colorectal cancer (CRC) ranks third among the most common cancer-related deaths worldwide, with wide geographical variation in incidence and mortality across the world. Most patients die of metastatic disease. Second to lymph nodes, the liver is the most common site of metastases (CRCLM), and this occurs in 60% of CRC patients [1–3].

Colorectal cancer hepatic metastases represent the final stage of a multi-step biological process with a series of mutations in colonic epithelial cells that detach from the large intestine and disseminate through the blood and, finally, attached to the hepatic sinusoids. There it interacts with the sinusoidal endothelial cells, Kupffer cells, stellate cells, and pit cells. It invades, adapts to, and colonizes the liver [4].

If left alone and untreated, their natural history is short, with a median survival rate varying from 6 to 13 months, depending on the extent of the disease at initial presentation [5].

The 5FU- and leucovorin-based regimens of the eighth and ninth decades were inefficient, and it took a while until resection of liver metastases was recognized to be a chance for long-term survival. Until recently, only 10–20% of these patients were considered for resection [5, 6].

The second half of the twentieth century saw advances in different medical fields that have led to better patient prognosis and resectability assessments, as well as to new and better surgical and oncological treatments.

Survival rates for unresectable liver metastases nowadays have reached previously unthinkable heights. Patients with unresectable colorectal liver metastases (without EHD) survive longer if they are treated with a combination of systemic treatment and

M. M. Correia (✉)
National Cancer Institute, Rio de Janeiro, Brazil

Department of Surgery, UNIVERSIDADE DO GRANDE RIO, Duque de Caxias, Brazil

M. M. Correia et al. (eds.), *Colorectal Cancer Liver Metastases*,
https://doi.org/10.1007/978-3-030-25486-5_10

local treatment with radiofrequency ablation and with or without resection. According to the final results of the CLOCC study, the overall survival rate for the combined treatment group was 43.1% for 5 years and 35.9% for 8 years [7].

Surgical indications have widened and subsequent results are presently associated with 5-year overall survival rates of 30% for patients with ten or more liver metastases (R0/R1 resection associated with at least an additional favorable factor) [8].

The LiverMetSurvey registry shows a 42% 5-year survival rate after liver resection in 23,607 nonselected patients [9].

Nevertheless, the emergence of so many different treatment options has managed to end with some controversies and created others. Just to mention: resection in the existence of tumor progression; chemotherapy for resectable liver metastases; best choice for first-line chemotherapeutic regimen; what to do with "vanishing" metastases; number of nodules and resection; what to do with limited extra hepatic disease (EHD); what cases can be converted; age and fitness for surgery; molecular profile, open or minimally invasive surgery; ideal surgical strategy, use of ablation therapies and so on.

Expert reviews and multidisciplinary international consensuses have tried to develop recommendations for the management of patients with liver metastases from colorectal cancer, but not always they have been in consensus with one another [10–13].

The MDT

In the absence of clear prospective evidence under some patient-specific circumstances, a panel discussion in multidisciplinary case conferences (MCC) is essential to optimize outcomes. The goal for patients with stage IV CLC is a multidisciplinary approach aiming to decrease perioperative morbidity and mortality, as well as to increase the number of resectable patients for potential R0 resections that will lead to longer overall survival (OS) [14–23].

The original article of YE Ying-jiang showed that the inception of MDT working improved the diagnostic accuracy and MDT was one of the predictors of OS of CRC patients (*p* 0.002 and HR 0.621) [24].

This strategy is associated with better management and outcomes. This group is so-called "Multidisciplinary Team" (MDT) and should include surgeons with expertise in colorectal and liver surgery, oncologists, hepatologists, diagnostic and interventional radiologists, pathologists, and clinical nurse specialists. The patient should be thoroughly informed and have the final word when it comes the time to decide for the treatment option.

In fact, MDT cancer management of all patients has become a mandatory legal requirement in the UK, France, Belgium, Spain, and a number of other European countries [10].

The EU Parliament and Council has also expressed support for these teams as a way to cope with coordination and communication issues associated with the implementation and organization of cancer care and access across countries [25].

Two areas have been emphasized, namely patients' rights and empowerment and policy support. Both should be considered as key elements of the quality of care.

The National Health Research Institutes in Taiwan initiated a certification program on the quality of cancer care in hospitals in 2008. Establishing MDTs is required to fulfill the criteria for public and private reimbursements [16].

National and regional authorities and professional organizations should also prioritize this issue on their agendas and promote specific guidance, stressing the importance of MDTs as a cornerstone of modern cancer care.

Component Roles

- Surgeons need to be experts in CRC, hepatobiliary, and vascular surgery. If one does not possess all expertise, then a collaborative work will be needed. He or she will need to be familiar with intraoperative ultrasonography, hepatic ablation therapies, and maximal and minimally invasive surgery. Most of all, the surgeon will have to be good at discriminating which patients are readily resectable; which ones can be downstaged ("converted") and which ones are clearly suitable for palliation or best supportive care only. The surgeon is the main responsible for defining the ideal timing for colon and liver resection.
- The Medical Oncologist, in the case of need for conversion chemotherapy, should select the most active treatment for the shortest time combining chemotherapy to targeted drugs, in order to reduce tumor size damaging the least the normal liver and, at the same time, preventing the nodules to vanish completely. Take part in the evidence-based discussion for every case, regarding the need for neoadjuvant, adjuvant, or no chemotherapy at all.
- Radiologists will have to be experts in diagnostic and interventional radiology, if not two different experts will be necessary. They must be domain multidetector row helical CT, MRI with Gadolinium and liver-specific contrast media and Positron Emission Tomography. In terms of interventions, biopsies, chemo and bland embolizations, portal vein embolizations, SIRT, catheter placement for hepatic artery chemotherapy infusion and tumor ablation techniques should be part of their armamentarium. It is expected that the radiologists provide information regarding response based on size, morphological and metabolic criteria, assessment of steatosis, and portal hypertension. The acceptable future liver remnant volume should be estimated by a radiologist and a liver surgeon.
- The Pathologist assesses the responses (Tumor Regression Grade) to preoperative chemotherapy for both the primary and metastases. He provides information on the tumor, margin size and status, micrometastases, grade of fibrosis and necrosis. It is also important to inform the tumor growth pattern and the presence of residual viable cells at the periphery of the metastases ("dangerous halo"), which represent the need for enough surgical margin despite tumor downsizing. The presence of RAS (NRAS and KRAS) mutations and other predictive biomarkers should be informed. At last, but not least, the pathologist should determine the effects of the chemotherapy on normal liver parenchyma (CASH and "Blue Liver") [9].

- The Clinical Nurses or Case Manager Nurses are important in the patient's management, because they provide indications on the follow-up and assistance, as well as collaborating continuously for the reassurance of the patient, adequate communication within the group and data care.
- The patients' quality of life is impacted by treatment decisions. No treatment should be provided without giving clear and thorough information to the patient. There must be proper and fluid communication of the MDT with patients and relatives at every stage of the care process, so that they can exert their preferences for treatment and/or care whenever possible and appropriate. Also, patients should have access to second opinions and be able to choose from different treatment providers. Written and digital materials regarding toxicities should be provided, as well as information about community resources and patient support groups.
- Residents – Should study the cases in advance, consult evidence in the literature, opinate in the cases, and keep register of the decisions and track down the patients. If necessary, they should provide requests for further studies/interventions. Their expertise gain should be monitored to identify gradual progress in the understanding and domain of treatment indications.
- The Coordinator should ensure efficient discussion, professionals' attendance, preparation of patients' list, involvement of other specialists as needed, and implementation of the decisions taken by the team. This position should be temporary and the nomination process transparent. Ideally, a rotation system should be in place [19].

MDT and Treatment Algorithms

The clinical scenarios are multiple:

- The asymptomatic CRC and resectable synchronous CRLM
- The asymptomatic CRC and nonresectable synchronous CRLM
- The symptomatic CRC and resectable synchronous CRLM
- The symptomatic CRC and nonresectable synchronous CRLM
- Resectable metachronous CRLM
- Nonresectable metachronous CRLM
- Recurrent CRLM

Furthermore, the MDT must take into consideration many other prognostic factors such as presence, absence, and sort of EHD; primary location in the colon or rectum; obstructive or not; right or left colon; RAS family mutated or wild types; low or high disease volume; low or high CEA levels; age; and patient's decision.

It is not an easy task, and the collective decision-making process must be based on solid evidence. It has become clear that stage 4 patients comprise groups with different prognosis, varying from incurable to potentially curable. Regarding distant disease, the latest version of AJCC Cancer Staging system classifies stage IV into three different prognostic sub-groups, with declining survival expectations [26]:

- Stage IV a – It has spread to one distant organ (such as the liver or lung) or distant set of lymph nodes but not to distant parts of the peritoneum (the lining of the abdominal cavity) (M1a).
- Stage IV b – It has spread to more than one distant organ (such as the liver or lung) or distant set of lymph nodes but not to distant parts of the peritoneum (the lining of the abdominal cavity) (M1b).
- Stage IV c – It has spread to distant parts of the peritoneum (the lining of the abdominal cavity) and may or may not have spread to distant organs or lymph nodes (M1c).

After thorough analysis and discussion of the case, based on the European Society for Medical Oncology Clinical Practice Guidelines for Metastatic Colorectal Cancer, the MDT should classify patients into one of the three defined groups and define the treatment strategy [15]:

- 0: primarily technically R0-resectable liver metastases
- 1: potentially resectable metastatic disease with curative intention
- 2: disseminated disease, technically "never"/unlikely resectable.

Treatment indication algorithms represent the usual available options, such as that given in Fig. 10.1:

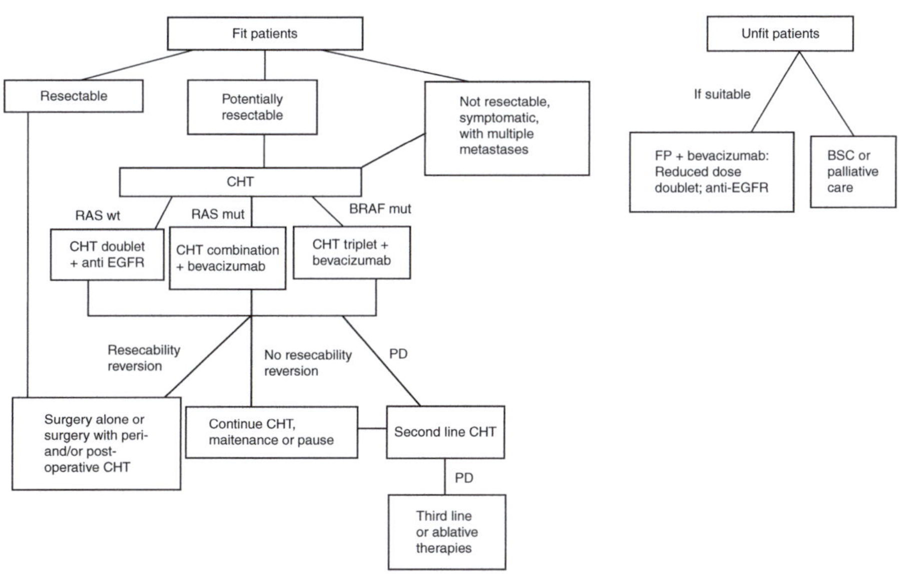

Fig. 10.1 Treatment indications for CRCLM patients [27]

Is There Evidence that MDT Really Makes a Difference?

Kruger and colleagues studied the evolution in the surgical management of CRCLM using a propensity score matching analysis to estimate the impact the establishment of a MDT. Comparing two different eras (before and after MDT), they concluded that the survival rates were similar, suggesting that the biological behavior was the most important factor [28].

Renstsch and Schiergens have stated that, despite MCC being the standard of care for placing emphasis on the individualized decision-making process, no proof of a true link between MDT activity and subsequent patient benefit had, to their knowledge, been established in a large cohort until the publication of the paper of Wanis and colleagues [29].

This group compared patients with CRLM presented to an MDT with those not presented. The cases discussed at the MCC were more exposed to more radical approaches and a trend toward increased use of chemotherapy [30].

Jones and Poston managed to emphasize the importance of the participation of a liver surgeon in the decision-making process for deciding on resectability in clinical trials. They realized that oncologists and surgeons differ widely in their perception of which cases should be resected and highlighted the critical importance of joint decision-making. Among seven seminal clinical trials with cytotoxic and targeted biological agents in patients with initially unresectable CRCLM, only four had had the participation of a liver surgeon in the decision-making process on resectability. The mean resectability rate for those without surgeons was 9.7% and to those with surgeons the same rate was 38.8%. It emphasizes not only the importance of an MDT but also the importance of the right composition of such teams [31].

The interesting work of YE in which he compared two cohorts of patients with CRC referred to his hospital between 1999 and 2006, stratified into those before (297 pts) and after (298 pts) the introduction of the MDT concluded for beneficial effect of the MDT. CT TNM staging was more accurate, recurrence rate was lower, overall survival was longer and MDT itself alone was an independent favorable risk factor ($P < 0.001$) [18].

Yuan-Tzu Lan and colleagues came to the same conclusion regarding the beneficial effects of an MDT. A significantly improved 3-year survival rate was found for Stage IV patients discussed in MDTs (from 25.6% to 38.2% – $P < 0.001$). After the implementation of the MDT, the resection rate increased from 19.6% to 35.2% [16].

Others have also proved prolonged survival rates in cohorts exposed to MDTs and other benefits are reduced number of interventions, shorter delays in care, better control of chemotherapy, and decreased postoperative mortality [14, 32–35].

Conclusion

The establishment and operation of an MDT may be challenging. Conflicts regarding leadership, insufficient support, poor or inexistent data management, and lack of commitment from staff are ubiquitous. However, if the group members overcome these initial obstacles, they might experiment the opportunities for sharing and building collective knowledge and cross-training.

For the patient, the implementation of MDTs warrants greater accuracy of disease staging, fewer treatment and referral delays, higher resection rates, lower mortality rates, individualized evidence-based continuous practice, enhanced quality of life, and OS.

References

1. Schreuders EH, Ruco A, Rabeneck L, Schoen RE, Sung JJ, Young GP, Kuipers EJ. Colorectal cancer screening: a global overview of existing programmes. Gut. 2015;64(10):1637–49.
2. Patanaphan V, Salazar OM. Colorectal cancer: metastatic patterns and prognosis. South Med J. 1993;86(1):38–41.
3. Bartolini I, Ringressi MN, Melli F, Risaliti M, Brugia M, Mini E, et al. Analysis of prognostic factors for resected synchronous and metachronous liver metastases from colorectal cancer. Gastroenterol Res Pract. 2018;2018:5353727.
4. Paschos KA, Majeed AW, Bird NC. Natural history of hepatic metastases from colorectal cancer: pathobiological pathways with clinical significance. World J Gastroenterol. 2014;20(14):3719–37.
5. Nesbitt C, Glendinning RJ, Byrne C, Poston GJ. Factors that influence treatment strategies in advanced colorectal cancer. Eur J Surg Oncol. 2007;33(Suppl 2):S88–94.
6. Wanebo HJ, Semoglou C, Attiyeh F, Stearns MJ Jr. Surgical management of patients with primary operable colorectal cancer and synchronous liver metastases. Am J Surg. 1978;135(1):81–5.
7. Ruers T, Van Coevorden F, Punt CJ, Pierie JE, Borel-Rinkes I, Ledermann JA, et al. Local treatment of unresectable colorectal liver metastases: results of a randomized phase II trial. J Natl Cancer Inst. 2017;109(9):1–10.
8. Allard MA, Adam R, Giuliante F, Lapointe R, Hubert C, Ijzermans JNM, et al. Long-term outcomes of patients with 10 or more colorectal liver metastases. Br J Cancer. 2017;117(5):604–11.
9. Andres A, Majno P, Terraz S, Morel P, Roth A, Rubbia-Brandt L, et al. Management of patients with colorectal liver metastasis in eleven questions and answers. Expert Rev Anticancer Ther. 2016;16(12):1277–90.
10. Adam R, de Gramont A, Figueras J, Kokudo N, Kunstlinger F, Loyer E, et al. Managing synchronous liver metastases from colorectal cancer: a multidisciplinary international consensus. Cancer Treat Rev. 2015;41(9):729–41.
11. Abdalla EK, Bauer TW, Chun YS, D'Angelica M, Kooby DA, Jarnagin WR. Locoregional surgical and interventional therapies for advanced colorectal cancer liver metastases: expert consensus statements. HPB (Oxford). 2013;15(2):119–30.
12. Adams RB, Aloia TA, Loyer E, Pawlik TM, Taouli B, Vauthey JN, et al. Selection for hepatic resection of colorectal liver metastases: expert consensus statement. HPB (Oxford). 2013;15(2):91–103.

13. Coimbra FJ, Ribeiro HS, Marques MC, Herman P, Chojniak R, Kalil AN, et al. First brazilian consensus on multimodal treatment of colorectal liver metastases, module 1: pre-treatment evaluation. Arq Bras Cir Dig. 2015;28(4):222–30.
14. Lordan JT, Karanjia ND, Quiney N, Fawcett WJ, Worthington TR. A 10-year study of outcome following hepatic resection for colorectal liver metastases: the effect of evaluation in a multidisciplinary team setting. Eur J Surg Oncol. 2009;35(3):302–6.
15. Engstrand J, Kartalis N, Strömberg C, Broberg M, Stillström A, Lekberg T, et al. The impact of a hepatobiliary multidisciplinary team assessment in patients with colorectal cancer liver metastases: a population-based study. Oncologist. 2017;22(9):1067–74.
16. Lan YT, Jiang JK, Chang SC, Yang SH, Lin CC, Lin HH, et al. Improved outcomes of colorectal cancer patients with liver metastases in the era of the multidisciplinary teams. Int J Color Dis. 2016;31(2):403–11.
17. Adam R, De Gramont A, Figueras J, Guthrie A, Kokudo N, Kunstlinger F, et al. The oncosurgery approach to managing liver metastases from colorectal cancer: a multidisciplinary international consensus. Oncologist. 2012;17(10):1225–39.
18. Nordlinger B, Vauthey JN, Poston G, Benoist S, Rougier P, Van Cutsem E. The timing of chemotherapy and surgery for the treatment of colorectal liver metastases. Clin Colorectal Cancer. 2010;9(4):212–8.
19. Weledji EP. Centralization of liver cancer surgery and impact on multidisciplinary teams working on stage IV colorectal cancer. Oncol Rev. 2017;11(2):331.
20. Thillai K, Repana D, Korantzis I, Kane P, Prachalias A, Ross P. Clinical outcomes for patients with liver-limited metastatic colorectal cancer: arguing the case for specialist hepatobiliary multidisciplinary assessment. Eur J Surg Oncol. 2016;42(9):1331–6.
21. Österlund P, Isoniemi H, Scheinin T, Ristimäki A, Lantto E. Multidisciplinary tailoring of therapy of metastatic colon cancer. Duodecim. 2016;132(12):1177–84.
22. Li H, Du X, Xia S, Li S, Xu J, Zou G, Hu S. Application of multidisciplinary treatment in patients with liver metastasis of colorectal cancer. Zhonghua Wei Chang Wai Ke Za Zhi. 2016;19(10):1124–8.
23. Schiergens TS, von Einem J, Thomas MN, Albertsmeier M, Giessen-Jung C, Dörsch M, et al. Multidisciplinary treatment of colorectal liver metastases. Minerva Med. 2017;108(6):527–46.
24. Ye YJ, Shen ZL, Sun XT, Wang ZF, Shen DH, Liu HJ, et al. Impact of multidisciplinary team working on the management of colorectal cancer. Chin Med J. 2012;125(2):172–7.
25. Borras JM, Albreht T, Audisio R, Briers E, Casali P, Esperou H, et al. Policy statement on multidisciplinary cancer care. Eur J Cancer. 2014;50(3):475–80.
26. American Cancer Society [Homepage]. Colorectal cancer stages: how is the stage determined?. [Acess ago 20 2018]. Available from: https://www.cancer.org/cancer/colon-rectal-cancer/detection-diagnosis-staging/staged.html.
27. Fiorentini G, Sarti D, Aliberti C, Carandina R, Mambrini A, Guadagni S. Multidisciplinary approach of colorectal cancer liver metastases. World J Clin Oncol. 2017;8(3):190–202.
28. Krüger JAP, Fonseca GM, Makdissi FF, Jeismann VB, Coelho FF, Herman P. Evolution in the surgical management of colorectal liver metastases: propensity score matching analysis (PSM) on the impact of specialized multidisciplinary care across two institutional eras. J Surg Oncol. 2018;118:50.
29. Rentsch M, Schiergens TS. Treatment plan improvement by multidisciplinary case conferences for patients with colorectal cancer and synchronous liver metastases. Hepatobiliary Surg Nutr. 2018;7(2):147–8.
30. Wanis KN, Pineda-Solis K, Tun-Abraham ME, Yeoman J, Welch S, Vogt K. Management of colorectal cancer with synchronous liver metastases: impact of multidisciplinary case conference review. Hepatobiliary Surg Nutr. 2017;6(3):162–9.
31. Jones RP, Poston GJ. Resection of liver metastases in colorectal cancer in the era of expanding systemic therapy. Annu Rev Med. 2017;68:183–96.

32. Adam R, Haller DG, Poston G, Raoul JL, Spano JP, Tabernero J, Van Cutsem E. Toward optimized front-line therapeutic strategies in patients with metastatic colorectal cancer: an expert review from the International Congress on Anti-Cancer Treatment (ICACT) 2009. Ann Oncol. 2010;21(8):1579–84.
33. Goyer P, Karoui M, Vigano L, Kluger M, Luciani A, Laurent A, et al. Singlecenter multidisciplinary management of patients with colorectal cancer and resectable synchronous liver metastases improves outcomes. Clin Res Hepatol Gastroenterol. 2013;37(1):47–55.
34. Vigano L, Langella S, Ferrero A, Russolillo N, Sperti E, Capussotti L. Colorectal cancer with synchronous resectable liver metastases: monocentric management in a hepatobiliary referral center improves survival outcomes. Ann Surg Oncol. 2013;20(3):938–45.
35. De Greef K, Rolfo C, Russo A, Chapelle T, Bronte G, Passiglia F, et al. Multisciplinary management of patients with liver metastasis from colorectal cancer. World J Gastroenterol. 2016;22(32):7215–25.

Defining Resectability of Colorectal Cancer Liver Metastases: Technical and Oncologic Perspectives

11

Rebecca K. Marcus and Thomas A. Aloia

Overview

While over 50% of colorectal cancer (CRC) patients will develop liver metastases during the course of their disease, less than 25% of patients with colorectal liver metastases (CRLM) are thought to be resectable at presentation. Currently, multimodality therapy including margin negative resection is the only treatment strategy associated with 5-year survival rates of 50% [1, 2]. Thus, efforts at increasing the resectability rates of patients with CRLM are warranted. At present, these efforts include aggressive multidisciplinary management with chemotherapy, innovative surgical strategies, and interventional techniques.

Resectability of CRLM should be defined along three separate domains, and adherence to a stepwise protocol for preoperative evaluation of patients with CRLM is critical to proper patient selection (Fig. 11.1). As part of this stepwise evaluation, all patients must undergo thorough preoperative evaluations in which they are considered operative candidates first from a medical standpoint, then from an oncologic standpoint, and finally from a technical standpoint to define their resectability. Proper patient selection, in combination with detail-oriented care, enables performance of both successful and safe hepatectomies.

R. K. Marcus · T. A. Aloia (✉)
Department of Surgical Oncology, The University of Texas MD Anderson Cancer Center, Houston, TX, USA
e-mail: rmarcus@mcw.edu; taaloia@mdanderson.org

M. M. Correia et al. (eds.), *Colorectal Cancer Liver Metastases*,
https://doi.org/10.1007/978-3-030-25486-5_11

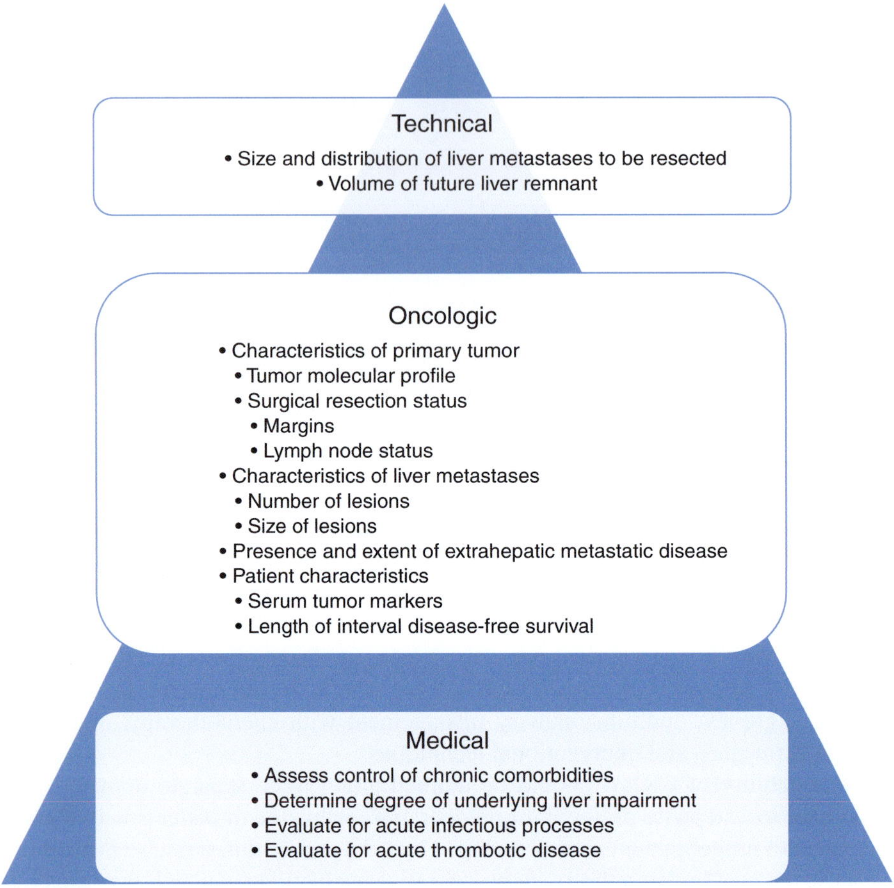

Fig. 11.1 Core components to the stepwise evaluation of resectability in patients with colorectal liver metastases

Components of a Structured Determination of Resectability

Core Medical Evaluation

The first step in the evaluation of CRLM patients is to assess medical, or physiologic, resectability. Specifically, a patient's ability to safely undergo general anesthesia for one or more major abdominal operations, thereby enabling complete resection of his/her liver disease, is determined. Important factors to consider include chronic comorbidities, underlying liver impairment, and acute infectious or thrombotic processes. As it is increasingly recognized that patients with multiple controlled comorbidities can tolerate modern hepatic operations, following a systems-based review of all known comorbidities, individual assessment of the identified comorbidities should be performed to determine how well controlled each is. A history of cardiac and/or pulmonary disease is of particular importance, given the cardiovascular demands of low central venous pressure anesthesia and portal pedicle clamping encountered during many hepatectomies. Such comorbidities must be thoroughly investigated because poorly controlled cardiac or pulmonary disease places patients at significant risk for both intra- and postoperative complications.

The presence of any underlying liver disease is also important to consider. A history of chronic liver dysfunction and/or cirrhosis secondary to hepatitis, alcohol use/abuse, or obesity (i.e., non-alcoholic fatty liver disease) should be elicited. More acutely, the effect of previous therapy on liver function should be assessed. In particular, certain systemic chemotherapy regimens are known to cause liver dysfunction (e.g., oxaliplatin-induced vascular changes and irinotecan-induced steatosis) [3–6]. Depending on the severity of a patient's liver dysfunction, preoperative risk factor modifications and/or increased intraoperative precautions may be required to ensure a safe operation with low risk of postoperative hepatic insufficiency. In some cases, a patient's poor liver function may result in the determination of unresectability.

Finally, the presence of acute processes such as infections or thromboembolic disease should be determined. As these processes may increase the risk of undergoing anesthesia and surgery, treatment should be considered. Treatment is not an exclusively benign process, however, given that the risk of progression while delaying operative intervention to treat acute processes is not insignificant.

Advances in prehabilitation and perioperative medicine have helped increase the number of CRLM patients who are deemed resectable from a medical standpoint. Furthermore, increased utilization of minimally invasive techniques and enhanced recovery after surgery (ERAS) protocols have enabled surgery to be safer in general [7]. That said, patient selection remains paramount, and adjuncts to the above-described preoperative exam exist (e.g., multiple risk calculators and frailty indices) to help appropriately identify patients with adequate performance status to undergo major surgery with acceptably low risks of perioperative adverse events [8–10].

The Consideration of Patient Age

Previous studies have demonstrated that age is not a significant prognostic variable for long-term survival in CRLM patients [11–13]. Thus, age itself should not be considered a contraindication to resection in the absence of other prohibitory medical factors. Instead, age should be viewed as a warning sign since older patients tend to have increased numbers of comorbidities and so are at increased risk of having poorly controlled comorbidities that may deem them unresectable from a medical standpoint [11, 12, 14]. In general, exceptionally vigilant screening and selection of older patients for surgery is necessary.

While a thorough preoperative medical evaluation of any CRLM patient being considered for surgical resection should include assessment of baseline physical, cognitive, and nutritional statuses, these are especially important factors to assess in patients of more advanced age. These are typically evaluated using a combination of screening tools that can be easily utilized in the surgery clinic (e.g., grip strength,

Timed Up and Go test, and Mini-Cog test) and laboratory assessments. The purpose of these evaluations is to detect frailty, which has been demonstrated to predict increased perioperative risk, delayed postoperative recovery, and prolonged periods of time between surgery and resumption of further oncologic therapy (RIOT) [15]. These screening tools may also help identify easily remediable risk factors, ultimately enabling more CRLM patients to undergo resection. Identification of non-remediable risk factors is also important, as patients should be made aware of this information in order to provide completely informed consent regarding the risks of hepatectomy.

Assessment of Oncologic Resectability

After establishing medical fitness for surgery, the next step in the evaluation of CRLM patients is to determine oncologic resectability. This refers to the selection of patients likely to benefit from surgery based on their underlying tumor biology. While all patients with CRLM are classified as stage IV in the tumor-node-metastasis (TNM) staging system, considerable survival heterogeneity is observed within this population of patients. This heterogeneity is related to several factors, including patient characteristics, primary tumor, and intra- and extrahepatic metastatic diseases. In general, patients considered candidates for CRLM resection should have minimal extrahepatic disease and, if they received preoperative systemic chemotherapy, should demonstrate stable or responding disease on imaging with corresponding improvement in serum tumor markers [16].

Assessment of oncologic resectability involves evaluation of serum tumor markers and complete radiological staging, potentially including endoscopic evaluation. Trends in serum tumor markers, most commonly serum carcinoembryonic antigen (CEA), can reflect the extent of disease or response to preoperative therapy. Marked elevations of the preoperative CEA level (i.e., >200 ng/mL) indicate a high risk of early recurrence [17]. Similarly, sharply rising CEA during preoperative chemotherapy suggests poorly controlled disease and likely represents a contraindication to resection, whereas reduction in CEA levels over the course of therapy portends a more favorable prognosis [16]. Unfortunately, up to 30% of patients with CRLM do not produce measurable quantities of CEA.

Radiologic staging and endoscopic evaluation are important for evaluation of both the primary tumor and metastatic disease. With respect to the primary tumor, radiographic and endoscopic evaluations help determine whether the primary tumor site has been completely treated or, if not, whether it is amenable to resection. Of note, neither the location of the primary tumor nor the histologic grade has been shown to affect patient outcomes or to be significant predictors of long-term survival in patients with CRLM; however, the stage of the primary tumor is useful in risk stratification of metastatic disease. In particular, patients with positive regional lymph nodes associated with their primary tumor are more likely to recur after liver metastasectomy [18–21].

Radiologic staging is also utilized to quantify the number and location of hepatic metastasis and extrahepatic disease. In patients treated with preoperative systemic therapy, radiologic studies are additionally helpful for assessing response to therapy. Negative prognostic factors of CRLM include higher number of liver metastases (i.e., >3–5), bilateral disease, and maximal tumor size greater than 5 cm [22]. The timing of diagnosis of liver metastases relative to that of the primary tumor is also a key prognostic factor. Specifically, synchronous presentation, typically defined as liver metastasis diagnosis less than 1 year from diagnosis of the primary tumor, is associated with shorter survival than metachronous presentation [23–25].

Extrahepatic disease is well recognized as one of the most informative surgical prognostic factors, and, in recent years, the approach to management of such disease has undergone reevaluation [22, 23, 26]. For example, historically, non-pulmonary extrahepatic disease has been considered to be a contraindication to hepatectomy [22, 26]. However, a high-volume French group with experience in both hyperthermic perfusion and liver resection found that the number of sites of extrahepatic disease was more prognostic than the actual location(s) [27]. Additionally, the presence of low-volume pulmonary metastases, regardless of resectability status, is no longer considered a contraindication to hepatic resection. The rationale for this is that morbidity and mortality in these patients are rarely related to pulmonary failure [28, 29]. Two large studies evaluating the impact of concomitant liver and lung CRC metastases investigated the impact of simultaneous resection of both types of metastases and found 5-year survival rates of 30% [28, 30].

In contrast, the presence of metastatic disease to the portal lymph nodes is a particularly poor prognostic factor with disease recurrence occurring in almost all patients with positive resected portal lymph nodes [31]. At the same time, consensus statements on the management of extrahepatic disease have concluded that there is no convincing data to suggest that therapeutic portal lymphadenectomy for metastatic CRC improves survival [18, 26]. In highly selected patients, there does appear to be a role for hepatic resection in conjunction with metastases to other extrahepatic sites. This has been examined in the form of several large retrospective studies evaluating resections of the peritoneum, mesentery, retroperitoneal lymph nodes, and multiple solid organs [31–33]. These studies reported 5-year survival rates ranging from 20% to 28%, and, based on their results, hepatectomy combined with surgical resection of extrahepatic disease is believed to be appropriate in selected patients.

Lastly, tumor molecular profiling is a rapidly evolving area that is becoming essential to consider when determining resectability. Early data demonstrating poor response to EGFR inhibitors in *KRAS*-mutated tumors is well documented [34–38]. More recent studies indicate that various sites of mutation within the *KRAS* gene predict different clinical behavior and recurrence patterns [39–41]. Tumors with *KRAS* mutations in combination with *TP53* or *PIKC3A* mutations have also been investigated; the results showed that tumors with *TP53* or *PIKC3A* mutations demonstrated inferior response to systemic therapy and decreased survival in comparison to tumors with only *KRAS* mutations [42, 43] Finally, studies of BRAF mutations in CRLM patients, while less common, indicated an aggressive clinical course associated with very early recurrence after surgical intervention. In the future, an increased understanding of the impact of tumor mutational status may enable truly personalized medical and surgical treatments based on tumor mutational profiles [44].

Predictive Models and Clinical Risk Calculators

Applying the oncologic risk factors described above, multiple retrospective studies have developed predictive models to stratify survival after metastasectomy [17, 22, 45–49]. In the series by Fong et al., seven parameters were found to be independent predictors of an unfavorable prognosis: (1) presence of extrahepatic disease, (2) positive resection margin, (3) nodal metastases associated with primary CRC tumor, (4) disease-free survival less than 1 year, (5) largest liver metastasis greater than 5 cm, (6) more than one liver metastasis, and (7) a serum CEA greater than 200 ng/mL [22]. The subsequently derived MSKCC preoperative clinical risk score (CRS) system utilizes equal weighting of the last five factors, with each positive criterion counting as one point. The presence of 0–2 of these factors is associated with favorable outcomes and 5-year survival of 47%. Thus, the authors suggest that CRLM patients with CRS of 0–2 are good candidates for early hepatectomy, while patients with CRS ≥3 should be considered for nonoperative interventions and, potentially, surgery in the future [22]. This system has proven useful in selecting patients for additional radiologic staging [50], diagnostic laparoscopy [51], neoadjuvant treatment, ablation, and stratification in clinical trials.

Recently, more sophisticated predictive models have been developed, including a complex nomogram [45] and a multifactorial predictive index [46]. The increased accuracy of these models must be balanced against their requirement for more labor-intensive data manipulation and calculation. Furthermore, at present, while systems that discriminate outcomes and provide additional prognostic information are helpful, they rarely can provide absolute data to support the decision to deny an otherwise-resectable patient an operation, even if found to be at high risk for recurrence. These systems can currently be used for clinical trial eligibility and to facilitate comparisons across clinical studies.

Determination of Technical Resectability

Only after confirmation of medical and oncological resectability should technical resectability be addressed. Technical resectability is the ability to remove all metastases with negative microscopic margins and preservation of adequate functional liver volume. In general, this requires retention of two contiguous liver segments with adequate vascular inflow, outflow, and biliary drainage. To assess technical resectability, both liver-specific imaging for volumetric analysis and a clear understanding of the operative techniques and approaches that can be performed are required.

As the number and fidelity of available imaging modalities has increased, the sensitivity and specificity for detection of intra- and extrahepatic CRC metastases larger than 1 cm have significantly improved. With these imaging enhancements, however, comes the identification of sub-centimeter indeterminate lesions that may complicate surgical decision-making. Computed tomographic (CT) scanning is indispensable in the evaluation of patients with CRLM given its low cost, rapid acquisition, and the ability to image the lungs, solid intraabdominal organs, lymph nodes, and soft tissues. While MRI is more expensive and less patient-friendly than CT, the use of MRI with hepatocyte-specific contrast agents in difficult cases (e.g., diagnostic uncertainty, steatotic liver, disappearing lesions following systemic therapy) should be considered.

Over the past several years, there has been exponential growth in the knowledge of and experience with operative management of CRLM. Surgical options now include anatomic hepatectomy, one-stage parenchymal-sparing hepatectomy, traditional two-stage hepatectomy (TSH) with or without portal vein embolization (PVE), associated liver partition and portal vein ligation for staged hepatectomy (ALPPS), local ablative techniques, and hepatic arterial infusion therapy (HAI). Additionally, advances in diagnostic imaging, future liver remnant (FLR) augmentation (e.g., PVE), perioperative anesthesia and medicine, and patient selection have made liver surgery safer and enabled operative intervention for patients previously defined as unresectable [52, 53].

While the number of operative approaches has increased, studies demonstrating superiority of one approach compared with another are lacking. As such, controversy persists about the optimal operative management of patients with CRLM. Because CRLM represent an increasingly common and challenging problem for hepatobiliary surgeons, it is our school of thought that they should not constrain themselves to a single treatment strategy. Instead, surgeons should rely on a multidisciplinary team approach and utilization of all surgical tools available, thereby permitting extension of curative-intent treatments to the greatest number of patients. To accomplish this, a tailored approach to determining technical resectability that takes advantage of all available surgical tools and individually applies them based on an algorithmic assessment of the extent and distribution of metastatic disease has been proposed [54]. This conceptual framework is best understood by classifying the burden of intrahepatic disease in two dimensions with assessment of the right versus left hemilivers and peripheral versus central distribution of disease (Fig. 11.2).

Bilobar Peripheral Disease

For patients with bilobar CRLM that are all peripheral, a one-stage parenchymal-sparing hepatectomy (PSH) is indicated. With this approach, intraoperative ultrasound guidance is used to perform multiple nonanatomic partial hepatectomies. Advantages of this approach are its single-stage nature and preservation of

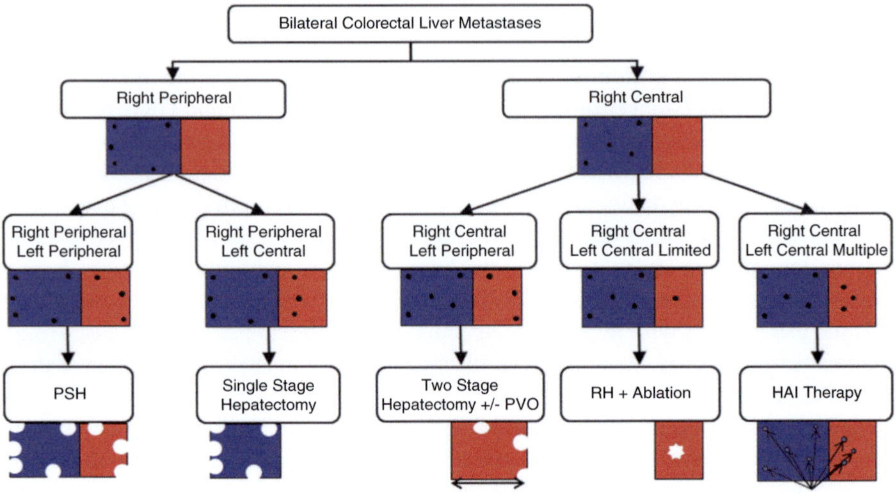

Fig. 11.2 Algorithm for assessing the distribution and extent of colorectal liver metastases to inform operative treatment strategies. For each scenario, the right liver is modeled in blue and left liver in red. Tumors are represented as closed circles, parenchymal sparing resections as open circles, and ablations as open stars. (*PVO* portal vein occlusion, *RH* right hepatectomy)

uninvolved liver tissue. Studies have disproven early concerns of greater rates of local and intrahepatic recurrence with PSH and have shown similar rates of recurrence and survival in PSH versus more extensive resection techniques [55, 56]. Moreover, the preservation of uninvolved liver enabled by PSH is associated with greater rates of salvageability and survival in the event of subsequent liver-limited recurrences [2].

In preparation for a PSH, fiducial markers may be utilized to help localize metastases that are small and deeply located. Metastases with these characteristics are at high risk for disappearing during the course of preoperative systemic therapy [57]. Depending on disease extent and distribution, as well as provider experience and comfort, PSH can be performed via a minimally invasive approach utilizing laparoscopic ultrasound. Importantly, the sensitivities and specificities of open and laparoscopic intraoperative ultrasound for identification of small CRLM have been demonstrated to be similar [58]. Hand-assisted approaches have the same recovery benefits as totally laparoscopic approaches with extraction incisions, with the added benefit of liver palpation for radiographically occult lesions.

Right Liver-Peripheral, Left Liver-Central Disease

For patients with CRLM in the peripheral right hemiliver and central left hemiliver, a formal left hepatectomy may be combined with one or more PSH of the right liver. In the situation of only a single central left metastasis, consideration could also be given to ablation of the central left tumor with PSH or anatomic partial hepatectomy for the right-sided lesions. Either of these approaches can be performed in a single-stage fashion. The latter demonstrates how local ablation techniques used in conjunction with surgical resection extend treatment options for patients with bilobar CRLM. Although inferior to resection of all disease, a strategy of resection and ablation is associated with superior results compared with nonoperative therapies [59]. Optimal ablation results are achieved when tumors are smaller than 3 cm and separate from major vessels [60, 61]. Regarding ablation technique, although cryotherapy has been used historically, most centers currently utilize radiofrequency ablation or the emerging technology of microwave ablation [62].

Right Liver-Central, Left Liver-Peripheral Disease

When CRLM patients have metastases in the central right liver, a right hepatectomy is typically required. Given the volume differential between the right and left livers, the need to perform a formal right hepatectomy and additional left-sided resections places this cohort of patients at the greatest risk of postoperative liver insufficiency. In the setting of dominant right-liver metastases and peripheral left metastases, a staged approach is usually required to achieve resection of all CRLM while leaving adequate FLR. Either a traditional TSH or the ALPPS procedure can be used to accomplish this. In its early form, TSH was performed without PVE and was predictably associated with high postoperative mortality rates, most commonly due to liver insufficiency [16]. The addition of PVE between stages to induce hypertrophy of the FLR decreased postoperative morbidity and mortality following the second-stage procedure [63]. Specifically, those patients who demonstrate adequate hypertrophy on CT volumetry performed 3–4 weeks status-post PVE undergo a second-stage operation. This is typically a right hepatectomy with possible extension to include all or part of segment IV. Portal vein ligation at the time of first-stage operation as an alternative to PVE has also been described, but the liver regeneration induced by this maneuver is inferior to that of PVE with embolic microspheres and coils [64, 65].

In 2012, the ALPPS approach to staged hepatectomy was introduced [66]. In the first stage of this novel procedure, right portal vein ligation is combined with parenchymal transection and clearance of disease from the FLR. The second stage is performed during the same hospitalization, 1–2 weeks after the first stage. It has been demonstrated that ALPPS is associated with rapid and significant hypertrophy of the FLR, as well as high completion rates of both stages of surgery. However, perioperative morbidity and mortality rates for ALPPS are greater than that with a traditional TSH approach [67, 68]. Furthermore, there is evidence that the rapid hypertrophy seen after the first stage of ALPPS is less reliably linked with adequate liver function compared with the hypertrophy experienced following PVE. Finally, early oncologic outcomes suggest lower recurrence-free and overall survival (OS) rates following ALPPS compared with other approaches, but long-term follow-up data is not yet available [69, 70]. As it has consistently demonstrated high completion rates, low perioperative morbidity and mortality, and good survival outcomes, the current standard of care for this distribution of CRLM remains TSH with PVE [1, 71].

Bilobar Central Liver Disease

CRLM patients with this distribution of disease are not typically amenable to R0 resection. If left-sided metastases are limited, consideration may be given to a right hepatectomy combined with ablation. The presence of multiple bilobar, centrally located metastases represents truly unresectable disease and is an indication for HAI therapy. Compared to systemic alternatives, arterial-based therapies allow for a greater concentration of cytotoxic drugs and/or radiation to be delivered directly to metastases while decreasing potential systemic toxicities. When used as first-line therapy, chemotherapy administered via a HAI pump has been found to result in tumor response rates of 40–50% [72]. Response rates have been demonstrated to be even greater when use of HAI pumps is combined with systemic chemotherapy, or when pumps are utilized after failure of first-line systemic chemotherapy [73–75]. Furthermore, the use of HAI therapy in initially unresectable patients may result in tumor downsizing and subsequent resection in some patients [76]. Current consensus guidelines recommend that HAI therapy should be delivered as part of a multidisciplinary program at experienced centers [77]. Other hepatic artery–based therapies (e.g., radioembolization and transcatheter arterial chemoembolization) should also be given therapeutic consideration [78].

Further Evaluation of High-Risk Patients

For patients found to be high-risk surgical candidates based on their initial preoperative evaluation, repeat evaluation following receipt of nonoperative intervention(s) is warranted because some patients will convert to operative candidates. Two commonly encountered circumstances among CRLM patients that warrant repeat surgical assessment are when there is concern for adequate FLR or a large burden of disease. As discussed previously, PVE has high technical and clinical success rates and ultimately enables many CRLM patients with initially small remnant livers to develop adequate FLR. The exact timing of the PVE (i.e., preoperatively versus between staged procedures) depends on the extent and distribution of the patient's disease burden. Regardless of timing, repeat imaging is always obtained within a few weeks of PVE to assess for compensatory hypertrophy and potential disease progression, and to calculate new FLR volumes. If the volumes are found to be adequate, and the patient is otherwise a surgical candidate from medical, oncologic, and technical perspectives, they may proceed with resection.

CRLM patients may also be deemed to be a very high-risk group for surgery because of a large burden of disease, which decreases the potential for R0 resection and increases the chance of early recurrence. In these situations, preoperative systemic therapy is the treatment of choice. There are several benefits to chemotherapy, all of which may help to ultimately achieve surgical resection. With respect to liver disease itself, systemic therapy may decrease the disease burden, thereby making R0 resection possible and also contributing to improved margin control at the time of surgery. This improved margin control has been found to translate into improved disease-free survival (DFS) [5, 16, 79, 80]. Systemic therapy may also be utilized to treat any extrahepatic disease that is present.

Perhaps most important is that administering preoperative chemotherapy to high-risk patients provides the test of time. More than a decade ago, it was noted that progression on preoperative systemic therapy correlated with poor postoperative DFS. Specifically, Adams et al. found a DFS of only 3% in patients who had tumor progression, as opposed to DFS of 20–21% in patients who had stable disease or a disease response [16]. Other groups subsequently corroborated this finding. At the 2012 AHPBA/SSO/SSAT Consensus Conference on the Management of Colorectal Liver Metastases, the criteria for resectability in this scenario were further refined. Specifically, given their differential outcomes, patients with minimal growth (i.e., growth that does not alter the magnitude of required hepatic resection) of existing disease while receiving systemic therapy were advised to proceed to resection. In contrast, patients who develop new lesions during preoperative treatment should be referred for alternative nonoperative therapy in an effort to achieve disease control prior to any potential surgery [81].

Patients with a positive response to preoperative systemic therapy have been demonstrated to experience a more favorable prognosis. In fact, in cases of complete pathological response (defined as greater than 50% of the tumor area that consists of nonviable tumor cells), OS approaches 75% at 5 years [82]. Furthermore, pathological response to preoperative systemic therapy has been found to be the strongest predictor of long-term survival after CRC metastasis resection [82]. One caveat is that even though a significant percentage of tumor cells succumb to effective systemic therapy, CRC metastases may not concentrically shrink. As the RECIST and modified RECIST criteria are largely based on changes in measured maximal tumor diameters, these criteria may not provide an appropriate surrogate for pathological response [83]. An alternative CT imaging response criteria based on tumor shrinkage, border clarity, and contrast enhancement have been developed to overcome the limitations of the RECIST criteria [84]. These response criteria have been shown to correlate with pathological response and long-term outcomes in both surgically and medically treated CRLM patients [85]. A final benefit of providing preoperative systemic therapy is that it predicts tolerance for breaks in chemotherapy, which are inevitable if a patient undergoes surgery, and also predicts tolerance for potential adjuvant therapy that may be recommended by the multidisciplinary treatment team.

Conclusion

For patients with CRLM, hepatic resection is the standard of care. Orderly definition of resectability along physiologic, oncologic, and technical domains is necessary to identify those patients most suited for surgical intervention. It is important to keep in mind the potential barriers to adequately defining patient resectability including inadequate surgical treatment of the primary tumor and overtreatment with preoperative systemic therapy, which may result in hepatoxicity and/or systemic toxicity that prohibits surgery. Low-quality imaging is also an important barrier throughout the process of defining CRLM patient resectability, as surgery will not be offered for CRLM that are not detected and because poor pre- and intra-operative metastases detection inhibits safe R0 resection.

In this chapter, a framework for the stepwise determination of patient resectability was described. In appropriately selected patients, hepatic metastasectomy can be performed by experienced surgeons with acceptable morbidity and mortality. Furthermore, surgery results in prolonged survival in most patients and offers the best possibility for cure. Looking forward, the advent of more effective biologic and cytotoxic therapies will continue to extend therapeutic options and increase the number of patients who might benefit from resection.

References

1. Brouquet A, Abdalla EK, Kopetz S, et al. High survival rate after two-stage resection of advanced colorectal liver metastases: response-based selection and complete resection define outcome. J Clin Oncol. 2011;29:1083–90.
2. Mise Y, Aloia TA, Brudvik KW, et al. Parenchymal-sparing hepatectomy in colorectal liver metastasis improves salvageability and survival. Ann Surg. 2016;263:146–52.
3. Aloia T, Sebagh M, Plasse M, et al. Liver histology and surgical outcomes after preoperative chemotherapy with fluorouracil plus oxaliplatin in colorectal cancer liver metastases. J Clin Oncol. 2006;24:4983–90.
4. Kooby DA, Fong Y, Suriawinata A, et al. Impact of steatosis on perioperative outcome following hepatic resection. J Gastrointest Surg. 2003;7:1034–44.
5. Parikh AA, Gentner B, Wu TT, et al. Perioperative complications in patients undergoing major liver resection with or without neoadjuvant chemotherapy. J Gastrointest Surg. 2003;7:1082–8.
6. Rubbia-Brandt L, Audard V, Sartoretti P, et al. Severe hepatic sinusoidal obstruction associated with oxaliplatin-based chemotherapy in patients with metastatic colorectal cancer. Ann Oncol. 2004;15:460–6.
7. Day RW, Cleeland CS, Wang XS, et al. Patient-reported outcomes accurately measure the value of an enhanced recovery program in liver surgery. J Am Coll Surg. 2015;221:1023–1030 e1021–1022.
8. Bilimoria KY, Liu Y, Paruch JL, et al. Development and evaluation of the universal ACS NSQIP surgical risk calculator: a decision aid and informed consent tool for patients and surgeons. J Am Coll Surg. 2013;217:833–842.e831–833.
9. Reddy S, Contreras CM, Singletary B, et al. Timed stair climbing is the single strongest predictor of perioperative complications in patients undergoing abdominal surgery. J Am Coll Surg. 2016;222:559–66.
10. Wagner D, Buttner S, Kim Y, et al. Clinical and morphometric parameters of frailty for prediction of mortality following hepatopancreaticobiliary surgery in the elderly. Br J Surg. 2016;103:e83–92.
11. Ballantyne GH, Quin J. Surgical treatment of liver metastases in patients with colorectal cancer. Cancer. 1993;71:4252–66.
12. Cady B, Stone MD, WV MD Jr, et al. Technical and biological factors in disease-free survival after hepatic resection for colorectal cancer metastases. Arch Surg. 1992;127:561–8; discussion 568–569
13. Tzeng CW, Cooper AB, Vauthey JN, et al. Predictors of morbidity and mortality after hepatectomy in elderly patients: analysis of 7621 NSQIP patients. HPB (Oxford). 2014;16:459–68.

14. Tzeng CW, Cooper AB, Vauthey JN, et al. Predictors of morbidity and mortality after hepatectomy in elderly patients: analysis of 7621 NSQIP patients. HPB (Oxford). 2013;15:773.
15. Aloia TA, Zimmitti G, Conrad C, et al. Return to intended oncologic treatment (RIOT): a novel metric for evaluating the quality of oncosurgical therapy for malignancy. J Surg Oncol. 2014;110:107–14.
16. Adam R, Pascal G, Castaing D, et al. Tumor progression while on chemotherapy: a contraindication to liver resection for multiple colorectal metastases? Ann Surg. 2004;240:1052–61; discussion 1061-1054
17. Nordlinger B, Guiguet M, Vaillant JC, et al. Surgical resection of colorectal carcinoma metastases to the liver. A prognostic scoring system to improve case selection, based on 1568 patients. Association Francaise de Chirurgie. Cancer. 1996;77:1254–62.
18. Adam R, de Haas RJ, Wicherts DA, et al. Is hepatic resection justified after chemotherapy in patients with colorectal liver metastases and lymph node involvement? J Clin Oncol. 2008;26:3672–80.
19. Nanji S, Tsang ME, Wei X, Booth CM. Regional lymph node involvement in patients undergoing liver resection for colorectal cancer metastases. Eur J Surg Oncol. 2017;43:322–9.
20. Okuno M, Goumard C, Mizuno T, et al. Prognostic impact of perihepatic lymph node metastases in patients with resectable colorectal liver metastases. Br J Surg. 2018;105:1200.
21. Pulitano C, Bodingbauer M, Aldrighetti L, et al. Colorectal liver metastasis in the setting of lymph node metastasis: defining the benefit of surgical resection. Ann Surg Oncol. 2012;19:435–42.
22. Fong Y, Fortner J, Sun RL, et al. Clinical score for predicting recurrence after hepatic resection for metastatic colorectal cancer: analysis of 1001 consecutive cases. Ann Surg. 1999;230:309–18; discussion 318–321
23. Rosen CB, Nagorney DM, Taswell HF, et al. Perioperative blood transfusion and determinants of survival after liver resection for metastatic colorectal carcinoma. Ann Surg. 1992;216:493–504. discussion 504-495
24. Scheele J, Stang R, Altendorf-Hofmann A, Paul M. Resection of colorectal liver metastases. World J Surg. 1995;19:59–71.
25. Vibert E, Bretagnol F, Alves A, et al. Multivariate analysis of predictive factors for early postoperative death after colorectal surgery in patients with colorectal cancer and synchronous unresectable liver metastases. Dis Colon Rectum. 2007;50:1776–82.
26. Abdalla EK, Adam R, Bilchik AJ, et al. Improving resectability of hepatic colorectal metastases: expert consensus statement. Ann Surg Oncol. 2006;13:1271–80.
27. Elias D, Liberale G, Vernerey D, et al. Hepatic and extrahepatic colorectal metastases: when resectable, their localization does not matter, but their total number has a prognostic effect. Ann Surg Oncol. 2005;12:900.
28. Miller G, Biernacki P, Kemeny NE, et al. Outcomes after resection of synchronous or metachronous hepatic and pulmonary colorectal metastases. J Am Coll Surg. 2007;205:231–8.
29. Mise Y, Kopetz S, Mehran RJ, et al. Is complete liver resection without resection of synchronous lung metastases justified? Ann Surg Oncol. 2015;22:1585–92.
30. Headrick JR, Miller DL, Nagorney DM, et al. Surgical treatment of hepatic and pulmonary metastases from colon cancer. Ann Thorac Surg. 2001;71:975–9; discussion 979–980.
31. Carpizo DR, Are C, Jarnagin W, et al. Liver resection for metastatic colorectal cancer in patients with concurrent extrahepatic disease: results in 127 patients treated at a single center. Ann Surg Oncol. 2009;16:2138–46.
32. Minagawa M, Makuuchi M, Torzilli G, et al. Extension of the frontiers of surgical indications in the treatment of liver metastases from colorectal cancer: long-term results. Ann Surg. 2000;231:487–99.
33. Elias D, Ouellet JF, Bellon N, et al. Extrahepatic disease does not contraindicate hepatectomy for colorectal liver metastases. Br J Surg. 2003;90:567–74.
34. Bos JL, Fearon ER, Hamilton SR, et al. Prevalence of ras gene mutations in human colorectal cancers. Nature. 1987;327:293–7.

35. Amado RG, Wolf M, Peeters M, et al. Wild-type KRAS is required for panitumumab efficacy in patients with metastatic colorectal cancer. J Clin Oncol. 2008;26:1626–34.
36. Karapetis CS, Khambata-Ford S, Jonker DJ, et al. K-ras mutations and benefit from cetuximab in advanced colorectal cancer. N Engl J Med. 2008;359:1757–65.
37. Van Cutsem E, Kohne CH, Hitre E, et al. Cetuximab and chemotherapy as initial treatment for metastatic colorectal cancer. N Engl J Med. 2009;360:1408–17.
38. Peeters M, Price TJ, Cervantes A, et al. Randomized phase III study of panitumumab with fluorouracil, leucovorin, and irinotecan (FOLFIRI) compared with FOLFIRI alone as second-line treatment in patients with metastatic colorectal cancer. J Clin Oncol. 2010;28:4706–13.
39. Pereira AA, Rego JF, Morris V, et al. Association between KRAS mutation and lung metastasis in advanced colorectal cancer. Br J Cancer. 2015;112:424–8.
40. Vauthey JN, Kopetz S, Aloia TA, Andreou A. KRAS mutation in colorectal cancer metastases after adjuvant FOLFOX for the primary. Br J Cancer. 2012;107:1442–3; author reply 1444.
41. Vauthey JN, Zimmitti G, Kopetz SE, et al. RAS mutation status predicts survival and patterns of recurrence in patients undergoing hepatectomy for colorectal liver metastases. Ann Surg. 2013;258:619–26; discussion 626–617.
42. Chun YS, Passot G, Yamashita S, et al. Deleterious effect of RAS and evolutionary high-risk TP53 double mutation in colorectal liver metastases. Ann Surg. 2019;269(5):917–23.
43. Yamashita S, Chun YS, Kopetz SE et al. APC and PIK3CA mutational cooperativity predicts pathologic response and survival in patients undergoing resection for colorectal liver metastases. Ann Surg. 2017. PMID: 28379870. [Epub ahead of print].
44. Vauthey JN, Kopetz SE. From multidisciplinary to personalized treatment of colorectal liver metastases: 4 reasons to consider RAS. Cancer. 2013;119:4083–5.
45. Kattan MW, Gonen M, Jarnagin WR, et al. A nomogram for predicting disease-specific survival after hepatic resection for metastatic colorectal cancer. Ann Surg. 2008;247:282–7.
46. Rees M, Tekkis PP, Welsh FK, et al. Evaluation of long-term survival after hepatic resection for metastatic colorectal cancer: a multifactorial model of 929 patients. Ann Surg. 2008;247:125–35.
47. Iwatsuki S, Dvorchik I, Madariaga JR, et al. Hepatic resection for metastatic colorectal adenocarcinoma: a proposal of a prognostic scoring system. J Am Coll Surg. 1999;189:291–9.
48. Malik HZ, Prasad KR, Halazun KJ, et al. Preoperative prognostic score for predicting survival after hepatic resection for colorectal liver metastases. Ann Surg. 2007;246:806–14.
49. Zakaria S, Donohue JH, Que FG, et al. Hepatic resection for colorectal metastases: value for risk scoring systems? Ann Surg. 2007;246:183–91.
50. Schussler-Fiorenza CM, Mahvi DM, Niederhuber J, et al. Clinical risk score correlates with yield of PET scan in patients with colorectal hepatic metastases. J Gastrointest Surg. 2004;8:150–7; discussion 157–158.
51. Jarnagin WR, Conlon K, Bodniewicz J, et al. A clinical scoring system predicts the yield of diagnostic laparoscopy in patients with potentially resectable hepatic colorectal metastases. Cancer. 2001;91:1121–8.
52. Chun YS, Vauthey JN, Ribero D, et al. Systemic chemotherapy and two-stage hepatectomy for extensive bilateral colorectal liver metastases: perioperative safety and survival. J Gastrointest Surg. 2007;11:1498–504; discussion 1504-1495.
53. Passot G, Chun YS, Kopetz SE, et al. Predictors of safety and efficacy of 2-stage hepatectomy for bilateral colorectal liver metastases. J Am Coll Surg. 2016;223:99–108.
54. Cloyd JM, Aloia TA. Hammer versus Swiss Army knife: developing a strategy for the management of bilobar colorectal liver metastases. Surgery. 2017;162:12–7.
55. Gold JS, Are C, Kornprat P, et al. Increased use of parenchymal-sparing surgery for bilateral liver metastases from colorectal cancer is associated with improved mortality without change in oncologic outcome: trends in treatment over time in 440 patients. Ann Surg. 2008;247:109–17.
56. Torzilli G, Procopio F, Botea F, et al. One-stage ultrasonographically guided hepatectomy for multiple bilobar colorectal metastases: a feasible and effective alternative to the 2-stage approach. Surgery. 2009;146:60–71.

57. Passot G, Odisio BC, Zorzi D, et al. Eradication of missing liver metastases after fiducial placement. J Gastrointest Surg. 2016;20:1173–8.
58. Vigano L, Ferrero A, Amisano M, et al. Comparison of laparoscopic and open intraoperative ultrasonography for staging liver tumours. Br J Surg. 2013;100:535–42.
59. Abdalla EK, Vauthey JN, Ellis LM, et al. Recurrence and outcomes following hepatic resection, radiofrequency ablation, and combined resection/ablation for colorectal liver metastases. Ann Surg. 2004;239:818–25; discussion 825-817.
60. Berber E, Pelley R, Siperstein AE. Predictors of survival after radiofrequency thermal ablation of colorectal cancer metastases to the liver: a prospective study. J Clin Oncol. 2005;23:1358–64.
61. Kennedy TJ, Cassera MA, Khajanchee YS, et al. Laparoscopic radiofrequency ablation for the management of colorectal liver metastases: 10-year experience. J Surg Oncol. 2013;107:324–8.
62. Stang A, Fischbach R, Teichmann W, et al. A systematic review on the clinical benefit and role of radiofrequency ablation as treatment of colorectal liver metastases. Eur J Cancer. 2009;45:1748–56.
63. Jaeck D, Oussoultzoglou E, Rosso E, et al. A two-stage hepatectomy procedure combined with portal vein embolization to achieve curative resection for initially unresectable multiple and bilobar colorectal liver metastases. Ann Surg. 2004;240:1037–49; discussion 1049-1051.
64. Broering DC, Hillert C, Krupski G, et al. Portal vein embolization vs. portal vein ligation for induction of hypertrophy of the future liver remnant. J Gastrointest Surg. 2002;6:905–13; discussion 913.
65. Wilms C, Mueller L, Lenk C, et al. Comparative study of portal vein embolization versus portal vein ligation for induction of hypertrophy of the future liver remnant using a mini-pig model. Ann Surg. 2008;247:825–34.
66. Schnitzbauer AA, Lang SA, Goessmann H, et al. Right portal vein ligation combined with in situ splitting induces rapid left lateral liver lobe hypertrophy enabling 2-staged extended right hepatic resection in small-for-size settings. Ann Surg. 2012;255:405–14.
67. Ratti F, Schadde E, Masetti M, et al. Strategies to increase the resectability of patients with colorectal liver metastases: a multi-center case-match analysis of ALPPS and conventional two-stage hepatectomy. Ann Surg Oncol. 2015;22:1933–42.
68. Schadde E, Ardiles V, Robles-Campos R, et al. Early survival and safety of ALPPS: first report of the international ALPPS registry. Ann Surg. 2014;260:829–36; discussion 836-828.
69. Alvarez FA, Ardiles V, de Santibanes M, et al. Associating liver partition and portal vein ligation for staged hepatectomy offers high oncological feasibility with adequate patient safety: a prospective study at a single center. Ann Surg. 2015;261:723–32.
70. Oldhafer KJ, Donati M, Jenner RM, et al. ALPPS for patients with colorectal liver metastases: effective liver hypertrophy, but early tumor recurrence. World J Surg. 2014;38:1504–9.
71. Wicherts DA, Miller R, de Haas RJ, et al. Long-term results of two-stage hepatectomy for irresectable colorectal cancer liver metastases. Ann Surg. 2008;248:994–1005.
72. Kemeny N, Daly J, Reichman B, et al. Intrahepatic or systemic infusion of fluorodeoxyuridine in patients with liver metastases from colorectal carcinoma. A randomized trial. Ann Intern Med. 1987;107:459–65.
73. Boige V, Malka D, Elias D, et al. Hepatic arterial infusion of oxaliplatin and intravenous LV5FU2 in unresectable liver metastases from colorectal cancer after systemic chemotherapy failure. Ann Surg Oncol. 2008;15:219–26.
74. Ducreux M, Ychou M, Laplanche A, et al. Hepatic arterial oxaliplatin infusion plus intravenous chemotherapy in colorectal cancer with inoperable hepatic metastases: a trial of the gastrointestinal group of the Federation Nationale des Centres de Lutte Contre le Cancer. J Clin Oncol. 2005;23:4881–7.
75. Kemeny N, Gonen M, Sullivan D, et al. Phase I study of hepatic arterial infusion of floxuridine and dexamethasone with systemic irinotecan for unresectable hepatic metastases from colorectal cancer. J Clin Oncol. 2001;19:2687–95.
76. Kemeny NE, Melendez FD, Capanu M, et al. Conversion to resectability using hepatic artery infusion plus systemic chemotherapy for the treatment of unresectable liver metastases from colorectal carcinoma. J Clin Oncol. 2009;27:3465–71.

77. Karanicolas PJ, Metrakos P, Chan K, et al. Hepatic arterial infusion pump chemotherapy in the management of colorectal liver metastases: expert consensus statement. Curr Oncol. 2014;21:e129–36.
78. Zacharias AJ, Jayakrishnan TT, Rajeev R, et al. Comparative effectiveness of hepatic artery based therapies for unresectable colorectal liver metastases: a meta-analysis. PLoS One. 2015;10:e0139940.
79. Nordlinger B, Sorbye H, Glimelius B, et al. Perioperative chemotherapy with FOLFOX4 and surgery versus surgery alone for resectable liver metastases from colorectal cancer (EORTC Intergroup trial 40983): a randomised controlled trial. Lancet. 2008;371:1007–16.
80. Allen PJ, Kemeny N, Jarnagin W, et al. Importance of response to neoadjuvant chemotherapy in patients undergoing resection of synchronous colorectal liver metastases. J Gastrointest Surg. 2003;7:109–17.
81. Adams RB, Aloia TA, Loyer E, et al. Selection for hepatic resection of colorectal liver metastases: expert consensus statement. HPB (Oxford). 2013;15:91–103.
82. Blazer DG 3rd, Kishi Y, Maru DM, et al. Pathologic response to preoperative chemotherapy: a new outcome end point after resection of hepatic colorectal metastases. J Clin Oncol. 2008;26:5344–51.
83. Tuma RS. Sometimes size doesn't matter: reevaluating RECIST and tumor response rate endpoints. J Natl Cancer Inst. 2006;98:1272–4.
84. Shindoh J, Loyer EM, Kopetz S, et al. Optimal morphologic response to preoperative chemotherapy: an alternate outcome end point before resection of hepatic colorectal metastases. J Clin Oncol. 2012;30:4566–72.
85. Chun YS, Vauthey JN, Boonsirikamchai P, et al. Association of computed tomography morphologic criteria with pathologic response and survival in patients treated with bevacizumab for colorectal liver metastases. JAMA. 2009;302:2338–44.

Algorithms for Patients with Colorectal Liver Metastasis

12

Orlando Jorge Martins Torres, Marcos Belotto de Oliveira, Paulo Cezar Galvão do Amaral, Eliza Dalsasso Ricardo, Agnaldo Soares Lima, Alexandre Prado de Resende, and Renata D'Alpino Peixoto

Introduction

We introduce a few concepts and their definitions that will be used in this chapter.

Moment of Diagnosis

Colorectal cancer is a potentially lethal disease in which the liver is the most common site of metastasis. By definition, synchronous metastasis (SM) is a condition

O. J. M. Torres (✉)
Department of Gastrointestinal Surgery, Hepatopancreatobiliary Unit—Federal University of Maranhão, São Luís, Brazil

M. B. de Oliveira
Medical Sciences University—Santa Casa de Misericórdia de São Paulo, São Paulo, Brazil

Medical member of Pancreas MDT of the Santa Casa de Misericórdia de São Paulo, São Paulo, Brazil

P. C. G. do Amaral
Department of Gastrointestinal Surgery, San Rafael Hospital, Salvador, Brazil

E. D. Ricardo
Clinical Oncologist, Osvaldo Cruz Hospital, São Paulo, Brazil

A. S. Lima
Department of Gastrointestinal Surgery, Hepatopancreatobiliary Unit, Federal University of Minas Gerais, Belo Horizonte, Brazil
e-mail: agnaldo@gold.com.br

A. P. de Resende
Department of Gastrointestinal Surgery, Mater Dei Hospital, Belo Horizonte, Brazil
e-mail: aresende@gold.com.br

R. D'Alpino Peixoto
Coordinator of Gastrointestinal and Neuroendocrine tumor, Osvaldo Cruz Hospital, São Paulo, Brazil

M. M. Correia et al. (eds.), *Colorectal Cancer Liver Metastases*,
https://doi.org/10.1007/978-3-030-25486-5_12

when the patient presents with metastatic liver disease at the same time of presentation of the primary disease. SM represents unfavorable disease with poor long-term survival. For these patients, the standard approach comprises resection of the colorectal primary tumor, adjuvant chemotherapy, and then resection of the liver tumor. Other approaches are concomitant approach and reverse strategy (Fig. 12.1).

Metachronous liver metastases are classified as *early* metachronous metastases or *late* metachronous metastases depending on whether they have been detected within or more than 12 months after diagnosis or after undergoing a primary colorectal tumor surgery. Resectable metachronous liver metastases may be resected straightforward without the need for chemotherapy, specially when small in size and number. The traditional strategy of treatment is presented in Fig. 12.2.

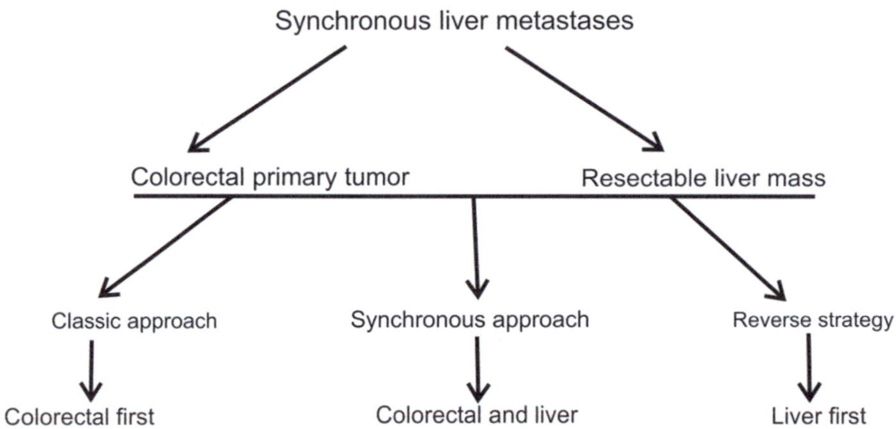

Fig. 12.1 Treatment for synchronous liver metastases

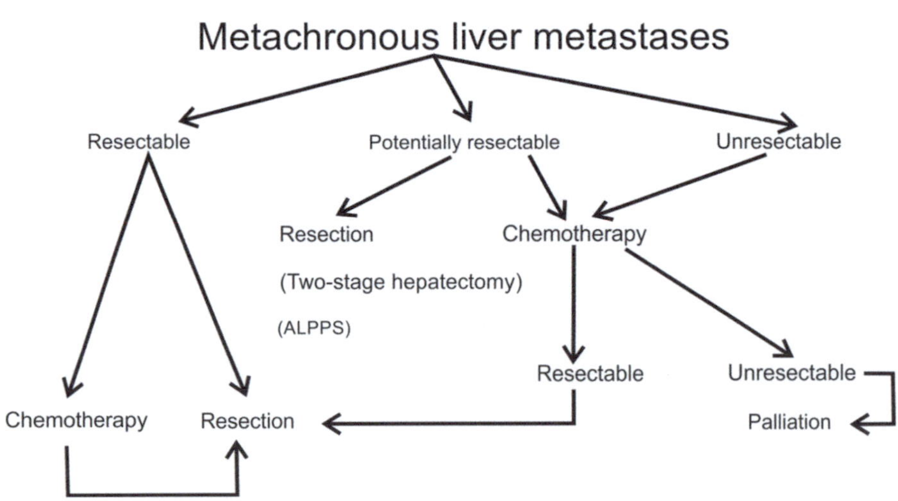

Fig. 12.2 Treatment for metachronous liver metastases

Resectability

Patients with colorectal liver metastasis are classified into three categories at the time of presentation: *resectable, potentially resectable,* and *unresectable*. Each condition is addressed in the following sections.

Synchronous Hepatic Metastases

At the time of diagnosis of colorectal cancer, 20–25% of patients present with metastatic disease [1–4], with the liver being the dominant metastatic site. Synchronous hepatic metastases occur in 15–20% of patients [5], with 70–80% of these cases being liver-limited metastases [6]. The distinction between synchronous and metachronous metastases is not straightforward as most patients who develop metastases after the treatment of primary tumor might have already had them at the time of diagnosis. In fact, by definition, all metastases are synchronous, irrespective of whether they are occult or detectable at the time of diagnosis. Therefore, synchronous colorectal metastases should be defined as those "synchronously" detected with primary tumor.

It has been well known that synchronously detected colorectal metastatic disease carries a worse prognosis [7–9]. Overall survival is lower for patients who are diagnosed with metastases at or within 1 month versus more than 12 months after the primary tumor diagnosis [10, 11]. Indeed, presence of synchronous metastases has been incorporated in prognostic scoring systems for hepatic metastases resection, such as the Fong score [8]. In addition to conferring a more aggressive course than metachronous disease, synchronous liver metastases also add complexity in terms of surgical approach, when indicated. Patients may undergo simultaneous resection of both primary tumor and liver metastases or a staged resection, which includes either colorectal-first (classic) or liver-first (reverse) approach. When simultaneous resection is performed, the liver resection is typically performed first. If, during the liver procedure, a major complication (such as bleeding or clinical instability) occurs or hepatic resection would be greater than planned, the colorectal resection should be postponed and a staged approach adopted instead. When a major hepatectomy is performed (resection of >3 segments), simultaneous resection carries higher morbidity (36.1% versus 15.1%) and mortality (8.3% versus 1.4%) than staged resection. However, several studies have shown that the length of hospital stay and perioperative mortality are similar between simultaneous and staged colorectal metastatic liver resection [12–15]. In addition, simultaneous approach is associated with a significantly lower total cost [16]. Both strategies ensure similar oncological outcomes.

Unfortunately, there is no data from randomized studies to help guide treatment decisions in synchronous colorectal liver metastases that may be candidate for surgery. There is only one general agreement among specialists: multidisciplinary discussion is always necessary. Many factors come into play in synchronous disease, such as disease burden, acuity of symptoms, liver metastases resectability, location of primary tumor, RAS and BRAF status, comorbidities, and age [17]. They may all influence the timing and sequence of surgical resection of the primary tumor and metastases as well as the choice of the chemotherapy regimen.

Most oncologists consider initial chemotherapy for a recently diagnosed resectable synchronous disease in order to assess the cancer biology prior to a surgical attempt. Patients who develop progressive disease during systemic treatment do not benefit from surgery and are consequently spared from it.

In the absence of randomized controlled trials, most recommendations come from experts' opinions, biological rationale, and personal experience [10].

Scenarios

There are six scenarios of synchronous colorectal liver metastases, depending on liver resectability, primary tumor location, and presence of primary tumor symptoms:

Clearly Unresectable—(Not Candidate to Conversion Therapy)—Asymptomatic Primary TUMOR

- Colon or upper rectal cancer: These patients are typically treated with systemic therapy, taking into consideration the choice of chemotherapeutic regimen, the RAS status, BRAF status, performance status, age, and adverse events profile [10]. Primary tumor resection is only indicated for those who develop symptoms, such as bleeding, obstruction, or perforation. Previous studies have demonstrated that 7–20% of patients with metastatic colorectal cancer will eventually require emergent surgical intervention of the primary tumor [18–20]. Nonetheless, there is still no available data from randomized trials regarding the benefits of primary resection in the context of unresectable metastatic disease.
- Middle or lower rectal cancer: The same concepts of systemic therapies apply to rectal primary tumors. In the majority of cases, initiation of chemotherapy should not be postponed in favor of local therapy, given the high response rates with systemic treatment and rarity of rapid progression through first-line regimens. The exception is for patients with a low burden of metastatic disease and a bulky (yet) asymptomatic rectal tumor, in which case there is a high likelihood of long-term overall survival and, therefore, patient may benefit from initial treatment of the primary tumor to prevent symptoms from progressive pelvic disease. In this scenario, traditional chemoradiotherapy with a fluoropyrimidine or short-course radiotherapy is reasonable before initiation of systemic treatment with consideration of surgery at some point. On the other hand, patients with high-volume systemic metastases and a small, asymptomatic rectal tumor are more likely to die of their systemic disease before the primary tumor causes significant symptoms. In such patients, systemic chemotherapy is usually most appropriate, with local pelvic therapy reserved only for palliation, if needed (Fig. 12.3).

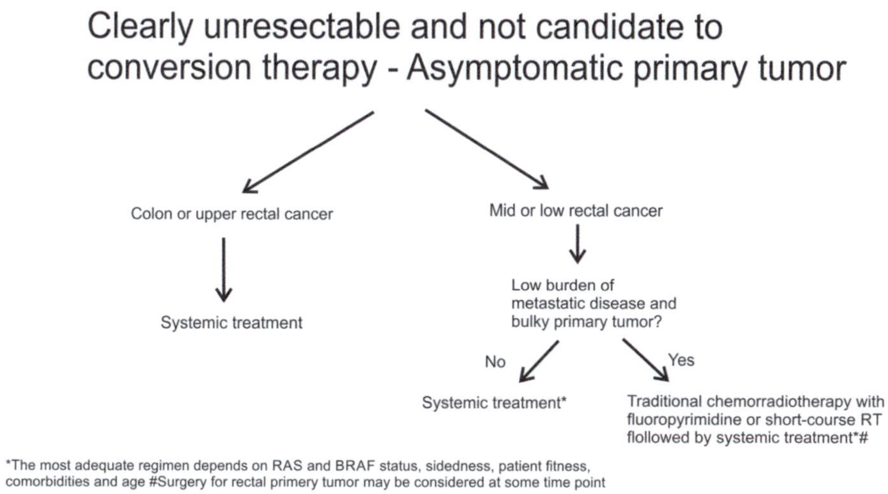

Fig. 12.3 Treatment for clearly unresectable asymptomatic primary tumor

Clearly Unresectable (Not Candidate to Conversion Therapy)—Symptomatic Primary TUMOR

- Colon or upper rectal cancer: These patients should undergo resection of the primary tumor before considering initiation of systemic treatment in order to avoid complications related to the primary tumor. After surgery, systemic chemotherapy is indicated according to RAS status, BRAF status, performance status, age, and adverse events profile [10]. When bevacizumab is considered, there should be at least 6 weeks from surgery to its use due to healing problems.
- Middle or lower rectal cancer: In patients with perforated tumors, immediate surgery is necessary followed by systemic treatment. For those with excessive bleeding, initial chemoradiotherapy or short-course radiotherapy (RT) followed or not by surgery might be preferred before initiation of systemic treatment. However, for patients with obstructive symptoms, the type of surgical intervention depends on the volume of systemic disease. For those with high volume of metastases, confection of a diversion colostomy followed by aggressive systemic treatment is indicated. On the other hand, those with low volume of systemic disease, short-course RT followed by radical surgery and then systemic treatment may be preferred due to better future pelvic control. After primary tumor treatment, systemic therapy should be initiated (Fig. 12.4).

Unresectable (But Potentially Convertible to Resectable)—Asymptomatic Primary Tumor

- Colon or upper rectal cancer: These patients should undergo optimal chemotherapy first (doublets or triplets in combination with biological agents). The best systemic combination therapy depends on RAS and BRAF status, as well as presence of bilaterality. For fit patients and for those with RAS- or

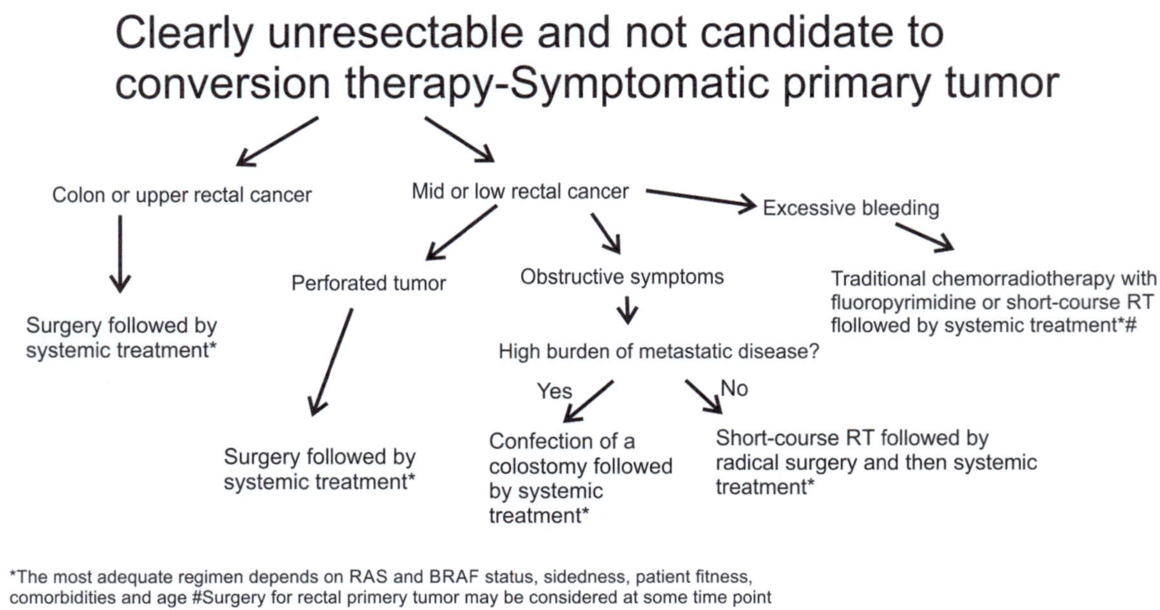

Fig. 12.4 Treatment for clearly unresectable symptomatic primary tumor

BRAF-mutated tumors, a triplet (FOLFOXIRI) with or without bevacizumab is associated with higher response rates. For those with RAS and BRAF wild-type cancers, either a doublet along with anti-EGFR therapy or FOLFOXIRI with or without bevacizumab is indicated [17]. Although data with FOLFOXIRI plus anti-EGFR therapy is very promising for RAS and BRAF wild-type tumors, more studies with this combination are necessary, and so far, it cannot be routinely indicated. Optimal timing for assessment of response to chemotherapy is probably every 8 weeks [17]. As soon as (and if) the liver metastases become resectable, surgery should be performed in order to avoid chemotherapy-induced liver toxicity, which include nonalcoholic steatohepatitis (NASH), steatosis, centrilobular necrosis, and sinusoidal changes [21, 22]. Liver resection should be delayed at least 4 weeks after completion of chemotherapy and panitumumab or cetuximab, and 6–8 weeks if bevacizumab was a component of therapy. The recommendation is for a *reverse* surgical strategy, with resection of the liver metastases before the primary tumor, mainly due to extensive hepatic involvement in this scenario. One-stage surgery should not be performed unless there is limited hepatic disease and an "easy-to-resect" primary tumor. In most retrospective studies, simultaneous procedures included fewer, smaller, and more often unilobar synchronous colorectal liver metastases, which have led to the recommendation that simultaneous procedures should only be pursued when they involve minor hepatic resections, which is usually not the case in patients with initially unresectable disease [23]. Simultaneous procedures with major hepatectomies should be performed only in very carefully selected patients and by an experienced hepatobiliary team.

If complete resection is achieved, most oncologists prefer to complete a total of 6 months of systemic therapy. The only drugs associated with overall survival benefit for micrometastases are fluoropyrimidines and oxaliplatin. Therefore, even though irinotecan and/or targeted therapies were used preoperatively, following surgery we complete 6 months with FOLFOX or XELOX. However, although there are no evidence-based data to support the use of targeted therapies after resection, if a regimen is highly effective in the preoperative setting, the same regimen is used postoperatively.

- Middle or lower rectal cancer: The same concepts of systemic therapies apply to rectal primary tumors. For cT1–2 cN0 rectal primaries, RT is not necessary and the same concepts of colon cancer apply here. However, for bulky, yet asymptomatic rectal primary tumors, as soon as liver metastases become resectable, short-course RT followed by reverse strategy (liver-first surgery followed by primary rectal resection) should be used in order to decrease local recurrence risks. Because rectal procedures are technically more challenging than colon procedures, with a higher risk of morbidity and mortality, most groups prefer a liver-first strategy followed by rectal tumor resection. However, some studies have demonstrated that combined rectal and hepatic resection is safe in high-volume centers [24–26] (Fig. 12.5).

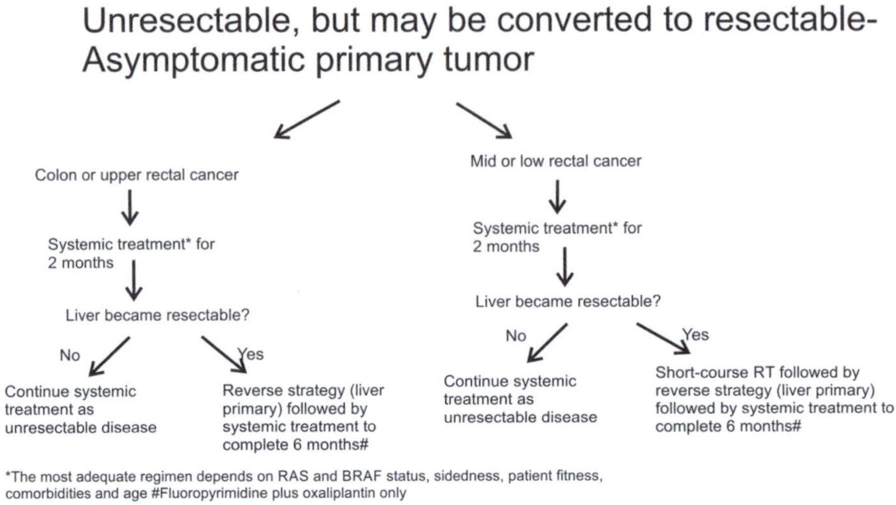

Fig. 12.5 Treatment for unresectable (may be converted to resectable) asymptomatic primary tumor

Unresectable (But Potentially Convertible to Resectable)—Symptomatic Primary Tumor

- Colon or upper rectal cancer: These patients should undergo resection of the primary tumor before considering initiation of conversion systemic treatment in order to avoid complications related to the primary tumor. As soon as liver metastases become resectable, surgery is indicated followed by chemotherapy with fluoropyrimidine and oxaliplatin for a total of 6 months. Simultaneous hepatic resections should not be performed during an emergent colorectal resection for bleeding, perforation, or obstruction, because apart from increased morbidity, they may also lead to a higher chance of distant metastases [26–28].
- Middle or lower rectal cancer: In patients with perforated tumors, immediate surgery is necessary followed by systemic treatment. For those with excessive bleeding, initial chemoradiotherapy or short-course radiotherapy (RT) followed or not by surgery might be preferred before initiation of systemic treatment. However, for patients with obstructive symptoms, the type of surgical intervention depends on the volume of systemic disease. For those with high volume of metastases, confection of a colostomy followed by aggressive systemic treatment is indicated. On the other hand, for those with low volume of systemic disease, short-course RT followed by radical surgery and then systemic treatment may be preferred due to better future pelvic control. After primary tumor treatment, systemic therapy should be initiated (Fig. 12.6).

Resectable Liver Disease and Asymptomatic Primary Tumor

- Colon or upper rectal cancer: There is no "right" approach to integrating systemic chemotherapy with surgical resection of hepatic colorectal metastases that

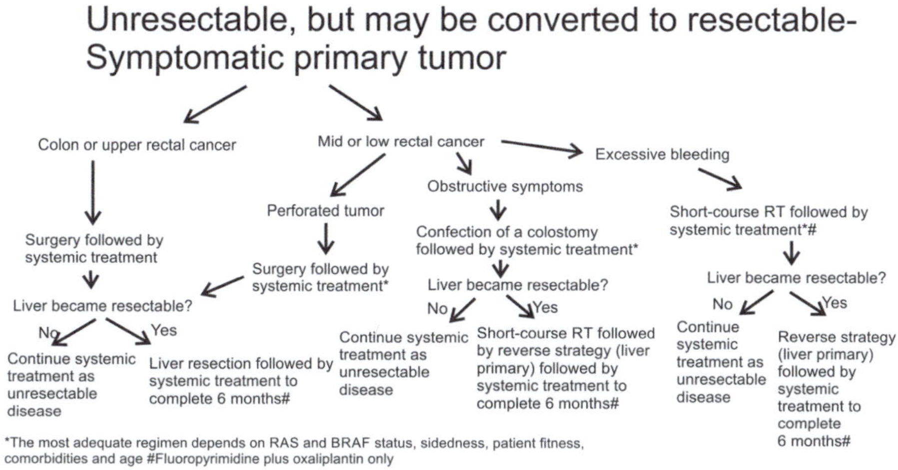

Fig. 12.6 Treatment for unresectable (may be converted to resectable) symptomatic primary tumor

are resectable upfront. At some centers, if the hepatic metastases are resectable and the patient has an asymptomatic primary colon cancer, upfront surgical resection rather than initial chemotherapy may be offered for medically fit patients with fewer metastases. On the other hand, most centers prefer to deliver systemic treatment before surgery, especially in patients who have more than four metastases (unless all are localized to a single lobe), radiographic suspicion for portal node involvement, or bilobar disease [27]. The strategy of starting with systemic treatment (fluoropyrimidine and oxaliplatin) instead of surgery allows the evaluation of the biological behavior of the tumor and futile surgeries are avoided. Patients whose disease progresses while on chemotherapy or who develop extrahepatic disease have biologically aggressive tumors that would not benefit from resection. For resectable liver metastases, most oncologists prescribe a fluoropyrimidine (either 5-FU or capecitabine) with oxaliplatin based on the EORTC trial for a total of 6 months [28–31]. Although the authors study used six cycles of chemotherapy before and after surgery, most oncologists and liver surgeons prefer to deliver four cycles preoperatively followed by restaging in order to avoid chemotherapy-induced liver toxicity. If the disease proves to stabilize or if it responds, surgery is recommended.

- Middle or lower rectal cancer: Initially, patients with cT3/cT4 and/or lymph node positive tumors are preferentially treated with systemic therapy. If patients show partial response or stable disease after three to four cycles of chemotherapy and if liver disease remains resectable, then these patients may be considered candidates for short-course radiotherapy followed by reverse surgical strategy (liver-first approach) and systemic treatment until completing 6 months of treatment. On the other hand, patients with cT1/cT2 and negative lymph node tumors should be initially treated with systemic treatment (fluoropyrimidine and

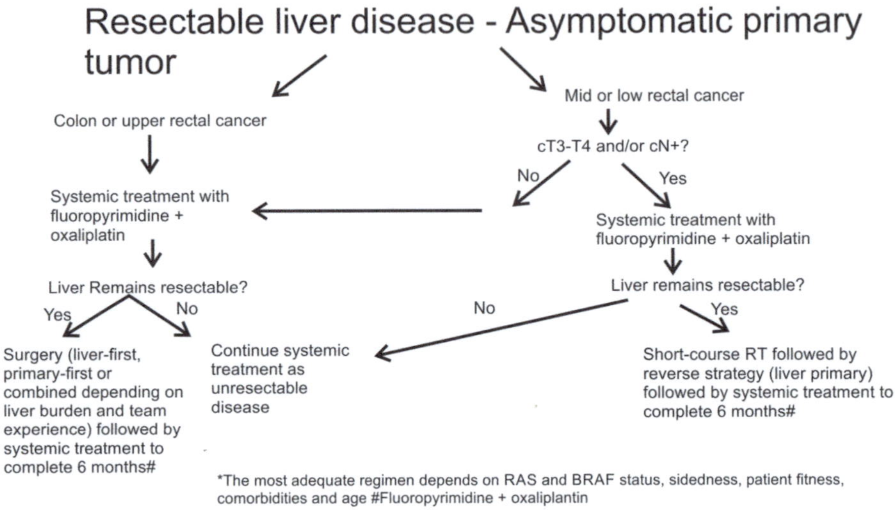

Fig. 12.7 Treatment for resectable liver disease—asymptomatic primary tumor

oxaliplatin). If patients show partial response or stable disease after three to four cycles of chemotherapy and if liver disease remains resectable, then these patients may be considered candidates for reverse surgical strategy (liver-first approach) followed by systemic chemotherapy until completing 6 months of treatment (Fig. 12.7).

Resectable Liver Disease and Symptomatic Primary Tumor

- Colon or upper rectal cancer: These patients should undergo resection of the primary tumor before considering initiation of systemic treatment with fluoropyrimidine and oxaliplatin in order to avoid complications related to the primary tumor. Liver resection can be performed concomitantly in "easy cases"—low burden, colonic primary, or easily resectable upper rectum cases. In other cases, CT should be started after resection of the primary tumor. If there is no progression of the disease after three or four cycles of chemotherapy, then liver metastasectomy should be performed followed by completion of systemic treatment for up to 6 months. Utilizing the liver-first approach may delay resection of the primary tumor and increase the risk of developing complications related to the colorectal tumor [18, 19, 31–33].
- Middle or lower rectal cancer: If the patient presents with a perforated tumor, immediate surgery of the primary lesion should be performed followed by systemic treatment with fluoropyrimidine and oxaliplatin. If there is no evidence of failure to control the disease after three to four cycles of chemotherapy, hepatic metastasectomy should be performed followed by completion of 6 months of chemotherapy. However, if the initial presentation is an obstructive tumor, a diversion colostomy should be performed immediately followed by systemic treatment. If there is no disease progression after three to four cycles of

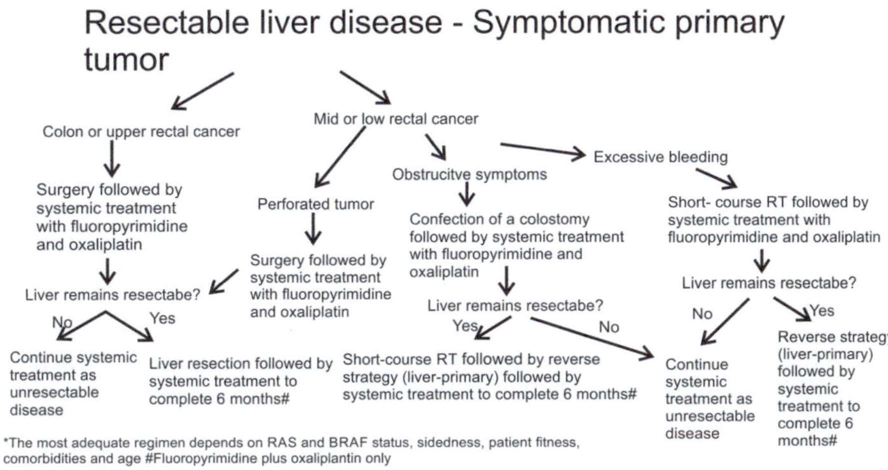

Fig. 12.8 Treatment for resectable liver disease—symptomatic primary tumor

chemotherapy, short-course radiotherapy should be indicated. After that, a reverse strategy (liver-first approach and then the primary tumor) should be performed and, at last, systemic treatment with fluoropyrimidine and oxaliplatin should be carried out until the completion of 6 months. On the other hand, if the main symptom is excessive bleeding, then short-course radiotherapy followed by systemic treatment with fluoropyrimidine and oxaliplatin is preferable. However, if the metastatic disease in the liver remains resectable, the patient should undergo surgery with a reverse strategy (liver-first approach and then the rectal primary tumor) followed by systemic treatment until the completion of 6 months (Fig. 12.8).

References

1. Lykoudis PM, O'Reilly D, Nastos K, Fusai G. Systematic review of surgical management of synchronous colorectal liver metastases. Br J Surg. 2014;101(6):605–12.
2. Nordlinger B, Van Cutsem E, Gruenberger T, Glimelius B, Poston G, Rougier P, et al. Combination of surgery and chemotherapy and the role of targeted agents in the treatment of patients with colorectal liver metastases: recommendations from an expert panel. Ann Oncol. 2009;20(6):985–92.
3. Nordlinger B, Van Cutsem E, Rougier P, Köhne CH, Ychou M, Sobrero A, et al. Does chemotherapy prior to liver resection increase the potential for cure in patients with metastatic colorectal cancer? A report from the European Colorectal Metastases Treatment Group. Eur J Cancer. 2007;43(14):2037–45.
4. Simmonds PC, Primrose JN, Colquitt JL, Garden OJ, Pos-ton GJ, Rees M. Surgical resection of hepatic metastases from colorectal cancer: a systematic review of published studies. Br J Cancer. 2006;94(7):982–99.
5. Borner MM. Neoadjuvant chemotherapy for unresectable liver metastases of colorectal cancer–too good to be true? Ann Oncol. 1999;10(6):623–6.

6. Manfredi S, Lepage C, Hatem C, Coatmeur O, Faivre J, Bouvier AM. Epidemiology and management of liver metastases from colorectal cancer. Ann Surg. 2006;244(2):254–9.
7. Nordlinger B, Guiguet M, Vaillant JC, Balladur P, Boudjema K, Bachellier P, et al. Surgical resection of colorectal carcinoma metastases to the liver. A prognostic scoring system to improve case selection, based on 1568 patients. Association Française de Chirurgie. Cancer. 1996;77(7):1254–62.
8. Fong Y, Fortner J, Sun RL, Brennan MF, Blumgart LH. Clinical score for predicting recurrence after hepatic resection for metastatic colorectal cancer: analysis of 1001 consecutive cases. Ann Surg. 1999;230(3):309–18.
9. Iwatsuki S1, Dvorchik I, Madariaga JR, Marsh JW, Dodson F, Bonham AC, et al. Hepatic resection for metastatic colorectal adenocarcinoma: a proposal of a prognostic scoring system. J Am Coll Surg. 1999;189(3):291–9.
10. Adam R, de Gramont A, Figueras J, Kokudo N, Kunstlinger F, Loyer E, et al. Managing synchronous liver metastases from colorectal cancer: a multidisciplinary international consensus. Cancer Treat Rev. 2015;41(9):729–41.
11. Andres A, Toso C, Adam R, Barroso E, Hubert C, Capus- sotti L, et al. A survival analysis of the liver-first reversed management of advanced simultaneous colorectal liver metastases: a Liver- MetSurvey-Based Study. Ann Surg. 2012;256(5):772–9.
12. Martin R, Paty P, Fong Y, Grace A, Cohen A, DeMatteo R, et al. Simultaneous liver and colorectal resections are safe for synchronous colorectal liver metastasis. J Am Coll Surg. 2003;197(2):233.
13. Lyass S, Zamir G, Matot I, Goitein D, Eid A, Jurim O. Combined colon and hepatic resection for synchronous colorectal liver metastases. J Surg Oncol. 2001;78(1):17.
14. Martin RC 2nd, Augenstein V, Reuter NP, Scoggins CR, McMasters KM. Simultaneous versus staged resection for synchronous colorectal cancer liver metastases. J Am Coll Surg. 2009;208(5):842.
15. Reddy SK, Pawlik TM, Zorzi D, Gleisner AL, Ribero D, Assumpcao L, et al. Simultaneous resections of colorectal cancer and synchronous liver metastases: a multi-institutional analysis. Ann Surg Oncol. 2007;14(12):3481.
16. Le Souder EB, Azin A, Hirpara DH, Walker R, Cleary S, Quereshy F. Considering the cost of a simultaneous versus staged approach to resection of colorectal cancer with synchronous liver metastases in a publicly funded healthcare model. J Surg Oncol. 2018;117(7):1376–85.
17. Van Cutsem E, Cervantes A, Adam R, Sobrero A, Van Krieken JH, Aderka D, et al. ESMO consensus guidelines for the management of patients with metastatic colorectal cancer. Ann Oncol. 2016;27(8):1386–422.
18. Poultsides GA, Servais EL, Saltz LB, Patil S, Kemeny NE, Guillem JG, et al. Outcome of primary tumor in patients with synchronous stage IV colorectal cancer receiving combination chemotherapy without surgery as initial treatment. J Clin Oncol. 2009;27(20):3379–84.
19. McCahill LE, Yothers G, Sharif S, Petreli NJ, Lai LL, Bechar N, et al. Primary mFOLFOX6 plus bevacizumab without resection of the primary tumor for patients presenting with surgically unresectable metastatic colon cancer and an intact asymptomatic colon cancer: definitive analysis of NSABP trial C-10. J Clin Oncol. 2012;30(26):3223–8.
20. Ruo L, Gougoutas C, Paty PB, Guillem JG, Cohen AM, Wong WD. Elective bowel resection for incurable stage IV colorectal cancer: prognostic variabelsfor asymptomatic patients. J Am Coll Surg. 2003;196(5):722–8.
21. Karoui M, Penna C, Amin-Hashem M, Mitry E, Benoist S, Franc B, et al. Influence of preoperative chemotherapy on the risk of major hepatectomy for colorectal liver metastases. Ann Surg. 2006;243(1):1–7.
22. Nordlinger B, Benoist S. Benefits and risks of neoadjuvant therapy for liver metastases. J Clin Oncol. 2006;24(31):4954–5.
23. Mentha G, Majno P, Terraz S, Rubbia Brandt L, Gervaz P, Andres A, et al. Treatment strategies for the management of advanced colorectal liver metastases detected synchronously with the primary tumour. Eur J Sur Oncol. 2007;33(2):S76–83.

24. Boostrom SY, Vassiliki LT, Nagorney DM, Wolff BG, Chua HK, et al. Synchronous rectal and hepatic resection of rectal metastatic disease. J Gastrointest Sur. 2011;15(9):1583–8.
25. Martin R, Paty PB, Fong Y, Grace A, DeMatteo R, et al. Simultaneous liver and colorectal resections are safe for synchronous colorectal liver metastasis. J Am Coll Surg. 2003;197(2):233–42.
26. Adam R. Colorectal cancer with synchronous liver metastases. Br J Sur. 2007;94(2):129–31.
27. Kopetz S, Vauthey JN. Perioperative chemotherapy for resectable hepatic metastases. Lancet. 2008;371(9617):963–5.
28. Nordlinger B, Sorbye H, Glimelius B, Poston GL, Schlag PM, Rougier P, et al. Perioperative chemotherapy with FOLFOX4 and surgery versus surgery alone for resectable liver metastases from colorectal cancer (EORTC Intergroup trial 40983): a randomised controlled trial. Lancet Oncol. 2013;14(12):1208–15.
29. Coimbra FJF, Ribeiro HSC, Marques MC, Herman P, Chojniak R, Kali AN, Wiermann EG, Cavallero SRA, Coelho FF, Fernandes PHS, Silvestrini AA, Almeida MFA, Araujo ALE, Pitombo M, Teixeira HB, Waechter FL, Ferreira FG, Diniz AL, D'Ippolito G, Begnami MDFS, Prolla G, Balzan SMP, Oliveira TB, Szultan LA, Lendoire J, Torres OJM. First Brazilian consensus on multimodal treatment of colorectal liver metastases. Module 1: pre-treatment evaluation. ABCD Arq Bras Cir Dig. 2015;28(4):222–30.
30. Ribeiro HSC, Torres OJM, Marques MC, Herman P, Kalil AN, Fernandes ESM, Oliveira FF, Castro LS, Hanriot R, Oliveira SCR, Boff MF, Costa Junior WL, Gil RA, Pfiffer TEF, Makdissi FF, Rocha MS, Amaral PCG, Costa LAGA, Aloia TA, D'Albuquerque LAC, Coimbra FJF. First Brazilian consensus on multimodal treatment of colorectal liver metastases. Module 2: approach to resectable metastases. ABCD Arq Bras Cir Dig. 2016;29(1):9–13.
31. Torres OJM, Marques MC, Santos FN, Farias IC, Coutinho AK, Oliveira CVC, Kalil AN, Mello CAL, Kruger JAP, Fernandes GS, Quireze Junior C, Murad AM, Barros e Silva MJ, Zurstrassen CE, Freitas HC, Cruz MR, Weschenfelder R, Linhares MM, Castro LS, Volmmer C, Dixon E, Ribeiro HSC, Coimbra FJF. First Brazilian consensus on multimodal treatment of colorectal liver metastases. Module 3: controversies and unresectable metastases. ABCD Arq Bras Cir Dig. 2016;29(3):173–9.
32. Jegatheeswaran S, Mason JM, Hancock HC, Siriwardena AK. The liver-first approach to the management of colorectal cancer with synchronous hepatic metastases. JAMA Surg. 2013;148(4):385–91.
33. Temraz S, Mukherji D, Shamseddine A. Sequencing of treatment in metastatic colorectal cancer: where to fit the target? World J Gastroenterol. 2014;20(8):1993–04.

Treatment Options for Resectable Colorectal Liver Metastases in the Presence of Extrahepatic Disease

13

Kimberly A. Bertens, Jad Abou Khalil, and Guillaume Martel

Traditionally, extrahepatic disease (EHD) was considered a contraindication to resection of colorectal liver metastases (LM) [1, 2]. Nevertheless, widespread improvement in surgical morbidity and mortality, as well as improved efficacy of chemotherapeutic agents, has driven increased interest in surgical metastasectomy with the intent of improved survival and potential cure [3, 4]. In patients that undergo complete resection of LM and EHD, recurrence is expected 80–95% of the time [5–8]. Therefore, recurrence is the norm, and care must be taken to select patients who are most likely to benefit from surgical resection. However, recent evidence has shown that long-term survival is possible in selected patients with resected LM and EHD.

Various factors have been found to be predictive of a poor outcome in this patient population. Having multiple sites of EHD predicts worse survival, and the total number of metastatic lesions (both within the liver and outside) is inversely related to survival [3, 5, 9]. Other factors that have been shown to be negative predictors of long-term survival in patients with LM and synchronous EHD are size of LM > 3 cm, more than five LM, and disease progression on neoadjuvant therapy [6]. In the largest meta-analysis to date, patients with more than one site of EHD had a median survival of only 17 months, which is comparable to chemotherapy alone [9]. Incomplete surgical resection with both microscopic (R1) and grossly (R2) positive margins also precludes long-term survival and should be avoided [5, 8, 9].

This chapter endeavors to review the clinical evidence behind metastasectomy in the setting of LM and EHD and to provide clinical guidelines on when surgery should be considered.

K. A. Bertens (✉) · J. Abou Khalil · G. Martel
Department of Surgery, The Ottawa Hospital, Ottawa, ON, Canada
e-mail: kbertens@toh.ca; jaboukhalil@toh.ca; gumartel@toh.ca

M. M. Correia et al. (eds.), *Colorectal Cancer Liver Metastases*,
https://doi.org/10.1007/978-3-030-25486-5_13

Pulmonary Metastases

Background

The lung is the second most common location of metastases in patients with colorectal cancer (CRC) after the liver, and the most common extra-abdominal site. During the course of their disease, 10–20% of patients will develop pulmonary metastases (PM), with synchronous presentation being most common [10–12]. Isolated PM is a less common situation occurring only 2–8% of the time [11, 13]. Patients with rectal cancer have a higher likelihood of developing lung metastases in comparison to those with a colon primary. It is important to note that only a small proportion of patients with PM have disease amenable to surgical resection, as the majority present with multiple, bilateral nodules, or have limited pulmonary function that impedes their ability to tolerate extensive surgery.

Evidence for Pulmonary Metastasectomy

Historically, untreated patients with metastatic CRC have a median survival of 8 months [14]. Although modern chemotherapy has prolonged the median overall survival (OS) to 24–28 months, 5-year survival in the absence of surgery remains rare [15]. These less-than ideal results generated interest in surgical metastasectomy in patients with isolated PM from CRC [16]. A multitude of predominantly retrospective studies have demonstrated favorable 5-year OS of 27–68% in patients who underwent pulmonary metastasectomy for isolated PM [17–20]. However, it deserves mention that pulmonary metastasectomy for CRC has been criticized by some individuals who raise concerns regarding the inherent selection bias of small retrospective series, and a positive citation bias, with studies that show benefit being cited more frequently [21–23]. There is no doubt that the patients with CRC who benefit from pulmonary resection are a highly selected group, and meticulous patient selection likely factors in the positive results seen with PM. In an attempt to better address the question of whether pulmonary metastasectomy is beneficial to the population at large, a multicenter, randomized control trial of lung resection versus active monitoring is currently underway, with an estimated completion date of 2020 [24, 25].

Pulmonary and Hepatic Metastases

The focus of this chapter is the management of LM in the setting of EHD. Traditionally, extrapulmonary sites of disease were considered a contraindication to lung resection. However, over the past decade, this dogma has been challenged. Therefore, it is worthwhile to review the evidence for lung resection specifically in the setting of synchronous or metachronous liver metastases (LM) (Table 13.1). The 5-year OS for patients with resected liver and lung metastases ranged from 20% to 61% (all studies in the table).

In a study using the LiverMetSurvey registry, patients with resected, isolated LM were compared to those who had both LM and PM resected, and those who had LM resected with unresected PM. There was no statistically significant difference in 5-year

Table 13.1 Retrospective studies of patients undergoing resection for metastatic CRC to both liver and lungs

First author	Year	Sample size (*n*)	Median survival (months)	5-year overall survival (%)
Kobayashi [26]	1999	47	NR	31
Nagakura [27]	2001	27	NR	27
Mineo [28]	2003	29	41	51
Shah [29]	2006	39	42	NR
Miller [30]	2007	131	40	31
Takahashi [31]	2007	30	39	58
Lee [32]	2008	32	NR	61
Barlow [33]	2009	16	17	20
Neeff [34]	2009	44	NR	42
Limmer [35]	2010	17	98	55
Brouquet [36]	2011	112	NR	50
Gonzalez [37]	2012	27	46	39
Andres [38]	2015	149	NR	45
Leung [6]	2017	57	54	32
Rajakannu [7]	2018	150	76	60

NR not reported

OS between the patients with resected liver-only disease and those with resected lung and liver metastases (51.5% versus 44.5%, $p = 0.08$); however, the patients with unresected PM had a significantly worse 5-year OS (14.3%, $p = 0.001$) [38]. A recent meta-analysis by Hwang et al. summarized the outcomes of patients with CRC and EHD. The authors demonstrated that patients with PM had a median survival of 45 months, which was superior to that for patients with peritoneal carcinomatosis (PC) (29 months) and lymph nodes outside of the primary drainage basin (26 months) [39].

Patients with hepatic and pulmonary metastases that are limited and amenable to resection have a favorable outcome, which is comparable to patients with resected isolated liver disease. Nevertheless, recurrence is common, which explains the discrepancy between disease-free survival (DFS) and OS in many studies [7, 28]. A 10-year OS of up to 35% has been reported, and recent studies have demonstrated that 20% of patients undergoing both hepatic and pulmonary resection for CRC can achieve long-term cure [7].

Mediastinal and/or Hilar Lymph Node Metastases

Generally, most surgeons do not undertake systematic lymph node dissection at the time of pulmonary metastasectomy [40]. The prevalence of lymph node metastases (LNM) in patients undergoing PM is 22.4% [41]. LNM are more often detected in patients with rectal cancer as compared to colon cancer, patients requiring anatomical lung resections, and those with greater number of lung metastases [20, 41]. There are conflicting results with regards to whether having LNM independently portends a worse survival, and there is no compelling evidence that removal of clinically negative nodes improves survival in patients undergoing PM [20, 41]. Still, many studies demonstrate inferior outcomes in patients with clinically positive mediastinal or hilar lymph nodes, and surgical resection should be recommended with caution in this patient population [20, 41].

Prognostic Factors

Various prognostic indicators for poor survival in the setting of PM have been reported in the literature. Significant discrepancy between the various small retrospective studies exists, and a universally accepted risk score has not been established. Rectal primary has been shown to be predictive of worse OS than colon primary [20, 41, 42]. The timing of disease presentation is important, with both synchronous disease and a short disease-free interval (<24 months) between the first and second metastasectomies being independently predictive of worse survival [7, 30, 31]. An elevated pre-lung resection carcinoembryonic antigen (CEA) level has been demonstrated to be negatively prognostic in both isolated PM and hepatic and pulmonary metastases, although the absolute cut-off value differs between studies [7, 31, 42, 43]. There have been conflicting results regarding the significance of the number of lung metastases, with some studies demonstrating equitable survival regardless of the number of lung lesions [29, 32, 41, 43, 44]. In a recent study of 150 patients with both PM and LM, no LM-related factor was independently predictive of survival, indicating that PM, being the more distant metastases, may be the driving factor of prognosis [7].

Conclusion

In the setting of previously resected or resectable LM, surgery should be offered to patients with limited pulmonary metastases that are amenable to surgical metastasectomy. Recurrence postsurgery is commonplace, but nevertheless, cure can be achieved in this patient population [7]. Although not an absolute contraindication to surgical resection, patients with mediastinal lymph node metastases, multiple bilateral pulmonary nodules, short disease-free interval, and more than one site of EHD should be cautiously considered prior to embarking on surgical resection. In patients with risk factors predicting poor outcome, chemotherapy should be considered prior to selection for surgery. If a patient presents with synchronous lung and liver metastases, there is no evidence to recommend which organ should be resected first. However, it would be reasonable to recommend resecting the organ with the greatest burden of disease first, because if an R0 resection cannot be achieved, resection of the other site is strongly discouraged.

Peritoneal Metastases

Background

Both the peritoneal surface and the liver are common sites of spread of colon cancer; however, only a small subset of patients present with both peritoneal carcinomatosis (PC) and LM. In a Dutch review of patients with CRC, only 2% had both PC and LM [45]. It is more common for patients with PC to also have LM (34%), whereas only 11% of those with LM had concomitant PC [45]. The median OS in the patient population with both LM and PC in the absence of curative-intent treatment is 5 months [45].

Evidence for Resection of Peritoneal Disease

Within the medical community, concern has been raised about the paucity of phase III trials to support benefit to cytoreductive surgery and hyperthermic intraperitoneal chemotherapy (HIPEC). There has been one randomized trial published consisting of 105 patients comparing standard approach (systemic chemotherapy +/−palliative surgery) to aggressive cytoreduction with HIPEC followed by systemic chemotherapy [46]. This trial demonstrated improved survival in those who underwent cytoreduction and HIPEC (22.3 versus 12.6 months, $p = 0.032$); however, the authors cautioned that patients with involvement of six or more regions of the abdominal cavity, and those who had grossly inadequate cytoreduction, had a dismal prognosis [46]. The PRODIGE 7 trial, which as of the time of print, has only been published in abstract form is a randomized trial comparing cytoreductive surgery and HIPEC with oxaliplatin to cytoreductive surgery alone. The authors report no difference in median OS between the HIPEC and non-HIPEC arms (41.7 versus 41.2 months, $p = 0.995$) [47]. Despite the scarcity of randomized trials, a multitude of observational trials support the principle that in highly selected patients, resection of PC combined with HIPEC results in increased survival over palliative treatments alone, and median OS of 21–63 months has been reported [48, 49]. The American Society of Peritoneal Surface Malignancies (ASPSM) multi-institutional study reported a median OS of up to 86 months and a 5-year OS of 58% in patients with favorable histology and minimal burden of disease [48]. Liver resection of CRC metastasis has also been demonstrated to increase survival over palliative treatments and is accepted as standard of care. However, the treatment of LM in the setting of PC still presents a clinical conundrum.

Peritoneal Disease in the Presence of Hepatic Metastases

There are no randomized trials to inform clinicians on the benefit of resection of LM and PC in patients with CRC, but observational series suggest a potential benefit over palliative treatments in select patients. Leung et al. identified 33 patients with concomitant LM and PC treated over a 10-year time period—the median OS was 40 months and the 5-year OS was 42% [6]. In a case–control study, 37 patients with both PC and LM treated with liver resection, and cytoreductive surgery with HIPEC, were matched to 61 patients with PC alone. The 3-year OS was significantly lower in those with both LM and PC (40% versus 66%. $p = 0.04$) [50]. In this small series, independent predictors of lower survival included a high peritoneal carcinomatosis index (PCI) (>12), the presence of LM, positive nodal status, and patients not receiving adjuvant chemotherapy [50]. The authors concluded that patients with limited PC and less than three LM stood to benefit the most from an attempt at curative surgical resection. Conversely, a small non-matched comparison of 16 patients with treated PC and LM and 39 patients with treated PC without hepatic involvement showed no difference in survival between the groups (median OS 36 months) [51]. However, the lower PCI scores and shorter procedural duration in the group with hepatic involvement reveal the highly selected nature of this cohort and significant potential for selection bias. A similar study comparing 36 patients with treated PC and LM and 42 patients with treated PC in the absence of LM showed median OS of 24 and 46 months, respectively, with more than three LM and more than seven PCI being associated with decreased survival [52]. A systematic review and meta-analysis of these and other published cohorts failed to demonstrate a statistically significant improved OS in patients with PC and LM from CRC treated with curative-intent surgery compared to palliative chemotherapy (HR 1.24, 95%CI 0.96–1.60) [53].

The unexpected finding of PC at the time of a planned liver resection of LM from CRC is another clinical conundrum for which high-level evidence to guide clinical decision-making is lacking. A French study suggested that intraoperative discovery of unexpected PC occurs in 3% of patients undergoing liver resection for CRC [54]. In this series, only patients found to have very minimal peritoneal disease (PCI < 2) underwent curative-intent surgery; this highly selected group had a median OS of 42 months and 5-year OS of 18% [54].

Conclusion

Although long-term survival is possible with curative-intent treatment of PC and LM, the benefit of aggressive surgical intervention appears to be limited to a highly selected group of patients with minimal disease burden. Although clinical factors such as less than 12 PCI and less than three liver metastases have been proposed as selection criteria, the exact criteria beyond which the survival benefit of curative-intent surgery exceeds the risk of added morbidity have yet to be defined or prospectively validated.

Metastases to Abdominal Lymph Nodes

Background

Colorectal cancer LM can spread to locoregional lymph nodes, including porta hepatis nodes, and from there to more distant celiac, para-aortic and retroperitoneal lymph nodes [55]. This phenomenon of "remetastasis" has traditionally been associated with extremely poor prognosis and has largely been considered a contraindication to curative hepatic resection [56, 57]. With the advent of modern chemotherapeutic regimens, numerous investigators have reexamined the role of curative liver resection in the context of lymph node metastasis (LNM). More specifically, the recent literature has focused upon three main questions: (1) the role of routine porta hepatis lymphadenectomy, (2) the management of macroscopic porta hepatis LNM identified preoperatively, or intraoperatively, and (3) the management of celiac, para-aortic and retroperitoneal LNM.

Occult Porta Hepatis Lymph Node Metastases

The incidence of occult microscopic porta hepatis LNM from metastatic CRC has been estimated at 11–27% [58–62]. These data have been derived largely from series where a prophylactic porta hepatis lymphadenectomy was carried out systematically in all patients undergoing liver resection. Elias et al. conducted one of the first such studies, where 100 consecutive patients underwent curative liver resection and wide lymphadenectomy along the porta hepatis and celiac artery [58]. None of these patients had macroscopic or palpable metastatic lymph nodes. The authors reported that 14% of patients had microscopically involved metastatic lymph nodes, most commonly along the transverse portion of the common hepatic artery. Microscopic lymph node involvement was noted to be associated with the number of liver metastases, a higher CEA level, and the extent of hepatectomy required.

Similarly, Laurent et al. reported a 15% incidence of occult lymph node metastasis among 156 patients undergoing curative-intent liver resection for colorectal metastasis [63]. Disease recurrence occurred in 91% among those with microscopic lymph node disease, compared to 59% among those without lymph node involvement ($p = 0.003$). The 5-year overall survival was significantly worse among those with lymph node involvement (43% vs. 5%, $p < 0.001$).

In contrast to the above data, Grobmyer et al. examined perihepatic lymph nodes in 100 consecutive patients with both LM and primary hepatic tumors, some of whom had preoperative suspicion of nodal involvement [60]. Among those, 15% had metastatic lymph nodes, of which 87% had suspicion of involvement on preoperative CT and/or PET scan, while the other 13% were clinically palpable at surgical exploration. Among those patients with negative preoperative CT and PET scans, as well as negative manual exploration, none had microscopically involved lymph nodes. Thus, the authors argued against routine lymph node harvest in the context of negative preoperative CT and PET scans. Rather, a recommendation for selective sampling was made. These recommendations must be interpreted in the context of a more recent multicenter randomized controlled trial that demonstrated that the routine use of PET scan prior to liver resection was largely ineffective at altering surgical management [64].

Portal Versus Retroperitoneal Lymph Node Metastases

The oncologic outcomes of liver resection for colorectal metastasis with concomitant metastatic lymph node excision have been widely studied. In a recent systematic review, Hadden et al. identified 21 relevant publications pertaining to 559 patients with nodal disease [9]. Proportional meta-analysis of these manuscripts revealed pooled 3-year and 5-year OS of 35% (95% CI 29–41%, $I^2 = 15\%$) and 15% (95% CI 11–20%, $I^2 = 27\%$), respectively. The authors argued that these data support the use of radical surgery for colorectal liver metastases with concomitant LNM, as pooled survival outcomes exceeded those reported in modern series of patients receiving systemic chemotherapy alone. An acknowledged limitation of this paper was the inability to pool for oncologic differences between distinct lymph node basins (i.e., portal pedicle vs. para-aortic).

More recently, Leung et al. have reported their 10-year data on 219 patients who underwent liver resection with concurrent EHD treated with resection [6]. A total of 40 (18%) patients had portal LNM, defined as nodes along the hepatic artery proper, portal vein, and common hepatic artery. In this series, patients with portal LNM had a median OS of 24 months, as well as 3- and 5-year OS rates of 32% and 14%, respectively. No patient survived to 10 years following resection. Portal LNM was identified as an extrahepatic disease site carrying a particularly poor prognosis. A clinical risk score was devised, including liver metastases >3 cm, having more than five liver metastases, and site of EHD (portal/retroperitoneal nodes or multiple sites). Patients with 3/3 clinical risk points all died or recurred within 6 months and had a median recurrence-free survival of 1.4 months. The authors of this paper thus argued that liver resection with concurrent EHD resection should be highly selected, particularly as it pertains to patients with metastatic portal lymph nodes. It may be particularly inadvisable to pursue resection in patients with 3/3 clinical risk points.

Jaeck et al. were the first to differentiate oncologic outcomes between those with metastatic lymph nodes located in the porta hepatis and celiac axis, arguing that liver resection should only be considered among those with porta hepatis nodal involvement and not among those with celiac disease (3-year overall survival 38% versus 1-year OS 0%) [61]. Similarly, Adam et al. reported on 47 patients who had concurrent liver resection and regional LNM [65]. Not surprisingly, OS was significantly worse among patients with LNM (5-year overall survival 53% versus 18%, $p < 0.001$). More importantly, lymph node location strongly affected survival: those with porta hepatis lymph nodes achieved a 5-year overall survival of 25% compared to those with both celiac and para-aortic nodes, whose overall survival is 0% ($p = 0.001$).

Another multi-institutional study reported data on 171 patients who had a liver resection and extrahepatic metastasectomy [5]. Among those, 41 had portal LNM, leading to a median OS of 23 months and 3-year and 5-year OS of 43% and 27%, respectively. Most importantly, this study separated portal from aortocaval LNM, reporting a significantly different median survival of 13 months, 3-year OS of 22%, and 5-year OS of 7% ($p = 0.001$). In light of the above series, it is interesting to note that the recent series by Leung et al. did not find a difference in survival between patients who had portal versus retroperitoneal LNM [6]. This finding is inconsistent with that of other series. It may be related to varying definitions of anatomic lymph node locations, as it can sometimes be difficult to differentiate between lymph node sites within retrospective surgical datasets.

Conclusion

In summary, the possibility of LNM, particularly within the porta hepatis, should be considered in every patient undergoing liver resection for CRC metastases. A thorough preoperative imaging assessment of lymph nodes draining the liver is recommended for every patient. Routine systematic lymph node harvest is unlikely to be necessary in the context of modern imaging techniques. Liver resection should be considered selectively in patients with porta hepatis LNM who also have a limited disease burden within the liver and no additional sites of EHD. Liver resection cannot be recommended in the context of retroperitoneal/para-aortic/celiac lymph node metastases, or among patients with additional sites of EHD.

Other Sites of Disease

Background

CRC metastases to distant solid organs, outside of the lung and liver, are rare, and as such, robust clinical recommendations are not possible. Much of the literature existing on rare sites of EHD is based on case series or single institution retrospective reviews, both of which are significantly impacted by substantial selection bias. The largest meta-analysis on surgical resection of EHD examined 2308 patients who underwent resection for EHD, and only 4% had metastases to infrequent sites such as bone, brain, ovary, and adrenal gland [9].

Adrenal Gland

The adrenal gland is an uncommon location for CRC to metastasize, and it is seldom the only metastatic site of disease [66]. The current literature consists primarily of case reports of CRC metastases and case series of adrenal metastases from all tumor types. One such case series reported 3-year OS and 5-year OS of 50% and 40%, respectively, in patients undergoing adrenalectomy for metastases from all primary sites, of which the majority were non-small-cell lung cancer and RCC [66]. Only 10.3% of patients in this study had CRC metastases to the adrenal gland. In the absence of robust data, recommendations for or against adrenal metastasectomy for CRC cannot be made. However, a survival benefit in select patients without other sites of EHD can be reasonably inferred.

Ovary

Ovarian metastases occur in approximately 2–8% of women with CRC, and 50–70% of these patients also have extra-ovarian metastases [67, 68]. There is some evidence that ovarian metastases may be less responsive to chemotherapy when compared to other sites of CRC metastases [69]. The reported prognosis is highly variable, with median OS ranging from 28 to 82 months [6, 8, 68]. Historically, some surgeons advocated for prophylactic oophorectomy in all postmenopausal women undergoing bowel resection for CRC. However, this practice has not been demonstrated to impact survival, and in the absence of clinical indications, prophylactic oophorectomy is not recommended [70, 71]. Given the relatively low surgical morbidity, and the potential for long-term survival, resection of ovarian metastases in the setting of resectable LM is indicated, especially if an ovarian metastasis is the only site of EHD.

Bone

The reported incidence of bone metastases in CRC is in the range of 5–7%, with signet-ring cell subtype of CRC more commonly behaving in this fashion [72, 73]. Bone metastases are rarely an isolated site of CRC disease, and the median OS is between 5 and 7 months [74, 75]. The prognosis is highly variable in patients with isolated bone metastases, and treatment with radiation or surgery can be considered, especially for symptom control on a case-by-case basis.

Brain

Brain metastases from CRC is fortuitously rare, with a reported incidence of only 0.3–0.6%, and this is more common when the primary disease is located in the rectum [76, 77]. Typically, brain metastases occur late in the disease course when patients often have numerous other sites of metastatic CRC and as such confer a uniformly dismal prognosis. In patients with CRC brain metastases, only 2–10% have isolated brain lesions [78–80]. The decision to pursue local treatment depends on the patient's performance status, number and location of lesions, the presence of leptomeningeal disease, and whether or not there are other sites of disease [81]. In general, however, even with aggressive local treatment consisting of whole brain radiation, stereotactic radiation, or surgery, the OS is dismal ranging from 12 to 15 months, and long-term survival greater than 5 years is observed in less than 4% [82–86]. Often times, the decision to treat brain metastases is driven by objectionable symptoms than an intention to alter survival. In the absence of more compelling survival benefit, routine cerebral metastasectomy in the setting of LM cannot be recommended.

Summary

There has been increasing enthusiasm for surgical resection in patients with both resectable LM and EHD, despite having been previously considered a contraindication to surgery. Certainly, it has been demonstrated that in carefully selected patients, medium- to long-term survival, and even cure, can be achieved. However, much of the surgical evidence for resection of EHD in the setting of resectable hepatic disease is based upon single-center, retrospective studies, and as such, the possibility of significant selection and publication bias exists. Patients with metastatic CRC should be always discussed in a multidisciplinary setting prior to embarking on treatment. Moreover, patients should be properly informed that the majority of individuals who undergo aggressive surgical treatment of LM in the setting of EHD will recur. Surgical resection should be offered to selected patients who are the most likely to benefit from metastasectomy. Those individuals with poor prognostic indicators such as multiple sites of EHD, a high metastatic burden, retroperitoneal or celiac axis LNM, brain or bone metastases, progression on neoadjuvant systemic therapy, and short disease-free intervals should not be offered resection.

References

1. Scheele J, Stangl R, Altendorf-Hofmann A, Gall FP. Indicators of prognosis after hepatic resection for colorectal secondaries. Surgery. 1991;110(1):13–29.
2. Fong Y, Cohen AM, Fortner JG, Enker WE, Turnbull AD, Coit DG, et al. Liver resection for colorectal metastases. J Clin Oncol. 1997;15(3):938–46.

3. Elias D, Sideris L, Pocard M, Ouellet JF, Boige V, Lasser P, et al. Results of R0 resection for colorectal liver metastases associated with extrahepatic disease. Ann Surg Oncol. 2004;11(3):274–80.
4. Elias D, Ouellet JF, Bellon N, Pignon JP, Pocard M, Lasser P. Extrahepatic disease does not contraindicate hepatectomy for colorectal liver metastases. Br J Surg. 2003;90(5):567–74.
5. Pulitano C, Bodingbauer M, Aldrighetti L, de Jong MC, Castillo F, Schulick RD, et al. Liver resection for colorectal metastases in presence of extrahepatic disease: results from an international multi-institutional analysis. Ann Surg Oncol. 2011;18:1380–8.
6. Leung U, Gonen M, Allen PJ, Kingham TP, DeMatteo RP, Jarnagin WR, et al. Colorectal cancer liver metastases and concurrent extrahepatic disease treated with resection. Ann Surg. 2017;265:158–65.
7. Rajakannu M, Magdeleinat P, Vibert E, Ciacio O, Pittau G, Innominato P, et al. Is cure possible after sequential resection of hepatic and pulmonary metastases from colorectal cancer. Clin Colorectal Cancer. 2018;17(1):41–9.
8. Carpizo D, Are C, Jarnagin W, DeMatteo R, Fong Y, Gonen M, et al. Liver resection for metastatic colorectal cancer in patients with concurrent extrahepatic disease: results in 127 patients treated at a single center. Ann Surg Oncol. 2009;16:2138–46.
9. Hadden WJ, de Reuver PR, Brown K, Mittal A, Samra JS, Hugh TJ. Resection of colorectal liver metastases and extra-hepatic disease: a systematic review and proportional meta-analysis of survival outcomes. HPB. 2016;18:209–20.
10. August DA, Ottow RT, Sugarbaker PH. Clinical perspectives of human colorectal cancer metastasis. Cancer Metastasis Rev. 1983;3(4):303–24.
11. Mitry E, Guiu B, Cosconea S, Jooste V, Faivre J, Bouvier AM. Epidemiology, management and prognosis of colorectal cancer with lung metastases: a 30-year population-based study. Gut. 2010;59(10):1383–8.
12. Labianca R, Beretta GD, Kildani B, Milesi L, Merlin F, Mosconi S, et al. Colon cancer. Crit Rev Oncol Hematol. 2010;74(2):106–33.
13. Tan KK, Lopes Gde L, Sim R. How uncommon are isolated lung metastases in colorectal cancer? A review from database of 754 patients over 4 years. J Gastrointest Surg. 2009;13(4):642–8.
14. Simmonds PC. Palliative chemotherapy for advanced colorectal cancer: systematic review and meta-analysis. Colorectal Cancer Collaborative Group. BMJ. 2000;321(7260):531–5.
15. Bendell J. Optimum chemotherapy for metastatic colorectal cancer. Lancet. 2006;368(9552):2039–41.
16. Thomford NR, Woolner LB, Clagett OT. The surgical treatment of metastatic tumors in the lungs. J Thorac Cardiovasc Surg. 1965;49:357–63.
17. Inoue M, Ohta M, Iuchi K, Matsumura A, Ideguchi K, Yasumitsu T, et al. Benefits of surgery for patients with pulmonary metastases from colorectal carcinoma. Ann Thorac Surg. 2004;78(1):238–44.
18. McCormack PM, Burt ME, Bains MS, Martini N, Rusch VW, Ginsberg RJ. Lung resection for colorectal metastases. 10-year results. Arch Surg. 1992;127(12):1403–6.
19. Gonzalez M, Poncet A, Combescure C, Robert J, Ris HB, Gervaz P. Risk factors for survival after lung metastasectomy in colorectal cancer patients: a systematic review and meta-analysis. Ann Surg Oncol. 2013;20(2):572–9.
20. Meimarakis G, Spelsberg F, Angele M, Preissler G, Fertmann J, Crispin A, et al. Resection of pulmonary metastases from colon and rectal cancer: factors to predict survival differ regarding to the origin of the primary tumor. Ann Surg Oncol. 2014;21:2563–72.
21. Primrose J, Treasure T, Fiorentino F. Lung metastasectomy in colorectal cancer: is this surgery effective in prolonging life? Respirology. 2010;15(5):742–6.
22. Van Raemdonck D. Pulmonary metastasectomy: common practice but is it also best practice? Future Oncol. 2015;11(2 Suppl):11–4.
23. Treasure T. Metastasectomy for colorectal cancer: are there clothes on the emperor? J R Soc Med. 2017;100(6):227–30.
24. Migliore M, Milosevic M, Lees B, Treasure T, Di Maria G. Finding the evidence for pulmonary metastasectomy in colorectal cancer: the PulMiCC trial. Furture Oncol. 2015;11(2 Suppl):15–8.

25. ClinicalTrials.gov [Internet] A randomized trial of pulmonary metastasectomy in colorectal cancer (PulMiCC) Available from: https://clinicaltrials.gov/ct2/show/NCT01106261.
26. Kobayashi K, Kawamura M, Ishihara T. Surgical treatment for both pulmonary and hepatic metastases from colorectal cancer. J Thorac Cardiovasc Surg. 1999;118(6):1090–6.
27. Nagakura S, Shirai Y, Yamato Y, Yokoyama N, Suda T, Hatakeyama K. Simultaneous detection of colorectal carcinoma liver and lung metastases does not warrant resection. J Am Coll Surg. 2001;193(2):153–60.
28. Mineo TC, Ambrogi V, Tonini G, et al. Long term results after resection of simultaneous and sequential lung and liver metastases from colorectal carcinoma. J Am Coll Surg. 2003;197:386–91.
29. Shah SA, Haddad R, Al-Sukhni W, Kim RD, Greig PD, Grant DR, et al. Surgical resection of hepatic and pulmonary metastases from colorectal carcinoma. J Am Coll Surg. 2006;202(3):468–75.
30. Miller G, Biernacki P, Kemeny NE, Gonen M, Downey R, Jarnagin WR, et al. Outcomes after resection of synchronous or metachronous hepatic and pulmonary colorectal metastases. J Am Coll Surg. 2007;205(2):231–8.
31. Takahashi S, Nagai K, Saito N, Konishi M, Nakagohri T, Gotohda N, et al. Multiple resections for hepatic and pulmonary metastases of colorectal carcinoma. Jpn J Clin Oncol. 2007;37(3):186–92.
32. Lee WS, Yun HR, Yun SH, Chun HK, Lee WY, Kim SJ, et al. Treatment outcomes of hepatic and pulmonary metastases from colorectal carcinoma. J Gastroenterol Hepatol. 2008;23(8pt2):e367–72.
33. Barlow AD, Nakas A, Pattenden C, Martin-Ucar AE, Dennison AR, Berry DP, et al. Surgical treatment of combined hepatic and pulmonary colorectal cancer metastases. Eur J Surg Oncol. 2009;35(3):307–12.
34. Neeff H, Horth W, Makowiec F, Fischer E, Imdahl A, Hopt UT, et al. Outcome after resection of hepatic and pulmonary metastases of colorectal cancer. J Gastrointest Surg. 2009;13(10):1813–20.
35. Limmer S, Oevermann E, Killaitis C, Kujath P, Hoffmann M, Bruch HP. Sequential surgical resection of hepatic and pulmonary metastases from colorectal cancer. Langenbeck's Arch Surg. 2010;395(8):1129–38.
36. Brouquet A, Vauthey JN, Contreras CM, Walsh GL, Vaporciyan AA, Swisher SG, et al. Improved survival after resection of liver and lung colorectal metastases compared with liver-only metastases: a study of 112 patients with limited lung metastatic disease. J Am Coll Surg. 2011;213(1):62–9.
37. Gonzalez M, Robert JH, Halkic N, et al. Survival after lung metastasectomy in colorectal cancer patients with previously resected liver metastases. World J Surg. 2012;36(2):386–91.
38. Andres A, Mentha G, Adam R, Gerstel E, Skipenko OG, Barroso E, et al. Surgical management of patients with colorectal cancer and simultaneous liver and lung metastases. BJS. 2015;102:691–9.
39. Hwang M, Jayakrishnan TT, Green DE, George B, Thomas JP, Groeschl RT, et al. Systematic review of outcomes of patients undergoing resection for colorectal liver metastases in the setting of extra hepatic disease. E J Cancer. 2014;50(10):1747–57.
40. Internullo E, Cassivi SD, Van Raemdonck D, Friedel G, Treasure T, ESTS Pulmonary Metastasectomy Working Group. Pulmonary metastasectomy: a survey of current practice amongst members of the European Society of Thoracic Surgeons. J Thorac Oncol. 2008;3:1257–66.
41. Bolukbas S, Sponholz S, Kudelin N, Eberlein M, Schirren J. Risk factors for lymph node metastases and prognosticators of survival in patients undergoing pulmonary metastasectomy for colorectal cancer. Ann Thorac Surg. 2014;97:1926–32.
42. Suzuki H, Kiyoshima M, Kitahara M, Asato Y, Amemiya R. Long-term outcomes after surgical resection of pulmonary metastases from colon cancer. Ann Thorac Surg. 2015;99:434–40.
43. Yokoyama S, Mitsuoka M, Kinugasa T, Hashiguchi T, Matsumoto R, Murakami D, et al. Survival after initial lung metastasectomy for metastatic colorectal cancer in the modern chemotherapeutic era. BMC Surg. 2017;17(1):54.
44. Reddy RH, Kumar B, Shah R, Mirsadraee S, Papagiannopoulous K, Lodge P, et al. Staged pulmonary and hepatic metastasectomy in colorectal cancer—is it worth it? Eur J Cardiothorac Surg. 2004;25:151–4.
45. Thomassen I, van Gestel YR, Lemmens VE, de Hingh IH. Incidence, prognosis, and treatment options for patients with synchronous peritoneal carcinomatosis and liver metastases from colorectal origin. Dis Colon Rectum. 2013;56(12):1373–80.

46. Verwaal VJ, van Ruth S, de Bree E, van Sloothen GW, van Tinteren H, Boot H, et al. Randomized trial of cytoreduction and hyperthermic intraperitoneal chemotherapy versus systemic chemotherapy and palliative surgery in patients with peritoneal carcinomatosis of colorectal cancer. J Clin Oncol. 2003;21(20):3737–43.
47. Quenet F, Elias D, Roca L, Goere D, Ghouti L, Pocard M, Facy O, Arvieux C, Lorimier G, Pezet D, Marchal F, Loi V, Meeus P, De Forges H, Stanbury T, Paineau J, Glehen O. A UNICANCER phase III trial of hyperthermic intra-peritoneal chemotherapy (HIPEC) for colorectal peritoneal carcinomatosis (PC): PRODIGE 7. J Clin Oncol. 2018;36(18_suppl):LBA3503.
48. Esquivel J, Lowy AM, Markman M, Chua T, Pelz J, Baratti D, et al. The American Society of Peritoneal Surface Malignancies (ASPSM) multiinstitution evaluation of the Peritoneal Surface Disease Severity Score (PSDSS) in 1,013 patients with colorectal cancer with peritoneal carcinomatosis. Ann Surg Oncol. 2014;21(13):4195–201.
49. Huang CQ, Min Y, Wang SY, Yanf XJ, Liu Y, Xiong B, et al. Cytoreductive surgery plus hyperthermic intraperitoneal chemotherapy improves survival for peritoneal carcinomatosis from colorectal cancer: a systematic review and meta-analysis of current evidence. Oncotarget. 2017;l8(33):55657–83.
50. Maggiori L, Goere D, Viana B, Tzanis D, Dumont F, Honore C, et al. Should patients with peritoneal carcinomatosis of colorectal origin with synchronous liver metastases be treated with a curative intent? A case-control study. Ann Surg. 2013;258(1):116–21.
51. Chua TC, Yan TD, Zhao J, Morris DL. Peritoneal carcinomatosis and liver metastases from colorectal cancer treated with cytoreductive surgery perioperative intraperitoneal chemotherapy and liver resection. Eur J Surg Oncol. 2009;35(12):1299–305.
52. Alzahrani N, Ung L, Valle SJ, Liauw W, Morris DL. Synchronous liver resection with cytoreductive surgery for the treatment of liver and peritoneal metastases from colon cancer: results from an Australian Centre. ANZ J Surg. 2017;87(11):E167–E72.
53. de Cuba EMV, Kwakman R, Knol DL, Bonjer HJ, Meijer GA, te Velde EA. Cytoreductive surgery and HIPEC for peritoneal metastases combined with curative treatment of colorectal liver metastases. Cancer Treat Rev. 2013;39(4):321–7.
54. Allard MA, Adam R, Ruiz A, Vibert E, Paule B, Levi F, et al. Is unexpected peritoneal carcinomatosis still a contraindication for resection of colorectal liver metastases? Eur J Surg Oncol. 2013;39(9):981–7.
55. Moszkowicz D, Cauchy F, Dokmak S, Belghiti J. Routine pedicular lymphadenectomy for colorectal liver metastases. J Am Coll Surg. 2012;214:e39–45.
56. August DA, Sugarbaker PH, Schneider PD. Lymphatic dissemination of hepatic metastases: implications for follow-up and treatment of patients with colorectal cancer. Cancer. 1985;55:1490–4.
57. Carpizo DR, D'Angelica M. Liver resection for metastatic colorectal cancer in the presence of extrahepatic disease. Lancet Oncol. 2009;10:801–9.
58. Elias D, Saric J, Jaeck D, Arnaud JP, Gayet B, Rivoire M, et al. Prospective study of microscopic lymph node involvement of the hepatic pedicle during curative hepatectomy for colorectal metastases. Br J Surg. 1996;83:942–5.
59. Ercolani G, Grazi GL, Ravaioli M, Grigioni WF, Cescon M, Gardini A, et al. The role of lymphadenectomy for liver tumors: further considerations on the appropriateness of treatment strategy. Ann Surg. 2004;239:202–9.
60. Grobmyer SR, Wang L, Gonen M, Fong Y, Klimstra D, D'Angelica M, et al. Perihepatic lymph node assessment in patients undergoing partial hepatectomy for malignancy. Ann Surg. 2006;244:260–4.
61. Jaeck D, Nakano H, Bachellier P, Inoue K, Weber JC, Oussoulzoglou E, et al. Significance of hepatic pedicle lymph node involvement in patients with colorectal liver metastases: a prospective study. Ann Surg Oncol. 2002;9:430–8.
62. Pindak D, Pavlendova J, Tomas M, Dolnik J, Duchon R, Pechan J. Selective versus routine lymphadenectomy in the treatment of liver metastasis from colorectal cancer: a retrospective cohort study. BMC Surg. 2017;17(1):34.
63. Laurent C, Sa Cunha A, Rullier E, Smith D, Rullier A, Saric J. Impact of microscopic hepatic lymph node involvement on survival after resection of colorectal liver metastasis. J Am Coll Surg. 2004;198:884–91.
64. Moulton CA, Gu CS, Law CH, Tandan VR, Hart R, Quan D, et al. Effect of PET before liver resection on surgical management for colorectal adenocarcinoma metastases: a randomized controlled trial. JAMA. 2014;311:1863–9.

65. Adam R, de Haas RJ, Wicherts DA, Aloia TA, Delvart V, Azoulay D, et al. Is hepatic resection justified after chemotherapy in patients with colorectal liver metastases and lymph node involvement? J Clin Oncol. 2008;26:3672–80.
66. Rosso AE, Untch BR, Kris MG, Chou JF, Capanu M, Coit DG. Adrenal metastasectomy in the presence and absence of extraadrenal metastatic disease. Ann Surg. 2019;270(2):373–7.
67. Banerjee S, Kapur S, Moran BJ. The role of prophylactic oophorectomy in women undergoing surgery for colorectal cancer. Color Dis. 2005;7(3):214–7.
68. Lee SJ, Lee J, Lim HY, Kang WK, Choic CH, Lee JW, et al. Survival benefit from ovarian metastasectomy in colorectal cancer patients with ovarian metastasis: a retrospective analysis. Cancer Chemother Pharmacol. 2010;66(2):229–35.
69. Goere D, Daveau C, Elias D, Boige V, Tomasic G, Bonnet S, et al. The differential response to chemotherapy of ovarian metastases from colorectal carcinoma. Eur J Surg Oncol. 2008;34:1335–9.
70. Sielezneff I, Salle E, Antoine K, Thirion X, Brunet C, Sastre B. Simultaneous bilateral oophorectomy does not improve prognosis of postmenopausal women undergoing colorectal resection for cancer. Dis Colon Rectum. 1997;40(11):1299–302.
71. Young-Fadok TM, WolV BG, Nivatvongs S, Metzger PP, Ilstrup DM. Prophylactic oophorectomy in colorectal carcinoma: preliminary results of a randomized, prospective trial. Dis Colon Rectum. 1998;1:277–83.
72. Katoh M, Unakami M, Hara M, Fukuchi S. Bone metastasis from colorectal cancer in autopsy cases. J Gastroenterol. 1995;30:615–8.
73. Kanthan R, Loewy J, Kanthan SC. Skeletal metastases in colorectal carcinomas: a Saskatchewan profile. Dis Colon Rectum. 1999;42:1592–7.
74. Roth ES, Fetzer DT, Barron BJ, Joseph UA, Gayed IW, Wan DQ. Does colon cancer ever metastasize to bone first? A temporal analysis of colorectal cancer progression. BMC Cancer. 2009;9:274.
75. Nozue M, Oshiro Y, Kurata M, Seino K, Koike N, Kawamoto T, et al. Treatment and prognosis in colorectal cancer patients with bone metastasis. Oncol Rep. 2002;9:109–12.
76. Cascino TL, Leavengood JM, Kemeny N, Posner JB. Brain metastases from colon cancer. J Neuro-Oncol. 1983;1:203–20.
77. Schouten LJ, Rutten J, Huveneers HA, Twijnstra A. Incidence of brain metastases in a cohort of patients with carcinoma of the breast, colon, kidney, and lung and melanoma. Cancer. 2002;94:2698–705.
78. Alden TD, Gianino JW, Saclarides TJ. Brain metastases from colorectal cancer. Dis Colon Rectum. 1996;39:541–5.
79. Damiens K, Ayoub JP, Lemieux B, Aubin F, Saliba W, Campeau MP, et al. Clinical features and course of brain metastases in colorectal cancer: an experience from a single institution. Curr Oncol. 2012;19:254–8.
80. Kye BH, Kim HJ, Kang WK, Cho HM, Hong YK, Oh ST. Brain metastases from colorectal cancer: the role of surgical resection in selected patients. Color Dis. 2012;14:e378–85.
81. Vatandoust S, Price TJ, Karapetis CS. Colorectal cancer: metastases to a single organ. World J Gastroenterol. 2015;21(41):11767–76.
82. Hammoud MA, McCutcheon IE, Elsouki R, Schoppa D, Patt YZ. Colorectal carcinoma and brain metastasis: distribution, treatment, and survival. Ann Surg Oncol. 1996;3:453–63.
83. Farnell GF, Buckner JC, Cascino TL, O'Connell MJ, Schomberg PJ, Suman V. Brain metastases from colorectal carcinoma. The long term survivors. Cancer. 1996;78:711–6.
84. Suzuki Y, Yamaguchi T, Matsumoto H, Nakano D, Honda G, Shinoura N, et al. Prognostic factors and treatment effects in patients with curatively resected brain metastasis from colorectal cancer. Dis Colon Rectum. 2014;57:56–3.
85. Aprile G, Zanon E, Tuniz F, Iaiza E, De Pauli F, Pella N, et al. Neurosurgical management and postoperative whole-brain radiotherapy for colorectal cancer patients with symptomatic brain metastases. J Cancer Res Clin Oncol. 2009;135:451–7.
86. Wronski M, Arbit E. Resection of brain metastases from colorectal carcinoma in 73 patients. Cancer. 1999;85:1677–85.

Anatomical, Physiological, and Kinetic Evaluation of the Future Liver Remnant of CRLM After Portal Vein Embolisation

14

D. Asano, D. Ban, and M. Tanabe

Introduction

During the past decade, the introduction of effective systemic therapies and increasing use of major hepatectomy have led to significant improvements in the long-term survival of patients with colorectal liver metastases (CRLM) [1].

Improvements in chemotherapy have led to more aggressive strategies for the treatment for CRLM. In terms of surgical treatment, hepatectomy has played a greater role in the comprehensive treatment of CRLM. Increasing numbers of patients are receiving resection for synchronous or metachronous CRLM and the numbers who have conversion surgery after chemotherapy also are increasing. Because repeat hepatectomy can prolong the survival of patients with CRLM [2], it is important to assess the future liver remnant (FLR), especially regarding major hepatectomy for patients with huge or multiple CRLM.

When FLR is considered to be insufficient, portal vein embolization (PVE) may be carried out preoperatively. Preoperative portal vein embolization was introduced by Kinoshita et al. in 1986 as a countermeasure to portal tumor thrombi [3]. They found permanent hypertrophy of the liver that may be useful as a means of preparation for surgery. This led Makuuchi et al. [4] to use PVE to initiate future liver remnant hypertrophy, prior to extended resection for hilar bile duct cancer. Preoperative PVE of the liver has been suggested to induce ipsilateral atrophy and contralateral compensatory hypertrophy of the remnant liver, thus preventing postoperative liver failure, because liver failure is the major cause of mortality following liver resection.

The aim of this chapter is to discuss the method of FLR and the role of PVE.

D. Asano · D. Ban · M. Tanabe (✉)
Department of Hepatobiliary and Pancreatic Surgery, Graduate School of Medicine, Tokyo Medical and Dental University, Tokyo, Japan
e-mail: d-asano.msrg@tmd.ac.jp; d-ban.msrg@tmd.ac.jp; tana.msrg@tmd.ac.jp

M. M. Correia et al. (eds.), *Colorectal Cancer Liver Metastases*,
https://doi.org/10.1007/978-3-030-25486-5_14

How to Calculate the Standardized FLR

Considering the required volume of the FLR, it is necessary to clarify how to evaluate the liver volume. Computed tomography (CT) is the cornerstone of surgical planning; it can reproducibly and accurately measure liver volume. The standard technique is one that measures resected and total liver volumes and estimates the "normal liver" by subtracting the tumor volume: (resected volume ± tumor volume)/(total liver volume ± tumor volume).

With multiple tumors, this technique is demanding and the calculations become imprecise because of the cumulative errors associated with multiple measurements. In addition, the method does not account for the actual functional liver volume when the bile ducts are dilated or the liver parenchyma is compromised by vascular obstruction. An alternative method, known as standardized FLR, allows for a more accurate assessment of the FLR and comparison of outcomes data between patients of varying sizes. Using this method, the future liver remnant is measured directly by CT, but the total liver volume is calculated using a formula [5]. The ratio of future liver remnant to the total estimated liver is calculated. The formula is derived from the close association between the total liver volume and body surface area (BSA), as described previously (total liver volume = 706.2 × BSA + 2.4). This alternative method allows for a uniform comparison of the remnant volume before extended resection, with or without preoperative PVE. Based on this method, a correlation between the future liver remnant volume and operative outcome has been established. A recent meta-analysis that compared 12 TLV formulas [6] revealed that the least biased and most precise formula for predicting TLV is −794.41 + 1267.28 × BSA [7].

Indication of PVE

Many previous studies have discussed the indications of preoperative PVE. In 1997, Kubota et al. [8] reported that individuals with normal liver function (ICGR15 < 10%) could undergo resection of up to 60% of the nontumorous parenchyma without the need for PVE. Although in 2000 Vauthey et al. [5] indicated an increase in major complications for FLR ≤25%, recent studies reported that an FLR >20% is sufficient for safe hepatic resection and an FLR of 20.1–30% is not an indication for preoperative PVE [9]. In addition, patients who underwent PVE before surgery to increase their standardized FLR from <20% to >20% had statistically equivalent rates of liver insufficiency to patients with >20% at baseline [9].

PVE is useful for injured liver, as well as for normal liver. Although Azoulay et al. [10] performed PVE for patients with hepatocellular carcinoma in an injured liver, there were no deaths or complications related to PVE and the long-term survival rates were comparable to those after resection without PVE. In their study, patients with FLR <40% underwent PVE. In another study [11, 12] of hepatectomy for CRLM after chemotherapy, FLR ≤30% was an independent predictor of postoperative hepatic insufficiency (PHI). Zorzi et al. [13] previously described the minimal necessary FLR volume as greater than 20% for patients with normal livers, greater than 30% for patients with extensive preoperative chemotherapy or with histopathologic injuries, and greater than 40% for patients with cirrhosis.

Belghiti [14] strongly advocated including PVE in the management of patients with chronic liver disease or with injured livers (i.e., after chemotherapy or with major steatosis or cholestasis) before any major liver resection [15]. In these patients, the absence of hypertrophy of the nonembolized liver following successful PVE should be considered as an indicator of the absence of liver capacity to regenerate and, therefore, a contraindication for major liver resection [16].

Anatomical Evaluation of FLR

Azoulay et al. reported that PVE increased the FLR from 26% ± 6% to 37% ± 8% ($P < 10^{-4}$) (gain 43% ± 14%, range 14–71%, median 42%) and increased the number of patients who underwent hepatectomy for CRLM by 19% [17]. In another current series, 31 patients underwent preoperative PVE and all had an increase in the FLR before extended resection [18].

In a recent meta-analysis [19] involving 1088 patients who underwent PVE before major hepatectomy, 85% of patients underwent the planned hepatectomy ($n = 930$). Only 18 patients (0.02%) could not undergo resection because of inadequate hypertrophy of the remnant liver. The calculated range of percentage increase of future liver remnant volume following portal vein embolization was 8–27% in their analysis.

Physiological Evaluation of FLR

Hypertrophy of the FLR is the most important effect of PVE; however, controversy remains as to whether PVE induces only volume change, rather than functional gain. Because there is no absolute predictor for the function of the FLR, we usually try to predict this using various physiological markers, such as the Child–Pugh score, cholinesterase level, and indocyanine green (ICG) clearance test. Although these markers reflect the function of the entire liver, what is important is the function of the FLR. Uesaka et al. [20] reported the functional increase of FLR after PVE by demonstrating a significant increase in ICG excretion and bile volume from the unembolized lobe.

Others have suggested that radiocolloid liver scintigraphy with technetium-99 m-galactosyl human serum albumin (99mTc-GSA) is more accurate than ICG clearance for predicting the function of FLR [21]. 99mTc-GSA has affinity for the asialoglycoprotein receptor, which is expressed only in the hepatocyte membranes of mammals. Because levels of this receptor are reduced in various liver diseases, liver scintigraphy with 99mTc-GSA is a good diagnostic tool for evaluation of functional liver volume [22]. Indeed, 99mTc-GSA scintigraphy has been reported to be more accurate for the evaluation of liver function than the ICG clearance test [23,

24]. Furthermore, the uptake of 99mTc-GSA, as assessed with SPECT imaging, can be used to evaluate partial liver function [25], and uptake by the left lobe before and after embolization of the right portal branch can be calculated with 99mTc-GSA SPECT scintigraphy. There was no correlation between the degree of hypertrophy measured with CT and that assessed by 99mTc-GSA uptake. This means that morphologic hypertrophy and 99mTc-GSA uptake, a marker of liver function, do not always coincide [21]. Patients with a small liver volume (<35%) and a low 99mTc-GSA uptake (<25%) in the nonembolized lobe after PVE tend to develop postoperative liver failure. CT volumetry and 99mTc-GSA scintigraphy constitute a useful tool for the prediction of postoperative liver failure [21].

99mTc-labeled mebrofenin hepatobiliary scintigraphy (HBS) with SPECT has been validated recently as a quantitative method for evaluating liver function, as well as liver functional volume. 99mTc-mebrofenin HBS measures total liver (uptake) function, as well as FLR function, and can be used before surgery to predict postoperative liver failure. 99mTc-GSA scintigraphy and 99mTc-mebrofenin HBS are both nuclear imaging techniques but are based on different principles. 99m Tc-GSA scintigraphy measures the binding of 99mTc-GSA to its receptor, which is expressed on functional hepatocytes. 99mTc-mebrofenin HBS measures the kinetic process of uptake and excretion of 99mTc-mebrofenin by hepatocytes [26].

Kinetic Evaluation of FLR

Although the anatomical cut-off values of sFLR discussed above are useful guides, they do not consistently predict surgical outcome. Shindoh et al. [27] advocated a new concept, kinetic growth rate (KGR), which was defined as the degree of hypertrophy at initial volume assessment divided by the number of weeks since PVE. In their study, KGR was the most accurate predictor among sFLR volume, degree of hypertrophy, and KGR. A KGR of less than 2% per week versus ≥2% per week correlates with rates of hepatic insufficiency (21.6% vs. 0%, $p = 0.0001$) and liver-related 90-day mortality (8.1% vs. 0%, $P = 0.04$).

The risk of PHI is increased among patients with significant post-chemotherapy hepatic atrophy. Even in high-risk patients with ≥10% degree of atrophy from preoperative chemotherapy, KGR ≥2% mitigates the deleterious effects of hepatic atrophy and significantly reduces PHI to almost zero [28]. In addition to its role in sFLR augmentation, PVE represents a critical dynamic test of regenerative capacity. For example, patients who experience less than a 5% absolute degree of hypertrophy are more likely to experience inadequate liver regeneration following hepatectomy, resulting in PHI and mortality [29].

Optimal Timing of Surgery After PVE

It is important, when we perform hepatectomy after PVE, to consider the degree of hypertrophy and the progression of the tumor(s). The risk of tumor growth obviously demands the minimum waiting time possible. This interval is determined mostly by the time required to attain sufficient FRL volume. The average interval for the CT volumetric study from portal vein embolization to surgery was 29 days in a large meta-analysis, including 1088 patients [19]. Ribero et al. [29] indicated that the days 22–56 after PVE constitute the plateau period, which is consistent with that meta-analysis.

One study separately assessed biliary excretion of ICG by the embolized and nonembolized liver lobes and concluded that the functional gain in the nonembolized lobes was greater than the volumetric increase [20]. Another study confirmed that the increase in FRL function after PVE, measured by 99mTc-GSA or 99mTc-mebrofenin scintigraphy, exceeds the increase in volume in cirrhotic and noncirrhotic patients [21, 26]. This implies that the required waiting time before surgery may be shorter than that suggested by volumetric studies, which is more favorable considering the risk of tumor progression after PVE.

Postoperative Results and Complications After PVE

It is said that complications of PVE are rare (0–10%) [30]. Minor complications include abdominal discomfort or pain, fever, nausea or vomiting, ileus, overflow of embolization materials, and coil displacement. Major complications, which are very rare, include liver abscess, cholangitis, main or left portal vein thrombosis, subscapular hematoma, portal hypertension, and septic necrosis from hepatic artery injury [19].

Some studies revealed that there was no significant difference in the incidence of perioperative mortality and morbidity between those who did and did not undergo PVE [16, 30, 31]. Farges et al. reported that PVE in patients with chronic liver disease significantly decreased the risk of postoperative complications, as well as the time in the intensive care unit and total hospital stay after right hepatectomy [16].

Azoulay et al. reported, in originally nonresectable CRLM, a 40% 5-year actuarial survival rate after resection following PVE compared with a 38% 5-year actuarial survival rate following resection, in a cohort with a similar extent of resection without PVE [17].

Chemotherapy-Related Hepatic Injury

Chemotherapy-induced liver injury is a major factor in the surgical treatment of CRLM. Systemic chemotherapy has been used increasingly in the preoperative setting before liver resection because of several theoretical advantages. These include the potential to reduce the size of tumors preoperatively, to increase curative resection rates, and to convert some patients from having unresectable to resectable disease. Use of preoperative therapy in patients at high risk of recurrence may assist in identifying responders, so that therapy can be tailored postoperatively, based on the preoperative response. In addition, patients with multiple tumors who progress during preoperative chemotherapy, and who, therefore, may not benefit from resection, can be spared nontherapeutic surgery [32].

When we plan hepatectomy for CRLM after systemic chemotherapy, hepatic injury associated with chemotherapy should be taken under consideration. Steatosis or steatohepatitis induced by irinotecan and sinusoidal dilation induced by oxaliplatin are the best recognized liver injuries after systemic chemotherapy [13, 33, 34]. It is also said that hepatic steatosis may occur after treatment with 5-fluorouracil [13].

Steatosis and steatohepatitis due to irinotecan are known as "yellow liver" (Fig. 14.1). In one previous study, two of the three patients with steatohepatitis had received irinotecan preoperatively [34]. Vauthey et al. [33] reported that patients with steatohepatitis had an increased 90-day mortality, compared with patients who did not have steatohepatitis (14.7% vs. 1.6%, respectively; $P = 0.001$; OR = 10.5; 95% CI, 2.0–36.4), and the effect was more pronounced in patients with a higher BMI. Patients with steatohepatitis also had a higher risk of death specifically from postoperative liver failure (5.8%) versus all other patients (0.8%; $P = 0.01$; OR = 7.7; 95% CI, 1.24–47.7).

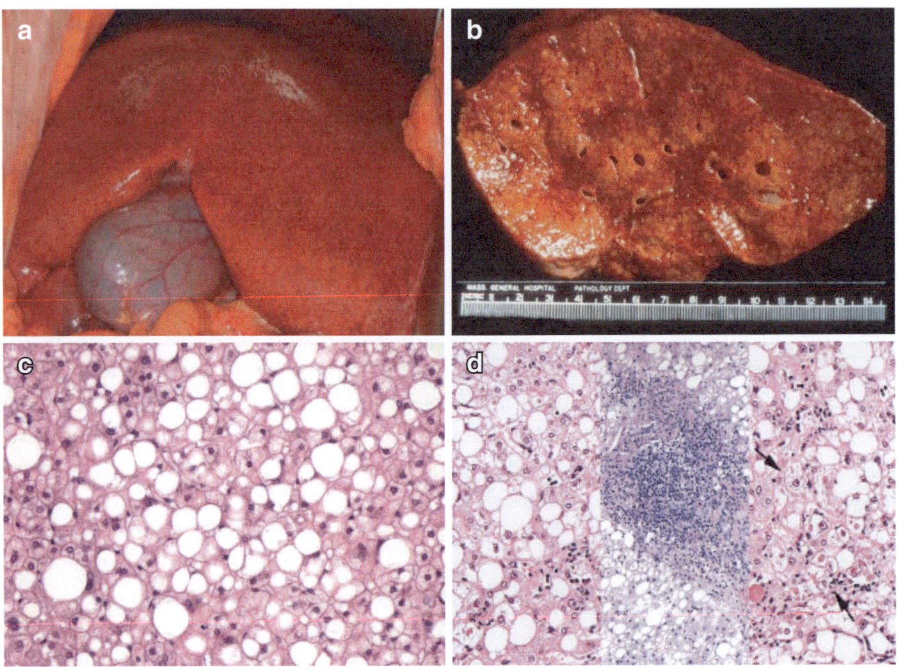

Fig. 14.1 Spectrum of nonalcoholic fatty liver disease (NAFLD). (**a**, **b**) Macroscopic aspect of fatty ("yellow") liver. The steatotic liver is enlarged, soft, and appears yellow in color because of fatty infiltration. (**c**) Simple steatosis, the mildest manifestation of NAFLD, denotes the accumulation of large globules of fat in the hepatocytes (macrovesicular steatosis) (hematoxylin and eosin; magnification × 400). (**d**) Histopathological spectrum of nonalcoholic steatohepatitis. Various degrees of inflammation can be seen scattered throughout the lobule as well as in portal tracts. Hepatocyte damage is demonstrated by scattered ballooned (arrows) and apoptotic cells (hematoxylin and eosin; magnification ×200 for the right and left fields, ×125 for the center). (Used with permission from Zorzi et al. [13])

Sinusoidal dilation due to chemotherapy is known as "blue liver" (Fig. 14.2) and is also recognized as sinusoidal obstruction syndrome (SOS). Rubbia-Brandt et al. [35] were the first to report oxaliplatin-associated SOS in the nontumorous liver specimens of patients undergoing hepatic resection following treatment with oxaliplatin. Perisinusoidal injuries, including dilatation and congestion with fibrosis and venous occlusion, were present in 78% of patients treated with oxaliplatin [13]. In contrast to steatohepatitis, some studies reported that this injury was not associated with increased morbidity or mortality rates [13, 33]. It is said that bevacizumab reduces the incidence and severity of SOS [36, 37].

PVE may provide an important functional test of liver reserve in patients with marginal remnants. Patients with liver remnants that are inadequate, based on systematic liver volumetry, are candidates for such embolization. In addition to the absolute liver volume, hypertrophy of the FLR in response to embolization predicts outcome after hepatectomy [29]. PVE may provide information about the functional hepatic reserve to help determine whether major resection will be safe. If adequate hypertrophy occurs, hepatectomy may be safe. Continuing

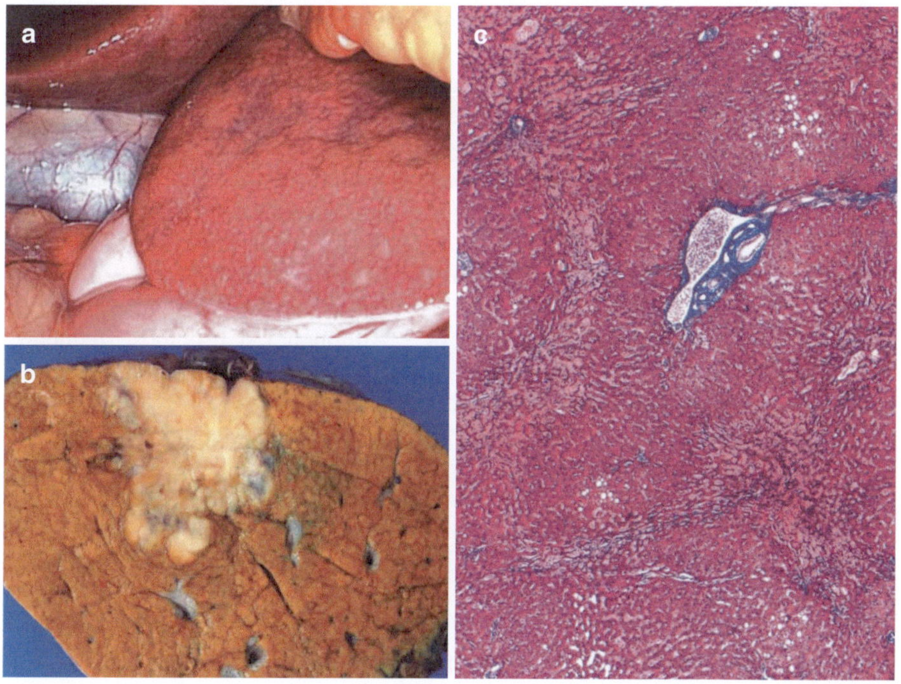

Fig. 14.2 Spectrum of oxaliplatin-associated sinusoidal obstruction syndrome (SOS). (**a**, **b**) Macroscopic aspect of liver with oxaliplatin-associated injury ("blue" liver). The distended sinusoids lead to entrapment of erythrocytes that in turn makes the liver blue in color ((**b**) courtesy of Dr. 1. Brown, Brisbane, Queensland, Australia). (**c**) Microscopic demonstration of centrilobular sinusoidal dilatation with only scattered macrovesicular steatosis (trichrome; magnification ×100). (Used with permission from Zorzi et al. [13])

chemotherapy while embolization is performed does not impair hepatic hypertrophy in response to portal vein embolization [38]. The minimum FLR that must remain after resection in patients with various types of chemotherapy-related liver injury remains unknown. However, the general consensus is as follows: portal vein embolization is indicated when the FLR volume is 20% or less of the total liver volume (TLV) in patients with normal liver, 30% or less of the TLV in patients who have had extensive chemotherapy, and 40% or less of the TLV in patients with well-compensated cirrhosis [39]. Shindoh et al. reported that FLR >30% is needed for patients after >12 weeks of chemotherapy to safely reduce PHI and mortality risk [11].

Contraindications to PVE

Contraindications to PVE include FLR volume larger than the cut-off volumes specified above and tumor invasion of the portal vein to be resected, because, in such cases, portal flow is already diverted. Relative contraindications to PVE include tumor extension to the FLR, uncorrectable coagulopathy, biliary dilatation in the FLR (if the biliary tree is obstructed, drainage is recommended), portal hypertension, and renal failure [39].

The most important problem is acceleration of tumor progression due to PVE [40]. High rates of unresectable disease have been described after PVE, ranging from 6.4% to 33% [41]. The tumor growth rate calculated from imaging was more rapid in the PVE group than the controls (control: 0.05 ± 0.25 ml/day, PVE: 0.36 ± 0.68 ml/day, $P = 0.06$). The mitotic rate was higher post-PVE, as was the proliferation index Ki67 ($P = 0.04$). This showed that the tumor growth rate increased following PVE and that this is related to increased tumor cell division [42].

To prevent tumor progression after PVE, sequential TACE with preoperative PVE or post-PVE chemotherapy is suggested [41]. Although TACE is most frequently used in patients with hepatocellular carcinoma, there are also reports indicating its use for other liver tumors, including colorectal metastases [43, 44]. This suggests that sequential TACE with preoperative PVE could also be potentially beneficial in patients with colorectal metastases.

If preoperative PVE is required, chemotherapy is discontinued several weeks prior to embolization until surgery 3–4 weeks thereafter, because of its alleged negative influence on the hypertrophy response. This allows tumor progression to occur during the period in which chemotherapy is discontinued, in addition to the possible tumor stimulatory effects of PVE. Belghiti's group recently found no significant difference in the hypertrophy response or postoperative complications when chemotherapy was continued after PVE [38]. They therefore recommended not to disrupt a successful chemotherapy course in patients with colorectal metastases, prior to or after portal vein occlusion. Another study showed that post-PVE chemotherapy was associated not only with prevention of tumor growth but also with improved survival [45].

Chemotherapy does not retard the growth of the liver after PVE and may prevent cancer progression. Thus, the combination of PVE and chemotherapy may enhance both oncologic and operative safety.

Conclusion

PVE is safe and effective prior to hepatectomy for patients with CRLM. The minimum necessary FLR volume is greater than 20% for patients with normal livers, greater than 30% for patients with extensive preoperative chemotherapy or with histopathologic injuries, and greater than 40% for patients with cirrhosis. We should not hesitate to perform PVE for those with CRLM because many of them might have received multiple chemotherapies. Progression of tumors is the problem to be solved for PVE.

References

1. Kopetz S, Chang GJ, Overman MJ, Eng C, Sargent DJ, Larson DW, et al. Improved survival in metastatic colorectal cancer is associated with adoption of hepatic resection and improved chemotherapy. J Clin Oncol. 2009;27(22):3677–83.
2. Yan TD, Sim J, Black D, Niu R, Morris DL. Systematic review on safety and efficacy of repeat hepatectomy for recurrent liver metastases from colorectal carcinoma. Ann Surg Oncol. 2007;14(7):2069–77.
3. Kinoshita H, Sakai K, Hirohashi K, Igawa S, Yamasaki O, Kubo S. Preoperative portal vein embolization for hepatocellular carcinoma. World J Surg. 1986;10(5):803–8.
4. Makuuchi M, Thai BL, Takayasu K, Takayama T, Kosuge T, Gunven P, et al. Preoperative portal embolization to increase safety of major hepatectomy for hilar bile duct carcinoma: a preliminary report. Surgery. 1990;107(5):521–7.
5. Vauthey JN, Chaoui A, Do KA, Bilimoria MM, Fenstermacher MJ, Charnsangavej C, et al. Standardized measurement of the future liver remnant prior to extended liver resection: methodology and clinical associations. Surgery. 2000;127(5):512–9.
6. Johnson TN, Tucker GT, Tanner MS, Rostami-Hodjegan A. Changes in liver volume from birth to adulthood: a meta-analysis. Liver Transplant. 2005;11(12):1481–93.
7. Vauthey JN, Abdalla EK, Doherty DA, Gertsch P, Fenstermacher MJ, Loyer EM, et al. Body surface area and body weight predict total liver volume in Western adults. Liver Transplant. 2002;8(3):233–40.
8. Kubota K, Makuuchi M, Kusaka K, Kobayashi T, Miki K, Hasegawa K, et al. Measurement of liver volume and hepatic functional reserve as a guide to decision-making in resectional surgery for hepatic tumors. Hepatology (Baltimore, Md). 1997;26(5):1176–81.
9. Kishi Y, Abdalla EK, Chun YS, Zorzi D, Madoff DC, Wallace MJ, et al. Three hundred and one consecutive extended right hepatectomies: evaluation of outcome based on systematic liver volumetry. Ann Surg. 2009;250(4):540–8.
10. Azoulay D, Castaing D, Krissat J, Smail A, Hargreaves GM, Lemoine A, et al. Percutaneous portal vein embolization increases the feasibility and safety of major liver resection for hepatocellular carcinoma in injured liver. Ann Surg. 2000;232(5):665–72.
11. Shindoh J, Tzeng CW, Aloia TA, Curley SA, Zimmitti G, Wei SH, et al. Optimal future liver remnant in patients treated with extensive preoperative chemotherapy for colorectal liver metastases. Ann Surg Oncol. 2013;20(8):2493–500.

12. Yamashita S, Shindoh J, Mizuno T, Chun YS, Conrad C, Aloia TA, et al. Hepatic atrophy following preoperative chemotherapy predicts hepatic insufficiency after resection of colorectal liver metastases. J Hepatol. 2017;67(1):56–64.
13. Zorzi D, Laurent A, Pawlik TM, Lauwers GY, Vauthey JN, Abdalla EK. Chemotherapy-associated hepatotoxicity and surgery for colorectal liver metastases. Br J Surg. 2007;94(3):274–86.
14. Belghiti J. Arguments for a selective approach of preoperative portal vein embolization before major hepatic resection. J Hepatobiliary Pancreat Surg. 2004;11(1):21–4.
15. Tanaka H, Hirohashi K, Kubo S, Shuto T, Higaki I, Kinoshita H. Preoperative portal vein embolization improves prognosis after right hepatectomy for hepatocellular carcinoma in patients with impaired hepatic function. Br J Surg. 2000;87(7):879–82.
16. Farges O, Belghiti J, Kianmanesh R, Regimbeau JM, Santoro R, Vilgrain V, et al. Portal vein embolization before right hepatectomy: prospective clinical trial. Ann Surg. 2003;237(2):208–17.
17. Azoulay D, Castaing D, Smail A, Adam R, Cailliez V, Laurent A, et al. Resection of nonresectable liver metastases from colorectal cancer after percutaneous portal vein embolization. Ann Surg. 2000;231(4):480–6.
18. Vauthey JN, Pawlik TM, Abdalla EK, Arens JF, Nemr RA, Wei SH, et al. Is extended hepatectomy for hepatobiliary malignancy justified? Ann Surg. 2004;239(5):722–30; discussion 30–2.
19. Abulkhir A, Limongelli P, Healey AJ, Damrah O, Tait P, Jackson J, et al. Preoperative portal vein embolization for major liver resection: a meta-analysis. Ann Surg. 2008;247(1):49–57.
20. Uesaka K, Nimura Y, Nagino M. Changes in hepatic lobar function after right portal vein embolization. An appraisal by biliary indocyanine green excretion. Ann Surg. 1996;223(1):77–83.
21. Hirai I, Kimura W, Fuse A, Suto K, Urayama M. Evaluation of preoperative portal embolization for safe hepatectomy, with special reference to assessment of nonembolized lobe function with 99mTc-GSA SPECT scintigraphy. Surgery. 2003;133(5):495–506.
22. Vera DR, Stadalnik RC, Krohn KA. Technetium-99 m galactosyl-neoglycoalbumin: preparation and preclinical studies. J Nucl Med. 1985;26(10):1157–67.
23. Mitsumori A, Nagaya I, Kimoto S, Akaki S, Togami I, Takeda Y, et al. Preoperative evaluation of hepatic functional reserve following hepatectomy by technetium-99 m galactosyl human serum albumin liver scintigraphy and computed tomography. Eur J Nucl Med. 1998;25(10):1377–82.
24. Kwon AH, Ha-Kawa SK, Uetsuji S, Inoue T, Matsui Y, Kamiyama Y. Preoperative determination of the surgical procedure for hepatectomy using technetium-99 m-galactosyl human serum albumin (99mTc-GSA) liver scintigraphy. Hepatology (Baltimore, Md). 1997;25(2):426–9.
25. Sugai Y, Komatani A, Hosoya T, Yamaguchi K. Response to percutaneous transhepatic portal embolization: new proposed parameters by 99mTc-GSA SPECT and their usefulness in prognostic estimation after hepatectomy. J Nucl Med. 2000;41(3):421–5.
26. de Graaf W, van Lienden KP, van den Esschert JW, Bennink RJ, van Gulik TM. Increase in future remnant liver function after preoperative portal vein embolization. Br J Surg. 2011;98(6):825–34.
27. Shindoh J, Truty MJ, Aloia TA, Curley SA, Zimmitti G, Huang SY, et al. Kinetic growth rate after portal vein embolization predicts posthepatectomy outcomes: toward zero liver-related mortality in patients with colorectal liver metastases and small future liver remnant. J Am Coll Surg. 2013;216(2):201–9.
28. Omichi K, Yamashita S, Cloyd JM, Shindoh J, Mizuno T, Chun YS, et al. Portal vein embolization reduces postoperative hepatic insufficiency associated with postchemotherapy hepatic atrophy. J Gastrointest Surg. 2018;22(1):60–7.
29. Ribero D, Abdalla EK, Madoff DC, Donadon M, Loyer EM, Vauthey JN. Portal vein embolization before major hepatectomy and its effects on regeneration, resectability and outcome. Br J Surg. 2007;94(11):1386–94.
30. Abdalla EK, Hicks ME, Vauthey JN. Portal vein embolization: rationale, technique and future prospects. Br J Surg. 2001;88(2):165–75.

31. Abdalla EK, Barnett CC, Doherty D, Curley SA, Vauthey JN. Extended hepatectomy in patients with hepatobiliary malignancies with and without preoperative portal vein embolization. Arch Surg (Chicago, Ill: 1960). 2002;137(6):675–80; discussion 80–1.
32. Adam R, Pascal G, Castaing D, Azoulay D, Delvart V, Paule B, et al. Tumor progression while on chemotherapy: a contraindication to liver resection for multiple colorectal metastases? Ann Surg. 2004;240(6):1052–61; discussion 61–4.
33. Vauthey JN, Pawlik TM, Ribero D, Wu TT, Zorzi D, Hoff PM, et al. Chemotherapy regimen predicts steatohepatitis and an increase in 90-day mortality after surgery for hepatic colorectal metastases. J Clin Oncol. 2006;24(13):2065–72.
34. Pawlik TM, Olino K, Gleisner AL, Torbenson M, Schulick R, Choti MA. Preoperative chemotherapy for colorectal liver metastases: impact on hepatic histology and postoperative outcome. J Gastrointest Surg. 2007;11(7):860–8.
35. Rubbia-Brandt L, Audard V, Sartoretti P, Roth AD, Brezault C, Le Charpentier M, et al. Severe hepatic sinusoidal obstruction associated with oxaliplatin-based chemotherapy in patients with metastatic colorectal cancer. Ann Oncol. 2004;15(3):460–6.
36. Ribero D, Wang H, Donadon M, Zorzi D, Thomas MB, Eng C, et al. Bevacizumab improves pathologic response and protects against hepatic injury in patients treated with oxaliplatin-based chemotherapy for colorectal liver metastases. Cancer. 2007;110(12):2761–7.
37. Hubert C, Sempoux C, Humblet Y, van den Eynde M, Zech F, Leclercq I, et al. Sinusoidal obstruction syndrome (SOS) related to chemotherapy for colorectal liver metastases: factors predictive of severe SOS lesions and protective effect of bevacizumab. HPB. 2013;15(11):858–64.
38. Goere D, Farges O, Leporrier J, Sauvanet A, Vilgrain V, Belghiti J. Chemotherapy does not impair hypertrophy of the left liver after right portal vein obstruction. J Gastrointest Surg. 2006;10(3):365–70.
39. Abdalla EK, Adam R, Bilchik AJ, Jaeck D, Vauthey JN, Mahvi D. Improving resectability of hepatic colorectal metastases: expert consensus statement. Ann Surg Oncol. 2006;13(10):1271–80.
40. Kokudo N, Tada K, Seki M, Ohta H, Azekura K, Ueno M, et al. Proliferative activity of intrahepatic colorectal metastases after preoperative hemihepatic portal vein embolization. Hepatology (Baltimore, Md). 2001;34(2):267–72.
41. de Graaf W, van den Esschert JW, van Lienden KP, van Gulik TM. Induction of tumor growth after preoperative portal vein embolization: is it a real problem? Ann Surg Oncol. 2009;16(2):423–30.
42. Pamecha V, Levene A, Grillo F, Woodward N, Dhillon A, Davidson BR. Effect of portal vein embolisation on the growth rate of colorectal liver metastases. Br J Cancer. 2009;100(4):617–22.
43. Vogl TJ, Mack MG, Balzer JO, Engelmann K, Straub R, Eichler K, et al. Liver metastases: neoadjuvant downsizing with transarterial chemoembolization before laser-induced thermotherapy. Radiology. 2003;229(2):457–64.
44. Vogl TJ, Zangos S, Eichler K, Yakoub D, Nabil M. Colorectal liver metastases: regional chemotherapy via transarterial chemoembolization (TACE) and hepatic chemoperfusion: an update. Eur Radiol. 2007;17(4):1025–34.
45. Fischer C, Melstrom LG, Arnaoutakis D, Jarnagin W, Brown K, D'Angelica M, et al. Chemotherapy after portal vein embolization to protect against tumor growth during liver hypertrophy before hepatectomy. JAMA Surg. 2013;148(12):1103–8.

Systemic Therapy for Colorectal Cancer Liver Metastases: Sorting Through the Options

15

Bhavana P. Singh, Benjamin A. Weinberg, Sunnie S. Kim, and John L. Marshall

Introduction

Colorectal cancer (CRC) is the third most common cancer worldwide, and approximately 1,361,000 new cases are diagnosed each year [1]. Up to 25% of patients have liver metastases at presentation, and liver metastases are detected in 40–50% of patients diagnosed with CRC globally every year [2].

Previously, the standard of care was to treat colorectal liver metastases (CLMs) with systemic chemotherapy. Recent advances in chemotherapy and surgical techniques have led to liver metastasectomy being a standard treatment option in selected patients with resectable CLMs. As a result, surgery is the ultimate standard of treatment for resectable CLMs. Multiple unfavorably located CLMs can now be resected, leading to complex hepatic resections and, in many cases, improved patient outcomes. Liver resection is the only potential curative therapeutic option for CLMs, but only around 20% of the patients with CLMs can be offered surgery with curative intent. When surgical resection of these metastases is possible, 5-year overall survival (OS) approaches 35% [3]. However, disease recurrence is common and occurs in majority of patients.

In addition to surgical resection, systemic chemotherapy remains a mainstay in the treatment of CLMs. This chapter reviews various chemotherapeutic strategies in the neoadjuvant and/or adjuvant settings. Neoadjuvant chemotherapy may benefit patients with initially resectable CLMs and allow initially unresectable CLM patients to have a chance for future resection. Furthermore, chemotherapy can decrease overall tumor burden and prolonged survival. Effective chemotherapeutic agents include 5-fluorouracil/leucovorin (5-FU/LV), capecitabine, oxaliplatin, and

B. P. Singh · B. A. Weinberg · S. S. Kim · J. L. Marshall (✉)
The Ruesch Center for the Cure of Gastrointestinal Cancers, Lombardi Comprehensive Cancer Center, Georgetown University Medical Center, Washington, DC, USA
e-mail: Bhavana.P.Singh@medstar.net; Baw12@gunet.georgetown.edu; Sunnie.kim@gunet.georgetown.edu; marshalj@georgetown.edu

M. M. Correia et al. (eds.), *Colorectal Cancer Liver Metastases*,
https://doi.org/10.1007/978-3-030-25486-5_15

irinotecan [4]. There are also data supporting the role of biologics in the treatment of CLMs, such as the anti-vascular endothelial growth factor (VEGF) monoclonal antibody bevacizumab and the anti-epidermal growth factor receptor (EGFR) monoclonal antibodies cetuximab and panitumumab.

Another mainstay of treatment of CLMs is liver-directed therapy. Locoregional therapies such as chemoembolization, radioembolization, thermal ablation, and arterial infusion chemotherapy are additional therapeutic options beyond surgical resection and remain an option in patients who are not operative candidates. Given the diversity of therapeutic modalities, the optimal management of hepatic metastases should be individually tailored and directed by a multidisciplinary team, including medical oncologists, surgeons, radiation oncologists, and interventional radiologists.

Neoadjuvant Chemotherapy for Resectable Liver Metastases

There are several advantages to using neoadjuvant chemotherapy as a primary approach in the eradication of CLMs. These advantages include downstaging of large liver lesions, increasing the likelihood of resectability, and treating micrometastases [5–7]. In addition, patients who rapidly progress on neoadjuvant chemotherapy demonstrate an aggressive clinical phenotype and should be spared a likely ineffective liver surgery. That being said, there is still debate regarding the utility of neoadjuvant chemotherapy for resectable liver metastases [8].

The main argument against the use of neoadjuvant therapy is the potential delay to surgical treatment, which may lead to an increase in the risk of disease progression and loss of the window of resectability. Moreover, neoadjuvant chemotherapy may induce hepatic changes, such as steatohepatitis, hepatic sinusoidal obstruction, and periportal inflammation, negatively affecting patient outcome and increasing the risk of liver failure and death after major liver resection [9]. Steatohepatitis may also mask metastases on preoperative imaging, observed in 5–25% of cases [10]. Chemotherapy can also be "too" effective, rendering CLMs difficult to locate by imaging and complicating surgical resections [10, 11].

The sentinel EORTC 40983 trial examined the utility of neoadjuvant chemotherapy in CLMs [12]. This study was a multicenter, randomized trial comparing upfront surgery alone versus perioperative chemotherapy (Table 15.1) in which 364 patients were randomized 1:1 to either upfront surgery or six cycles of preoperative and postoperative FOLFOX4 (LV, 5-FU, and oxaliplatin). There were no significant differences in median overall survival (mOS, 54.3 vs. 61.3 months with FOLFOX4; hazard ratio [HR] 0.88, 95% confidence interval [CI] 0.68–1.14; $P = 0.34$). Nevertheless, progression-free survival (PFS) was 7.3% higher at 3 years in the perioperative chemotherapy group (28.1% vs. 35.4%; HR 0.79, 95% CI 0.62–1.02; $P = 0.058$). In an extended analysis by Sorbye et al., elevated serum carcinoembryonic antigen (CEA) levels above 5 ng/mL were predictive of benefit from perioperative chemotherapy. The 3-year PFS rate was 35% with perioperative FOLFOX4 compared to 20% with surgery alone for patients with CEA levels above

Table 15.1 Selected clinical trials

First author (Year)	Phase	N	Population	Treatment	Outcomes
Nordlinger (2013) [12]	3	364	Resectable CLMs (up to 4 liver metastases)	Surgery vs. Periop FOLFOX4	mOS 54.3 vs. 61.3 months (*P* = 0.34)
Nasti (2013) [14]	2	39	Resectable CLMs	FOLFIRI/Bev	ORR 66.7%, R0 84.6%, mPFS 14 mo, mOS 38 mo
Delaunoit (2005) [17]	3	795	Untreated mCRC	IFL vs. FOLFOX4 vs. IROX	24 (3.3%) underwent liver resection, 11 with FOLFOX4, 11 with IROX, 2 with IFL
Kishi (2010) [20]	R	219	CLMs that underwent resection	Periop FOLFOX4 or FOLFOX4/Bev × 1–8 vs. ≥ 9 cycles	ORR 57% vs. 55% (*P* = 0.738)
Barone (2007) [23]	2	40	Unresectable CLMs	mFOLFIRI	ORR 47.5%, R0 33%
Alberts (2005) [24]	2	42	Unresectable CLMs	FOLFOX4	ORR 60%, R0 40%
Takahashi (2013) [25]	2	36	Unresectable CLMs	mFOLFOX6	ORR 50%, R0 36%
Masi (2006) [26]	2	74	Unresectable CLMs	FOLFOXIRI	ORR 72%, R0 16%
Ychou (2013) [27]	2	122	Unresectable CLMs	FOLFIRI/FOLFOX4 vs. FOLFIRI-HD/ FOLFOX7/ FOLFIRINOX	ORR 33% vs. 49%, R0 23% vs. 26%
Skof (2009) [28]	2	87	Unresectable CLMs	CAPIRI vs. FOLFIRI	ORR 49% vs. 48% (*P* = 0.76), R0 24% vs. 24%
Wong (2011) [29]	2	45	Unresectable high-risk CLMs	CAPOX/Bev	ORR 78%, R0 20%
Snoeren (2017) [48]	3	79	Resected CLMs	CAPOX/Bev vs. CAPOX	1-year DFS 79% vs. 68% (*P* = 0.89)
Ychou (2009) [50]	3	306	Resected CLMs	5-FU/LV vs. FOLFIRI	mDFS 21.6 vs. 24.7 mo (*P* = 0.44)
Bertolini (2011) [30]	2	21	Non-optimally resectable CLMs	FOLFOX/Bev	ORR 57%
Uetake (2015) [31]	2	45	Unresectable CLMs	mFOLFOX6/Bev	ORR 56%, R0 44%
Carrato (2017) [32]	2	77	Unresectable CLMs, *KRAS* WT	FOLFOX4/Pan vs. FOLFIRI/Pan	ORR 74% vs. 67% (*P* = 0.501), R0/R1 34% vs. 46%
Leone (2013) [33]	2	46	Unresectable CLMs	CAPOX/Pan	ORR 54%, *KRAS* WT ORR 65%, R0 22%
Folprecht (2010) [7]	2	111	Unresectable CLMs	FOLFOX6/Cet vs. FOLFIRI/Cet	ORR 68% vs. 57%, R0 38% vs. 30%, *KRAS* WT ORR 70% vs. 41

(continued)

Table 15.1 (continued)

First author (Year)	Phase	N	Population	Treatment	Outcomes
Ji (2013) [35]	2	73	Unresectable CLMs, *KRAS* WT	mFOLFOX6/Cet	ORR 73%, R0 27%
Ye (2013) [36]	2	138	Unresectable CLMs, *KRAS* WT	mFOLFOX6 or FOLFIRI + Cet vs. mFOLFOX6 or FOLFIRI	ORR 57% vs. 29% (*P* < 0.01), R0 25.7% vs. 7.4% (*P* < 0.01)
Primrose (2014) [38]	3	257	Resectable or suboptimally resectable CLMs, *KRAS* WT	mFOLFOX6 or FOLFIRI or CAPOX + Cet vs. mFOLFOX6 or FOLFIRI or CAPOX	mPFS 14.1 vs. 20.5 mo (*P* = 0.03), ORR 70% vs. 62% (*P* = 0.59)
Wasan (2017) [65]	3	1103	Unresectable CLMs	FOLFOX/SIRT vs. FOLFOX	mOS 22.6 vs 23.3 mo (*P* = 0.61)

Abbreviations: *5-FU* 5-fluorouracil; *Bev* bevacizumab; *CAPIRI* capecitabine and irinotecan, *CAPOX* capecitabine and oxaliplatin, *Cet* cetuximab, *CLMs* colorectal cancer liver metastases, *FOLFIRI* leucovorin, 5-FU, and irinotecan, *FOLFOX* leucovorin, 5-FU, and oxaliplatin, *FOLFOXIRI/FOLFIRINOX* leucovorin, 5-FU, oxaliplatin, and irinotecan, *HD* high dose, *IFL* irinotecan, bolus 5-FU, and leucovorin, *IROX* irinotecan and oxaliplatin, *LV* leucovorin, *mCRC* metastatic colorectal cancer, *mo* month, *mDFS* median disease-free survival, *mOS* median overall survival, *mPFS* median progression-free survival, *ORR* objective response rate, *Pan* panitumumab, *R* retrospective, *R0* microscopic margin negative resection, *SIRT* selective internal radiotherapy, *WT* wild type

5 ng/mL. Perioperative FOLFOX4 benefitted patients with resectable disease and elevated CEA regardless of the number of metastatic lesions (1 vs. 2–4, interaction HR = 0.98) [13].

The integration of biologic agents into the neoadjuvant treatment of resectable or borderline resectable CLMs is an area of active interest. In a study by Nasti et al., 39 patients with resectable CLMs received FOLFIRI plus bevacizumab, and the objective response rate (ORR) was 66.7% (95% CI 49.8%–80.9%) [14]. Thirty-seven patients (94.9%) underwent surgery with an R0 resection rate of 84.6%. Median PFS and OS were 14 months (95% CI 11–24) and 38 months (95% CI 28—not reached [NR]), respectively. In another study by Stremitzer et al., 125 patients with resectable or borderline resectable CLMs were treated with 3 months of neoadjuvant and 3 months of adjuvant bevacizumab-based combination chemotherapy and underwent liver resection with curative intent [15]. Their analysis of 42 primary tumor specimens from this study demonstrated that higher intratumoral mRNA levels of pro-angiogenic genes (including *VEGFA* and *VEGFB*) were associated with lower recurrence-free survival (RFS) and OS rates. Future studies should consider stratifying patients undergoing liver resections for CLMs based on their tumors' angiogenic protein expression signature.

In practice, patients undergo either upfront resection of the CLM followed by adjuvant therapy (see below) or neoadjuvant chemotherapy (usually FOLFOX or CAPOX [capecitabine and oxaliplatin], often with bevacizumab). While either approach is acceptable, the National Comprehensive Cancer Network (NCCN) guidelines prefer neoadjuvant therapy for 2–3 months for the reasons outlined above, followed by an additional 3–4 months of adjuvant therapy following surgery [16]. Bevacizumab needs to be held for at least 6 weeks prior to any planned surgery due to impaired wound healing and bleeding risk associated with this agent.

Neoadjuvant "Conversion" Chemotherapy for Unresectable Liver Metastases

Defining the resectability of CLMs is not standardized and needs to be part of a multidisciplinary discussion. Neoadjuvant chemotherapy has been used to decrease the size of liver lesions to make them more amenable to surgical resection. Initially described in patients treated on the Intergroup N9741 study, resection of metastatic disease after chemotherapy was possible in a small but important subset of patients with initially unresectable CLMs [17]. More recent data suggest that only 12–33% of patients with initially unresectable hepatic metastases treated with neoadjuvant chemotherapy develop a significant response enabling surgical resection [18]. The degree at which these patients achieve a complete pathologic response is also variable but is low overall (between 4% and 9%) [19].

The duration of neoadjuvant therapy has also been examined. In a pivotal study by Kishi et al., neoadjuvant chemotherapy consisting of nine cycles or greater was not associated with an increase in complete or major pathologic response (short vs. long duration: 57% vs. 55%; $P = 0.74$) [20]. Instead, the type of chemotherapy used, in this case FOLFOX with bevacizumab, had a greater impact on response than the duration of treatment. Furthermore, this research team documented a higher incidence of liver injury in the group with the longer duration of therapy (4% vs. 11%; $P = 0.035$). Even after a complete response on imaging, there are likely residual microscopic tumor foci, and many believe that resections should include all original sites of disease [10]. One study documented persistent macroscopic or microscopic residual disease or early recurrence in situ in 83% of these patients [11]. This finding may explain why only 20–50% of patients achieve long-term remission among those treated with systemic therapy and liver resection.

The choice of chemotherapy has been researched extensively, and no optimal regimen for conversion therapy has been established. Instead, many physicians pick a regimen based on a high objective response rate. There is a strong correlation between response rate and subsequent resection rate in patients with initially unresectable metastatic disease [21]. Commonly used regimens include FOLFOX, CAPOX, FOLFIRI (LV, 5-FU, and irinotecan), and FOLFOXIRI (LV, 5-FU, oxaliplatin, and irinotecan), which are all regimens used in metastatic CRC.

Several studies have examined the efficacy of different first-line combination chemotherapy regimens for CLMs. In a study using neoadjuvant FOLFIRI, investigators reported that 32.7% of patients with CRC with initially unresectable liver metastases were able to undergo a potentially curative surgical resection [22]. In an updated analysis in 2007, 47.5% of the patients achieved an objective response and 33% underwent resection [23]. After a median follow-up of 56 months, mOS was 31.5 months for all patients, 24 months for non-resected patients, and was not reached for resected patients. Median time to progression (mTTP) was 14.3 and 5.2 months for all and non-resected patients, respectively. Median disease-free survival (mDFS) in resected patients was 52.5 months. FOLFOX4 was also found to have a high response rate in patients with liver-only metastases from CRC in a study by Alberts et al. [24] Of note, this study also documented a high recurrence rate after surgery (73%). In the Japanese ROOF trial, mFOLFOX6 regimen was safely administered to 36 patients, resulting in 18 partial responses (50%), 12 with stable disease, and 4 with progressive disease [25]. Similar antitumor activity was also demonstrated with FOLFOXIRI [26].

In an attempt to perform head-to-head analyses, the METHEP trial randomized 125 patients to either standard (FOLFIRI/FOLFOX4) or intensified chemotherapy (FOLFIRI-HD/FOLFOX7/FOLFIRINOX) [27]. ORR was 33%, 47%, 43%, and 57% after the first four cycles of FOLFIRI/FOLFOX4, FOLFIRI-HD, FOLFOX7, and FOLFIRINOX, respectively. FOLFIRINOX offered the best conversion rate to resectability (67%). Additionally, CAPIRI (capecitabine and irinotecan) was compared to FOLFIRI by Skof et al., and CAPIRI showed a similar ORR to FOLFIRI in the neoadjuvant treatment of CLMs [28]. In addition, the CAPIRI regimen resulted in similar PFS and OS with acceptable toxicity compared to the FOLFIRI regimen.

Role of Biologics

There is a growing body of evidence examining the role of biologically active compounds in the treatment of CLMs. These agents include anti-angiogenic drugs such as bevacizumab and anti-EGFR agents, such as cetuximab and panitumumab.

As mentioned above, bevacizumab is a recombinant humanized monoclonal antibody that blocks angiogenesis by inhibiting VEGF-A. It was the first angiogenesis inhibitor to be approved by the US Food and Drug Administration (FDA). The rationale for the use of bevacizumab in addition to chemotherapy is that recurrence after resection of CLMs may be caused by VEGF-mediated outgrowth of micrometastases, and inhibiting VEGF could prevent this recurrence. An earlier study examined perioperative CAPOX plus bevacizumab in patients with high-risk CLMs not selected for upfront resection [29]. Following neoadjuvant CAPOX plus bevacizumab, the ORR was 78% (95% CI 63%–89%). This study also showed that metachronous unresectable CLMs could be converted to resectable disease in 40% of patients.

Another study by Bertollini et al. showed an objective response in 12 patients (57.1%) receiving FOLFOX6 and bevacizumab [30]. This study also indicated that the combination does not increase postsurgical complications and yields high rates of resectability, a finding that was confirmed by Uetake et al. and Takatsuki et al. in studies that demonstrated similar response rates [25, 31]. Despite the ongoing concern regarding bevacizumab-induced impaired wound healing after resection, several studies have demonstrated the safety of this agent in CLM treatment.

Anti-EGFR agents are active in *RAS* and *BRAF* wild-type (WT) left-sided metastatic colorectal cancer, and there have been several studies examining their role in the treatment of patients with CLMs. In the PLANET-TTD trial, panitumumab was added to FOLFOX4 or FOLFIRI as first-line treatment of patients with *KRAS* exon 2 WT colorectal cancer and CLMs [32]. The ORR was 74% with panitumumab-FOLFOX4 and 67% with panitumumab-FOLFIRI, and 45% and 59% of patients, respectively, underwent surgical resection. The activity of panitumumab in combination with CAPOX was also demonstrated, with an ORR of 54% [33]. In patients with *KRAS* WT tumors, the ORR reached 65% (2 CRs and 19 PRs), which allowed 15 patients with initially unresectable liver metastasis to be converted to resectable disease.

Cetuximab has also been studied extensively in this population. In the CELIM trial, which compared first-line FOLFOX plus cetuximab and FOLFIRI plus cetuximab, both regimens demonstrated responses in 57–68% of patients, and resectability rates increased from 32% (22 of 68 patients) at baseline to 60% (41 of 68) after chemotherapy [7]. In a follow-up survival analysis, this study confirmed a favorable long-term survival for patients with initially unresectable colorectal liver metastases who responded to conversion therapy and underwent resection [34]. In this study, both FOLFOX plus cetuximab and FOLFIRI plus cetuximab appeared to be appropriate regimens for conversion treatment in patients with *KRAS* WT tumors. Similar activity with cetuximab combined with FOLFOX6 or FOLFIRI has been shown in several other studies [35, 36]. In Japan, the KSCC group examined the use of S-1 and oxaliplatin (SOX) plus cetuximab in 33 patients (see section *Adjuvant Therapy Following Resection of Liver Metastases* for further discussion of S-1). They found an overall response rate of 63.6% (95% CI 45.1%–79.6%), and liver resection was possible in 16 of 33 (48%) patients [37].

Conversely, the New EPOC trial demonstrated that chemotherapy (FOLFOX, CAPOX, or FOLFIRI) plus cetuximab for resectable or suboptimally resectable CLMs in *KRAS* exon 2 WT patients resulted in shorter mPFS compared to chemotherapy alone [38]. Anti-EGFR therapies are thought to be more efficacious in CRC with left-sided primary tumors [39–42]; however, most of the patients in this study had left-sided primary tumors, so tumor sidedness does not explain the discrepancy in PFS seen following the addition of cetuximab to chemotherapy. Pugh et al. have suggested that study patients with tumors low in microRNA (miR)-31-3p expression were not adversely affected by the addition of cetuximab [43]. However, future studies will need to further investigate which *RAS* WT patients benefit from cetuximab in the context of CLM resection.

Recently, several studies have compared anti-VEGF and anti-EGFR therapies. In the BECK trial, 35 patients with unresectable CLMs were enrolled, and patients with *KRAS* WT tumors were assigned to mFOLFOX6 plus cetuximab while those with *KRAS*-mutant (MT) tumors were assigned to mFOLFOX6 plus bevacizumab [44]. The conversion rate was 72.7% in patients with WT tumors and 33.3% in patients with MT tumors ($P = 0.03$). In 58.8% of patients overall, hepatectomy was performed, according to protocol, and the ORR was 64.7%. Examining the different histologies of metastases following patient treatment with bevacizumab versus cetuximab, Stremitzer et al. found that the addition of bevacizumab to combination chemotherapy showed more necrosis but less fibrosis of metastases, along with a trend toward higher histological and radiological response and longer recurrence-free survival compared to cetuximab [45].

Tumor Sidedness

In summary, multiple studies in patients with *RAS* WT metastatic CRC have demonstrated that patients with left-sided primary tumors who are treated with anti-EGFR therapies plus chemotherapy have improved OS compared to chemotherapy alone or chemotherapy plus bevacizumab, whereas patients with right-sided primary tumors generally have inferior outcomes but do benefit from bevacizumab [39–42]. Patients with right-sided primary tumors have inferior OS compared to patients with left-sided primaries. In an interesting retrospective study of 725 patients who had resected CLMs after neoadjuvant chemotherapy, those with primary tumors of midgut origin (right-sided: cecum to proximal transverse colon) had worse RFS (15% vs. 27%; $P < 0.001$) and OS at 3 years (46% vs. 68%; $P < 0.001$) than patients with tumors of hindgut origin (left-sided: distal transverse colon to rectum), independent of *RAS* mutational status [46].

For patients with unresectable CLMs, neoadjuvant chemotherapy remains the preferred approach. In our practice, we typically use FOLFOX/CAPOX in the first-line setting, often in combination with bevacizumab or cetuximab/panitumumab (*RAS* and *BRAF* WT in patients with left-sided primaries only), although FOLFIRI or FOLFIRINOX, both plus a biological agent, are appropriate alternatives.

Adjuvant Therapy Following Resection of Liver Metastases

Several trials examined the role of adjuvant chemotherapy following the resection of CLMs. In an early study of 5-FU/LV, adjuvant intravenous systemic chemotherapy provided a significant DFS benefit to patients with resected CLMs [47]. This result was further supported by the HEPATICA study by Snoeren et al. [48]. This study compared CAPOX plus bevacizumab to CAPOX alone as adjuvant treatment and found no significant difference in toxicity between the two arms.

Pooling data from two large trials, Mitry et al. found that using adjuvant chemotherapy after resection of liver metastases provided minor benefit [49]. This research group combined data from the Federation Francophone de Cancerologie Digestive Trial 9002 and the European Organisation for Research and Treatment of Cancer/National Cancer Institute of Canada Clinical Trials Group/Gruppo Italiano di Valutazione Interventi in Oncologia trial, both of which used 5-FU-based regimens. The pooled analysis included 278 patients, and mPFS was 27.9 months in the chemotherapy arm compared to 18.8 months in the surgery-alone arm (HR 1.32, 95% CI, 1.00–1.76; $P = 0.058$). mOS was 62.2 months in the chemotherapy arm compared to 47.3 months in the surgery arm (HR 1.32, 95% CI, 0.95–1.82;

$P = 0.095$). Adjuvant chemotherapy was also independently associated with both PFS and OS in the multivariable analysis. Shortly thereafter, Ychou et al. compared adjuvant therapy with 5-FU/LV versus FOLFIRI. There was no statistically significant improvement in mDFS with the use of FOLFIRI (24.7 vs. 21.6 months with 5-FU/LV; HR 0.89, 95% CI 0.66–1.119; $P = 0.44$) [50].

In an attempt to determine if the use of less-toxic regimens had an impact on OS and recurrence, Hasegawa et al. examined the role of oral uracil-tegafur (a prodrug that is converted by cells to 5-FU) and leucovorin (UFT/LV) in combination with surgery versus surgery alone [51, 52]. The researchers found that the median RFS in the UFT/LV-treated group was 1.45 years compared to 0.70 years following surgery alone (HR = 0.56; 95%, CI 0.38–0.83; $P = 0.003$). This study was followed by a phase II investigation of the efficacy of S-1 (Taiho Pharmaceutical, Tokyo, Japan) in patients with resected CLMs. S-1 is an oral preparation combining tegafur, gimeracil (an inhibitor of dihydropyrimidine dehydrogenase, which degrades 5-FU), and oteracil (which inhibits the phosphorylation of 5-FU in the gastrointestinal tract). S-1 often does not have the same gastrointestinal toxic effects of 5-FU. It is currently the standard of care for patients with gastric cancer in Japan, and its approval has been expanded to colon cancer. Initially, researchers found a therapy-completion rate of 58.3%, and the most common reason for cessation of therapy was disease relapse [53]. The study demonstrated 3-year DFS and OS rates of 47.4% and 80.0%, respectively [54]. These prodrugs are useful in the treatment of patients who are unwilling or unable to receive traditional intravenous therapies.

For patients with resectable metachronous CLMs, options include local therapy (e.g., radiofrequency ablation [RFA], selective internal radiation therapy [SIRT], or stereotactic body radiation therapy [SBRT]), upfront resection, or neoadjuvant chemotherapy followed by resection. Generally, resection is preferred to local therapy because resection is thought to have a higher curative potential, but limited data exist to compare these methodologies head-to-head. For those patients who receive upfront resection, adjuvant FOLFOX or CAPOX is preferred if the patient has never received chemotherapy previously, whereas observation alone is preferred for patients who have received prior oxaliplatin-based chemotherapy [16]. Those patients who received neoadjuvant chemotherapy prior to liver resection can continue with the same regimen after surgery (adjuvant), undergo observation alone, or switch to an alternative chemotherapy regimen after surgery if there was evidence of tumor growth while on neoadjuvant therapy. Again, there are limited data to guide therapeutic selection in this setting; thus, a shared decision-making model—between oncologist and patient—is preferred.

The duration of adjuvant chemotherapy following CLM resection is controversial, especially in light of the findings from the International Duration of Adjuvant Therapy (IDEA) collaboration which showed that 3 months of adjuvant FOLFOX/CAPOX is non-inferior to 6 months of treatment for patients with lower risk (T1-3N1), resected stage-3 CRC in terms of RFS at 3 years [55]. For now, 6 months of adjuvant (or total combined neoadjuvant/adjuvant) chemotherapy for patients with resected CLMs should remain the standard of care given the high-risk nature of recurrent CRC in a patient with stage-IV disease.

Combination Chemotherapy and Liver-Directed Therapy

The use of chemotherapy in conjunction with liver-directed therapy has also been researched extensively. Initially in the CALGB 9481 trial, Kemeny et al. compared hepatic arterial infusion (HAI) treatment with floxuridine (FUDR) and LV plus dexamethasone (Dex) versus systemic 5-FU/LV [56]. It was found that mOS was significantly longer for HAI versus systemic treatment (24.4 vs. 20 months; $P = 0.0034$), as were the response rate (47% vs. 24%; $P = 0.012$) and time to hepatic progression (9.8 vs. 7.3 months; $P = 0.034$). Time to extrahepatic progression (7.7 vs. 14.8 months; $P = 0.029$) was significantly shorter in the HAI group. This study demonstrated the need for further research to address the benefit of adding systemic chemotherapy to HAI. Bolton et al. expanded on these data, examining HAI alternating with systemic therapy after surgical resection and found that this approach may improve survival following surgery. The estimated median DFS and hepatic DFS rates were 1.2 years (95% CI 0.9–2.1) and 1.8 years (95% CI 1.8–NR), respectively.

Chen et al. later added to these initial data by researching the role of HAI with irinotecan, oxaliplatin, and floxuridine as a first-line treatment of patients with unresectable CLMs [57]. They found an ORR of 61.3% and a mOS of 24.8 months, and the median time to tumor progression was 10.1 months. Similarly, the Japan Clinical Oncology Group Trial 0208-DI conducted a phase I/II study of HAI using 5-FU plus systemic irinotecan [58]. This research group found that patients had a response rate of 72% and a mOS of 49.8 months (95% CI 27.5–78.1 months). Later, House et al. evaluated the benefit of adding HAI-FUDR/Dex to adjuvant systemic chemotherapy (5-FU/leucovorin plus oxaliplatin or irinotecan) administered after resection of CLMs [59]. Compared to adjuvant chemotherapy alone (125 patients), adding HAI-FUDR (125 patients) was associated with an improved 5-year liver RFS, overall RFS, and disease-specific survival (DSS): respectively 75%, 48%, and 79% vs. 55%, 25%, and 55% ($P < 0.01$).

D'Angelica et al. examined the addition of bevacizumab to HAI plus systemic chemotherapy [60]. They found an ORR of 76% (four complete responses). Twenty-three patients (47%) achieved conversion to hepatic resection at a median of 6 months after treatment initiation. mOS and mPFS for all patients were 38 months (95% CI 28-NR) and 13 months (95% CI 7–16), respectively. The study group also found that bevacizumab administration did not impact outcome. Levi et al. explored the effect of adding cetuximab to adjuvant chemotherapy in the OPTILIV study [61]. The primary study endpoint was reached in that R0-R1 hepatectomy was achieved for 29.7% (95% CI 18.5%–40.9%) of patients compared to 15% in historical controls (adjuvant chemotherapy alone). The objective response rate was 40.6% (95% CI 28.6%–52.3%). Median PFS and OS reached 9.3 months (95% CI 7.8–10.9) and 25.5 months (95% CI 18.8–32.1), respectively.

Several groups have examined the role of chemotherapy in individuals receiving transarterial chemoembolization (TACE) and RFA for CLM treatment. In the EORTC Intergroup phase II study, the researchers set out to determine the role of RFA plus chemotherapy in treating CLMs. The primary objective was to achieve a 30-month OS rate that was greater than 38% [62]. In fact, the 30-month OS rate was

61.7% (95% CI 48.2%–73.9%) for RFA combined with chemotherapy, although the 30-month OS for the comparative group (chemotherapy alone) was also high (much higher than expected) at 57.6% (95% CI 44.1%–70.4%). The mPFS was 16.8 months (95% CI 11.7–22.1) with the combination versus 9.9 months (95% CI 9.3–13.7) with systemic treatment alone. mOS was longer in the combination arm (45.3 vs. 40.5 months; $P = 0.22$), but this was not statistically significant. This study failed to prove the superiority of RFA compared to chemotherapy alone. Furthermore, the study started out as a phase III trial but was redesigned as a phase II trial due to poor patient accrual.

Iezzi et al. studied the safety and efficacy of drug-eluting beads loaded with irinotecan (DEBIRI) in combination with capecitabine in the treatment of CLMs [63]. During a mean follow-up of 11 months, two partial responses (PRs) were reported with overall disease control of 60% (2 PRs, 10 with stable disease). mPFS and mOS were 4 and 7.3 months, respectively. Thereby, the study investigators determined that DEBIRI was a safe modality to deliver liver-directed therapy. Martin et al. examined FOLFOX plus DEBIRI versus FOLFOX plus bevacizumab as a first-line treatment for unresectable CLMs [64]. The ORR was greater in the FOLFOX-DEBIRI arm versus the FOLFOX/bevacizumab arm at 6 months (76% vs. 60%; $P = 0.05$). There was significantly more tumor downsizing to resection in the FOLFOX-DEBIRI arm versus the FOLFOX/bevacizumab arm (35% vs. 16%; $P = 0.05$), and there was improved median PFS (15.3 vs. 7.6 months). Further studies are needed to determine the efficacy of these approaches.

The role of selective internal radiation therapy (SIRT) using yttrium-90 microspheres (Y-90) in combination with systemic chemotherapy was evaluated in the FOXFIRE, FOXFIRE-Global, and SIRFLOX studies. These randomized clinical trials were designed to study whether Y-90 in combination with FOLFOX chemotherapy as first-line therapy for CRC could improve overall survival compared with FOLFOX alone in patients with liver-only or liver-dominant metastases [65]. Although there was a significantly lower cumulative incidence of liver progression with Y-90 (HR 0.51, 95% CI 0.43–0.62; $P < 0.0001$), there was no significant difference in mOS (22.6 vs. 23.3 months with chemotherapy alone; HR 1.04, 95% CI 0.90–1.19; $P = 0.61$). Importantly, the odds of undergoing a resection were not significantly different between the study groups (odds ratio [OR] 1.07, 95% CI 0.78–1.48; $P = 0.67$). Based on these data, researchers concluded that first-line use of Y-90 in combination with chemotherapy in unselected patients with metastatic CRC cannot be recommended.

Non-chemotherapy Systemic Therapies

There have been several studies looking at the effect of systemic therapies other than chemotherapy on patients with CLMs. Although uptake of these therapies into clinical practice has been limited, research results are promising. Specifically, several studies have investigated the role of anti-idiotype monoclonal antibody vaccines in the metastatic setting. These vaccines are developed in the hope that they will overcome the host immune system's tolerance to tumor-associated antigens by transforming epitope structures into idiotypic determinants expressed on the surface of antibodies. One multi-institutional phase II prospective trial studied the use of anti-idiotype monoclonal antibody vaccines to the tumor-associated antigens CEA (CeaVac) and human milk fat globule (TriAb) after curative resection of CLMs [66]. Unfortunately, anti-idiotype monoclonal antibody vaccine therapy with CeaVac and TriAb did not improve 2-year RFS rate over and above the 40% reported for hepatic resection alone. Researchers were able to demonstrate that it was well tolerated but did not achieve the expected endpoint.

There have also been several studies focused on the role of radio-immunotherapy (RIT) with native or radiolabeled monoclonal antibodies. In one study, Ychou et al. studied the role of ^{131}I-anti-CEA F(ab′)2 in the adjuvant treatment of CLMs [67]. At a median follow-up of 127 months, mDFS was 12 months and the mOS was 50 months. Major grade 3 and 4 adverse events included neutropenia and thrombocytopenia. Sahlmann et al. elaborated on these results in 2017 [68]. Thus the mTTP, mOS, and median cause-specific survival (CSS) for all patients receiving RIT using anti-CEA ^{131}I-labetuzumab were 16, 55, and 60 months, respectively. Patients were subdivided into two subgroups: "truly adjuvant" if they had no suspicious lesions postoperatively on PET or CT and if serum CEA levels were normal (less than 5 ng/mL) or "possibly nonadjuvant" if these conditions were not met. The "truly adjuvant" patients ($N = 39$) had an improved mTTP (NR vs. 6.1 months; HR 0.12; $P < 0.001$), mOS (75.6 vs. 33.4 months; HR 0.44; $P = 0.014$), and CSS (NR vs. 41.4 months; HR 0.42; $P = 0.014$) compared with "possibly nonadjuvant" patients ($N = 24$). Repeat RIT with ^{131}I-labetuzumab potentially improved survival but was associated with significant and often dose-limiting hematotoxicity.

Finally, Morse et al. studied the use of modified autologous dendritic cells (DCs) in 74 patients with no evidence of disease following CLM resection and perioperative chemotherapy [69]. In this phase II study, patients were randomized 1:1 to receive DCs modified with the poxvector vaccine PANVAC (encoding the antigens CEA and MUC1 that are overexpressed on CRC cells) or PANVAC in combination with granulocyte-macrophage colony-stimulating factor (GM-CSF). RFS at 2 years was similar in both arms (47% with DC/PANVAC vs. 55% with PANVAC/GM-CSF; $P = 0.48$), and there was a significant increase in mOS when both arms were compared to a contemporary control group that was not vaccinated (NR vs. 44.1 months; $P < 0.0001$).

Sequencing of Therapies for Rectal Cancer with Synchronous Liver Metastases

Although surgery remains the hallmark of treatment for liver metastases, there is still great debate about the timing of adjuvant chemotherapy and radiation therapy in rectal cancer specifically. The reason for this debate is due to the fact that radiation is often used with radiosensitizers, such as 5-FU, to downsize the primary tumor and reduce the risk of locoregional failure after resection [70]. 5-FU monotherapy often has a limited effect on systemic metastases, thereby adding to the question about the appropriate sequencing of therapies. Chemoradiotherapy with a fluoropyrimidine prior to surgery induces tumor downstaging, thereby allowing for a more complete removal of the tumor. A "liver-first" approach has been proposed by some researchers, which includes systemic chemotherapy followed by resection of CLMs and subsequent surgery for the primary rectal tumor [71]. The issue with this approach is that it often requires two surgical procedures and may delay systemic therapy which must be held around each surgery. In one study, van Dijk et al. used a treatment sequence including preoperative short-course pelvic radiotherapy of five fractions of 5 Gy each, followed by CAPOX/bevacizumab [72]. They found that the 2-year overall survival rate was 80% (95% CI 66.3%–90.0%) and the 2-year recurrence rate was 64% (95% CI 49.8%–84.5%). The conclusion was that surgical treatment of all tumor sites carried out after short-course radiotherapy and CAPOX/bevacizumab combination therapy is a feasible and potentially curative approach. In another study, Kim et al. evaluated the efficacy and safety of upfront mFOLFOX6 followed by short-course radiotherapy and surgery in patients with locally advanced rectal cancer and liver-only metastases [73]. One of the major endpoints was resectability, and they found that surgical resection of the rectum and liver was possible in 78% of patients. Local tumor downstaging was observed in 54% of patients. mOS and mPFS were 38 and 9 months, respectively. Given the multiple modalities used in the management of rectal cancer, the optimal sequence of therapies for patients with rectal cancer and resectable CLMs should be the focus of multidisciplinary discussions between medical oncologists, radiation oncologists, and surgeons.

Ongoing Clinical Trials

There are ongoing clinical trials examining new therapeutics for the treatment of CLMs. To determine the appropriate sequence of therapy, the CHARISMA trial randomizes individuals to either surgery alone (standard treatment, arm A) or to six cycles of neoadjuvant oxaliplatin-based chemotherapy, followed by surgery (arm B) [74]. In the CAIRO 5 trial (NCT02162563), researchers plan to test for *RAS* and *BRAF* tumor mutation status and select patients based on the location of the primary tumor [75]. Patients with *RAS* or *BRAF* MT and/or right-sided tumors will be randomized between doublet chemotherapy (FOLFOX or FOLFIRI) plus bevacizumab, and triple chemotherapy (FOLFOXIRI) plus bevacizumab. Patients with *RAS* and *BRAF* WT left-sided primary tumors will be randomized between doublet chemotherapy (FOLFOX or FOLFIRI) plus either bevacizumab or panitumumab. The primary outcome is mPFS and secondary outcomes include secondary resection rate, mOS, ORR, pathological complete response rate, and toxicity. Finally, several studies are examining the role of novel therapies such as immunotherapy in the treatment of CLMs. In a phase I trial, an experimental anti-cancer immunotherapy called NKR-2 (modified T cells) will be administered transarterially into the liver to treat unresectable CLMs (NCT03370198). There is another study examining tremelimumab (an anti-cytotoxic T-lymphocyte-associated protein 4

[CTLA-4] antibody) in combination with durvalumab (an anti-programmed death ligand 1 [PD-L1] antibody) in patients with CLMs (NCT02754856). There are also several studies looking at novel procedures for CLMs. In the COLLISION trial, a prospective multicenter phase III randomized controlled trial, researchers aim to prove non-inferiority of thermal ablation compared to hepatic resection in patients with at least one resectable and ablatable CLM smaller than 3 cm and no extrahepatic disease (NCT03088150). The studies highlighted here are just a few of the numerous trials underway that are examining the optimal treatment of CLMs.

Conclusion

Advancements in the treatment of CLMs have resulted in longer patient OS due to downstaging of CLMs and increased number of subsequent metastasectomies. There is ongoing debate regarding the timing of appropriate therapy; however, neoadjuvant chemotherapy is widely accepted as an appropriate upfront treatment, often followed by adjuvant chemotherapy after surgery. Surgical resection remains the hallmark of treatment. There is also an emerging role for locoregional therapies in terms of preventing disease progression, although this strategy is not commonly used in the first-line setting due to lack of OS benefit. Continued research is necessary to develop more standardized algorithms of care for patients with CLMs.

Acknowledgment We would like to thank Marion Hartley, PhD, for her edits and suggestions during the composition of this chapter.

References

1. Ferlay J, Soerjomataram I, Dikshit R, Eser S, Mathers C, Rebelo M, et al. Cancer incidence and mortality worldwide: sources, methods and major patterns in GLOBOCAN 2012. Int J Cancer. 2015;136(5):E359–86.
2. McMillan DC, McArdle CS. Epidemiology of colorectal liver metastases. Surg Oncol. 2007;16(1):3–5.
3. Manfredi S, Lepage C, Hatem C, Coatmeur O, Faivre J, Bouvier AM. Epidemiology and management of liver metastases from colorectal cancer. Ann Surg. 2006;244(2):254–9.
4. Brandi G, De Lorenzo S, Nannini M, Curti S, Ottone M, Dall'Olio FG, et al. Adjuvant chemotherapy for resected colorectal cancer metastases: literature review and meta-analysis. World J Gastroenterol. 2016;22(2):519–33.
5. Bismuth H, Adam R, Levi F, Farabos C, Waechter F, Castaing D, et al. Resection of nonresectable liver metastases from colorectal cancer after neoadjuvant chemotherapy. Ann Surg. 1996;224(4):509–20; discussion 520-502
6. Nordlinger B, Benoist S. Benefits and risks of neoadjuvant therapy for liver metastases. J Clin Oncol. 2006;24(31):4954–5.
7. Folprecht G, Gruenberger T, Bechstein WO, Raab HR, Lordick F, Hartmann JT, et al. Tumour response and secondary resectability of colorectal liver metastases following neoadjuvant chemotherapy with cetuximab: the CELIM randomised phase 2 trial. Lancet Oncol. 2010;11(1):38–47.

8. Chua TC, Saxena A, Liauw W, Kokandi A, Morris DL. Systematic review of randomized and nonrandomized trials of the clinical response and outcomes of neoadjuvant systemic chemotherapy for resectable colorectal liver metastases. Ann Surg Oncol. 2010;17(2):492–501.
9. Fernandez FG, Ritter J, Goodwin JW, Linehan DC, Hawkins WG, Strasberg SM. Effect of steatohepatitis associated with irinotecan or oxaliplatin pretreatment on resectability of hepatic colorectal metastases. J Am Coll Surg. 2005;200(6):845–53.
10. Bischof DA, Clary BM, Maithel SK, Pawlik TM. Surgical management of disappearing colorectal liver metastases. Br J Surg. 2013;100(11):1414–20.
11. Benoist S, Brouquet A, Penna C, Julie C, El Hajjam M, Chagnon S, et al. Complete response of colorectal liver metastases after chemotherapy: does it mean cure? J Clin Oncol. 2006;24(24):3939–45.
12. Nordlinger B, Sorbye H, Glimelius B, Poston GJ, Schlag PM, Rougier P, et al. Perioperative FOLFOX4 chemotherapy and surgery versus surgery alone for resectable liver metastases from colorectal cancer (EORTC 40983): long-term results of a randomised, controlled, phase 3 trial. Lancet Oncol. 2013;14(12):1208–15.
13. Sorbye H, Mauer M, Gruenberger T, Glimelius B, Poston GJ, Schlag PM, et al. Predictive factors for the benefit of perioperative FOLFOX for resectable liver metastasis in colorectal cancer patients (EORTC Intergroup Trial 40983). Ann Surg. 2012;255(3):534–9.
14. Nasti G, Piccirillo MC, Izzo F, Ottaiano A, Albino V, Delrio P, et al. Neoadjuvant FOLFIRI+bevacizumab in patients with resectable liver metastases from colorectal cancer: a phase 2 trial. Br J Cancer. 2013;108(8):1566–70.
15. Stremitzer S, Zhang W, Yang D, Ning Y, Sunakawa Y, Matsusaka S, et al. Expression of genes involved in vascular morphogenesis and maturation predicts efficacy of bevacizumab-based chemotherapy in patients undergoing liver resection. Mol Cancer Ther. 2016;15(11):2814–21.
16. National Comprehensive Cancer Network. NCCN guidelines version 2.2018 Colon Cancer. 2018.; https://www.nccn.org/professionals/physician_gls/pdf/colon.pdf. Accessed May 10, 2018.
17. Delaunoit T, Alberts SR, Sargent DJ, Green E, Goldberg RM, Krook J, et al. Chemotherapy permits resection of metastatic colorectal cancer: experience from Intergroup N9741. Ann Oncol. 2005;16(3):425–9.
18. Adam R, Wicherts DA, de Haas RJ, Ciacio O, Levi F, Paule B, et al. Patients with initially unresectable colorectal liver metastases: is there a possibility of cure? J Clin Oncol. 2009;27(11):1829–35.
19. Adam R, Wicherts DA, de Haas RJ, Aloia T, Levi F, Paule B, et al. Complete pathologic response after preoperative chemotherapy for colorectal liver metastases: myth or reality? J Clin Oncol. 2008;26(10):1635–41.
20. Kishi Y, Zorzi D, Contreras CM, Maru DM, Kopetz S, Ribero D, et al. Extended preoperative chemotherapy does not improve pathologic response and increases postoperative liver insufficiency after hepatic resection for colorectal liver metastases. Ann Surg Oncol. 2010;17(11):2870–6.
21. Folprecht G, Grothey A, Alberts S, Raab HR, Kohne CH. Neoadjuvant treatment of unresectable colorectal liver metastases: correlation between tumour response and resection rates. Ann Oncol. 2005;16(8):1311–9.
22. Pozzo C, Basso M, Cassano A, Quirino M, Schinzari G, Trigila N, et al. Neoadjuvant treatment of unresectable liver disease with irinotecan and 5-fluorouracil plus folinic acid in colorectal cancer patients. Ann Oncol. 2004;15(6):933–9.
23. Barone C, Nuzzo G, Cassano A, Basso M, Schinzari G, Giuliante F, et al. Final analysis of colorectal cancer patients treated with irinotecan and 5-fluorouracil plus folinic acid neoadjuvant chemotherapy for unresectable liver metastases. Br J Cancer. 2007;97(8):1035–9.
24. Alberts SR, Horvath WL, Sternfeld WC, Goldberg RM, Mahoney MR, Dakhil SR, et al. Oxaliplatin, fluorouracil, and leucovorin for patients with unresectable liver-only metastases from colorectal cancer: a North Central Cancer Treatment Group phase II study. J Clin Oncol. 2005;23(36):9243–9.

25. Takahashi T, Shibata Y, Tojima Y, Tsuboi K, Sakamoto E, Kunieda K, et al. Multicenter phase II study of modified FOLFOX6 as neoadjuvant chemotherapy for patients with unresectable liver-only metastases from colorectal cancer in Japan: ROOF study. Int J Clin Oncol. 2013;18(2):335–42.
26. Masi G, Cupini S, Marcucci L, Cerri E, Loupakis F, Allegrini G, et al. Treatment with 5-fluorouracil/folinic acid, oxaliplatin, and irinotecan enables surgical resection of metastases in patients with initially unresectable metastatic colorectal cancer. Ann Surg Oncol. 2006;13(1):58–65.
27. Ychou M, Rivoire M, Thezenas S, Quenet F, Delpero JR, Rebischung C, et al. A randomized phase II trial of three intensified chemotherapy regimens in first-line treatment of colorectal cancer patients with initially unresectable or not optimally resectable liver metastases. The METHEP trial. Ann Surg Oncol. 2013;20(13):4289–97.
28. Skof E, Rebersek M, Hlebanja Z, Ocvirk J. Capecitabine plus irinotecan (XELIRI regimen) compared to 5-FU/LV plus irinotecan (FOLFIRI regimen) as neoadjuvant treatment for patients with unresectable liver-only metastases of metastatic colorectal cancer: a randomised prospective phase II trial. BMC Cancer. 2009;9:120.
29. Wong R, Cunningham D, Barbachano Y, Saffery C, Valle J, Hickish T, et al. A multicentre study of capecitabine, oxaliplatin plus bevacizumab as perioperative treatment of patients with poor-risk colorectal liver-only metastases not selected for upfront resection. Ann Oncol. 2011;22(9):2042–8.
30. Bertolini F, Malavasi N, Scarabelli L, Fiocchi F, Bagni B, Del Giovane C, et al. FOLFOX6 and bevacizumab in non-optimally resectable liver metastases from colorectal cancer. Br J Cancer. 2011;104(7):1079–84.
31. Uetake H, Yasuno M, Ishiguro M, Kameoka S, Shimada Y, Takahashi K, et al. A multicenter phase II trial of mFOLFOX6 plus bevacizumab to treat liver-only metastases of colorectal cancer that are unsuitable for upfront resection (TRICC0808). Ann Surg Oncol. 2015;22(3):908–15.
32. Carrato A, Abad A, Massuti B, Gravalos C, Escudero P, Longo-Munoz F, et al. First-line panitumumab plus FOLFOX4 or FOLFIRI in colorectal cancer with multiple or unresectable liver metastases: a randomised, phase II trial (PLANET-TTD). Eur J Cancer. 2017;81:191–202.
33. Leone F, Artale S, Marino D, Cagnazzo C, Cascinu S, Pinto C, et al. Panitumumab in combination with infusional oxaliplatin and oral capecitabine for conversion therapy in patients with colon cancer and advanced liver metastases. The MetaPan study. Cancer. 2013;119(19):3429–35.
34. Folprecht G, Gruenberger T, Bechstein W, Raab HR, Weitz J, Lordick F, et al. Survival of patients with initially unresectable colorectal liver metastases treated with FOLFOX/cetuximab or FOLFIRI/cetuximab in a multidisciplinary concept (CELIM study). Ann Oncol. 2014;25(5):1018–25.
35. Ji JH, Park SH, Lee J, Kim TW, Hong YS, Kim KP, et al. Prospective phase II study of neoadjuvant FOLFOX6 plus cetuximab in patients with colorectal cancer and unresectable liver-only metastasis. Cancer Chemother Pharmacol. 2013;72(1):223–30.
36. Ye LC, Liu TS, Ren L, Wei Y, Zhu DX, Zai SY, et al. Randomized controlled trial of cetuximab plus chemotherapy for patients with KRAS wild-type unresectable colorectal liver-limited metastases. J Clin Oncol. 2013;31(16):1931–8.
37. Oki E, Emi Y, Miyamoto Y, Kabashima A, Higashi H, Ogata Y, et al. Erratum to: phase II trial of S-1 and oxaliplatin plus cetuximab for colorectal cancer patients with initially unresectable or not optimally resectable liver metastases (KSCC1002). Ann Surg Oncol. 2015;22(Suppl 3):S1617.
38. Primrose J, Falk S, Finch-Jones M, Valle J, O'Reilly D, Siriwardena A, et al. Systemic chemotherapy with or without cetuximab in patients with resectable colorectal liver metastasis: the new EPOC randomised controlled trial. Lancet Oncol. 2014;15(6):601–11.
39. Venook AP, Niedzwiecki D, Innocenti F, Fruth B, Greene C, O'Neil BH, et al. Impact of primary tumor location on overall survival and progression-free survival in patients with metastatic colorectal cancer: analysis of CALGB/SWOB 80405 (Alliance). J Clin Oncol. 2016;34(suppl):abstr 3504.

40. Loupakis F, Yang D, Yau L, Feng S, Cremolini C, Zhang W, et al. Primary tumor location as a prognostic factor in metastatic colorectal cancer. J Natl Cancer Inst 2015;107(3):1–9. https://www.ncbi.nlm.nih.gov/pmc/articles/PMC4565528/pdf/dju427.pdf.
41. Brule SY, Jonker DJ, Karapetis CS, O'Callaghan CJ, Moore MJ, Wong R, et al. Location of colon cancer (right-sided versus left-sided) as a prognostic factor and a predictor of benefit from cetuximab in NCIC CO.17. Eur J Cancer. 2015;51(11):1405–14.
42. Schrag D, Weng S, Brooks G, Meyerhardt JA, Venook AP. The relationship between primary tumor sidedness and prognosis in colorectal cancer. J Clin Oncol. 2016;34(suppl):abstr 3505.
43. Pugh S, Thiebaut R, Bridgewater J, Grisoni ML, Moutasim K, Rousseau F, et al. Association between miR-31-3p expression and cetuximab efficacy in patients with KRAS wild-type metastatic colorectal cancer: a post-hoc analysis of the new EPOC trial. Oncotarget. 2017;8(55):93856–66.
44. Hatano E, Okuno M, Nakamura K, Ishii T, Seo S, Taura K, et al. Conversion to complete resection with mFOLFOX6 with bevacizumab or cetuximab based on K-ras status for unresectable colorectal liver metastasis (BECK study). J Hepatobiliary Pancreat Sci. 2015;22(8):634–45.
45. Stremitzer S, Stift J, Singh J, Starlinger P, Gruenberger B, Tamandl D, et al. Histological response, pattern of tumor destruction and clinical outcome after neoadjuvant chemotherapy including bevacizumab or cetuximab in patients undergoing liver resection for colorectal liver metastases. Eur J Surg Oncol. 2015;41(7):868–74.
46. Yamashita S, Brudvik KW, Kopetz SE, Maru D, Clarke CN, Passot G, et al. Embryonic origin of primary colon cancer predicts pathologic response and survival in patients undergoing resection for colon cancer liver metastases. Ann Surg. 2018;267(3):514–20.
47. Portier G, Elias D, Bouche O, Rougier P, Bosset JF, Saric J, et al. Multicenter randomized trial of adjuvant fluorouracil and folinic acid compared with surgery alone after resection of colorectal liver metastases: FFCD ACHBTH AURC 9002 trial. J Clin Oncol. 2006;24(31):4976–82.
48. Snoeren N, van Hillegersberg R, Schouten SB, Bergman AM, van Werkhoven E, Dalesio O, et al. Randomized phase III study to assess efficacy and safety of adjuvant CAPOX with or without bevacizumab in patients after resection of colorectal liver metastases: HEPATICA study. Neoplasia. 2017;19(2):93–9.
49. Mitry E, Fields AL, Bleiberg H, Labianca R, Portier G, Tu D, et al. Adjuvant chemotherapy after potentially curative resection of metastases from colorectal cancer: a pooled analysis of two randomized trials. J Clin Oncol. 2008;26(30):4906–11.
50. Ychou M, Hohenberger W, Thezenas S, Navarro M, Maurel J, Bokemeyer C, et al. A randomized phase III study comparing adjuvant 5-fluorouracil/folinic acid with FOLFIRI in patients following complete resection of liver metastases from colorectal cancer. Ann Oncol. 2009;20(12):1964–70.
51. Saiura A, Yamamoto J, Hasegawa K, Oba M, Takayama T, Miyagawa S, et al. A combination of oral uracil-tegafur plus leucovorin (UFT + LV) is a safe regimen for adjuvant chemotherapy after hepatectomy in patients with colorectal cancer: safety report of the UFT/LV study. Drug Discov Ther. 2014;8(1):48–56.
52. Hasegawa K, Saiura A, Takayama T, Miyagawa S, Yamamoto J, Ijichi M, et al. Adjuvant oral uracil-tegafur with leucovorin for colorectal cancer liver metastases: a randomized controlled trial. PLoS One. 2016;11(9):e0162400.
53. Uehara K, Maeda A, Sakamoto E, Hiramatsu K, Takeuchi E, Sakaguchi K, et al. Phase II trial of adjuvant chemotherapy with S-1 for colorectal liver metastasis. Ann Surg Oncol. 2013;20(2):475–81.
54. Kato T, Uehara K, Maeda A, Sakamoto E, Hiramatsu K, Takeuchi E, et al. Phase II multicenter study of adjuvant S-1 for colorectal liver metastasis: survival analysis of N-SOG 01 trial. Cancer Chemother Pharmacol. 2015;75(6):1281–8.
55. Grothey A, Sobrero AF, Shields AF, Yoshino T, Paul J, Taieb J, et al. Duration of adjuvant chemotherapy for stage III colon cancer. N Engl J Med. 2018;378(13):1177–88.
56. Kemeny NE, Niedzwiecki D, Hollis DR, Lenz HJ, Warren RS, Naughton MJ, et al. Hepatic arterial infusion versus systemic therapy for hepatic metastases from colorectal cancer: a

randomized trial of efficacy, quality of life, and molecular markers (CALGB 9481). J Clin Oncol. 2006;24(9):1395–403.
57. Chen Y, Wang X, Yan Z, Wang J, Luo J, Liu Q. Hepatic arterial infusion with irinotecan, oxaliplatin, and floxuridine plus systemic chemotherapy as first-line treatment of unresectable liver metastases from colorectal cancer. Onkologie. 2012;35(9):480–4.
58. Arai Y, Ohtsu A, Sato Y, Aramaki T, Kato K, Hamada M, et al. Phase I/II study of radiologic hepatic arterial infusion of fluorouracil plus systemic irinotecan for unresectable hepatic metastases from colorectal cancer: Japan Clinical Oncology Group Trial 0208-DI. J Vasc Interv Radiol. 2012;23(10):1261–7.
59. House MG, Kemeny NE, Gonen M, Fong Y, Allen PJ, Paty PB, et al. Comparison of adjuvant systemic chemotherapy with or without hepatic arterial infusional chemotherapy after hepatic resection for metastatic colorectal cancer. Ann Surg. 2011;254(6):851–6.
60. D'Angelica MI, Correa-Gallego C, Paty PB, Cercek A, Gewirtz AN, Chou JF, et al. Phase II trial of hepatic artery infusional and systemic chemotherapy for patients with unresectable hepatic metastases from colorectal cancer: conversion to resection and long-term outcomes. Ann Surg. 2015;261(2):353–60.
61. Levi FA, Boige V, Hebbar M, Smith D, Lepere C, Focan C, et al. Conversion to resection of liver metastases from colorectal cancer with hepatic artery infusion of combined chemotherapy and systemic cetuximab in multicenter trial OPTILIV. Ann Oncol. 2016;27(2):267–74.
62. Ruers T, Punt C, Van Coevorden F, Pierie JP, Borel-Rinkes I, Ledermann JA, et al. Radiofrequency ablation combined with systemic treatment versus systemic treatment alone in patients with non-resectable colorectal liver metastases: a randomized EORTC Intergroup phase II study (EORTC 40004). Ann Oncol. 2012;23(10):2619–26.
63. Iezzi R, Marsico VA, Guerra A, Cerchiaro E, Cassano A, Basso M, et al. Trans-arterial chemoembolization with irinotecan-loaded drug-eluting beads (DEBIRI) and capecitabine in refractory liver prevalent colorectal metastases: a phase II single-center study. Cardiovasc Intervent Radiol. 2015;38(6):1523–31.
64. Martin RC 2nd, Scoggins CR, Schreeder M, Rilling WS, Laing CJ, Tatum CM, et al. Randomized controlled trial of irinotecan drug-eluting beads with simultaneous FOLFOX and bevacizumab for patients with unresectable colorectal liver-limited metastasis. Cancer. 2015;121(20):3649–58.
65. Wasan HS, Gibbs P, Sharma NK, Taieb J, Heinemann V, Ricke J, et al. First-line selective internal radiotherapy plus chemotherapy versus chemotherapy alone in patients with liver metastases from colorectal cancer (FOXFIRE, SIRFLOX, and FOXFIRE-Global): a combined analysis of three multicentre, randomised, phase 3 trials. Lancet Oncol. 2017;18(9):1159–71.
66. Posner MC, Niedzwiecki D, Venook AP, Hollis DR, Kindler HL, Martin EW, et al. A phase II prospective multi-institutional trial of adjuvant active specific immunotherapy following curative resection of colorectal cancer hepatic metastases: cancer and leukemia group B study 89903. Ann Surg Oncol. 2008;15(1):158–64.
67. Ychou M, Azria D, Menkarios C, Faurous P, Quenet F, Saint-Aubert B, et al. Adjuvant radioimmunotherapy trial with iodine-131-labeled anti-carcinoembryonic antigen monoclonal antibody F6 F(ab')2 after resection of liver metastases from colorectal cancer. Clin Cancer Res. 2008;14(11):3487–93.
68. Sahlmann CO, Homayounfar K, Niessner M, Dyczkowski J, Conradi LC, Braulke F, et al. Repeated adjuvant anti-CEA radioimmunotherapy after resection of colorectal liver metastases: safety, feasibility, and long-term efficacy results of a prospective phase 2 study. Cancer. 2017;123(4):638–49.
69. Morse MA, Niedzwiecki D, Marshall JL, Garrett C, Chang DZ, Aklilu M, et al. A randomized phase II study of immunization with dendritic cells modified with poxvectors encoding CEA and MUC1 compared with the same poxvectors plus GM-CSF for resected metastatic colorectal cancer. Ann Surg. 2013;258(6):879–86.
70. Ceelen WP, Van Nieuwenhove Y, Van Belle S, Denys H, Pattyn P. Cytoreduction and hyperthermic intraperitoneal chemoperfusion in women with heavily pretreated recurrent ovarian cancer. Ann Surg Oncol. 2012;19(7):2352–9.

71. Verhoef C, van der Pool AE, Nuyttens JJ, Planting AS, Eggermont AM, de Wilt JH. The "liver-first approach" for patients with locally advanced rectal cancer and synchronous liver metastases. Dis Colon Rectum. 2009;52(1):23–30.
72. van Dijk TH, Tamas K, Beukema JC, Beets GL, Gelderblom AJ, de Jong KP, et al. Evaluation of short-course radiotherapy followed by neoadjuvant bevacizumab, capecitabine, and oxaliplatin and subsequent radical surgical treatment in primary stage IV rectal cancer. Ann Oncol. 2013;24(7):1762–9.
73. Kim KH, Shin SJ, Cho MS, Ahn JB, Jung M, Kim TI, et al. A phase II study of preoperative mFOLFOX6 with short-course radiotherapy in patients with locally advanced rectal cancer and liver-only metastasis. Radiother Oncol. 2016;118(2):369–74.
74. Ayez N, van der Stok EP, de Wilt H, Radema SA, van Hillegersberg R, Roumen RM, et al. Neo-adjuvant chemotherapy followed by surgery versus surgery alone in high-risk patients with resectable colorectal liver metastases: the CHARISMA randomized multicenter clinical trial. BMC Cancer. 2015;15:180.
75. Huiskens J, van Gulik TM, van Lienden KP, Engelbrecht MR, Meijer GA, van Grieken NC, et al. Treatment strategies in colorectal cancer patients with initially unresectable liver-only metastases, a study protocol of the randomised phase 3 CAIRO5 study of the Dutch Colorectal Cancer Group (DCCG). BMC Cancer. 2015;15:365.

Neoadjuvant Chemotherapy for Resectable Colorectal Cancer Liver Metastases: Indications and Results

16

Anna Ryan and John Bridgewater

Introduction

The improvements in efficacy and safety of systemic chemotherapy have facilitated its application in the neoadjuvant management of many malignancies including gastric, pancreatic and ovarian cancer. In this chapter we address whether NACT improves outcomes in the context of resectable colorectal liver metastases (CRLM).

Approximately a quarter of patients with colorectal cancer (CRC) develop CRLM within 5 years of diagnosis, and of these, between 20% and 30% have resectable disease for whom surgery confers best outcome. Five-year overall survival rates in the region of 30–40% are to be expected following CRLM resection, compared to 10% in unselected metastatic patients [1, 2]. Criteria for resectability have evolved, and more sophisticated surgical interventions are now feasible, meaning that a larger population of patients with CRLM are being managed curatively in addition to a larger number of patients "converted" to operability by systemic and local treatments (see Chap. 20). Despite this, the risk of recurrence remains significant, and approximately half of patients develop widespread metastatic recurrence within 3 years of resection. There is an unmet need to reduce recurrence rates and improve outcomes in this population of patients. The data on neoadjuvant chemotherapy in this setting are modest with only two extant phase III randomised controlled trials. Numerous smaller and retrospective studies have been published with heterogenous treatment protocols and outcomes.

A. Ryan · J. Bridgewater (✉)
University College London Hospital NHS Trust, London, UK
e-mail: anna.ryan4@nhs.net; j.bridgewater@ucl.ac.uk

M. M. Correia et al. (eds.), *Colorectal Cancer Liver Metastases*,
https://doi.org/10.1007/978-3-030-25486-5_16

Indications for Neoadjuvant Chemotherapy

The potential benefits of administering NACT in the management of resectable CRLM are fourfold:

1. Early treatment of micrometastases to reduce risk of recurrence
2. Reduction of tumour volume to facilitate more straightforward resection
3. Identification of patients with aggressive tumour biology who would not benefit from resection
4. Assessment of response to NACT with tumours in situ in order to guide adjuvant or future anticancer treatment in the event of recurrence

Potential risks of utilising NACT include:

1. Missing the window of opportunity for a curative resection
2. Toxicity from treatment including hepatotoxicity and increased risk of surgical morbidity
3. Reduced completion rate of adjuvant systemic treatment
4. In the event of complete response: difficulty of identifying site for hepatic resection intraoperatively (Box 16.1).

Box 16.1 Benefits and Risks of Neoadjuvant Chemotherapy for Resectable Colorectal Liver Metastases

Benefits of neoadjuvant chemotherapy for resectable colorectal liver metastases:

- Reduce risk of recurrence through eradication of micrometastases.
- Reduce tumour burden to facilitate R0 resection.
- Identify patients with rapid disease progression who will not benefit from surgery.
- Assess response to guide future management.

Risks of neoadjuvant chemotherapy for resectable colorectal liver metastases:

- Failure to proceed to potentially curative resection
- Failure to resect sites of metastases experiencing complete response
- Risk of chemotherapy-associated toxicity including hepatotoxicity
- Failure to complete planned adjuvant chemotherapy
- Treatment on basis of misdiagnosis

Table 16.1 Indications and contraindications for neoadjuvant chemotherapy in resectable colorectal liver metastases

Criteria	Description	Impact	Reference
Need to facilitate resection (anatomical factors)	Present	Indication	
Comorbidities precluding immediate resection	Present	Indication	
Unacceptable risk of chemotherapy-associated toxicity	Present	Contraindication	
Elevated CEA	>5 ng/mL	Predictive of benefit from NACT	Sorbye et al. [3]
	>70 ng/mL or > 200 ng/mL	Adverse prognostic	Creasy et al. [4]; John et al. [5]; Sasaki et al. [6]; Strowitzki et al. [7]
Increased number of liver metastases	Single vs multiple	Adverse prognostic; evidence of predictive value varies	Creasy et al. [4]; Sorbye et al. [3]
Performance status	Zero	Predictive of benefit from NACT	Sorbye et al. [3]
Body mass index	<30	Predictive of benefit from NACT	Sorbye et al. [3]
Prior chemotherapy	5FU	Not predictive	Sorbye et al. [3]
Size of largest liver metastasis	>3 cm	Not predictive	Sorbye et al. [3]
Resectable extrahepatic metastases	Present	Adverse prognostic	Creasy et al. [4]
Clinical risk score	Fong 3–5	Adverse prognostic and predictive of benefit	Ayez et al. [8]
BRAF mutation	Present	Adverse prognostic	Tol et al. [9]
Mismatch repair deficiency	Present	Favourable prognostic	Thibodeau et al. [10]
RAS mutation	Present	Adverse prognostic and predictive lack of benefit from EGFR-targeted agents	Sepulveda et al. [11]; Passot et al. [12]; Stremitzer et al. [13]

As a greater proportion of patients with metastatic disease are considered for resection, it becomes increasingly important to identify evidence-based criteria to guide patient selection for perioperative systemic therapy. Current indications for NACT are summarised in Table 16.1.

Surgical Factors

Patient selection for surgery is based on anatomical criteria of resectability and factors related to assessment of anaesthetic risk. Wide variation in referral patterns between surgeons and oncologists for consideration of liver resection exists [2]. In the UK this led to the National Institute for Clinical Excellence (NICE) stipulating that all patients with liver-limited metastatic disease should be discussed at a multidisciplinary meeting involving specialist liver surgeons. Criteria for resectability are considered in more detail in Chap. 13 but may include the following:

Resectable liver metastases are defined as metastases which can be totally resected by surgery:

- With one or several anatomical resections provided the amount of remnant liver parenchyma after surgery is not less than 30% of total functional parenchyma.
- With one or several wedge resections alone or in combination with anatomical resections.
- The clearance between the tumour and the cut surface of the liver should be 1 cm or more whenever possible.
- The number of independent liver metastases observed on preoperative imaging should not exceed four.

Liver metastases which are considered not resectable:

- Tumours invading right and left branches of hepatic artery or portal vein
- Tumours extended to the three main hepatic veins
- Tumours that cannot be totally resected due to their size, location or number of deposits

Oncological Factors

There are no accepted oncological criteria which specifically predict benefit of NACT with a sufficient evidence basis to select patients for NACT treatment. Prognostic oncological factors relating to risk of recurrence post-operatively are therefore currently used to stratify patients when considering preoperative treatment, with evidence suggesting that lower-risk patients derive less benefit from NACT. Over recent years, individual factors have been combined in various different clinical risk scoring (CRS) systems to predict patient outcomes. We consider both discrete risk factors and risk score systems below.

Serum Carcinoembryonic Antigen (CEA)

CEA levels are routinely used in surveillance of CRC and are increasingly recognised as having prognostic value [14]. Pre-hepatectomy CEA has been shown to be prognostic of overall survival in several studies (e.g. CEA > 70 ng/mL hazard ratio for survival, 4.84; CEA > 200 ng/mL 5-year OS 24% vs 45%, $p < 0.001$) [4–7]. An accepted significant boundary value has yet to be determined, and evidence suggests that even a moderately raised CEA (>5 ng/mL) is significant. However most frequently, CEA ≥200 ng/mL is utilised as a boundary, including in two CRS systems [15, 16]. Change in CEA during neoadjuvant chemotherapy is also prognostic of overall survival following resection of CRLM – a reduction of 50% during treatment, regardless of baseline level, is significantly associated with higher ORR and improved OS [17].

CEA may also be predictive of benefit from NACT. Subgroup analysis of the phase III randomised controlled trial EORTC-40983 demonstrated that patients with even a moderately elevated CEA (>5 ng/mL) were benefited by the administration of perioperative chemotherapy (3-year PFS 35% with NACT vs 20% surgery alone, HR 0.58, $p < 0.02$), whilst those with normal CEA did not benefit (HR 1.09) [3].

Number of Metastases

As may be expected, the presence of a high number of liver metastases is a negative prognostic factor [4]. Data from the LiverMetSurvey registry has suggested that NACT is not beneficial for patients with a single liver metastasis (5-year OS with NACT 45% vs without 58%) but does improve survival in those with >5 metastases (5-year OS 22% vs 12%) [18]. However in EORTC-40983, the benefit of NACT was not predicted by the number of metastases (1 vs 2–4), and benefit was shown even in a supplementary analysis only of patients with an isolated metachronous liver metastasis (3-year PFS improved from 33% to 46% with NACT) [3].

Other Predictive Factors

In the EORTC-40983 trial, patients with performance status (PS) 0 and a body mass index (BMI) lower than 30 gained benefit from NACT unlike those with PS 1 or BMI > 30; however the limited numbers in the poorer PS/high BMI categories limit the interpretation of these findings [3]. High BMI is a known risk factor for chemotherapy-associated steatohepatitis. The combination of increased risk and limited benefit from NACT suggests that those with a very high BMI are not recommended for NACT. Tolerance of NACT in those with a poorer performance may be impaired – in EORTC-40983, only 30% of those with PS 1 completed the protocol chemotherapy compared to 50% of those with PS 0.

Benefit from NACT in EORTC-40983 was not affected by prior adjuvant 5FU chemotherapy or by size of the largest liver metastasis (<3 vs >3 cm) [3].

The presence of extrahepatic disease, even if resectable, is consistent with the presence of more widespread micrometastases and is a negative prognostic marker [4]. Evidence from one study suggests that site (left vs right colon) of primary tumour may be prognostic for survival after resection of CRLM (median OS 3.2 vs 5.2 years, $p = 0.004$), but these factors have not been analysed for predictive value to date [19].

Clinical Risk Scores

Clinical risk scoring (CRS) systems have been generated which predict the survival of patients after resection of CRLM, although the most commonly utilised were established in cohorts of patients who did not receive neoadjuvant chemotherapy, and determining the value of CRS in the era of neoadjuvant therapy is important. The feasibility of applying CRS to select patients for NACT has not been prospectively tested.

A retrospective analysis of 466 patients performed by Zhu et al. [20] demonstrated that only patients with ≥2 independent prognostic risk factors derived benefit

Table 16.2 Clinical risk scoring systems in metastatic colorectal cancer

Reference	Criteria	Score
Nordlinger et al. [21]	Age ≥60	0–2 low risk
	Extension into serosa of primary tumour	3–4 intermediate risk
	Lymphatic spread of primary tumour	5–6 high risk
	Interval <2 years from primary tumour to metastases	
	Number of metastases ≥4	
	Size of largest liver metastasis ≥5 cm	
Fong et al. [15]	Number of liver metastases >1	0–2 low risk
	Preoperative CEA >200 ng/mL	3–5 high risk
	Size of the largest liver metastasis ≥5 cm	
	Lymph node-positive primary tumour	
	Interval <12 m from primary resection to diagnosis of liver metastases	
Nagashima et al. [22]	Extension into serosa of primary tumour	0–1 grade 1
	Lymph node-positive primary tumour	2–3 grade 2
	Number of liver metastases ≥2	≥4 grade 3
	Diameter of liver metastases ≥5 cm	
	Resectable extrahepatic metastases	
Konopke et al. [16]	Number of liver metastases ≥4	0 low risk
	CEA ≥200 ng/mL	1 intermediate risk
	Synchronous liver metastases	≥2 high risk

from NACT. Risk factors were primary tumour T4, ≥4 liver metastases, largest metastasis ≥5 cm, serum CEA ≥5 ng/mL. Those with ≥2 risk factors gained significant overall survival benefit (5-year OS 39% with NACT vs 33% surgery alone, $p = 0.028$).

A retrospective analysis of 4 CRS (Fong/MSKCC, Nordlinger, Nagashima and Konopke; see Table 16.2) was performed in 336 CRLM patients, of whom 81% were initially resectable [23]. All CRS except Konopke were significantly prognostic (for DFS and OS after resection) in the population who received NACT, and a change in score for two CRS (Fong/Nagashima) pre- to post-NACT was also prognostic. The most robust score predictive of benefit in the context of NACT was Nagashima [15, 16, 21, 22].

The most widely utilised CRS (Fong score) has been assessed in four further studies to determine prognostic value in the context of neoadjuvant chemotherapy [4, 7, 8, 24]. Creasy et al. found that high Fong score (3–5) was prognostic of survival in an analysis of over a thousand patients, of whom 92% received perioperative chemotherapy. Strowitzki et al. also found that high Fong score (3–5) was a strong predictor of overall survival in patients undergoing NACT prior to resection of CRLM; however, Schreckenbach et al. found that neither Fong nor Nordlinger CRS were prognostic for OS in those treated with chemotherapy. Ayez et al. found that high (3–5) Fong CRS score group ($n = 144$ with resectable CRLM, of whom 88 received NACT) was significantly predictive of benefit from NACT (OS 46 m with NACT vs 33 m surgery alone, $p = 0.004$), whilst those with low CRS score did not (OS 65 m vs 54 m $p = 0.31$).

To summarise these data indicated that Fong score ≥3 is likely to be predictive of benefit of NACT. Whether this can be utilised to select patients for treatment needs to be tested prospectively.

Tumour Biology

There are many studies investigating the most useful molecular biomarkers to guide management of colorectal cancer, but to date, no widely accepted predictive biomarkers have been identified which stratify patients for NACT. As with the oncological criteria discussed above, when considering whether to administer NACT, we must therefore consider markers which are prognostic of survival in general in order to identify patients at higher risk of recurrence, as well as any which may be specifically predictive of benefit from systemic therapy.

Prognostic Biomarkers

Guidelines on the use of molecular biomarkers in the evaluation of CRC recommend testing for two prognostic markers: BRAF and mismatch repair (MMR) status in all patients [11]. Mutations in BRAF are present in 5–10% of all colorectal cancers and are associated with poor prognosis [9]. Approximately 15% of CRC are MMR deficient (or have high microsatellite instability (MSI-H)); this is associated with good prognosis in curatively resected patients but a poor prognosis in those with advanced disease [10]. The Lynch syndrome is caused by germline mutations in MMR genes and accounts for approximately 5% of all CRC diagnoses. Patients with RAF mutation associated with MMR deficiency have a particularly poor prognosis.

Mutations in RAS genes are found in up to 50% of colorectal cancers and are associated with poorer outcomes [12]. RAS mutation may be a negative prognostic factor for recurrence and overall survival in patients with resected CRLM who received NACT [13]. Stromal PDL1 expression in CRC is prognostic for poorer PFS suggesting that targeting this receptor with trials of immunotherapy may be an appropriate strategy (see Novel agents discussed later) [25].

Currently molecular prognostic biomarkers are not routinely used to guide patient selection for NACT.

Predictive Biomarkers

Testing of RAS status is recommended as a predictive marker of benefit to epidermal growth factor receptor (EGFR)-targeted therapies, e.g. cetuximab. Where RAS is mutated downstream, activation of oncogenic pathways occurs regardless of EGFR inhibition by targeted agents; therefore only wild-type patients derive benefit [11].

Node-negative MMR-deficient tumours do not benefit from 5-fluorouracil chemotherapy in the adjuvant setting; however node-positive tumours do benefit from oxaliplatin-based therapy. Any planned NACT must include oxaliplatin in order to be of benefit to this cohort [26]. MMR status may be utilised to predict benefit of immunotherapy agents although these are not in routine use yet in resectable metastatic CRC.

The use of other biomarkers remains experimental. miR-31-3p (a micro-RNA which promotes colorectal cancer progression) has been postulated as a novel predictive biomarker of response to cetuximab in the metastatic setting [27]. Subgroup analysis of the New EPOC cohort found that those with low miR-31-3p expression were not harmed by the use of cetuximab in the neoadjuvant setting [28]. Overexpression of ERCC1 (a gene involved in DNA repair pathways) is predictive of poor response to oxaliplatin treatment in the adjuvant setting, and recent retrospective analyses also suggest reduced response to NACT in CRLM [29, 30]. Overexpression of other molecular markers including Polo-like kinase 1 (PLK1) and c-MET in CRLM has been shown to correlate with poorer outcomes following NACT in retrospective studies [31, 32]. Tumour fibrosis <40% and cellularity >10% were predictive of worse response to neoadjuvant therapy but did not impact on survival in one retrospective trial [33]. Other histopathological markers including microscopic biliary and perineural invasion have been assessed as potential predictive biomarkers and, whilst associated with higher tumour burden, are not predictive of survival or response to NACT [34].

To summarise, whilst these data suggest numerous avenues of future investigation, validated predictive molecular biomarkers which can select patients for NACT remain hypothetical, and prospective validation is required.

Efficacy of Neoadjuvant Chemotherapy

Two large-scale phase III trials and numerous smaller phase II/retrospective studies have been performed to address the question of how effective NACT is in improving outcomes for patients with resectable CRLM. These are summarised in Table 16.3. Interpretation of the data from this research is hindered by the heterogeneity of the NACT regimens utilised, the retrospective nature of the majority of the data and the natural evolution of surgical techniques over recent years.

Chemotherapy

The largest prospective trial of NACT in the management of resectable CRLM was presented in 2008 by Nordlinger et al. (EORTC-40983) [35]. A phase III randomised controlled trial of 364 patients with up to 4 resectable liver metastases comparing resection alone with surgery plus perioperative FOLFOX4 (six cycles neoadjuvant and six cycles adjuvant; see protocol in Box 16.2).

The overall response rate to NACT was 34% (complete response 3%, partial response 40%, stable disease 38% and disease progression 7%). Resection rate was unaffected by NACT, 83% successful resection vs 84% in surgery-alone group, and chemotherapy improved patient selection for resection, 5%

Table 16.3 Trials of neoadjuvant chemotherapy and biological therapy in resectable colorectal liver metastases

Study	Year	Design	*N*	Regimen	Results	Study	Year	Design	*N*	Regimen	Results
Tanaka	2003	Cohort	48	NACT	5-year OS 83.9%	Scarzotti	2011	Cohort	60	FOLFOX	ORR 44%
			23	Surgery	5-year OS 21.7%				44	Surgery	
Wein	2003	II	20	FOLFOX	ORR 100%, R0 rate 80%	Cucchetti	2012	Cohort	125	NACT	Post-operative morbidity HR 1.38
Lorenz	2003	II	42	FOLFOX	ORR 47.6%, R0 rate 80.9%				117	Surgery	
Taieb	2005	II	22	FOLFOX	ORR 77%, R0 rate 91%	Pinto	2012	Cohort	334	NACT	ORR 65%, 5-year OS 43%, 5-year DFS 13%
			25	Surgery					342	Surgery	5-year OS 55%, 5-year DFS 26%
Hewes	2007	Cohort	42	NACT	3-year OS 62%	Reddy	2012	Cohort	88	NACT	6 m recurrence rate 25.6%
			45	Surgery	3-year OS 80%				114	Surgery	6 m recurrence rate 14.9%
Sahajpal	2007	Cohort	53	NACT	Hepatic steatosis 57%	Spelt	2012	Cohort	97	NACT	R1 resection rate 24%
			43	Surgery	Hepatic steatosis 28%				36	Surgery	R1 resection rate 19%
Pawlik	2007	Cohort	153	NACT	Perioperative complications 35.3%	Araujo	2013	Cohort	175	NACT	R1 resection rate 12.6%, 5-year OS 56%
			59	Surgery	Perioperative complications 30.5%				236	Surgery	R1 resection rate 14.4%, 5-year OS 60%
Aloysius	2007	Cohort	25	NACT	Pathological CR 24%	Oh	2013	Cohort	15	FOLFOX	3-year OS 44%
			25	Surgery					15	Surgery	3-year OS 55.7%
Gruenberger	2008	II	56	CAPOX + Bev	ORR 73.2%, R0 rate 92%	Primrose	2014	III RCT	128	Chemo	ORR 62%, R0 rate 15%
Nordlinger	2008	III RCT	182	FOLFOX	ORR 43%, median OS 61.3 m, 5-year OS 51.2%				129	Chemo + Cetux	ORR 70%, R0 rate 15%
			182	Surgery	Median OS 54.3 m, 5-year OS 47.8%	Zhu	2014	Cohort	121	NACT	Median OS 60 m, 5-year OS 52%
Bathel	2009	II	35	FOLFIRI	ORR 40%, R0 rate 85.7%				345	Surgery	Median OS 53.4 m, 5-year OS 48%

(continued)

Table 16.3 (continued)

Study	Year	Design	*N*	Regimen	Results	Study	Year	Design	*N*	Regimen	Results
Boostrom	2009	Cohort	44	NACT	5-year OS 48%	Ayez	2015	Cohort	65	NACT	Median OS 57 m, 5-year OS 52%
			55	Surgery	5-year OS 45%				154	Surgery	Median OS 45 m, 5-year OS 46%
Lubezky	2009	Cohort	37	NACT	3-year OS 70%	Bonney	2015	Cohort	693	NACT	3-year OS 72%
			19	Surgery	3-year OS 84%				608	Surgery	3-year OS 74%
Scoggins	2009	Cohort	112	NACT	R1 resection rate 7%	Uetake	2015	II	19	FOLFOX + Bev	ORR 68.4%, R0 rate 84.2%
			74	Surgery	R1 resection rate 8%	Nagayama	2017	II	30	FOLFOX	ORR 53.6%, 3-year OS 81.9%
Adam	2010	Cohort	169	NACT	5-year OS 60%, 5-year DFS 46%	Pietrantonio	2017	II	31	CapeOxIri + cetuximab	ORR 87%, R0 rate 84%, median OS 62.5 m
			1302	Surgery	5-year OS 60%, 5-year DFS 42%						

non-therapeuticwlaparotomy vs 11% in the upfront surgery group. Post-operative complications were higher in chemotherapy group (25% vs 16% including hepatic failure, biliary fistula and infection); however mortality was not different.

The administration of NACT meant that up to a third of patients did not subsequently complete adjuvant chemotherapy (80/115: 70% completed 6 cycles of post-operative treatment) [35]. Most frequent reasons for omitting adjuvant treatment were patient choice, perioperative complications, toxicity from preoperative chemotherapy and disease progression.

The primary endpoint of EORTC-40983, improved 3-year PFS, was met with a benefit of 8·1% (from 28·1% [21·2–36·6] vs 36·2% [28·7–43·8], HR 0·77 [0·60–1·00], $p = 0·041$) (Fig. 16.1a). Median PFS was improved from 11.7 to 18.7 months. Five-year overall survival showed no significant difference (51% chemo vs 48% surgery alone, HR for death 0.88, 95% CI 0.68–1.14). Updated results presented in 2013 at 8.5-year follow-up showed a trend for improved 5-year PFS (38% vs 30%, HR 0.81, 95% CI 0.64–1.02, $p = 0.068$) and OS (HR 0.87, 95% CI 0.66–1.14, $p = 0.3$) in chemotherapy group [36]. Median overall survival was 61.3 months (95% CI 51.0–83.4) in the NACT group and 54.3 months in the surgery-alone group (95% CI 41.9–79.4), and at 8.5 years, 59% of the NACT group had died compared to 63% of the surgery-alone group. It is important to note that this study was not statistically powered to detect an overall survival advantage and that a 4% absolute survival advantage is consistent with trials of adjuvant therapy (e.g. MOSAIC) [37].

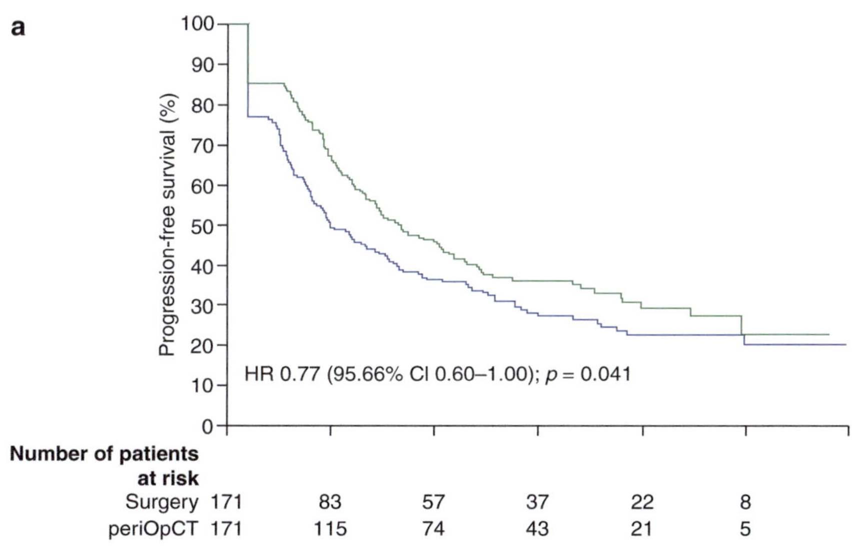

Fig. 16.1 Progression-free and overall survival in two randomised controlled trials of neoadjuvant chemotherapy in the management of colorectal liver metastases. (**a**) Progression-free survival of all eligible patients in EORTC-40983. (**b**) Progression-free survival of all patients in New EPOC trial. (**c**) Overall survival of all patients in New EPOC trials

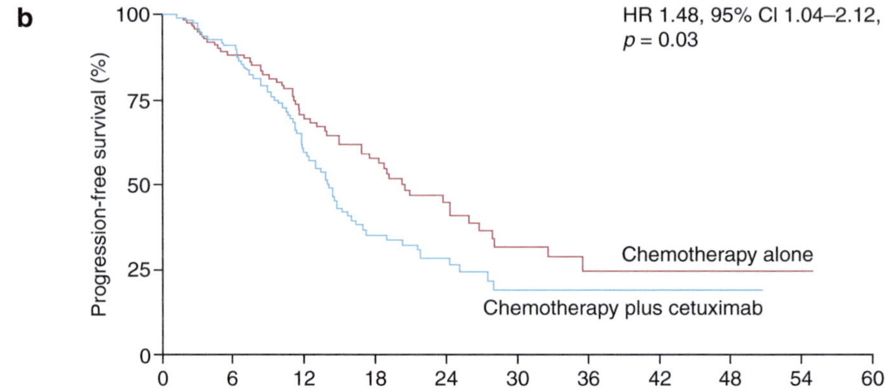

Number at risk

Chemotherapy	117	89	65	38	23	12	6	2	1	1	0
Chemotherapy plus cetuximab	119	87	53	24	23	5	3	2	1	0	0

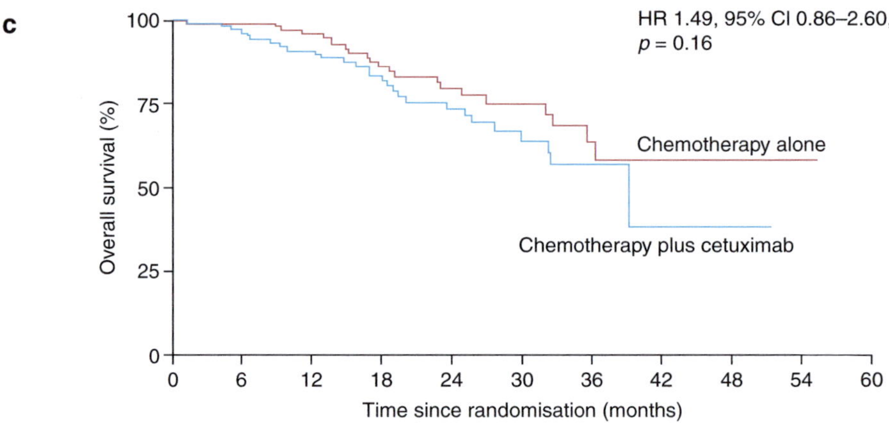

Number at risk

Chemotherapy	127	113	90	61	40	29	13	4	2	1	0
Chemotherapy plus cetuximab	127	99	81	55	38	22	7	2	1	0	0

Fig. 16.1 (continued)

Adjuvant chemotherapy provides overall survival benefit in the treatment of high-risk primary CRC [38], but the benefit of adjuvant chemotherapy following resection of liver metastases remains unclear. An improvement in disease-free survival at 5 years with adjuvant 5FU following resection of CRLM was reported in randomised multicentre study (33.5% vs 26.7%) [39], with no improvement in outcomes demonstrated through administration of doublet FOLFIRI chemotherapy adjuvantly [40]. The role of adjuvant chemotherapy is further discussed in Chap. 21.

Box 16.2 Neoadjuvant Chemotherapy Regimen Utilised in EORTC-40983: FOLFOX4

- Leucovorin 200 mg/m^2/day infusion over 2 hours
- 5-Fluorouracil 400 mg/m^2/day bolus plus 600 mg/m^2/day infusion over 22 hours
- Oxaliplatin 85 mg/m^2 infusion over 2 hours

Biological Agents

Cetuximab

The New EPOC study sought to demonstrate the benefit of adding cetuximab a monoclonal anti-EGFR antibody to perioperative FOLFOX chemotherapy [41]. It was a large-scale phase II trial involving 257 KRAS exon 2 wild-type patients with resectable or suboptimally resectable CRLM. Patients received chemotherapy (FOLFOX ($n = 156$), CAPOX ($n = 51$) or FOLFIRI ($n = 26$) regimens) with or without cetuximab for 12 weeks pre- and 12 weeks post-operatively. Median follow-up at interim analysis was 20.7 months when the trial was closed having met prespecified futility criteria.

There was a trend towards higher overall response rate in the cetuximab group (62% NACT versus 70% NACT+cetuximab, $p = 0.59$) (complete response 5% vs 6%, partial response 57% vs 64%, stable disease 21% vs 18%, progressive disease 8% vs 8%). The resection rate was not significantly different between the two groups (93% NACT vs 87% cetuximab). The number of R1 resections was relatively high (8% in the chemotherapy group and 12% in the cetuximab), and no evidence of tumour was present in 15% of resected specimens (despite imaging complete response in only 5–6% of cases).

There was a non-significantly higher grade 3–4 adverse event rate in the cetuximab group, primarily attributable to skin rash. At the time of analysis, 13% of the NACT and 16% of the cetuximab group had stopped their adjuvant treatment before completing the planned 12 weeks.

Progression-free survival with cetuximab was significantly poorer than with chemotherapy alone (14.1 m [95% CI 11.8–15.9] vs 20.5 m [95% CI 16.8–26.7], HR 1.48, $p = 0.03$) shown in Fig. 16.1b. Median overall survival (Fig. 16.1c) was 39.1 m (95% CI 23.6-not reached) in the cetuximab group but had not been reached in the chemotherapy group.

Subgroup analysis showed factors associated with lower-risk disease were associated with adverse effect of cetuximab (e.g. three or fewer metastases, absence of N2 disease, well or moderately differentiated primary tumour). The detrimental effect of cetuximab remained significant when only those who received FOLFOX as the backbone regimen were considered.

Pugh et al. analysed patterns of progression in 109 patients in a post hoc mortality analysis in 2012 [42]. They found that patterns of mortality were as expected for progression of micrometastatic disease rather than failure of local control due to inadequate resection. The pattern of progression did not differ significantly between the control and cetuximab arms aside from a significantly higher proportion of multisite recurrence in the cetuximab group in keeping with a failure of systemic disease control.

Cetuximab is effective in the context of metastatic CRC but has also failed to show a benefit in the adjuvant setting raising the possibility that EGFR-targeted biological therapies may have a different impact in the context of micro- vs macro-metastatic disease [43, 44]. EGFR inhibition may lead to upregulation of alternative signalling pathways leading to resistance, and translational studies are recommended to investigate these possibilities before any further clinical trials can be performed.

Bevacizumab

Bevacizumab is an antiangiogenic agent targeted against vascular endothelial growth factor (VEGF) which can be utilised in the KRAS mutant cohort of CRC patients. It is known to be of benefit in the advanced metastatic but not the adjuvant setting. Two studies have investigated concurrent bevacizumab with chemotherapy in the neoadjuvant setting [45, 46]. The phase II BOXER trial assessed CAPOX with bevacizumab perioperatively as conversion therapy for unresectable CRLM (including a subgroup of initially resectable high-risk patients $n = 15$). They found a high response rate (ORR 78%) and 40% rate of conversion to resectability within the total cohort [47]. Ten of the fifteen patients proceeded to resection, of whom six had R0 resection and four R1 resections. Of the remainder, one was still undergoing treatment at the time of reporting, and four did not undergo resection (one due to disease progression, three due to radiological complete response).

A second phase II study of 61 patients with resectable disease analysed the efficacy of 4 cycles of S1-oxaliplatin plus bevacizumab neoadjuvantly [48]. Chemotherapy completion rate was 82.0% and ORR 68.9%. In total 57/61 were resected (excluding 3 with disease progression, 4 due to toxicity and 1 patient choice), and 54 proceeded to have adjuvant chemotherapy (3 excluded due to non-CRC diagnosis). Of resected CRLM patients, 47/54 (87.0%) had R0 resection, with a pathological complete response rate of 13%.

To summarise, studies have demonstrated some evidence of improved response rates with the addition of bevacizumab to neoadjuvant protocols but no significant benefit in overall survival in unselected CRLM cohorts [49–51]. There is some evidence to suggest that bevacizumab may have greater benefit in those who have had resection of the primary tumour compared to those with the primary in situ, but the underlying biology of this hypothesis remains undetermined [52, 53].

Liver-Directed Therapies

Novel delivery mechanisms for chemotherapy have been introduced in recent years and may reduce the risk of increased surgical morbidity following systemic NACT and chemotherapy-associated liver injury. Transarterial chemoembolisation (TACE) with irinotecan (DEBIRI) was assessed in the PARAGON II trial [54]. Forty patients with resectable CRLM received DEBIRI 1 month prior to resection. No systemic chemotoxicity was noted, and all patients proceeded to surgery. R0 resection rate was 74% and 26% had R1 resections. Pathological response rate (complete response 17%, partial response 81%) did not correlate with radiological response rate (partial response 2.5%, stable disease 55%, progressive disease 27.5%). No patients received adjuvant chemotherapy. Median OS was 50.9 m. This study demonstrates the feasibility and safety of delivering liver-directed therapy prior to surgery for patients with resectable CRLM.

Ongoing Trials

CHARISMA is a Dutch multicentre randomised phase III RCT of poor prognosis (Fong score 3–5) resectable CRLM receiving six cycles of neoadjuvant CAPOX followed by surgery vs surgery alone [55]. Adjuvant therapy after R0 resection is not allowed. A target accrual of over 200 patients is expected for this study with a planned closure date in 2023. Details of this and other ongoing clinical trials in resectable CRLM are listed in Table 16.4.

Table 16.4 Ongoing trials of neoadjuvant chemotherapy in resectable colorectal liver metastases

Reference	Phase	*N*	Description	Intervention	Primary outcome	Location
NCT02453490	III	360	Randomised	NACT TOMOX vs TOMIRI vs FOLFOX vs FOLFIRI	ORR	China
EudraCT201300495239	III	224	Randomised	Surgery vs NACT oxaliplatin based	OS	Holland
NCT02087475	III	NR	Randomised	NACT FOLFIRI vs adjuvant FOLFIRI	PFS	China
EudraCT2006-005197-51	II	60	Randomised	NACT bevacizumab vs primary surgery	Change in SUV	Holland
NCT02688023	II	50	Single arm	NACT oxaliplatin + irinotecan + 5FU/Cape/S1	3-year DFS	China
NCT03487939	II	30	Single arm	NACT FOLFOXIRI	Tumour downstaging	China
EudraCT2012-000265-20	II	36	Single arm	NACT FOLFIRI + panitumumab	ORR	Austria

Retrospective Analyses

Several systematic reviews of available trial data have been performed; however these are hindered by the heterogeneity of trial cohorts, regimens and assessed outcome measures. Of the studies included in Table 16.3, for example, the cohort size varies from 15 to 1302 patients, and outcome measures include response rate, resection rate, perioperative complication rate as well as overall and progression-free survival. Furthermore changing views on surgical feasibility over recent years means that the profile of patient cohorts entered into studies of resectable disease has changed. Differences in quality of surgical interventions across different time periods and locations may also affect outcomes.

Liu et al. analysed data from 18 studies (6254 patients), of which 4 studies were included which are categorised by risk of recurrence. NACT appeared to increase the risk of death in the unselected cohort (hazard ratio 5-year survival 1.19) and improve survival of patients at high risk of recurrence (HR 0.69); however the two cohorts were mismatched, and those receiving NACT had a higher disease burden [56].

Sabanathan et al. analysed data from 11 studies involving 908 patients to determine the impact of adding biological agents to NACT, not limited to those with "resectable" metastases [57]. Significant heterogeneity of treatment regimens was noted (four oxaliplatin based, two irinotecan, five both; seven cetuximab, four bevacizumab). Combination biological therapy was associated with ORR 68% (95% CI 63–73%), and overall PFS was estimated at 14.4 m (bevacizumab group PFS 14 months (range 11–18), cetuximab group 13.6 months (range 9.8–16.5 months)).

Is Neoadjuvant Chemotherapy Better than Adjuvant?

Most of the presented data compares NACT to surgery alone, so identifying the optimal sequence of surgery and systemic treatment is difficult. To date three randomised controlled trials have been conducted investigating sequencing of treatment (AGITG ATTACHE, EPOC B and NSABP C-11). These compared 6 months of adjuvant chemotherapy (FOLFOX, FOLFIRI or CAPOX regimens) to 3 months pre- and 3 months post-operative treatment. All three trials struggled to recruit patients and were terminated early. Data collated from participants that were recruited (37 of a planned 948) will be published in 2019 (Thavaneswaran et al., in draft). The limited patient accrual in these studies may be indicative that despite overall international clinical equipoise, polarised views of individual clinicians regarding the role of NACT inhibit recruitment to randomised studies. This issue remains a challenge for future research.

Current Guidelines

Important sources of international guidance on the use of perioperative treatment in CRLM include the European Society of Medical Oncology (ESMO), National Comprehensive Cancer Network (NCCN, USA) and National Institute for Clinical

Table 16.5 Current guidelines in the use of neoadjuvant chemotherapy for resectable colorectal liver metastases

Publisher and date	Guidance
NCCN V2.2017	Workup: Determine RAS, BRAF, MMR/MSI status. Consider PET/CT if potentially resectable M1 disease. MDT evaluation including surgeon experienced in resection of hepatobiliary and lung metastases Synchronous or staged colectomy with liver resection and/or local therapy OR neoadjuvant therapy for 2–3 months (FOLFOX (preferred) or CAPOX (preferred) or FOLFIRI) vfollowed by synchronous/staged resection OR colectomy followed by chemotherapy and staged resection of metastatic disease Adjuvant treatment: Imaging to be performed prior to adjuvant treatment. FOLFOX or CAPOX or FLOX or Cape or 5FU/LV (6 m total perioperative treatment preferred) Biological therapy is not recommended in the neoadjuvant setting except as conversion therapy of unresectable metastases
ESMO 2016	Both technical criteria for resection and prognostic considerations define the need for systemic perioperative therapy In patients with clearly resectable disease and favourable prognostic criteria, perioperative treatment may not be necessary, and upfront resection is justified In patients with technically resectable disease where the prognosis is unclear or probably unfavourable, perioperative combination chemotherapy (FOLFOX or CAPOX) should be administered Targeted agents should not be used in resectable patients where the indication for perioperative treatment is prognostic in nature In situations where the criteria for prognosis and resectability are not sharply defined, perioperative therapy should be considered (as part of a continuum of treatment option). Patients with synchronous onset of metastases should be allocated to this group and therapeutic pathway In patients with favourable oncological and technical (surgical) criteria, who have not received perioperative chemotherapy, there is no strong evidence to support the use of adjuvant chemotherapy, whereas patients with unfavourable criteria may benefit from adjuvant treatment In patients who have not received any previous chemotherapy, adjuvant treatment with FOLFOX or CAPOX is recommended (unless patients were previously recently exposed to oxaliplatin-based adjuvant chemotherapy)
NICE 2011	Prioritise treatment to control symptoms If both primary and metastatic tumours are considered resectable, anatomical site-specific MDTs should consider initial systemic treatment followed by surgery The decision on whether the operations are done at the same time or separately should be made by the anatomical site-specific MDTs in consultation with the patient

Excellence (NICE, UK). A summary of the guidance within the most recent publications on the subject is given in Table 16.5. Details of guidance regarding criteria of resectability, surgical management and locally targeted therapies will be reviewed in detail in Chaps. 13, 24 and 28 and therefore are not considered further here.

NCCN guidelines have been recently updated [NCCN Colon Cancer v2.2018 March 2018]. It is recommended that 6 months of perioperative systemic therapy be considered for most patients undergoing resection of CRLM to increase the likelihood that residual microscopic disease will be eradicated. The recommendation is based upon an improvement in PFS (but not OS) demonstrated in the results of four meta-analyses [58–61]. The benefits of neoadjuvant vs adjuvant therapy are discussed, and NCCN conclude that the optimal sequencing of surgery and chemotherapy is unclear. If neoadjuvant chemotherapy is utilised, treatment should be limited to 2–3 months in order to avoid hepatotoxicity, and patients should be frequently monitored by the multidisciplinary team in order to facilitate an appropriately timed resection. Preferred cytotoxic regimens are FOLFOX or CAPOX. Biological therapy is not recommended in the neoadjuvant setting except in the initial therapy of unresectable disease which may be converted to resectability.

ESMO guidance was presented in July 2016 [62]. ESMO recommendations are based on categorising patients into groups based on surgical (technical) and oncological (prognostic) criteria regarding suitability for hepatic resection. Oncological criteria are concomitant extrahepatic disease (unresectable), number of lesions >5 and tumour progression. Patients with synchronous metastases are also included in this group.

In patients with favourable technical and oncological criteria, both upfront surgery and perioperative chemotherapy are recommended as options based on EORTC-40893 data showing no benefit in overall survival.

Perioperative chemotherapy is recommended where disease is resectable but prognostic criteria are unfavourable. Three months preoperative and 3 months postoperative chemotherapy is recommended. The recommended regimen is FOLFOX (or alternatively CAPOX), and biological agents are not routinely recommended. EGFR-targeted antibody treatment is not recommended due to New EPOC data, and bevacizumab is not recommended due to the lack of data available. However in patients with one or more unfavourable oncological and technical criteria resulting in a low chance of "curative" resection, either a triplet cytotoxic regimen (e.g. FOLFOXIRI) or the addition of bevacizumab may be considered.

NICE guidelines on the management of colorectal cancer were last published in 2011 and are currently under review with an update expected in October 2019. In 2011 limited data was available, and the recommendation was that if both primary and metastatic tumours are considered resectable, anatomical site-specific MDTs should consider initial systemic treatment followed by surgery, after full discussion with the patient.

Unanswered Questions

There are many uncertainties regarding the use of NACT in CRLM, in particular the role of biomarkers and predicting individual benefit of NACT and the selection of treatment agents.

Biomarkers and Tumour Biology

Despite being in the era of personalised molecular medicine, our current practice in the management of CRLM is based predominantly on anatomical criteria which have been familiar to physicians for decades. Current routine pathological testing is limited to mutations in RAS, BRAF and MMR/MSI status, and no molecular markers have been validated which can select CRLM patients for NACT. The impact of intra- and inter-tumoural heterogeneity in the context of NACT remains uncertain. Current management is often based on single biopsy samples or on pathology from a previously resected primary tumour, despite increasing understanding that tumour biology evolves over time and that different subclones of tumour cells are likely to seed heterogenous metastases [63].

In the near future, it is anticipated that insights into tumour biology from large-scale international collaborations (the International Cancer Genome Consortium/the Cancer Genome Atlas) will provide the tools for biological stratification of patients. Recently four novel consensus molecular subtypes (CMS) of colorectal cancer were characterised through analysis of TCGA datasets with the following key distinguishing features: CMS1 14% hypermutated, microsatellite unstable and strong immune activation; CMS2 37% canonical, marked WNT/MYC signalling activation; CMS3 (13%) epithelial, metabolic dysregulation; and CMS4 (23%) mesenchymal, TGF-beta activation, stromal invasion and angiogenesis [64]. These subtypes are likely to correspond to differences in prognosis and response to therapies and may form the basis of future molecularly guided management strategies.

Novel Agents and Choice of Cytotoxics

The optimal cytotoxic regimen and/or biological therapy remains to be determined. The only phase III randomised evidence to date for cytotoxic regimen is for FOLFOX, and as a proven first-line treatment in the adjuvant and palliative metastatic settings, it is strongly recommended. FOLFIRI is less likely to be effective, and there is no evidence of benefit as adjuvant treatment. However in the neoadjuvant setting, more intensive (triplet) regimens may be mandated to optimise response rates. The role of biological therapy remains uncertain, and carefully conducted research is required in this area to determine the safety and efficacy of combination or single-agent biological therapy.

Immunotherapy (in the form of the checkpoint inhibitor pembrolizumab) is effective for the palliative management of metastatic MMR-deficient/MSI-high CRC, but its role has not been determined in the neoadjuvant CRLM setting.

Other unanswered questions to be addressed include:

- Is the role of NACT equivalent for synchronous as for metachronous metastases?
- Does the benefit of NACT fall in patients who have previously received modern systemic chemotherapy compared to those who are chemotherapy-naïve?
- What is the minimum chemotherapy-free interval that should be achieved before considering neoadjuvant therapy?
- Is the benefit of NACT maintained in second or subsequent resections of CRLM?
- Does resection of primary tumour influence response to neoadjuvant treatment of the liver metastases?

Summary and Conclusions

The benefits of neoadjuvant chemotherapy include earlier treatment of micrometastatic disease, determination of responsiveness to therapy (which may be prognostic and help in planning post-operative treatment) and avoidance of surgical procedures for those patients with early disease progression. Potential disadvantages are missing "window of opportunity" for resection due to disease progression, chemotherapy toxicity contributing to increased surgical morbidity and reduced likelihood of completing adjuvant chemotherapy and the possibility of significant response which makes identifying the anatomical site for surgical resection challenging.

The current consensus is that NACT is of most benefit to moderate- or high-risk patients based on prognostic criteria such as a raised CEA level or high clinical risk score. There are no accepted predictive criteria or biomarkers which have been prospectively proven to select patients who will benefit from NACT.

There is no randomised controlled trial evidence of improved overall survival with NACT, but the key study was not powered to assess this and did prove a PFS benefit. FOLFOX is the most widely utilised regimen. Cetuximab is potentially harmful in the neoadjuvant setting, and bevacizumab may improve response rate in some cases but with no evidence of survival benefit to the population as a whole. Exploration of the role of liver-directed therapies and novel agents including immunotherapies is ongoing. NACT does not appear to increase the risk of perioperative death but may increase morbidity/complication rates. NACT reduces the chances of patients undergoing non-therapeutic laparotomy.

There are many unanswered questions relating to the role of NACT in the management of resectable CRLM. It is hoped that in the future, further data from well-designed clinical trials and molecular profiling research will translate to survival benefits in this group of patients (Box 16.3).

Box 16.3 Key Summary Points

- Neoadjuvant FOLFOX chemotherapy improves progression-free survival by 8% at 3 years, but there is no evidence of significant overall survival advantage.
- The greatest benefit is to patients at high risk of recurrence including those with elevated baseline CEA or a high Fong clinical risk score.
- Neoadjuvant chemotherapy increases the risk of perioperative morbidity but not mortality and reduces the risk of non-therapeutic laparotomy.
- Neoadjuvant cetuximab may be harmful and should only be administered in the context of a clinical trial.
- There is mixed evidence for the benefit of neoadjuvant bevacizumab, and it is not routinely recommended.

- The role of liver-directed therapies and novel agents including immunotherapies is unclear.
- Optimal sequencing of chemotherapy (neoadjuvant vs adjuvant) remains uncertain, and recruitment to randomised trials is challenging.
- Urgent progress in the identification of molecular biomarkers which predict benefit from neoadjuvant chemotherapy is required.

References

1. Kanas GP, et al. Survival after liver resection in metastatic colorectal cancer: review and meta-analysis of prognostic factors. Clin Epidemiol. 2012;4:283–301.
2. de Jong MC, et al. Rates and patterns of recurrence following curative intent surgery for colorectal liver metastasis: an international multi-institutional analysis of 1669 patients. Ann Surg. 2009;250(3):440–8.
3. Sorbye H, et al. Predictive factors for the benefit of perioperative FOLFOX for resectable liver metastasis in colorectal cancer patients (EORTC Intergroup Trial 40983). Ann Surg. 2012;255(3):534–9.
4. Creasy JM, et al. Actual 10-year survival after hepatic resection of colorectal liver metastases: what factors preclude cure? Surgery. 2018;163:1238.
5. John SK, et al. Prognostic factors and survival after resection of colorectal liver metastasis in the era of preoperative chemotherapy: an 11-year single-centre study. Dig Surg. 2013;30(4–6):293–301.
6. Sasaki K, et al. Pre-hepatectomy carcinoembryonic antigen (CEA) levels among patients undergoing resection of colorectal liver metastases: do CEA levels still have prognostic implications? HPB (Oxford). 2016;18(12):1000–9.
7. Strowitzki MJ, et al. Influence of neoadjuvant chemotherapy on resection of primary colorectal liver metastases: a propensity score analysis. J Surg Oncol. 2017;116(2):149–58.
8. Ayez N, et al. The use of neo-adjuvant chemotherapy in patients with resectable colorectal liver metastases: clinical risk score as possible discriminator. Eur J Surg Oncol. 2015;41(7):859–67.
9. Tol J, Nagtegaal ID, Punt CJ. BRAF mutation in metastatic colorectal cancer. N Engl J Med. 2009;361(1):98–9.
10. Thibodeau SN, Bren G, Schaid D. Microsatellite instability in cancer of the proximal colon. Science. 1993;260(5109):816–9.
11. Sepulveda AR, et al. Molecular biomarkers for the evaluation of colorectal cancer: guideline from the American society for clinical pathology, college of American pathologists, association for molecular pathology, and the American society of clinical oncology. J Clin Oncol. 2017;35(13):1453–86.
12. Passot G, et al. Prognostic factors after resection of colorectal liver metastases following preoperative second-line chemotherapy: impact of RAS mutations. Eur J Surg Oncol. 2016;42(9):1378–84.
13. Stremitzer S, et al. KRAS status and outcome of liver resection after neoadjuvant chemotherapy including bevacizumab. Br J Surg. 2012;99(11):1575–82.
14. Tarantino I, et al. Elevated preoperative CEA is associated with worse survival in stage I–III rectal cancer patients. Br J Cancer. 2012;107:266.
15. Fong Y, et al. Clinical score for predicting recurrence after hepatic resection for metastatic colorectal cancer: analysis of 1001 consecutive cases. Ann Surg. 1999;230(3):309–18; discussion 318-21

16. Konopke R, et al. Prognostic factors and evaluation of a clinical score for predicting survival after resection of colorectal liver metastases. Liver Int. 2009;29(1):89–102.
17. Stremitzer S, et al. CEA change after neoadjuvant chemotherapy including bevacizumab and clinical outcome in patients undergoing liver resection for colorectal liver metastases. Ann Surg Oncol. 2015;22(4):1315–23.
18. Adam R, et al. LiverMetSurvey: analysis of clinicopathologic factors associated with the efficacy of preoperative chemotherapy in 2,122 patients with colorectal liver metastases. J Clin Oncol. 2006;24(18_suppl):3521.
19. Creasy JM, et al. The impact of primary tumor location on long-term survival in patients undergoing hepatic resection for metastatic colon cancer. Ann Surg Oncol. 2018;25(2):431–8.
20. Zhu D, et al. Effect of neoadjuvant chemotherapy in patients with resectable colorectal liver metastases. PLoS One. 2014;9(1):e86543.
21. Nordlinger B, et al. Surgical resection of colorectal carcinoma metastases to the liver. A prognostic scoring system to improve case selection, based on 1568 patients. Association Française de Chirurgie. Cancer. 1996;77(7):1254–62.
22. Nagashima I, et al. Proposal of criteria to select candidates with colorectal liver metastases for hepatic resection: comparison of our scoring system to the positive number of risk factors. World J Gastroenterol. 2006;12(39):6305–9.
23. Wimmer K, et al. Impact of neoadjuvant chemotherapy on clinical risk scores and survival in patients with colorectal liver metastases. Ann Surg Oncol. 2017;24(1):236–43.
24. Schreckenbach T, et al. The clinical relevance of the Fong and the Nordlinger scores in the era of effective neoadjuvant chemotherapy for colorectal liver metastasis. Surg Today. 2015;45(12):1527–34.
25. D'Alterio C, et al. CXCR4-CXCL12-CXCR7, TLR2-TLR4, and PD-1/PD-L1 in colorectal cancer liver metastases from neoadjuvant-treated patients. Oncoimmunology. 2016;5(12):e1254313.
26. Ribic CM, et al. Tumor microsatellite-instability status as a predictor of benefit from fluorouracil-based adjuvant chemotherapy for colon cancer. N Engl J Med. 2003;349(3):247–57.
27. Mosakhani N, et al. MicroRNA profiling predicts survival in anti-EGFR treated chemorefractory metastatic colorectal cancer patients with wild-type KRAS and BRAF. Cancer Genet. 2012;205(11):545–51.
28. Pugh S, et al. Association between miR-31-3p expression and cetuximab efficacy in patients with KRAS wild-type metastatic colorectal cancer: a post-hoc analysis of the New EPOC trial. Oncotarget. 2017;8(55):93856–66.
29. Kim CY, et al. ERCC1 as a predictive marker for FOLFOX chemotherapy in an adjuvant setting. Ann Coloproctol. 2015;31(3):92–7.
30. Geva R, et al. The predictive role of ERCC1 status in oxaliplatin based neoadjuvant therapy for Metastatic Colorectal Cancer (mCRC) to the liver. Cancer Investig. 2015;33(4):89–97.
31. Lorenzon L, et al. Tumor regression grades, K-RAS mutational profile and c-MET in colorectal liver metastases. Pathol Res Pract. 2017;213(8):1002–9.
32. Fernández-Aceñero MJ, et al. PLK-1 expression is associated with histopathological response to neoadjuvant therapy of hepatic metastasis of colorectal carcinoma. Pathol Oncol Res. 2016;22(2):377–83.
33. Serrablo A, et al. Impact of novel histopathological factors on the outcomes of liver surgery for colorectal cancer metastases. Eur J Surg Oncol. 2016;42(9):1268–77.
34. Stift J, et al. Microscopic biliary and perineural invasion and clinical outcome after neoadjuvant bevacizumab-based chemotherapy and liver resection in patients with colorectal liver metastases. Eur J Surg Oncol. 2018;44(1):139–47.
35. Nordlinger B, et al. Perioperative chemotherapy with FOLFOX4 and surgery versus surgery alone for resectable liver metastases from colorectal cancer (EORTC Intergroup trial 40983): a randomised controlled trial. Lancet. 2008;371(9617):1007–16.
36. Nordlinger B, et al. Perioperative FOLFOX4 chemotherapy and surgery versus surgery alone for resectable liver metastases from colorectal cancer (EORTC 40983): long-term results of a randomised, controlled, phase 3 trial. Lancet Oncol. 2013;14(12):1208–15.

37. André T, et al. Improved overall survival with oxaliplatin, fluorouracil, and leucovorin as adjuvant treatment in stage II or III colon cancer in the MOSAIC trial. J Clin Oncol. 2009;27(19):3109–16.
38. André T, et al. Oxaliplatin, fluorouracil, and leucovorin as adjuvant treatment for colon cancer. N Engl J Med. 2004;350(23):2343–51.
39. Portier G, et al. Multicenter randomized trial of adjuvant fluorouracil and folinic acid compared with surgery alone after resection of colorectal liver metastases: FFCD ACHBTH AURC 9002 trial. J Clin Oncol. 2006;24(31):4976–82.
40. Ychou M, et al. A randomized phase III study comparing adjuvant 5-fluorouracil/folinic acid with FOLFIRI in patients following complete resection of liver metastases from colorectal cancer. Ann Oncol. 2009;20(12):1964–70.
41. Primrose J, et al. Systemic chemotherapy with or without cetuximab in patients with resectable colorectal liver metastasis: the New EPOC randomised controlled trial. Lancet Oncol. 2014;15(6):601–11.
42. Pugh SA, et al. Patterns of progression, treatment of progressive disease and post-progression survival in the New EPOC study. Br J Cancer. 2016;115(4):420–4.
43. Jonker DJ, et al. Cetuximab for the treatment of colorectal cancer. N Engl J Med. 2007;357(20):2040–8.
44. Alberts SR, et al. Effect of oxaliplatin, fluorouracil, and leucovorin with or without cetuximab on survival among patients with resected stage III colon cancer: a randomized trial. JAMA. 2012;307(13):1383–93.
45. Hurwitz H, et al. Bevacizumab plus irinotecan, fluorouracil, and leucovorin for metastatic colorectal cancer. N Engl J Med. 2004;350(23):2335–42.
46. Kerr RS, et al. Adjuvant capecitabine plus bevacizumab versus capecitabine alone in patients with colorectal cancer (QUASAR 2): an open-label, randomised phase 3 trial. Lancet Oncol. 2016;17(11):1543–57.
47. Wong R, et al. A multicentre study of capecitabine, oxaliplatin plus bevacizumab as perioperative treatment of patients with poor-risk colorectal liver-only metastases not selected for upfront resection. Ann Oncol. 2011;22(9):2042–8.
48. Mukai T, et al. Phase II trial of neoadjuvant chemotherapy with S-1 and oxaliplatin plus bevacizumab for colorectal liver metastasis (N-SOG 05 trial). Jpn J Clin Oncol. 2017;47(7): 597–603.
49. Cui CH, et al. Neoadjuvant chemotherapy (NCT) plus targeted agents versus NCT alone in colorectal liver metastases patients: a systematic review and meta-analysis. Oncotarget. 2015;6(41):44005–18.
50. Kataoka M, et al. The COMET open-label phase II study of neoadjuvant FOLFOX or XELOX treatment combined with molecular targeting monoclonal antibodies in patients with resectable liver metastasis of colorectal cancer. Ann Surg Oncol. 2017;24(2):546–53.
51. Bergeat D, et al. Preoperative bevacizumab and surgery for colorectal liver metastases: a propensity score analysis. Langenbeck's Arch Surg. 2017;402(1):57–67.
52. Cabart M, et al. Bevacizumab efficacy is influenced by primary tumor resection in first-line treatment of metastatic colorectal cancer in a retrospective multicenter study. Clin Colorectal Cancer. 2016;15(4):e165–74.
53. Lim C, et al. Bevacizumab improves survival in patients with synchronous colorectal liver metastases provided the primary tumor is resected first. Clin Transl Oncol. 2018;20:1274.
54. Jones RP, et al. PARAGON II – a single arm multicentre phase II study of neoadjuvant therapy using irinotecan bead in patients with resectable liver metastases from colorectal cancer. Eur J Surg Oncol. 2016;42(12):1866–72.
55. Ayez N, et al. Neo-adjuvant chemotherapy followed by surgery versus surgery alone in high-risk patients with resectable colorectal liver metastases: the CHARISMA randomized multicenter clinical trial. BMC Cancer. 2015;15:180.
56. Liu W, et al. The role of neoadjuvant chemotherapy for resectable colorectal liver metastases: a systematic review and meta-analysis. Oncotarget. 2016;7(24):37277–87.

57. Sabanathan D, Eslick GD, Shannon J. Use of neoadjuvant chemotherapy plus molecular targeted therapy in colorectal liver metastases: a systematic review and meta-analysis. Clin Colorectal Cancer. 2016;15(4):e141–7.
58. Ciliberto D, et al. Role of systemic chemotherapy in the management of resected or resectable colorectal liver metastases: a systematic review and meta-analysis of randomized controlled trials. Oncol Rep. 2012;27(6):1849–56.
59. Wang ZM, et al. Peri-operative chemotherapy for patients with resectable colorectal hepatic metastasis: a meta-analysis. Eur J Surg Oncol. 2015;41(9):1197–203.
60. Araujo RL, Gönen M, Herman P. Chemotherapy for patients with colorectal liver metastases who underwent curative resection improves long-term outcomes: systematic review and meta-analysis. Ann Surg Oncol. 2015;22(9):3070–8.
61. Khoo E, et al. Systematic review of systemic adjuvant, neoadjuvant and perioperative chemotherapy for resectable colorectal-liver metastases. HPB (Oxford). 2016;18(6):485–93.
62. Van Cutsem E, et al. ESMO consensus guidelines for the management of patients with metastatic colorectal cancer. Ann Oncol. 2016;27(8):1386–422.
63. Naxerova K, et al. Origins of lymphatic and distant metastases in human colorectal cancer. Science. 2017;357(6346):55–60.
64. Guinney J, et al. The consensus molecular subtypes of colorectal cancer. Nat Med. 2015;21(11):1350–6.

Management of Disappearing Liver Metastasis Following Preoperative Chemotherapy

17

Georgios Karagkounis and Michael A. Choti

Introduction

The past few decades have ushered a significant shift in the management of colorectal liver metastases (CRLM), as surgical resection is now offered to an increasing number of patients, with increasingly improved outcomes. While hepatectomy offers patients with CRLM the only reliable potential for cure, the treatment paradigm for this population has shifted due to the availability of increasingly effective chemotherapeutic regimens for advanced disease. For patients with metastatic disease limited to the liver, but who are anatomically not amenable to resection, chemotherapy can be used in some cases to "convert" patients to a resectable status [1]. In addition, even among patients with initially resectable disease, systemic chemotherapy can be offered prior to liver surgery, potentially improving outcomes by addressing potential micro-metastatic disease earlier. While this neoadjuvant approach has gained popularity, particularly among those patients at higher risk for recurrence, the impact of this strategy on long-term oncologic outcomes remains uncertain [2, 3].

The administration of systemic cytotoxic therapy prior to resection allows clinicians to observe the response of the macroscopic disease, offering insight into the biology of the patient's disease. Predictably, patients whose tumors demonstrate better response, radiologically and/or histopathologically, experience longer survival and have a higher probability of cure [1, 4–6]. Modern chemotherapeutic regimens offer patients objective response rates of 50% or greater [7–9]. While complete radiologic responses are uncommon [10], the complete disappearance of one or more CRLM following chemotherapy administration is more frequently observed,

G. Karagkounis
Department of General Surgery, Cleveland Clinic Foundation, Cleveland, OH, USA

M. A. Choti (✉)
Banner MD Anderson Cancer Center, Phoenix, AZ, USA
e-mail: Michael.Choti@bannerhealth.com

M. M. Correia et al. (eds.), *Colorectal Cancer Liver Metastases*,
https://doi.org/10.1007/978-3-030-25486-5_17

occurring in 10–25% of patients [12–18]. The natural history and prognostic impact of DLM is not completely understood; it is clear that a complete radiologic response does not consistently translate into pathologic complete response, necessitating their removal if resection/ablation of all known disease is the goal. Management of DLM is a common and particularly complex problem facing any multidisciplinary team caring for colorectal cancer patients, including the hepatic surgeon. This chapter discusses treatment options for patients at risk for DLM and addresses some of the more common controversies in their management.

Defining the Disappearing Liver Metastasis

Disappearing liver metastases (DLM) are defined as CRLM that are no longer detectable on cross-sectional imaging following therapy, most commonly the administration of systemic chemotherapy. The term typically refers to all preoperatively undetectable lesions, including those which can eventually be identified intraoperatively. Those that remain unidentified after exploration and are not resected are frequently termed "missing liver metastases" [11]. Considering that the definition of DLM relies on imaging quality and their detectability, it is therefore expected that their incidence and prognosis depends significantly on the imaging modalities used. Computed tomography (CT) remains the one most frequently used to diagnose and monitor CRLM due to its wide availability and less cost, while magnetic resonance imaging (MRI), positron emission tomography (PET), and ultrasonography (US) are also used in specific situations. The distinct sensitivity of each modality in detecting CRLM leads to different DLM rates, and, consequently, DLM outcomes reported by different centers are not inherently comparable.

Variation in imaging modalities is not the only reason data from various centers are difficult to compare and DLM are so hard to define. Most chemotherapeutic regimens currently in use for the treatment of CRLM are also affecting the hepatic parenchyma. For instance, treatment with 5-fluorouracil (5-FU) and irinotecan may result in hepatic steatosis, while oxaliplatin is associated with sinusoidal congestion. This leads to changes in the imaging characteristics of the liver surrounding the CRLM, typically decreasing its density on CT and increasing its echogenicity on US, limiting the contrast between hepatic parenchyma and CRLM and resulting in metastases that are harder to identify [19, 20]. Therefore, both the type of imaging modality used and the regimen of chemotherapy administered are critical components of the definition of DLM and should be taken into consideration when evaluating reports from different centers.

Considering these inherent difficulties in defining DLM, it is not surprising that their incidence, predictors, and prognostic impact vary significantly between reports [12–18]. A study by Tanaka et al. suggested that up to 18% of CRLM may disappear after chemotherapy [14], while van Vledder et al. found that approximately 25% of patients with CRLM who receive preoperative chemotherapy will have at least one DLM [16]. While better-quality preoperative imaging may result in improved lesion detection, the use of more effective chemotherapy regimens, along with an increasingly aggressive surgical and neoadjuvant approaches for patients with multiple metastases, will likely find the incidence of DLM increasing in the future. In order to mitigate the challenges presented by DLM, it is important to recognize the patients who are at greater risk for developing them. While significant variance may occur based on the choice of imaging, certain factors have been shown to predict development of DLM in multiple series. These include the presence of multiple CRLM (three or more) and smaller lesions (less than 2 cm), as well as patients who receive longer duration of preoperative chemotherapy [12, 16]. van Vledder et al. reported that the median pre-treatment diameter of DLM was 1 cm, compared to greater than 2 cm for those that did not disappear [16]. In addition, according to the same study, patients with DLM received, on average, two more cycles of chemotherapy compared to those who did not have a DLM (7.7 vs. 5.5 cycles, respectively). A study by Auer et al. identified a different set of factors that predicted DLM that were a true pathologic complete response (CR) after chemotherapy [15]. In this report, predictors of DLM with pathologic CR were those lesions not detectable on MRI, with a DLM following response to hepatic artery infusion (HAI) rather than systemic chemotherapy, and those patients with complete normalization of carcinoembryonic antigen (CEA) levels. This highlights the potential of MRI to uncover residual tumors that may have been otherwise classified as DLM. In addition, it suggests a role of HAI chemotherapy to achieve complete pathologic response in some cases.

Intraoperative Assessment of Disappearing Liver Metastases

An important tool for the hepatic surgeon in the surgical management of CRLM is the use of intraoperative ultrasonography (IOUS), particularly when faced with a patient with a DLM. Along with careful intraoperative visualization and palpation of the mobilized liver, IOUS improves the intraoperative detection rate for DLM and should be utilized whenever possible in hepatic surgery for CRLM. Whether liver surgery is performed with an open laparotomy or when done laparoscopically (where palpation and complete mobilization are more difficult), IOUS is the most sensitive method for avoiding the failure to identify a DLM during surgery. A report from Ferrero et al. noted that on open surgical exploration of patients with 67 DLM, only 6 were identified by physical examination of the liver alone, while an additional 39 lesions were detected by IOUS [17]. With a combination of these modalities, 11–67% of DLM can be expected to be identified intraoperatively [12–18]. The variability in the intraoperative detection rate can be explained by a combination of factors: the depth of each lesion and its proximity to anatomical landmarks, the contrast between the tumors and the surrounding parenchyma (determined by both inherent tumor characteristics and the degree of hepatic steatosis [20]), the sensitivity of preoperative assessment (i.e., contrast MRI), as well as the individual surgeon's experience in IOUS, which all contribute to the different rates reported in each series.

An approach that merits further discussion is the use of a contrast-enhanced IOUS (CE-IOUS). While in earlier reports CE-IOUS was performed using injectable carbon dioxide gas, currently most centers using this approach employ second-generation contrast agents, including SonoVue (sulfur hexafluoride microbubbles, Bracco, Milan, Italy) and Sonazoid (microspheres of perfluorobutane, GE Healthcare, Norway, and Daiichi Pharmaceutical Co., Tokyo, Japan). Initial reports suggest that CE-IOUS can improve the detection rate of CRLM, with a resultant change in the surgical management in up to 15% of cases [21]. In particular, a study by Arita et al. evaluated the use of CE-IOUS in DLM in 11 patients [22]. Among 32 lesions, 4 DLM were detected by IOUS alone, while the addition of contrast allowed the detection of 12 more lesions, 11 of which had residual malignant cells on pathology. Overall in this study, CE-IOUS identified 79% of the 19 DLM that were ultimately proven to harbor residual disease, while standard IOUS identified only 21% of them ($p = 0.004$). Based on these data, the authors suggested that CE-IOUS should become a standard component of the intraoperative assessment of DLM. However, in another series of 29 patients with 66 DLM, the majority of whom were evaluated with preoperative MRI, CE-IOUS had a more limited benefit, detecting only 1 additional lesion using this approach [23].

Resectability Following Chemotherapy: Can We Leave a Disappearing Liver Metastasis Behind?

A disappearing liver metastasis can have major implications for preoperative planning. The typical challenges facing the multidisciplinary team managing a patient with CRLM and lesions that disappeared after preoperative chemotherapy generally fall into one of three scenarios: (1) the DLM is in a location within the liver that will be resected to address the remaining disease (e.g., a right side DLM in a patient undergoing right hepatectomy); (2) the DLM is in a location that would otherwise not be resected (or there are no other lesions), but can be resected without compromising the future liver remnant; and (3) the DLM is at a location that would otherwise not be resected and, if it were to represent residual disease, the disease would be anatomically unresectable. Clearly, each of these scenarios has a distinct risk-benefit profile with regard to the management of DLM. While the first scenario requires no change in the operative planning and is relatively straightforward, the other two raise an important question: should we leave a DLM behind? The answer to this question centers on two important factors: the rate of true, pathologic complete response among DLM and the prognostic impact of leaving a DLM with residual disease behind. Both are harder to answer than it may first appear. The oncologic features of DLM vary widely depending on the quality of the preoperative imaging, type of chemotherapy regimen and route (e.g., systemic vs. HAI), and the methods of intraoperative assessment. In addition, the clinician needs to factor in whether, in case a DLM that is left behind recurs, this could be resected or ablated in the future (i.e., managed as a de facto staged resection)? When considering the assessment of a possible complete pathologic response in an unresected DLM, the durability of the DLM is important. Specifically, the longer duration of observation with no local recurrence increases any enthusiasm for considering this DLM truly

Table 17.1 Published reports of patients with Disappearing Liver Metastases (DLM) and the outcomes of these lesions

Authors (year)	No. of patients with DLM	No. of DLM evaluated	% DLM detected intraoperatively	% viable[a]
Benoist et al. (2006) [12]	38	66	30	83
Elias et al. (2007) [13]	16	69	Excluded	38
Tanaka et al. (2009) [14]	23	86	36	31
Auer et al. (2010) [15]	39	118	11	36
van Vledder et al. (2010) [16]	40	127	53	56
Ferrero et al. (2012) [17]	33	67	67	61
Ono et al. (2012) [18]	5	44	n.r.	18

DLM disappearing liver metastasis, *n.r.* not reported
[a]Includes microscopically viable tumor on pathology and locally recurring DLM

controlled. The overall true complete response rate can be estimated by combining both the pathologic CR rate in resected DLM and those DLM that were left in situ and remained durably without local recurrence (usually >1–2 years). As shown in Table 17.1, the rates range from 18% to 83%. As described earlier, several factors have been identified that predict durable complete response, among which are the inability to detect the lesion on preoperative MRI, the normalization of CEA levels following chemotherapy, and the use of HAI chemotherapy [13, 15]. The latter is very significant, as it has been reported by two independent groups and highlights the biologically distinct effects of HAI chemotherapy on CRLM, which appears to result in a greater rate of complete response compared to systemic chemotherapy alone (60–75% vs. 20–45%).

The prognostic impact of DLM left in situ is also unclear. One might assume that leaving residual viable disease behind fails to achieve complete eradication of all gross disease and fails at a curative intent approach. Indeed, reports find that DLM left behind are associated with local recurrences of 27% and 74% [12–18]. The vast majority of these recurrences occur within 12 months, with almost none beyond 18–24 months. Importantly, approximately half of patients with local recurrences at the untreated DLM will also recur at additional sites. In addition, among those with local-only recurrence, most are found to be candidates for repeat resection or ablation [11, 14, 16]. These findings in part explain why despite the apparently higher local recurrence rate of patients with DLM left in situ, their overall survival rates did not seem to differ compared to those patients undergoing resection of all initially detected disease [11, 12, 15, 16].

Based on our current understanding, a more cautious approach to the management of patients with more disseminated liver metastases should be promoted. Specifically, in patients with extensive disease in which DLM occur following a response to chemotherapy and result in now apparently resectable disease, but with DLM sites in clearly unresectable locations within the liver, a curative intent or surgical approach may not be prudent. In such cases, the use of contrast-enhanced MRI can be helpful. Considering a longer period of observation before considering a surgical approach may help to identify truly durable complete responses. For patients where all known sites of DLM can be resected at the time of the initial operation or in a staged approach, liver resection and/or operative ablation with curative intent should be considered.

Methods for Addressing or Avoiding Disappearing Liver Metastases

The key to optimizing the management of patients at risk for DLM development lies in a multidisciplinary approach, with an early involvement of the hepatic surgeon. As mentioned, it is critical to personalize a strategy for sequencing of therapies and duration of any preoperative therapy. For patients at the highest risk for DLM such as those with multiple, smaller CRLM, particularly in locations which would impact surgical planning, proceeding directly to surgery and administering chemotherapy postoperatively may be a reasonable option, avoiding the possibility of DLM development entirely. If the potential benefits of neoadjuvant therapy are desired, the cycles of chemotherapy administered should be limited. Importantly, studies have failed to show benefit of extended durations of preoperative chemotherapy for CRLM, [24, 25]. Therefore, neoadjuvant chemotherapy in patients with resectable CRLM should be administered for short duration (4–6 cycles). For patients with initially unresectable disease, chemotherapy should be continued until resectability has been achieved; a structured monitoring protocol with frequent cross-sectional imaging should ensure that chemotherapy is discontinued after that point, to avoid both undue hepatotoxicity and the potential for DLM development.

One strategy to consider in selected cases in order to help manage a lesion at risk for disappearing is the placement of markers ("fiducials") in the vicinity of at risk lesions, which are both radiopaque and detectable by IOUS [26]. These markers, placed prior to the initiation of chemotherapy by the interventional radiologist, using image guidance, remain in place and detectable in the event the lesion disappears. One study by Passot et al. evaluating the use of fiducials to localize 41 at-risk CRLM (19 of which disappeared following preoperative chemotherapy) found that marker-guided treatment (resection or ablation) was successful in all cases and there were no local recurrences noted on follow-up [27]. Problems with this technique include the added cost and inability to predict which lesions will disappear and would not be found intraoperatively. Moreover, the use of a metallic fiducial may present problems using MRI.

At the very core of the DLM challenge, however, remains preoperative imaging, as DLM essentially reflects the inability of preoperative (and intraoperative) imaging modalities to correctly differentiate complete from incomplete pathologic response to chemotherapy. Different cross-sectional imaging modalities have distinct sensitivities in identifying CRLM, resulting in different DLM definitions

[28–31]. Dual-phase, contrast-enhanced CT is the most widely used modality for the diagnosis and surveillance of CRLM and has a sensitivity of 70–85% and a specificity approaching 90% in this setting [28, 29]. However, the chemotherapy-induced hepatocellular changes, including steatosis, steatohepatitis, and sinusoidal congestion as discussed earlier, further limit the diagnostic capabilities of CT in the detection of lesions after induction chemotherapy, as they significantly decrease the contrast between the hypovascular CRLM and the surrounding hepatic parenchyma. Positron emission tomography (PET), alone or in combination with CT, can occasionally be useful in the metastatic workup of colorectal cancer. However, in the detection of DLM following chemotherapy, its value is limited, due to its relatively low sensitivity in detecting sub-centimeter lesions [32].

While PET does not offer an improvement over standard, dual-phase CT, MRI offers significant advantages and has become the imaging modality of choice in liver oncology. The sensitivity of MRI in detecting CRLM is 80–85%, with reported specificity of 90–95% and relatively less interference by chemotherapy-induced hepatic changes [30, 31]. Importantly, in studies directly comparing CT to contrast-enhanced MRI for the detection of CRLM, hepatic MRI has been shown to have consistently better sensitivity and specificity [33–35]. In a meta-analysis of previously published reports measuring the sensitivity of different modalities in detecting CRLM in patients who received neoadjuvant chemotherapy, van Kessel et al. reported that the pooled sensitivities of contrast-enhanced MRI, CT, PET, and PET-CT in this setting were 86%, 70%, 55%, and 52%, respectively, highlighting the superiority of MRI [36]. Yet, the use of preoperative MRI does not eliminate the problem of DLM. In a recent report by Owen et al., investigating 200 CRLM identified on baseline imaging, the authors found that contrast-enhanced MRI classified 77 (38.5%) of them as DLM, though eventually 55% of these disappearing lesions were viable (21 recurring locally and 21 having histologically residual disease) [37]. Finally, it should be noted that while obtaining MRI after the completion of chemotherapy can identify lesions that may have been classified as DLM by CT, it is less clear how the presence of a pre-chemotherapy MRI may influence this scenario. Due to the higher sensitivity of MRI, its use as a baseline assessment of CRLM burden typically identifies more lesions than a baseline CT scan and reveals smaller lesions, as well as those contrasting less with the surrounding hepatic parenchyma on CT. This, in turn, increases the number of lesions at risk of disappearance following chemotherapy, adding tumors with characteristics particularly prone to develop into DLM. This phenomenon highlights the variability in DLM definitions among the various reports and underscores the complex ways in which pre-chemotherapy and preoperative imaging can influence the incidence and eventual fate of DLM.

Ongoing research in new imaging modalities has promise for the future management of DLM. Image registration, with specific capability to fuse preoperative and intraoperative imaging to generate an image guidance system, may be able to assist the liver surgeon in localizing and targeting liver tumors. One study reported on the use of a navigation system that intraoperatively projects CT images using tracked IOUS [38]. Such systems may be useful for the intraoperative management of DLM.

Summary

The increasing use of preoperative chemotherapy in the management of CRLM has offered many advantages but has also led to the challenging situation of the DLM. This is not a rare event, occurring in 10–25% of patients receiving preoperative chemotherapy, with rates varying depending on the imaging modality, as well as the type and duration of therapy administered. Patients with multiple lesions, smaller lesions, and deep lesions are more susceptible to the development of a DLM, and in such cases, this occurrence should be anticipated. It is important that a multidisciplinary team is engaged early, including the hepatic surgeon. High-quality hepatic imaging is important when assessing these patients, using contrast liver MRI when possible. For patients with small lesions that are initially resectable, up-front surgery should be considered. Obtaining a post-chemotherapy MRI can in many cases reveal lesions that would otherwise be classified as DLM. Frequent communication among the care team should be maintained throughout the duration of preoperative chemotherapy, discontinuing therapy early and proceeding with resection if the development of DLM appears likely. While many DLM can be identified intraoperatively, particularly with IOUS, challenges remain regarding leaving undetected metastases behind. As most harbor residual viable tumor, an attempt to treat all original sites of disease should be made, when possible and safe, but situations may occur in which unidentified DLM will remain. In such cases, any eventual recurrence may be treated in the future. As when managing any patient with advanced colorectal cancer, an understanding of underlying disease biology, comprehensive preoperative staging, and thorough patient risk stratification is necessary to offer the optimal benefit.

Disclosures The authors have no relevant conflicts of interest to disclose.

References

1. Adam R, Delvart V, Pascal G, Valeanu A, Castaing D, Azoulay D, et al. Rescue surgery for unresectable colorectal liver metastases downstaged by chemotherapy: a model to predict long-term survival. Ann Surg. 2004;240(4):644–57; discussion 57–8.
2. Nordlinger B, Sorbye H, Glimelius B, Poston GJ, Schlag PM, Rougier P, et al. Perioperative chemotherapy with FOLFOX4 and surgery versus surgery alone for resectable liver metastases from colorectal cancer (EORTC Intergroup trial 40983): a randomised controlled trial. Lancet. 2008;371(9617):1007–16.
3. Nordlinger B, Sorbye H, Glimelius B, Poston GJ, Schlag PM, Rougier P, et al. Perioperative FOLFOX4 chemotherapy and surgery versus surgery alone for resectable liver metastases from colorectal cancer (EORTC 40983): long-term results of a randomised, controlled, phase 3 trial. Lancet Oncol. 2013;14(12):1208–15.
4. Adam R, Wicherts DA, de Haas RJ, Aloia T, Levi F, Paule B, et al. Complete pathologic response after preoperative chemotherapy for colorectal liver metastases: myth or reality? J Clin Oncol. 2008;26(10):1635–41.
5. Blazer DG 3rd, Kishi Y, Maru DM, Kopetz S, Chun YS, Overman MJ, et al. Pathologic response to preoperative chemotherapy: a new outcome end point after resection of hepatic colorectal metastases. J Clin Oncol. 2008;26(33):5344–51.

6. Chun YS, Vauthey J-N, Boonsirikamchai P, Maru DM, Kopetz S, Palavecino M, et al. Association of computed tomography morphologic criteria with pathologic response and survival in patients treated with bevacizumab for colorectal liver metastases. JAMA. 2009;302(19952320):2338–44.
7. de Gramont A, Bosset JF, Milan C, Rougier P, Bouche O, Etienne PL, et al. Randomized trial comparing monthly low-dose leucovorin and fluorouracil bolus with bimonthly high-dose leucovorin and fluorouracil bolus plus continuous infusion for advanced colorectal cancer: a French intergroup study. J Clin Oncol. 1997;15(2):808–15.
8. Douillard JY, Cunningham D, Roth AD, Navarro M, James RD, Karasek P, et al. Irinotecan combined with fluorouracil compared with fluorouracil alone as first-line treatment for metastatic colorectal cancer: a multicentre randomised trial. Lancet. 2000;355(9209):1041–7.
9. Tournigand C, Andre T, Achille E, Lledo G, Flesh M, Mery-Mignard D, et al. FOLFIRI followed by FOLFOX6 or the reverse sequence in advanced colorectal cancer: a randomized GERCOR study. J Clin Oncol. 2004;22(2):229–37.
10. Dy GK, Krook JE, Green EM, Sargent DJ, Delaunoit T, Morton RF, et al. Impact of complete response to chemotherapy on overall survival in advanced colorectal cancer: results from Intergroup N9741. J Clin Oncol. 2007;25(23):3469–74.
11. Elias D, Youssef O, Sideris L, Dromain C, Baton O, Boige V, et al. Evolution of missing colorectal liver metastases following inductive chemotherapy and hepatectomy. J Surg Oncol. 2004;86(1):4–9.
12. Benoist S, Brouquet A, Penna C, Julie C, El Hajjam M, Chagnon S, et al. Complete response of colorectal liver metastases after chemotherapy: does it mean cure? J Clin Oncol. 2006;24(24):3939–45.
13. Elias D, Goere D, Boige V, Kohneh-Sharhi N, Malka D, Tomasic G, et al. Outcome of posthepatectomy-missing colorectal liver metastases after complete response to chemotherapy: impact of adjuvant intra-arterial hepatic oxaliplatin. Ann Surg Oncol. 2007;14(11):3188–94.
14. Tanaka K, Takakura H, Takeda K, Matsuo K, Nagano Y, Endo I. Importance of complete pathologic response to prehepatectomy chemotherapy in treating colorectal cancer metastases. Ann Surg. 2009;250(6):935–42.
15. Auer RC, White RR, Kemeny NE, Schwartz LH, Shia J, Blumgart LH, et al. Predictors of a true complete response among disappearing liver metastases from colorectal cancer after chemotherapy. Cancer. 2010;116(6):1502–9.
16. van Vledder MG, de Jong MC, Pawlik TM, Schulick RD, Diaz LA, Choti MA. Disappearing colorectal liver metastases after chemotherapy: should we be concerned? J Gastrointest Surg. 2010;14(11):1691–700.
17. Ferrero A, Langella S, Russolillo N, Vigano L, Lo Tesoriere R, Capussotti L. Intraoperative detection of disappearing colorectal liver metastases as a predictor of residual disease. J Gastrointest Surg. 2012;16(4):806–14.
18. Ono T, Ishida H, Kumamoto K, Okada N, Ishibashi K. Outcome in disappearing colorectal cancer liver metastases during oxaliplatin-based chemotherapy. Oncol Lett. 2012;4(5):905–9.
19. Robinson PJ. The effects of cancer chemotherapy on liver imaging. Eur Radiol. 2009;19(7):1752–62.
20. van Vledder MG, Torbenson MS, Pawlik TM, Boctor EM, Hamper UM, Olino K, et al. The effect of steatosis on echogenicity of colorectal liver metastases on intraoperative ultrasonography. Arch Surg. 2010;145(7):661–7.
21. Takahashi M, Hasegawa K, Arita J, Hata S, Aoki T, Sakamoto Y, et al. Contrast-enhanced intraoperative ultrasonography using perfluorobutane microbubbles for the enumeration of colorectal liver metastases. Br J Surg. 2012;99(9):1271–7.
22. Arita J, Ono Y, Takahashi M, Inoue Y, Takahashi Y, Saiura A. Usefulness of contrast-enhanced intraoperative ultrasound in identifying disappearing liver metastases from colorectal carcinoma after chemotherapy. Ann Surg Oncol. 2014;21 Suppl 3:S390–7.
23. Sturesson C, Nilsson J, Lindell G, Andersson RG, Keussen I. Disappearing liver metastases from colorectal cancer: impact of modern imaging modalities. HPB (Oxford). 2015;17(11):983–7.

24. Karoui M, Penna C, Amin-Hashem M, Mitry E, Benoist S, Franc B, et al. Influence of preoperative chemotherapy on the risk of major hepatectomy for colorectal liver metastases. Ann Surg. 2006;243(1):1–7.
25. Kishi Y, Zorzi D, Contreras CM, Maru DM, Kopetz S, Ribero D, et al. Extended preoperative chemotherapy does not improve pathologic response and increases postoperative liver insufficiency after hepatic resection for colorectal liver metastases. Ann Surg Oncol. 2010;17(11):2870–6.
26. Zalinski S, Abdalla EK, Mahvash A, Vauthey JN. A marking technique for intraoperative localization of small liver metastases before systemic chemotherapy. Ann Surg Oncol. 2009;16(5):1208–11.
27. Passot G, Odisio BC, Zorzi D, Mahvash A, Gupta S, Wallace MJ, et al. Eradication of missing liver metastases after fiducial placement. J Gastrointest Surg. 2016;20(6):1173–8.
28. Kuszyk BS, Bluemke DA, Urban BA, Choti MA, Hruban RH, Sitzmann JV, et al. Portal-phase contrast-enhanced helical CT for the detection of malignant hepatic tumors: sensitivity based on comparison with intraoperative and pathologic findings. AJR Am J Roentgenol. 1996;166(1):91–5.
29. Kamel IR, Choti MA, Horton KM, Braga HJ, Birnbaum BA, Fishman EK, et al. Surgically staged focal liver lesions: accuracy and reproducibility of dual-phase helical CT for detection and characterization. Radiology. 2003;227(3):752–7.
30. Kondo H, Kanematsu M, Hoshi H, Murakami T, Kim T, Hori M, et al. Preoperative detection of malignant hepatic tumors: comparison of combined methods of MR imaging with combined methods of CT. AJR Am J Roentgenol. 2000;174(4):947–54.
31. Bhattacharjya S, Bhattacharjya T, Baber S, Tibballs JM, Watkinson AF, Davidson BR. Prospective study of contrast-enhanced computed tomography, computed tomography during arterioportography, and magnetic resonance imaging for staging colorectal liver metastases for liver resection. Br J Surg. 2004;91(10):1361–9.
32. Fong Y, Saldinger PF, Akhurst T, Macapinlac H, Yeung H, Finn RD, et al. Utility of 18F-FDG positron emission tomography scanning on selection of patients for resection of hepatic colorectal metastases. Am J Surg. 1999;178(4):282–7.
33. van Etten B, van der Sijp J, Kruyt R, Oudkerk M, van der Holt B, Wiggers T. Ferumoxide-enhanced magnetic resonance imaging techniques in pre-operative assessment for colorectal liver metastases. Eur J Surg Oncol. 2002;28(6):645–51.
34. Larson RE, Semelka RC, Bagley AS, Molina PL, Brown ED, Lee JK. Hypervascular malignant liver lesions: comparison of various MR imaging pulse sequences and dynamic CT. Radiology. 1994;192(2):393–9.
35. Oudkerk M, van den Heuvel AG, Wielopolski PA, Schmitz PI, Borel Rinkes IH, Wiggers T. Hepatic lesions: detection with ferumoxide-enhanced T1-weighted MR imaging. Radiology. 1997;203(2):449–56.
36. van Kessel CS, Buckens CF, van den Bosch MA, van Leeuwen MS, van Hillegersberg R, Verkooijen HM. Preoperative imaging of colorectal liver metastases after neoadjuvant chemotherapy: a meta-analysis. Ann Surg Oncol. 2012;19(9):2805–13.
37. Owen JW, Fowler KJ, Doyle MB, Saad NE, Linehan DC, Chapman WC. Colorectal liver metastases: disappearing lesions in the era of Eovist hepatobiliary magnetic resonance imaging. HPB (Oxford). 2016;18(3):296–303.
38. Kingham TP, Scherer MA, Neese BW, Clements LW, Stefansic JD, Jarnagin WR. Image-guided liver surgery: intraoperative projection of computed tomography images utilizing tracked ultrasound. HPB (Oxford). 2012;14(9):594–603.

Conversion Chemotherapy for CRLM-Best Associations, and Does Conversion Translate into Longer Survival?

18

Mariana Bruno Siqueira, João Paulo Fogacci,
Roberto de Almeida Gil, and Mauro Monteiro Correia

Introduction

Colorectal cancer (CRC) is the secondary tumor that most commonly affects the liver [1]. About 50% of patients diagnosed with CRC will develop liver metastases throughout the disease evolution [1]. Resection of hepatic metastases increases patient's survival rates from 10% in 5 years to 40%, and in some cases, this can translate into cure of the disease [1]. Unfortunately, approximately 80–90% of patients with stage IV CRC have liver disease which is considered unresectable at presentation [1].

Over the last decades, there has been a great advancement in systemic treatment of metastatic CRC, improving survival from 6 months to more than 30 months, combining chemotherapy (CT) regimens with higher response rates (RR) and better surgical techniques [1–3]. More effective CT protocols started to be used not only for palliative treatment but to facilitate the downsizing of CRC liver metastases (CRLM) and render initially unresectable metastases resectable with negative margins [1–3].

M. B. Siqueira
D'Or Institute of Research and Education (IDOR), Rio de Janeiro, Brazil

J. P. Fogacci
Hospital dos Servidores do Estado, Rio de Janeiro, Brazil

R. de Almeida Gil
Department of Medical Oncology, Instituto Nacional de Câncer (INCA), Rio de Janeiro, Brazil

M. M. Correia (✉)
National Cancer Institute, Rio de Janeiro, Brazil

Department of Surgery, UNIVERSIDADE DO GRANDE RIO, Duque de Caxias, Brazil

M. M. Correia et al. (eds.), *Colorectal Cancer Liver Metastases*,
https://doi.org/10.1007/978-3-030-25486-5_18

Discussion

Resectability criteria for CRLM are based on technical difficulties and oncological prognosis [2]. However, prospective evaluations do not exist either for oncological or for technical criteria, and for many of these, there is no international consensus [2]. Conversion CT is indicated to promote downsizing and render an unresectable disease for technical issues resectable [2, 3]. When the contraindication to hepatic resection is due to an oncological worse prognosis, just like in the presence of unresectable concomitant extrahepatic disease, CT treatment probably will not change the condition of the patient [2, 3].

Neoadjuvant or perioperative CT is indicated when technically the resection is feasible, but the oncological prognosis is dubious, like in the presence of more than five liver lesions (there is no consensus about that number), or when the patient has a progressive disease [2]. This can be indicated also when the oncological prognosis is favorable but to test in vivo CT response and to treat micrometastatic disease earlier [2]. In that case, when the patient has a resectable disease and a favorable prognosis, upfront surgery or perioperative CT are both options for disease management [2].

The evidence that support perioperative CT are the prospective trials EPOC and New EPOC [4, 5] (Table 18.1).

In the EORTC 40983 EPOC trial, 364 patients with CRLM initially resectable and up to 4 liver metastases were randomly assigned to upfront resection versus FOLFOX4 (5-fluorouracil, folinic acid, oxaliplatin) perioperatively (3 months before and 3 after surgery) [4]. The number of patients submitted to surgery was similar between the arms: 83% in CT arm and 84% in upfront resection arm. CT arm had 182 patients enrolled, and of that, 67 had partial or complete response by RECIST, and 11 had progressive disease [4]. There were more surgical complications in the CT arm, 25% versus 16% in resection-only arm, that included hepatic failure, biliary fistula, and intra-abdominal infection [4]. However, surgical mortality was comparable. After 8.5 years of follow-up, progression-free survival (PFS) was superior in CT arm versus surgical-alone arm (38 versus 30%, HR 0.81, $p = 0.068$), and statistical significance was achieved after exclusion of the uneligible for resection patients [4]. Median overall survival (OS) was 61.3 months in CT group versus 54.3 months in surgery-alone group, respectively, and this is not statistically different (HR 0.88, $p = 0.34$) [4]. Based on this trial, perioperative FOLFOX becomes standard of care and is widely indicated in clinical practice.

Following that, the addition of the monoclonal antibody anti-EGFR cetuximab to perioperative CT was tested in the same scenario, upfront resectable disease, at the New EPOC trial [5]. Two hundred seventy-two Kras exon 2 wild-type patients were randomised to perioperative CT versus CT plus cetuximab [5]. The CT backbone was allocated by the physician's choice between FOLFOX, FOLFIRI (5-fluorouracil, folinic acid, and irinotecan) and Capox (capecitabine and oxaliplatin). The result was disappointed, the addition of cetuximab to perioperative CT was detrimental, and PFS was 20.5 months in CT-alone arm versus 14.1 months in CT plus cetuximab arm [5]. Some hypotheses were raised after this unexpected result, and

Table 18.1 Conversion CT trials

Study	Protocol	Response rate	Metastasectomy	mPFS	mOS
EORTC 40983 EPOC trial Nordlinger B et al. 364 pt. Up to 4 liver metastases	FOLFOX4 perioperative vs. surgery alone	RR = 36%	FOLFOX4 83% vs. surgery alone 84%	FOLFOX4: 38% HR 0.81 $p = 0.068$ Surgery alone: 30%	FOLFOX4: 61.4 m Surgery alone: 54.3 m *1
New EPOC trial 272 pt. Primrose J et al. K-RAS with exon 2 WT Resectable or suboptimally resectable liver metastases	FOLFOX6 or XELOX perioperative vs. FOLFOX6 or XELOX + cetuximab	RR = 62% vs. RR = 70% $p = 0.59$	FOLFOX6 or XELOX perioperative: 93% FOLFOX6 or XELOX + cetuximab: 87% *2	FOLFOX6 or XELOX perioperative: 20.5 m HR = 1.48 $p = 0.030$ FOLFOX6 or XELOX + cetuximab: 14.1 m	FOLFOX6 or XELOX perioperative: 32.0 m HR = 1.49 $p = 0.16$ FOLFOX6 or XELOX + cetuximab: 39.1 m
GONO trial Fancone A et al. 244 pt. Unresectable colorectal cancer (included other sites besides liver)	FOLFOXIRI vs. FOLFIRI	RR = 66% vs. RR = 41% $p = 0.002$	R0 metastasectomy, in liver only: FOLFOXIRI 36% vs. FOLFIRI 12% $p = 0.017$	Triplet: 9.8 m HR = 0.63 $p = 0.0006$ Doublet = 6.9 m	Triplet: 22.6 m HR = 0.70 $p = 0.032$ Doublet: 16.7 m
TRIBE trial Cremolini C et al. 508 pt. Metastatic unresectable	FOLFOXIRI + bevacizumab vs. FOLFIRI + bevacizumab	Triplet + Bv = 65% vs. doublet + Bv = 54% $p = 0.013$	Triplet + Bv 12% vs. doublet + Bv 15%	Triplet + Bv: 12.3 m HR -0.77 $p = 0.006$ Doublet + Bv: 9.7 m	Triplet + Bv: 29.8 m HR = 0.80 $p = 0.03$ Doublet + Bv: 25.8 m
OLIVIA study Gruenberger T et al. 80 pt. Only unresectable liver metastases	FOLFOXIRI + bevacizumab vs. mFOLFOX6 + bevacizumab	RR = 81% vs. RR = 62%	Triplet + Bv 61% vs. doublet + Bv 49% Metastasectomy R0 49% vs. 23%	Triplet + Bv 18.6 m vs. doublet + Bv 11.5 m	X

(continued)

Table 18.1 (continued)

Study	Protocol	Response rate	Metastasectomy	mPFS	mOS
CELIM study Folprecht G et al. 111 pt. KRAS codon 12,13,61 WT Unresectable and/or 5 or more lesions in the liver	FOLFOX + cetuximab vs. FOLFIRI + cetuximab	RR = 68% vs. RR = 57% OR = 1.63 $p = 0.23$	R0 metastasectomy: 38% vs. 30%	FOLFOX + cetuximab: 10.8 m HR = 1.18 $p = 0.4$ FOLFIRI + cetuximab: 10.5 m	FOLFOX + cetuximab: 35.7 m HR = 1.03 $p = 0.9$ FOLFIRI + cetuximab: 29.0 m *3
Chinese trial Ye L et al. 138 pt. KRAS WT Only unresectable liver metastases	FOLFOX or FOLFIRI vs. FOLFOX or FOLFIRI + cetuximab	CHEMO alone RR = 29.4% vs CHEMO + cetuximab RR = 57.1% $p < 0.01$	R0 metastasectomy: CHEMO alone 6% vs. CHEMO + cetuximab 26% $p < 0.01$		CHEMO alone: 3-year OS 41% CHEMO + cetuximab: 3-year OS 18% $p = 0.013$
VOLFI trial Geissler M et al. pan-RAS WT 96 pt. Cohort I = irresectable Cohort II = conversion treatment	mFOLFOXIRI + panitumumab vs. mFOLFOXIRI	RR = 85.7% vs. RR = 54.5% $p = 0.0013$	Cohort II: 31 pt. CHEMO: 36.4% CHEMO + panitumumab: 60%		

*1. Long-term results, median follow-up 8.5 years

*2. Only 222 patients had surgical information available at the time of study publication

*3. In the CELIM trial, patients that reached a R0 metastasectomy had a better median OS than those who did not (53.9 m vs. 21.9 m, $p < 0.001$)

possible explanations include interactions between cetuximab and the chemotherapy backbone, further mutations in the EGFR pathway conferring insensitivity to EGFR inhibition, and upregulation of alternative signalling pathways in combination with surgery [5].

Therefore, despite the widely use of perioperative CT in clinical practice around the world, for patients with resectable metastases, the evidence available do not confirm improvement in OS with this strategy. This may be because, after recurrence, patients are exposed to more effective systemic treatments in the surgery-alone arm, promoting a spontaneous crossover and affecting the difference in OS rates [6]. Another key point is that monoclonal antibodies, like anti-EGFR or anti-VEGF, ca not be routinely indicated in this scenario, because of the New EPOC trial detrimental result [6].

Systemic CT can be used to convert unresectable metastases resectable, the conversion therapy. In the minority of patients, 5–15% will actually be operated, and they carry a worse prognosis than the patients with upfront resectable disease [6].

In the conversion scenario, we have to look for CT protocols that deliver a higher RR. Resection rates have been shown to be correlated with response to systemic therapy; however this correlation may be biased by the heterogeneity of the clinical trials, depending on the year of the trial, the patient selection criteria, and the resectability criteria used [2].

The use of CT protocols with two drugs (doublet) or three drugs (triplet) with or without the addition of monoclonal antibodies, targeting EGFR or VEGF, is the most frequent treatment indicated for conversion therapy [2].

The first relevant study in this case is the Italian GONO (Gruppo Oncologico del Nord Ovest) trial, performed by Falcone et al. [7]. The aim of the trial was to compare a doublet CT protocol (FOLFIRI) versus a triplet CT (FOLFOXIRI), which included 5-fluorouracil, oxaliplatin, and irinotecan at the same protocol, a more intense treatment. Two hundred forty-five patients were included, and all of them had upfront unresectable metastatic colorectal disease, randomly assigned to receive FOLFIRI versus FOLFOXIRI as first-line metastatic treatment. The primary endpoint was RR [7].

The final results of the trial favored the triplet protocol, and overall RR was 66% in the FOLFOXIRI arm versus 41% in the FOLFIRI arm ($p = 0.0002$) [7]. Secondary endpoints included complete surgical resection (R0 resection). The R0 resection rate was 15% in the triplet arm versus 6% in the doublet arm ($p = 0.033$), respectively [7]. In patients with only liver metastases, RO resection rate was 36% in FOLFOXIRI group versus 12% in FOLFIRI group ($p = 0.017$). The triplet protocol had more adverse events, especially peripheral neuropathy and afebrile neutropenia [7] (Table 18.1).

The TRIBE trial was conducted later and included 508 patients with metastatic unresectable disease that were randomised to receive FOLFIRI plus the antibody targeting VEGF bevacizumab versus FOLFOXIRI plus bevacizumab [8]. In this trial, the triplet plus bevacizumab treatment did not improve R0 resection rate in the ITT population (12% in doublet arm versus 15% in the triplet arm, $p = 0.327$) or in the liver-only metastases subgroup (28% in doublet arm versus 32% in triplet arm, $p = 0.823$) [8] (Table 18.1).

However, in the phase II trial OLIVIA, the results were divergent [9]. Eighty patients with unresectable liver metastases were randomised to FOLFOX plus bevacizumab versus FOLFOXIRI plus bevacizumab [9]. The primary endpoint was overall resection rate, and results showed superiority of the triplet schema for R0 resection, 54% versus 31% in the triplet arm and doublet arm, respectively. Major adverse events were diarrhea and neutropenia [9] (Table 18.1).

The evidence that support the association of CT and monoclonal antibody anti-EGFR in the conversion scenario are the following:

The phase II CELIM trial, where patients with unresectable metastatic disease or more than five liver lesions and KRAS exon 2 wild type were randomly assigned to receive FOLFIRI plus cetuximab versus FOLFOX plus cetuximab [10]. The overall RR was 70%, and 33% of the patients underwent R0 resection [10] (Table 18.1).

There is also a Chinese trial that enrolled 138 patients with unresectable liver metastases and KRAS wild type randomised to CT with FOLFOX or FOLFIRI versus CT plus cetuximab [11]. The addition of cetuximab increased R0 resection from 18/70 patients (26%) versus 5/68 patients (7%) in the CT-alone arm [11] (Table 18.1).

The recent study VOLFI, a phase II trial also, tested the combination of mFOLFOXIRI plus panitumumab versus mFOLFOXIRI alone in KRAS wild-type metastatic patients [12]. The overall RR was 85.7% in the experimental arm versus 54.5% in CT-alone arm, and the R0 resection rate was impressively 60% [12] (Table 18.1).

Other relevant subject is the adverse events associated with CT treatment, which included higher surgical morbidity compared with resection alone. Irinotecan is associated with hepatic steatosis (yellow liver), and the oxaliplatin-based CT is associated with hepatic sinusoidopathy (blue liver) and may cause noncirrhotic portal vein hypertension [2]. These side effects are related to the number of cycles of CT delivered to the patient before the surgical procedure [2]. The risk of developing this complications increases considerably after the sixth cycle of CT (2–3 months of CT) [2]. As mentioned before, in the EPOC trial, there were more postoperative complications in the CT arm, 25% versus 16% in resection-only arm [4]. The best strategy is to limit the number of cycles delivered to the patient preoperatively and to frequently access the radiological response to CT, especially in cases of conversion [2]. The recommendation of guidelines such as the European Society of Medical Oncology (ESMO) Guideline is to access every 2 months radiological response to treatment and as soon as feasible submit the patient to surgical procedure, and CT should not be maintained beyond 4 months [2]. Clinical detection of these alterations is difficult, and splenomegaly associated or not with thrombocytopenia may be a sign of oxaliplatin vascular injury [2, 6]. A general recommendation is to discontinue cytotoxic chemotherapy 4 weeks prior to surgery and anti-VEGF like bevacizumab, given the risk of bleeding, about 6–8 weeks before [2, 6]. Interestingly, the combination of oxaliplatin and bevacizumab appears to have some protective effect on sinusoidopathy [6].

Recently, new data have been published on the importance of localization of the primary tumor in the response to treatment with anti-EGFR monoclonal antibodies, in addition to its relation with the oncological prognosis and survival of patients with metastatic colorectal cancer [13]. In the CALGB/SWOG study 80405, 1137 KRAS exon 2 wild-type patients were randomized to receive chemotherapy of the investigator's choice (FOLFOX or FOLFIRI) with cetuximab versus chemotherapy with bevacizumab [14]. There was no statistical difference between the arms in terms of overall survival (31.2 months CT + bevacizumab versus 32 months CT + cetuximab after expanded RAS analysis, HR 0.9), nor in PFS [14]. The response rate was 55% in the bevacizumab group versus 59% in the cetuximab group [14]. However, after unplanned subgroup analysis, comparing primary tumors of the left colon and right colon, patients who had primary tumors on the left side and received CT plus cetuximab had a greater survival benefit than the group who received CT plus bevacizumab (39 months versus 32 months, respectively) [13]. In the case of tumors on the right side, CT plus bevacizumab was superior to CT plus cetuximab (29 months versus 13 months) [13]. As noticed, right-sided tumors were associated with extremely worst prognosis. Therefore, from these data and from the subsequent subgroup analysis of several comparative studies between CT plus cetuximab and isolated CT or CT plus bevacizumab, it is recommended that the first-line treatment of metastatic disease in the left side and wild-type RAS tumors is preferentially associated with the anti-EGFR antibody [13]. In the wild-type RAS right-sided tumors, the treatment of the first line may include an anti-VEGF antibody or even a triplet scheme, if the proposal is to increase the response rate for resection, as in cases of conversion CT [2].

In addition, more information on molecular tumor analysis is currently required to guide the conversion treatment of metastatic patients, such as the presence of mutation of the BRAF V600E gene and the presence of defects in the DNA repair pathway known as microsatellite instability (MSI-H) [15]. About 5–10% of patients with metastatic colorectal cancer have the BRAF V600E mutation, and this molecular alteration confers a reserved prognosis for these patients, in addition to being associated with a lower response to treatment with anti-EGFR antibody [15, 16]. MSI-H tumors are uncommon in the metastatic setting, accounting for less than 5% of patients, and the BRAF mutation is also more common in primary tumors of the right colon [15]. To date, they are not associated with response to monoclonal antibodies, but are associated with response to immunotherapy with checkpoint inhibitors [17].

Therefore, the choice of the best chemotherapy regimen for patients who are candidates for conversion therapy for subsequent resection of liver metastases should be individualized and take into account several factors, such as the reason that contraindicated the upfront surgery (technical or oncological), side of the primary tumor, and molecular analysis with at least information on the mutational status of the RAS and BRAF and preferably also information on the presence of microsatellite instability [2]. If the indication is oncological and it is desired to evaluate tumor sensitivity in vivo, oxaliplatin-based double chemotherapy should be the treatment of choice, with the addition of monoclonal antibodies not indicated in these cases [2]. If surgery is technically difficult and indication of the conversion treatment is to promote cytoreduction, treatments with a higher response rate should be indicated, in this case CT with doublet plus anti-EGFR scheme in the presence of wild RAS and BRAF and left colon [2]. In the case of right-sided tumors or in the presence of RAS or BRAF mutation, a triplet scheme with or without anti-VEGF or doublet with anti-VEGF should be used [2]. It is also recommended to take into account the adverse events associated with each regimen and to use the minimum number of cycles necessary to allow the resectability of the disease [2].

Conclusions

Clearly there is survival benefit for patients undergoing resection of liver metastases compared to exclusive palliative chemotherapy; however, to date, the perioperative chemotherapy strategy has not proven to be superior to isolated surgery in the case of resection of liver metastases. Taking into account that patients undergoing conversion chemotherapy would be patients ineligible for surgery and that the treatment-promoted cytoreduction increases the resectability rate and allows a greater number of patients to undergo surgical resection, treatment can be considered indirectly, beneficial to the survival of patients with colorectal cancer and liver metastases.

References

1. Nordlinger B, Van Cutsem E, Rougier P, et al. Does chemotherapy prior to liver resection increase the potential for cure in patients with metastatic colorectal cancer? A report from the European Colorectal Metastases Treatment Group. Eur J Cancer. 2007;43(14):2037–45.
2. Van Cutsem E, Cervantes A, Adam R, et al. ESMO consensus guidelines for the management of patients with metastatic colorectal cancer. Ann Oncol. 2016;27(8):1386–422.
3. Adam R, De Gramont A, Figueras J, et al. The oncosurgery approach to managing liver metastases from colorectal cancer: a multidisciplinary international consensus. Oncologist. 2012;17:1225–39.
4. Nordlinger B, Sorbye H, Glimelius B, et al. Perioperative FOLFOX4 chemotherapy and surgery versus surgery alone for resectable liver metastases from colorectal cancer (EORTC 40983): long-term results of a randomised, controlled, phase 3 trial. Lancet Oncol. 2013;14:1208–15.
5. Primrose J, Falk S, Finch-Jones M, et al. Systemic chemotherapy with or without cetuximab in patients with resectable colorectal liver metastasis: the new EPOC randomised controlled trial. Lancet Oncol. 2014;15:601–11.
6. DeVita VT Jr, Lawrence TS, Rosenberg SA. DeVita, Hellman and Rosenberg's cancer: principles and practice of oncology. 10th ed. Philadelphia: Wolters Kluwer; 2015.
7. Falcone A, Ricci S, Brunetti I, et al. Phase III trial of infusional fluorouracil, leucovorin, oxaliplatin, and irinotecan (FOLFOXIRI) compared with infusional fluorouracil, leucovorin, and irinotecan (FOLFIRI) as first-line treatment for metastatic colorectal cancer: the Gruppo Oncologico Nord Ovest. J Clin Oncol. 2007;25:1670–6.
8. Cremolini C, Loupakis F, Antoniotti C, et al. FOLFOXIRI plus bevacizumab versus FOLFIRI plus bevacizumab as first-line treatment of patients with metastatic colorectal cancer: updated overall survival and molecular subgroup analyses of the open-label, phase 3 TRIBE study. Lancet Oncol. 2015;16:1306–15.
9. Gruenberger T, Bridgewater J, Chau I, et al. Bevacizumab plus mFOLFOX-6 or FOLFOXIRI in patients with initially unresectable liver metastases from colorectal cancer: the OLIVIA multinational randomised phase II trial. Ann Oncol. 2014;26:702–8.

10. Folprecht G, Gruenberger T, Bechstein WO, et al. Tumour response and secondary resectability of colorectal liver metastases following neoadjuvant chemotherapy with cetuximab: the CELIM randomised phase 2 trial. Lancet Oncol. 2010;11:38–47.
11. Ye LC, Liu TS, Ren L, et al. Randomized controlled trial of cetuximab plus chemotherapy for patients with KRAS wild-type unresectable colorectal liver-limited metastases. J Clin Oncol. 2013;31:1931–8.
12. Geissler M, Riera-Knorrenschild J, Tannapfel A, et al. mFOLFOXIRI + panitumumab versus FOLFOXIRI as first line treatment in patients with RAS wild-type metastatic colorectal cancer (mCRC): a randomized phase II VOLFI trial of the AIO (AIO-KRK0109). J Clin Oncol. 2018;36(suppl):abstr 3509.
13. Holch JW, Ricard I, Stintzing S, et al. The relevance of primary tumour location in patients with metastatic colorectal cancer: a meta-analysis of first line clinical trials. Eur J Cancer. 2017;70:87–98.
14. Venook A, Niedzwiecki D, Lenz HJ, et al. CALGB/SWOG 80405: phase III trial of irinotecan/5-FU/leucovorin (FOLFIRI) or oxaliplatin/5-FU/leucovorin (mFOLFOX6) with bevacizumab (BV) or cetuximab (CET) for patients (pts) with KRAS wild-type (wt) untreated metastatic adenocarcinoma of the colon or rectum (MCRC). J Clin Oncol. 2014;32(15 Suppl):abstr LBA 3.
15. Tran B, Kopetz S, Tie J, et al. Impact of BRAF mutation and microsatellite instability on the pattern of metastatic spread and prognosis in metastatic colorectal cancer. Cancer. 2011;117:4623–32.
16. Rowland A, Dias MM, Wiese MD, et al. Meta-analysis of BRAF mutation as a predictive biomarker of benefit from anti-EGFR monoclonal antibody therapy for RAS wild-type metastatic colorectal cancer. Br J Cancer. 2015;112:1888–94.
17. Le DT, Durham JN, Smith KN, et al. Mismatch-repair deficiency predicts response of solid tumors to PD-1 blockade. Science. 2017;357(6349):409–13.

Adjuvant Chemotherapy for CRLM: Indications and Results

19

Carlos José Coelho de Andrade

Introduction

Colorectal cancer is the third most frequent malignant neoplasia in the world [13, 35]. Sixty percent of the cases will develop colorectal liver metastasis (CRLM), and 15–20% of them will be synchronous with the primary tumor [22, 23]. Unfortunately, only 20–30% of the patients with CRLM will be eligible for surgical resection, the only option for a long-term survival [19, 31, 43].

A retrospective analysis comparing patients with CRLM treated with surgery versus clinical interventions demonstrates considerable differences in 5-year survival (0% vs 30%) in which more than 20% of patients treated with surgery survived more than 10 years [14, 34, 41]. Although the comparison of surgery versus chemotherapy has never been dealt with by a prospective randomized study, there is a consensus that surgical resection is the treatment of choice for patients with CRLM [37]. Unfortunately, 70% of patients will relapse after complete resection of the liver metastasis at liver and extrahepatic sites [1, 9]. In order to improve this outcome, chemotherapy has been used in different ways: adjuvant, neoadjuvant, perioperative, systemically, and regionally by hepatic arterial infusion.

However, there are still controversies about the overall survival rates, the best chemotherapy regimens, and the eligibility of patients regarding chemotherapy. Although there are guidelines for adjuvant chemotherapy after complete resection [7, 29, 42], the evidence is weak.

This chapter will discuss the results of trials and highlight the limitations of evidence and the difficulties underlying the design and execution of an ideal trial and also propose a rational approach for eligible patients.

C. J. C. de Andrade (✉)
Instituto Nacional de Câncer, Americas Centro de Oncologia Integrado,
Hospital Pró-Cardíaco, Rio de Janeiro, Brazil

M. M. Correia et al. (eds.), *Colorectal Cancer Liver Metastases*,
https://doi.org/10.1007/978-3-030-25486-5_19

Adjuvant Systemic Chemotherapy

The main objective of adjuvant chemotherapy after complete resection of a colorectal liver metastasis is to eradicate micrometastatic disease. Why not then benefit resected liver limited stage IV disease in the same way as practiced for stage III disease after primary tumor resection.

Systemic palliative chemotherapy has been used in the treatment of advanced colorectal cancer, thus contributing to progression-free and overall survival [10, 36]. Also, adjuvant systemic chemotherapy increased the survival rate after primary surgery of colorectal cancer with improvements in disease-free and overall survival based on randomized controlled trials (RTC) [33]. It is important to acknowledge that a single or a combination chemotherapy treatment producing an increase in the overall survival in a palliative setting does not mean that the same improvement will occur within the adjuvant context. This is true for irinotecan and target therapies that although shown to be ineffective in adjuvant trials were beneficial in palliative treatments (CALGB 89803, PETACC-3, NSABP-C08, AVANT, NCCTG NO147, PETACC-8).

Regarding colorectal liver metastases in which a recurrence after a complete resection is a complicated issue, the use of adjuvant chemotherapy has been investigated as a means to improve outcome [25, 26, 28, 30, 45]. In this chapter we will focus only on systemic adjuvant and perioperative chemotherapy. The hepatic arterial infusions treatments will be described elsewhere in this book. Furthermore, only randomized controlled trials will be analyzed as shown in Table 19.1.

The first study evaluating the adjuvant strategy included not only patients with colorectal liver metastases but also those with lung metastases which were completely resected. In this survey we compared surgery alone versus surgery plus chemotherapy with 5FU/LV [25]. This was a collaborative study involving the European Organization for Research and Treatment of Cancer EORTC 40923, the National Cancer Institute of Canada Clinical Trial Group NCIC CTG CO.7, and the Gruppo Italiano di Valutazione Interventi in Oncologia GIVIO CO.3 (ENG Trial). This study had patient accrual problems because enrolment fell short of the target population. Only 107 patients were analyzed. Although there was a better disease-free and overall survival rate (4-year DFS 35% vs 45% and 4-year OS 47% vs 57%), there were no statistically significant differences for disease-free and overall survival. The p values were, respectively, $p = 0.35$ and $p = 0.39$. Another problem with this study was the inclusion of patients with lung metastases who might have had a different prognosis.

Another cooperative trial (Federation Francophone de Cancerologie Digestive Trial 9002, Association de Chirurgie Hepato-Biliaire et de Transplantation Hepatique, and Association Universitaire de Recherche en Chirurgie Vasculaire (FFCD-ACHBTH-AURC)) [28] was carried out. The authors evaluated the use of surgery alone vs surgery plus 5FU/LV in 173 patients with CRLM. After a follow-up lasting 87.4 months, there were no differences in OS (5-year OS 41.9% vs 51.1%, $p = 0.13$). After adjusting for negative prognostic factors (synchronous and multiple metastases), a benefit in disease-free survival was observed (17.6 vs 24.4 months,

Table 19.1 Prospective randomized trials on adjuvant and perioperative chemotherapy in resectable CRLM

Author/year	RCT	Sample	Arms	Outcome DFS/PFS	OS
Mitry et al. (2008) [25]	Yes	55 vs 52	Surg vs surg + 5FU/LV	4-year: 35% vs 45% ($p = 0.35$)	4-year: 47% vs 57% ($p = 0.39$)
Portier et al. (2006) [28]	Yes	86 vs 85	Surg vs surg + 5FU/LV	5-year: 33.5% vs 26.7% ($p = 0.028$)[a]	5-year: 51.1% vs 41.9% ($p = 0.13$)
Mitry et al. (2008) [25]	Yes (pooled 2 trials)	138 vs 140	Surg vs surg + 5FU/LV	Median DFS: 27.9 vs 18.8 months ($p = 0.058$)	Median OS: 62.2 vs 47.3 months ($p = 0.095$)
Ychou et al. (2009) [45]	Yes	153 vs 153	5FU/LV vs FOLFIRI	2-year: 46.2% vs 50.7% ($p = 0.44$)	3-year: 71.6% vs 72.7% ($p = 0.69$)
Nordlinger et al. (2013) [26]	Yes	171 vs 171	Surg vs peri-op FOLFOX + surg	3-year: 30.3% vs 38.2% ($p = 0.068$)	5-year: 47.8% vs 51.2% ($p = 0.34$)
Primrose et al. (2014) [30]	Yes	117 vs 119	FOLFOX/CAPOX vs FOLFOX/ CAPOX + cetuximab	Median PFS: 20.5 vs 14.1 months ($p = 0.03$)	Median OS: not reached vs 39.1 months ($p = 0.16$)
Kobayashi et al. (2014) [20]	Yes	89 vs 88	Surg vs surg + UFT/LV	3-year: PFS 32.3% vs 38.6% ($p = 0.03$)	3-year: 81.6% vs 82.8% ($p = 0.41$)

[a]After adjusting for negative prognostic factors

$p = 0.028$). Similar to the first study, the latter had problems with slow accrual (more than 10 years) and was therefore stopped, thus underlining the difficulties involved in trials conducted after liver resection of colorectal metastases.

Two years later [25], the pooled data of these 2 trials was published describing the analysis of 278 patients. A marginal benefit in progression of free and overall survival was observed (PFS 18.8 vs 27.9 months for surgery vs surgery plus chemotherapy, $p = 0.058$, and OS 43.7 vs 62.2 months, $p = 0.095$). Thus, although retrospective analysis has shown the benefit of adjuvant chemotherapy [9, 15, 27, 44], prospective trials using 5FU/LV did not succeed in demonstrating improvements in overall survival after liver resection.

Considering the benefit of combination of irinotecan and oxaliplatin with 5FU/LV over 5FU/LV alone in terms of progression-free and overall survival in metastatic disease [8, 11, 17, 32], a new phase began with studies that adopted modern chemotherapy combinations in the context of resectable CRLM. In a phase III trial [45], 306 patients were randomized to receive 5FU/LV or 5FU/LV plus irinotecan (FOLFIRI) after complete resection of CRLM. Although the experimental arm showed a difference in disease-free survival, this was not statistically significant (21.6 vs 24.7 months, $p = 0.44$). The conclusion was that FOLFIRI added no benefit over 5FU/LV.

Another modern combination with oxaliplatin was tested in a different study design in which perioperative chemotherapy was carried out in resectable colorectal liver metastases [26]. The long-term results of this trial that randomized 364 patients with resectable liver metastases receiving perioperative chemotherapy with FOLFOX (six cycles before and six after surgery) versus surgery alone showed a significant difference in 3-year disease-free survival (29.9% vs 39%, $p = 0.035$). However, there were no differences in the overall survival after 5 years (48.3% vs 52.4%, $p = 0.3$). Although this trial was reported as having no impact on the overall survival, the sample size was insufficient to detect survival differences. Some comments are relevant here: firstly, the trial was not designed to detect overall survival differences, and it must be emphasized that the lack of evidence of benefit is not evidence of its absence. Secondly, the control group had a better outcome than the experimental arm of the Mitry study which compared observation versus adjuvant chemotherapy with 5FU/LV. This may reflect a better patient selection to surgery, as well as a better surgical support. However, this could also represent a possible case of mixed phenomena. Thirdly, the clinical relevance of 4.1% in absolute survival difference in the 5-year follow-up was actually too close to the 6-year difference of 4.2% obtained in MOSAIC trial with 1347 patients randomized (almost four times bigger than the Nordlinger's trial). In this trial the adjuvant chemotherapy with FOLFOX given after surgery of the primary tumor became standard care as adjuvant treatment [4]. In summary, the benefit in overall survival may have been underestimated, and thus there is no clear evidence for the lack of benefit.

Furthermore, considering the benefits in metastatic disease, Primrose et al. [30] in a phase III trial randomized 257 WT KRAS patients to receive perioperative chemotherapy alone or perioperative chemotherapy with cetuximab. The primary analysis included 236 patients in which the progression-free survival in the experimental arm was lower than the control arm (14.1 vs 20.5 months). This showed a detrimental effect of cetuximab in perioperative setting of resectable and suboptimally resectable colorectal liver metastasis. With this study it became clear that the use of cetuximab should be avoided in the adjuvant context. Another phase III study randomized patients with complete resection of colorectal liver metastasis to receive capecitabine with oxaliplatin with or without bevacizumab. The study was discontinued by slow accrual, and no conclusions could be made (included only 40 patients per arm).

The use of oral fluoropyrimidine was also tested in a randomized trial comparing surgery with surgery plus uracil-tegafur with leucovorin (UFT/LV) in resectable CRLM. A phase III trial randomized 180 patients to receive surgery or surgery plus uracil-tegafur. The results were first published as an abstract [20]. There was a 3-year disease-free survival of 32.3% vs 38.6%, $p = 0.03$, but with no differences in overall survival (81.6% vs 82.8%, $p = 0.41$). The long-term results were again presented in the abstract format [18], with a median follow-up of 6 years. The 5-year RFS was 32.3% in the control versus 36.2% in the experimental arm, but the OS was 62.2% versus 65.3% with no statistical significance ($p = 0.54$).

Reasons for Different Results of Adjuvant Trials

To address these questions, some critical points should be raised.

The first one is the fact that the absence of evidence is not evidence for the absence of benefit. This reasoning was pointed out before [2, 3], stressing that one still has to pay attention to the meaning of a negative trial in which the sample size is not adequate to detect survival outcomes. Studies ill designed to detect differences in overall survival usually generate results with wide confidence intervals. While they are not statistically significant ($p > 0.05$), the intervention could actually offer a clinically relevant benefit which is not detected only because of the sample size. The right conclusion should not be one of a negative trial, but the acknowledgment of uncertainties around it. The best way to solve this hurdle is to design collaborative studies with a robust accrual capacity in order to achieve definitive conclusions. We need to accept that many guidelines recommend adjuvant chemotherapy after complete resection [7, 29, 42], although the level of evidence that support this contention is weak. This fact can create difficulties regarding accrual of patients in studies with an "only surgery" control arm [21].

The second point to be addressed is the heterogeneity of studied populations. When the control arm of one study has a better outcome than that of the experimental arm of another trial addressing the same problem, attention should be directed not only to the quality of the offered treatment but also to the inclusion criteria and potential prognostic differences of the patients. This is why it is extremely important to know the prognostic factors of population in order to evaluate the results of the adjuvant strategy ([16, 39, 40]). For example, the cooperative study published by Portier et al. [28] showed benefit only after adjusting the analysis to the worst prognostic group (synchronous and multiple metastasis). As in other diagnosis (breast, lung, and primary colon cancer), we saw the benefit of adjuvant chemotherapy in patients with a high-risk profile. In a retrospective analysis, Ayez et al. [6] evaluated patients with CRLM with a low versus high risk score in terms of benefit of chemotherapy associated with surgery. With a median follow-up of 47 months, the group of patients with low risk showed no significant differences in median overall survival between those who received and those who did not receive chemotherapy (65 vs 54 months, $p = 0.31$). In the high-risk group, there was a significant difference in overall survival between those who received or not the chemotherapy plus surgery (46 vs 33 months, $p = 0.004$). This raised the question about the potential benefit of the association of chemotherapy (adjuvant or perioperative) being restricted to the worst prognostic population. Based on that, future prospective studies should try to improve selection criteria and also a better stratification. The CHARISMA trial (EudraCT number: 2013-004952-39) is an example of a stricter selection study focusing on patients with a worst prognosis [5].

Dealing with Uncertainties and the Available Evidence

While we wait for better evidence to aid decision-making regarding patients with resectable CRLM, some rules of thumb could be useful to deal with uncertainties. Below there is a list of information that can guide the decision-making process.

1. Accept the uncertainties; this helps to share decisions with patients [24].
2. Whenever possible, ask the opinion of a multidisciplinary team; this improves the chances of getting a complete resection [12].
3. Whenever possible, also refer patients to clinical trials. This is the only way to build better evidence.
4. Irinotecan, cetuximab, and bevacizumab do not reflect the gains obtained in metastatic disease to adjuvant setting of resected CRLM [30, 38, 45].
5. Perioperative chemotherapy with FOLFOX has no detrimental effect on surgical mortality and improves disease-free survival, and it cannot unequivocally rule out the possible overall survival benefit for resectable disease [26].
6. When opting for adjuvant chemotherapy after resectable CRLM, choose the patients with the worst prognostic factors [6, 28].
7. Since guidelines give the option to offer adjuvant or perioperative chemotherapy in resectable CRLM [7, 29, 42], one should realize how difficult it is to include patients in clinical trials with a control arm containing surgery alone.

Future Directions

A better clinical trial design with a more specific population such as that of the CHARISMA study [5] will help us to refine the best group of patients to receive neoadjuvant chemotherapy in resectable CRLM. A cooperative effort is important to improve the accrual capacity of the studies. Clinical trials need to be very carefully designed, thus enabling the investigators to answer the important questions around the resectable CRLM issue. Also, the refinement of predictive and prognostic scores is a critical necessity to be addressed. Future attempts need to build newer models combining clinical and biological factors tested and validated in large populations before clinical use. The use of prognostic scores to select patients with high risk of relapse after CRLM resection combined with a more robust accrual capacity of cooperative group association could increase the ability to answer correctly the questions around CRLM approach.

Conclusions

Surgery is the standard of care for patients with resectable CRLM. The use of adjuvant or perioperative chemotherapy aiming at improving overall survival after surgery is controversial. Although there are robust data related to better disease-free survival, there is no clear evidence of overall survival benefit. In spite of the lack of evidence, the widespread use of adjuvant and perioperative chemotherapy is a reality. If it turns out to be real, the benefit is probably more visible in patients with worst prognoses. Better patient selection with a multidisciplinary team working in a patient-centered care should help to deal with uncertainties.

References

1. Abdalla EK, Vauthey JN, Ellis LM, Ellis V, Pollock R, Broglio KR, Hess K, Curley SA. Recurrence and outcomes following hepatic resection, radiofrequency ablation, and combined resection/ablation for colorectal liver metastases. Ann Surg. 2004;239:818–25; discussion 825–7.
2. Alderson P. Absence of evidence is not evidence of absence. BMJ. 2004;328:476–7.
3. Altman DG, Bland JM. Absence of evidence is not evidence of absence. BMJ. 1995;311:485.
4. Andre T, Boni C, Navarro M, Tabernero J, Hickish T, Topham C, Bonetti A, Clingan P, Bridgewater J, Rivera F, De Gramont A. Improved overall survival with oxaliplatin, fluorouracil, and leucovorin as adjuvant treatment in stage II or III colon cancer in the MOSAIC trial. J Clin Oncol. 2009;27:3109–16.
5. Ayez N, Van Der Stok EP, De Wilt H, Radema SA, Van Hillegersberg R, Roumen RM, Vreugdenhil G, Tanis PJ, Punt CJ, Dejong CH, Jansen RL, Verheul HM, De Jong KP, Hospers GA, Klaase JM, Legdeur MC, Van Meerten E, Eskens FA, Van Der Meer N, Van Der Holt B, Verhoef C, Grunhagen DJ. Neo-adjuvant chemotherapy followed by surgery versus surgery alone in high-risk patients with resectable colorectal liver metastases: the CHARISMA randomized multicenter clinical trial. BMC Cancer. 2015a;15:180.
6. Ayez N, Van Der Stok EP, Grunhagen DJ, Rothbarth J, Van Meerten E, Eggermont AM, Verhoef C. The use of neo-adjuvant chemotherapy in patients with resectable colorectal liver metastases: clinical risk score as possible discriminator. Eur J Surg Oncol. 2015b;41: 859–67.
7. Benson AB 3rd, Bekaii-Saab T, Chan E, Chen YJ, Choti MA, Cooper HS, Engstrom PF, Enzinger PC, Fakih MG, Fenton MJ, Fuchs CS, Grem JL, Hunt S, Kamel A, Leong LA, Lin E, May KS, Mulcahy MF, Murphy K, Rohren E, Ryan DP, Saltz L, Sharma S, Shibata D, Skibber JM, Small W Jr, Sofocleous CT, Venook AP, Willett CG, Gregory KM, Freedman-Cass DA. Metastatic colon cancer, version 3.2013: featured updates to the NCCN Guidelines. J Natl Compr Canc Netw. 2013;11:141–52; quiz 152.
8. De Gramont A, Figer A, Seymour M, Homerin M, Hmissi A, Cassidy J, Boni C, Cortes-Funes H, Cervantes A, Freyer G, Papamichael D, Le Bail N, Louvet C, Hendler D, De Braud F, Wilson C, Morvan F, Bonetti A. Leucovorin and fluorouracil with or without oxaliplatin as first-line treatment in advanced colorectal cancer. J Clin Oncol. 2000;18:2938–47.
9. De Jong MC, Pulitano C, Ribero D, Strub J, Mentha G, Schulick RD, Choti MA, Aldrighetti L, Capussotti L, Pawlik TM. Rates and patterns of recurrence following curative intent surgery for colorectal liver metastasis: an international multi-institutional analysis of 1669 patients. Ann Surg. 2009;250:440–8.
10. De Kort SJ, Willemse PH, Habraken JM, De Haes HC, Willems DL, Richel DJ. Quality of life versus prolongation of life in patients treated with chemotherapy in advanced colorectal cancer: a review of randomized controlled clinical trials. Eur J Cancer. 2006;42:835–45.
11. Douillard JY, Cunningham D, Roth AD, Navarro M, James RD, Karasek P, Jandik P, Iveson T, Carmichael J, Alakl M, Gruia G, Awad L, Rougier P. Irinotecan combined with fluorouracil compared with fluorouracil alone as first-line treatment for metastatic colorectal cancer: a multicentre randomised trial. Lancet. 2000;355:1041–7.
12. Engstrand J, Kartalis N, Stromberg C, Broberg M, Stillstrom A, Lekberg T, Jonas E, Freedman J, Nilsson H. The impact of a hepatobiliary multidisciplinary team assessment in patients with colorectal cancer liver metastases: a population-based study. Oncologist. 2017;22:1067–74.

13. Ferlay J, Soerjomataram I, Dikshit R, Eser S, Mathers C, Rebelo M, Parkin DM, Forman D, Bray F. Cancer incidence and mortality worldwide: sources, methods and major patterns in GLOBOCAN 2012. Int J Cancer. 2015;136:E359–86.
14. Fernandez FG, Drebin JA, Linehan DC, Dehdashti F, Siegel BA, Strasberg SM. Five-year survival after resection of hepatic metastases from colorectal cancer in patients screened by positron emission tomography with F-18 fluorodeoxyglucose (FDG-PET). Ann Surg. 2004;240:438–47; discussion 447–50.
15. Figueras J, Torras J, Valls C, Llado L, Ramos E, Marti-Rague J, Serrano T, Fabregat J. Surgical resection of colorectal liver metastases in patients with expanded indications: a single-center experience with 501 patients. Dis Colon Rectum. 2007;50:478–88.
16. George B, Kopetz S. Predictive and prognostic markers in colorectal cancer. Curr Oncol Rep. 2011;13:206–15.
17. Grothey A, Sargent D, Goldberg RM, Schmoll HJ. Survival of patients with advanced colorectal cancer improves with the availability of fluorouracil-leucovorin, irinotecan, and oxaliplatin in the course of treatment. J Clin Oncol. 2004;22:1209–14.
18. Hasegawa K, Saiura A, Takayama T, Miyagawa S, Yamamoto J, Bandai Y, Teruya M, Yoshimi F, Kawasaki S, Koyama H, Oba M, Takahashi M, Yamashita S, Mizunuma N, Matsuyama Y, Watanabe T, Makuuchi M, Kokudo N, Group TULS. Oral adjuvant chemotherapy using uracil-tegafur (UFT) with leucovorin (LV) after resection of colorectal cancer liver metastases: long-term survival results of the phase III UFT/LV study. J Clin Oncol. 2017;35:672.
19. Jiang Q, Yan X, Wang K, Bao Q, Sun Y, Wang H, Jin K, Xing B. [Evaluation of long-term survival after hepatic resection for metastatic colorectal cancer-a multifactorial model of 191 patients]. Zhonghua Wai Ke Za Zhi. 2014;52:171–4.
20. Kobayashi A, Hasegawa K, Saiura A, Takayama T, Miyagawa S, Yamamoto J, Bandai Y, Teruya M, Yoshimi F, Kawasaki S, Koyama H, Oba M, Takahashi M, Mizunuma N, Matsuyama Y, Watanabe T, Makuuchi M, Kokudo N. A randomized controlled trial evaluating efficacy of adjuvant oral uracil-tegafur (UFT) with leucovorin (LV) after resection of colorectal cancer liver metastases: the UFT/LV study. J Clin Oncol. 2014;32:3584.
21. Kokudo N, Hasegawa K, Makuuchi M. Control arm for surgery alone is needed but difficult to obtain in randomized trials for adjuvant chemotherapy after liver resection for colorectal metastases. J Clin Oncol. 2007;25:1299–300; author reply 1300.
22. Leporrier J, Maurel J, Chiche L, Bara S, Segol P, Launoy G. A population-based study of the incidence, management and prognosis of hepatic metastases from colorectal cancer. Br J Surg. 2006;93:465–74.
23. Manfredi S, Lepage C, Hatem C, Coatmeur O, Faivre J, Bouvier AM. Epidemiology and management of liver metastases from colorectal cancer. Ann Surg. 2006;244:254–9.
24. Mccahill LE, Hamel-Bissell BP. The patient lived experience for surgical treatment of colorectal liver metastases: a phenomenological study. Palliat Support Care. 2009;7:65–73.
25. Mitry E, Fields AL, Bleiberg H, Labianca R, Portier G, Tu D, Nitti D, Torri V, Elias D, O'Callaghan C, Langer B, Martignoni G, Bouche O, Lazorthes F, Van Cutsem E, Bedenne L, Moore MJ, Rougier P. Adjuvant chemotherapy after potentially curative resection of metastases from colorectal cancer: a pooled analysis of two randomized trials. J Clin Oncol. 2008;26:4906–11.
26. Nordlinger B, Sorbye H, Glimelius B, Poston GJ, Schlag PM, Rougier P, Bechstein WO, Primrose JN, Walpole ET, Finch-Jones M, Jaeck D, Mirza D, Parks RW, Mauer M, Tanis E, Van Cutsem E, Scheithauer W, Gruenberger T, EORTC Gastro-Intestinal Tract Cancer Group; Cancer Research UK; Arbeitsgruppe Lebermetastasen und–tumoren in der Chirurgischen Arbeitsgemeinschaft Onkologie (ALM-CAO); Australasian Gastro-Intestinal Trials Group (AGITG); Fédération Francophone de Cancérol. Perioperative FOLFOX4 chemotherapy and surgery versus surgery alone for resectable liver metastases from colorectal cancer (EORTC 40983): long-term results of a randomised, controlled, phase 3 trial. Lancet Oncol. 2013;14:1208–15.
27. Parks R, Gonen M, Kemeny N, Jarnagin W, D'Angelica M, Dematteo R, Garden OJ, Blumgart LH, Fong Y. Adjuvant chemotherapy improves survival after resection of hepatic colorectal

metastases: analysis of data from two continents. J Am Coll Surg. 2007;204:753–61; discussion 761–3.
28. Portier G, Elias D, Bouche O, Rougier P, Bosset JF, Saric J, Belghiti J, Piedbois P, Guimbaud R, Nordlinger B, Bugat R, Lazorthes F, Bedenne L. Multicenter randomized trial of adjuvant fluorouracil and folinic acid compared with surgery alone after resection of colorectal liver metastases: FFCD ACHBTH AURC 9002 trial. J Clin Oncol. 2006;24:4976–82.
29. Poston GJ, Tait D, O'Connell S, Bennett A, Berendse S, Guideline Development G. Diagnosis and management of colorectal cancer: summary of NICE guidance. BMJ. 2011;343:d6751.
30. Primrose J, Falk S, Finch-Jones M, Valle J, O'Reilly D, Siriwardena A, Hornbuckle J, Peterson M, Rees M, Iveson T, Hickish T, Butler R, Stanton L, Dixon E, Little L, Bowers M, Pugh S, Garden OJ, Cunningham D, Maughan T, Bridgewater J. Systemic chemotherapy with or without cetuximab in patients with resectable colorectal liver metastasis: the new EPOC randomised controlled trial. Lancet Oncol. 2014;15:601–11.
31. Rees M, Tekkis PP, Welsh FK, O'Rourke T, John TG. Evaluation of long-term survival after hepatic resection for metastatic colorectal cancer: a multifactorial model of 929 patients. Ann Surg. 2008;247:125–35.
32. Saltz LB, Douillard JY, Pirotta N, Alakl M, Gruia G, Awad L, Elfring GL, Locker PK, Miller LL. Irinotecan plus fluorouracil/leucovorin for metastatic colorectal cancer: a new survival standard. Oncologist. 2001;6:81–91.
33. Sargent D, Sobrero A, Grothey A, O'Connell MJ, Buyse M, Andre T, Zheng Y, Green E, Labianca R, O'Callaghan C, Seitz JF, Francini G, Haller D, Yothers G, Goldberg R, De Gramont A. Evidence for cure by adjuvant therapy in colon cancer: observations based on individual patient data from 20,898 patients on 18 randomized trials. J Clin Oncol. 2009;27:872–7.
34. Scheele J, Stangl R, Altendorf-Hofmann A. Hepatic metastases from colorectal carcinoma: impact of surgical resection on the natural history. Br J Surg. 1990;77:1241–6.
35. Siegel RL, Miller KD, Jemal A. Cancer statistics, 2015. CA Cancer J Clin. 2015;65:5–29.
36. Simmonds PC. Palliative chemotherapy for advanced colorectal cancer: systematic review and meta-analysis. Colorectal Cancer Collaborative Group. BMJ. 2000;321:531–5.
37. Simmonds PC, Primrose JN, Colquitt JL, Garden OJ, Poston GJ, Rees M. Surgical resection of hepatic metastases from colorectal cancer: a systematic review of published studies. Br J Cancer. 2006;94:982–99.
38. Snoeren N, Van Hillegersberg R, Schouten SB, Bergman AM, Van Werkhoven E, Dalesio O, Tollenaar RA, Verheul HM, Van Der Sijp J, Borel Rinkes IH, Voest EE, Hepatica Study Group. Randomized phase III study to assess efficacy and safety of adjuvant CAPOX with or without bevacizumab in patients after resection of colorectal liver metastases: HEPATICA study. Neoplasia. 2017;19:93–9.
39. Stintzing S, Stremitzer S, Sebio A, Lenz HJ. Predictive and prognostic markers in the treatment of metastatic colorectal cancer (mCRC): personalized medicine at work. Hematol Oncol Clin North Am. 2015;29:43–60.
40. Tejpar S, Stintzing S, Ciardiello F, Tabernero J, Van Cutsem E, Beier F, Esser R, Lenz HJ, Heinemann V. Prognostic and predictive relevance of primary tumor location in patients with RAS wild-type metastatic colorectal cancer: retrospective analyses of the CRYSTAL and FIRE-3 trials. JAMA Oncol. 2017;3(2):194–201.
41. Tomlinson JS, Jarnagin WR, Dematteo RP, Fong Y, Kornprat P, Gonen M, Kemeny N, Brennan MF, Blumgart LH, D'Angelica M. Actual 10-year survival after resection of colorectal liver metastases defines cure. J Clin Oncol. 2007;25:4575–80.
42. Van Cutsem E, Cervantes A, Adam R, Sobrero A, Van Krieken JH, Aderka D, Aranda Aguilar E, Bardelli A, Benson A, Bodoky G, Ciardiello F, D'Hoore A, Diaz-Rubio E, Douillard JY, Ducreux M, Falcone A, Grothey A, Gruenberger T, Haustermans K, Heinemann V, Hoff P, Kohne CH, Labianca R, Laurent-Puig P, Ma B, Maughan T, Muro K, Normanno N, Osterlund P, Oyen WJ, Papamichael D, Pentheroudakis G, Pfeiffer P, Price TJ, Punt C, Ricke J, Roth A, Salazar R, Scheithauer W, Schmoll HJ, Tabernero J, Taieb J, Tejpar S, Wasan H, Yoshino T, Zaanan A, Arnold D. ESMO consensus guidelines for the management of patients with metastatic colorectal cancer. Ann Oncol. 2016;27:1386–422.

43. Van Der Pool AE, De Wilt JH, Lalmahomed ZS, Eggermont AM, Ijzermans JN, Verhoef C. Optimizing the outcome of surgery in patients with rectal cancer and synchronous liver metastases. Br J Surg. 2010;97:383–90.
44. Wang X, Hershman DL, Abrams JA, Feingold D, Grann VR, Jacobson JS, Neugut AI. Predictors of survival after hepatic resection among patients with colorectal liver metastasis. Br J Cancer. 2007;97:1606–12.
45. Ychou M, Hohenberger W, Thezenas S, Navarro M, Maurel J, Bokemeyer C, Shacham-Shmueli E, Rivera F, Kwok-Keung Choi C, Santoro A. A randomized phase III study comparing adjuvant 5-fluorouracil/folinic acid with FOLFIRI in patients following complete resection of liver metastases from colorectal cancer. Ann Oncol. 2009;20:1964–70.

Surgical Outcome of Colorectal Cancer Liver Metastases in Our Facility: Efficacy of Conversion Surgery in Initially Unresectable Colorectal Liver Metastases

20

Shigeyuki Kawachi, Naokazu Chiba, Koichi Tomita, Toru Sano, and Motohide Shimazu

Introduction

Colorectal cancer (CRC) is one of the leading causes of cancer-related death, and the number of CRC-related deaths has markedly increased in recent years in Japan. Twenty-five percent (25%) of CRC patients have clinically detectable liver metastases at initial diagnosis, and approximately 50% of CRC patients develop liver metastases during the disease course [1]. The management of colorectal liver metastases (CLM) is crucial to improving the survival of CRC patients, and liver resection offers the only potential for cure. The prognosis of CLM patients treated with curative resection is excellent, with the 5-year survival approaching approximately 50% [2, 3].

After the introduction of new chemotherapeutic and targeted drugs, including oxaliplatin, irinotecan, bevacizumab, and cetuximab, the prognosis of CLM patients has notably improved, and some patients with initially unresectable CLM have converted to resectable CLM after downstaging chemotherapy. These patients had similar long-term survival rates as patients with initially resectable CLM, following curative hepatic resection (conversion surgery) [4].

We describe, herein, our experiences and strategy for patients with CLM and the surgical outcome of our patient series.

S. Kawachi (✉) · N. Chiba · K. Tomita · T. Sano
Department of Digestive and Transplantation Surgery,
Tokyo Medical University Hachioji Medical Center, Tokyo, Japan
e-mail: skawachi@tokyo-med.ac.jp

M. Shimazu
Tama Kyuryo Hospital, Machida, Japan

M. M. Correia et al. (eds.), *Colorectal Cancer Liver Metastases*,
https://doi.org/10.1007/978-3-030-25486-5_20

Patients and Methods

Consecutive 141 patients with CLM managed in our department in Tokyo Medical University Hachioji Medical Center during a 10-year period (2007–2017) were reviewed in this study. Our strategy for CLM patients is described in Fig. 20.1. Briefly, in metachronous CLM patients (CLM occurring >6 months from the primary lesion), upfront liver resection was performed if curative hepatectomy was technically possible (n = 18). Eight patients with resectable metachronous CLM received chemotherapy before hepatectomy because sustained adjuvant chemotherapy had been continued until diagnosis for CLM or because chemotherapy against concomitant distant metastases such as to the lung had been administered until CLM and/or lung metastasis resection. In synchronous CLM patients, upfront surgery was performed only in patients with solitary metastasis (n = 9). Neoadjuvant chemotherapy (NAC) such as four to six courses of FOLFOX was routinely performed in resectable synchronous multiple CLM cases (n = 30). Unresectable CLM cases in both synchronous (n = 52) and metachronous (n = 24) groups were administered FOLFOX chemotherapy regimen with targeted agents such as bevacizumab and panitumumab. Nine patients with unresectable synchronous CLM and three patients with unresectable metachronous CLM were converted to resectable CLM after downstaging chemotherapy (n = 12, conversion rate, 15.8%) and underwent curative hepatectomy.

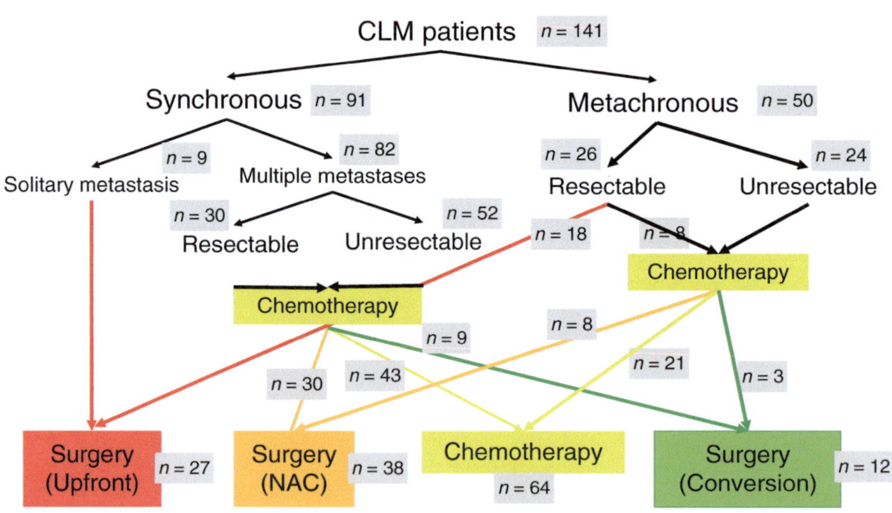

Fig. 20.1 The strategy for patients with CLM in our department

Results

According to our strategy for CLM patients, liver resection was performed in 77 patients (liver resection rate, 54.6%). Sixty-four patients were considered inoperable, and systemic chemotherapy with/without targeted agents was continued for as long as possible. The 3-year and 5-year overall survival (OS) of patients after CLM resection were 67.2% and 51.1%, respectively. The 3-year OS of inoperable patients was 15.7%, and none of these patients survived for up to 5 years (Fig. 20.2). The 3-year and 5-year disease-free survival (DFS) after resection of CLM were 30.5% and 26.7%, respectively.

In univariate analysis, DFS was affected by the disease-free interval from primary tumor to the detection of liver metastasis (synchronous or metachronous) and by the regional lymph node status of the primary tumor, whereas the number and size of liver metastases, serum carcinoembryonic antigen levels at diagnosis of liver metastases, gender, and differentiation were not predictors of adverse outcome in this series (Fig. 20.3). No prognostic factor was also observed regarding OS after liver resection. The median DFS time after liver resection was 25.6 and 7.2 months in the metachronous and synchronous groups, respectively.

Survival after different types of timing for liver resection is shown in Fig. 20.4. Whether patients received preoperative NAC had no significant effect on the OS and DFS after liver resection in CLM. It is noteworthy that 12 initially unresectable patients underwent surgery after conversion therapy with a 5-year OS of 51.1%, which was very similar to that seen in the upfront or NAC liver resection groups (50.5% and 55.7%, respectively).

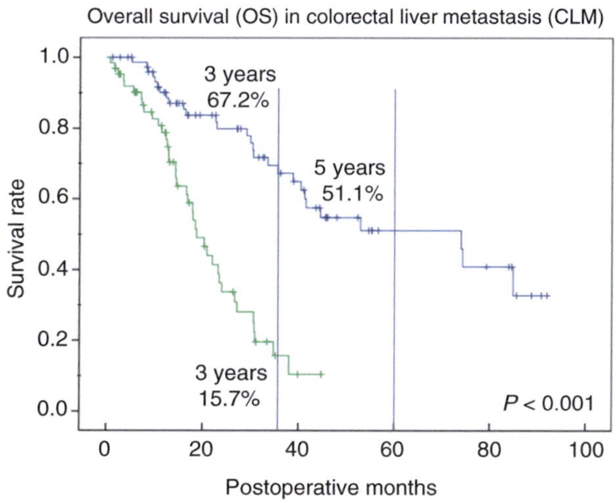

Fig. 20.2 Overall survival in CLM with/without liver resection. A significant difference was observed between the liver resection group and inoperable group ($P < 0.001$). Liver resection group – blue line. Inoperable group – green line

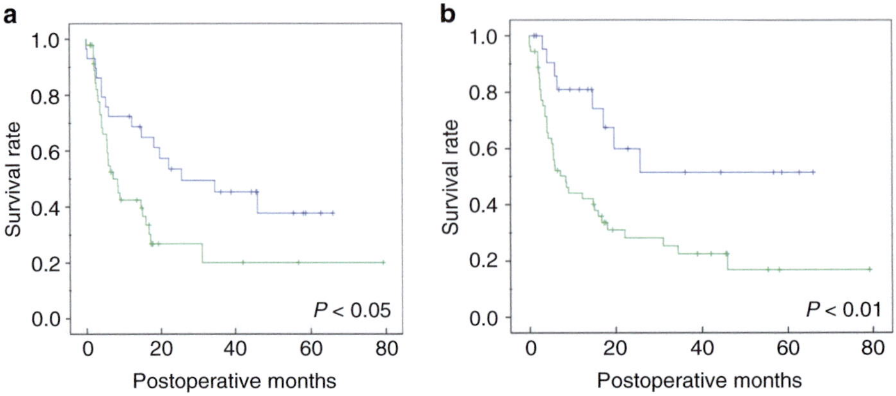

Fig. 20.3 DFS after liver resection in CLM. (**a**) Metachronous (blue line) vs synchronous (green line). (**b**) Lymph node negative (blue line) vs lymph node positive (green line). Only synchronous metastases and primary lymph node positivity were prognostic factors for adverse DFS

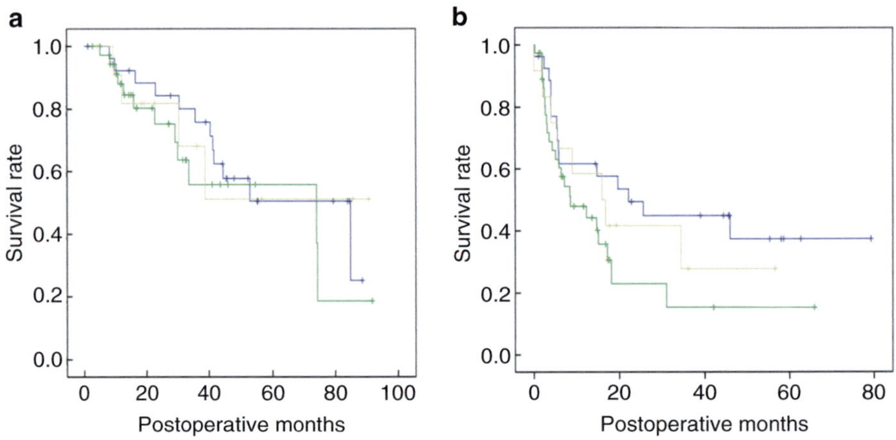

Fig. 20.4 OS (**a**) and DFS (**b**) in CLM patients after different types of liver resection. There was no significant difference in OS and DFS between upfront hepatectomy, neoadjuvant chemotherapy with hepatectomy, and conversion hepatectomy from initially unresectable CLM. Upfront – blue line. NAC – green line. Conversion – gray line

The timing of liver resection was especially controversial in synchronous CLM; survival after different types of the timing of liver resection is shown in Fig. 20.5. There was no significant difference in OS and DFS after liver resection, regardless of whether patients received upfront surgery or surgery after NAC. OS and DFS in the conversion group were also excellent in synchronous CLM and were comparable to rates in initially resectable patients.

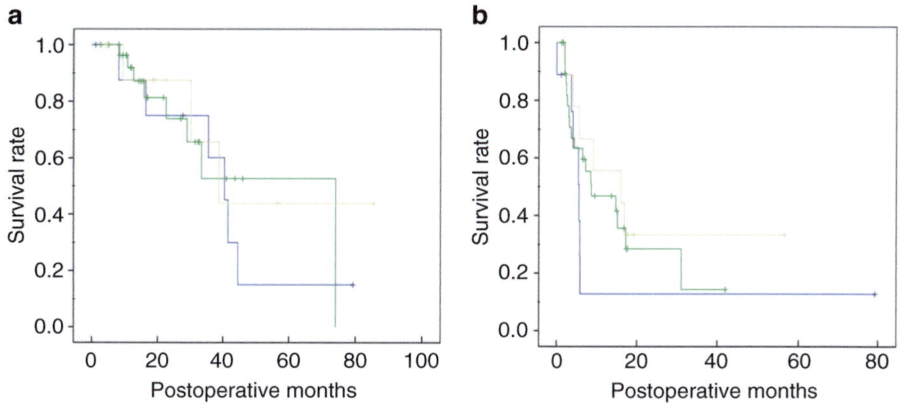

Fig. 20.5 OS (**a**) and DFS (**b**) in patients with synchronous CLM after different types of liver resection. There was no significant difference in OS and DFS between upfront hepatectomy, neoadjuvant chemotherapy, and conversion hepatectomy from initially unresectable CLM. Upfront – blue line. NAC – green line. Conversion – gray line

Case Presentation of a Patient that Received Conversion Therapy

A 54-year-old woman presented with sigmoid colon cancer and synchronous metastatic liver tumors in both lobes. Figure 20.6a shows the initial status of the liver metastases that we considered unresectable. Sigmoidectomy was performed, followed by systemic chemotherapy. After 8 cycles of FOLFOX + panitumumab administration, the CLM shrunk. However, the number of CLM was unchanged (Fig. 20.6b). Three-dimensional reconstruction of the computed tomography scans demonstrated shrunken multiple CLM and right trisectionectomy, and partial resection of the lateral segment was necessary to remove all CLM even after chemotherapy (Fig. 20.6c).

Because we predicted that the remnant liver volume (228 ml) would be too small if right trisectionectomy was performed directly and that portal vein embolization might be insufficient to regenerate such a small liver to a large enough size to meet hepatic demand after trisectionectomy, we performed associating liver partition and portal vein ligation for staged hepatectomy (ALPPS) (Fig. 20.6d).

In our department, 99mTc liver scintigraphy has been routinely used to estimate hepatic reserve, and remnant liver uptake 15 min after isotope administration (remnant LU15) >13 was the minimum requirement for performing hepatectomy [5].

Before the first hepatectomy, the remnant liver volume and LU15 were 228 ml and 8.89, respectively. Resection of three metastases in the lateral segment, liver

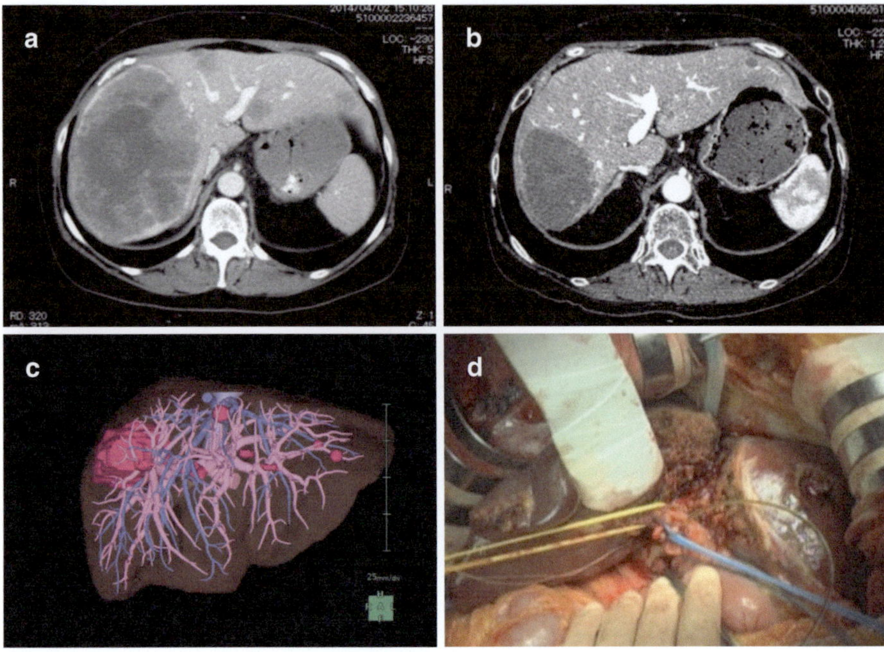

Fig. 20.6 (**a**) CT scan of sigmoid cancer and synchronous liver metastases at diagnosis. (**b**) CT scan after primary resection, followed by systemic chemotherapy (eight cycles of FOLFOX+panitumumab). (**c**) 3D reconstruction of liver metastases and hepatic vasculature by SYNAPSE VINCENT (Fujifilm Medical Co., Tokyo, Japan). (**d**) After partial resection of the left lateral segment, liver partitioning on the line of the right trisectionectomy and right portal vein ligation were performed

partitioning on the line of the right trisectionectomy, and right portal vein ligation were performed as the first hepatectomy. It was noteworthy that the subsequent remnant liver volume and LU15 were notably increased for only 3 days to the level of 466 ml (204% increase) and 17.3 (>13), respectively. The second hepatectomy (right trisectionectomy) was successfully performed 10 days after the first hepatectomy, and the patient was discharged 8 days after the second hepatectomy with no complication (Fig. 20.7). Although the DFS period was not relatively long, 4-year survival has been achieved to date.

Discussion

CLM is the major cause of death in CRC patients and is one of the most important and difficult issues in the treatment of these patients. It is widely accepted that surgical treatment is the only potentially curative therapy for patients with CLM. With the improvement of surgical techniques and the introduction of new chemotherapeutic and targeted drugs, including oxaliplatin, irinotecan, bevacizumab, cetuximab, ramucirumab, etc., the prognosis for CLM patients has markedly improved

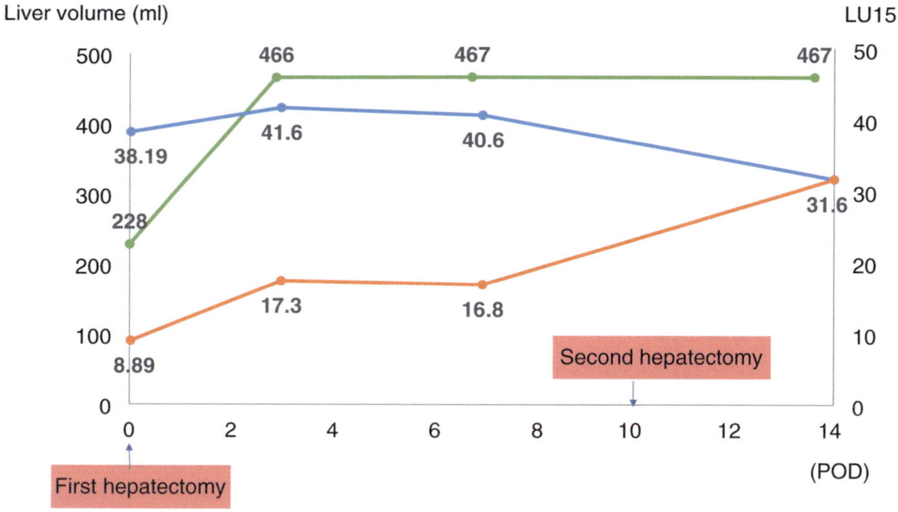

Fig. 20.7 The change in future remnant liver volume, total liver LU15, and remnant liver LU15 during the ALPPS procedure in a patient with initially unresectable CLM. The remnant liver volume and remnant LU15 were notably increased 3 days after the first ALPPS hepatectomy. Both the future remnant liver volume (466 ml) and remnant LU15 (17.3) were sufficient for a second hepatectomy (right trisectionectomy). Remnant liver volume – blue line. Total liver LU15 – green line. Remnant LU15 – red line

over the years. Fong et al. reported that the 5-year survival rate after hepatic resection for CLM was 37% in 1999 [2], whereas Dexiang et al. showed that the 5-year survival rate was 47% in 2012 [3]. In our study, the 5-year survival rate for patients with CLM after hepatectomy was 51%, which was satisfactory compared to other reports.

Previous reports have identified many prognostic factors including synchronous metastases, primary lymph node positivity, number of tumors, largest tumor diameter, poorly differentiated primary tumor, extrahepatic metastasis at hepatectomy, positive margin, and preoperative carbohydrate antigen 19-9 level [2, 3, 6, 7]. The number of tumors proposed as prognostic for high-risk groups has differed between reports, including >5, >4, and >1. Our study demonstrated that synchronous metastases and primary lymph node positivity were significant prognostic factors for DFS after hepatic resection. Although the limited number of patients in this single-center analysis may have affected these results, these two prognostic factors demonstrated a strong ability to predict poor survival.

The optimal timing for surgical resection for CLM has remained controversial, especially in synchronous CLM. Although there is no doubt that upfront liver resection is preferable for metachronous CLM, it is unclear whether the simultaneous or staged resection of the primary lesion and synchronous CLM should be adopted. It has been reported that preoperative chemotherapy may be preferred for patients who experience difficulty undergoing complete resection for multiple hepatic metastases [8], whereas the simultaneous resection strategy might be oncologically equivalent and more cost-efficient for patients with primary CRC presenting with resectable liver metastases [9]. Moreover, there is no evidence of increasing colorectal and hepatic complications in patients with simultaneous primary resection and major hepatectomy [10].

In our study, simultaneous resection of the primary lesion and CLM was performed for only synchronous solitary CLM; however, in synchronous multiple CLM, NAC was indicated after resection of the primary lesion. Our results indicated the lack of a significant difference between upfront and neoadjuvant strategy in both OS and DFS after liver resection in synchronous CLM. Considering that the number of CLM is a prognostic factors in many studies, NAC may be effective in patients with synchronous multiple CLM cases.

It was surprising that there was no significant difference between upfront, NAC, and conversion strategy regarding both OS and DFS after liver resection in all the CLM cases. Adam et al. reported that modern chemotherapy allows 12.5% of patients with unresectable CLM to be rescued by liver surgery and the 5-year OS rate was 33%. In our series, 15.8% of initially unresectable CLM cases were converted to resectable CLM by downstaging chemotherapy, and the 5-year OS and DFS rate were 51.1% and 27.8%, respectively. As this conversion group included two ALPPS procedures, we tried to perform a wide-as-possible hepatic resection according to the indication.

ALPPS should be used with extreme caution, giving special attention to postoperative complications and grade of functional liver regeneration [11]. Estimation of hepatic reserve using liver scintigraphy is effective, and we routinely performed liver scintigraphy before major liver resection [5]. In our presenting case, remnant LU15 was markedly increased for 3–4 days and reached within safety levels after the first hepatectomy of ALPPS. In our limited experience, ALPPS had a notable ability to regenerate the remnant liver, and a second hepatectomy can be safety performed if the remnant LU15 level is within safety levels like other major hepatectomies. Further observation and experience will be needed to define the surgical safety and oncological benefit of ALPPS in conversion hepatectomy.

Conclusion

Liver resection for CLM is the only potentially curative strategy, and recent changes in modern chemotherapy, targeted drugs, and expanded indications for hepatectomy have improved OS and DFS after hepatectomy for CLM. Our strategy for CLM was satisfactory and achieved 5-year OS and DFS of 51.1% and 26.7%, respectively. The efficacy of NAC in synchronous CLM is still controversial, and there may be still room to change the strategy for managing synchronous CLM and indications for the simultaneous resection of the primary lesion and synchronous CLM. Conversion hepatectomy for initially unresectable CLM was notably effective, with a similar OS and DFS as for initially resectable CLM. Although we noted above that the limited number of patients in this single-center analysis may have affected our findings, ALPPS seems effective for the challenging resection of advanced CLM, and further observation and experiences will be needed to define the safety and oncological benefit of ALPPS in conversion hepatectomy.

References

1. Garden OJ, Rees M, Poston GJ, Mirza D, Saunders M, Ledemann J, et al. Guidelines for resection of colorectal cancer liver metastases. Gut. 2006;55 Suppl 3:iii1–8. [PMID: 16835351]. https://doi.org/10.1136/gut.2006.098053.
2. Fong Y, Fortner J, Sun RL, Brennan MF, Blumgart LH. Clinical score for predicting recurrence after hepatic resection for metastatic colorectal cancer: analysis of 1001 consecutive cases. Ann Surg. 1999;230:309–18. [PMID: 10493478].
3. Dexiang Z, Li R, Ye W, Haifu W, Yunshi Z, Qinghai Y, et al. Outcome of patients with colorectal liver metastasis: analysis of 1613 consecutive cases. Ann Surg Oncol. 2012;19:2860–8. [PMID: 22526903]. https://doi.org/10.1245/s10434-012-2356-9.
4. Adam R, Delvart V, Pascal G, Valeanu A, Castaing D, Azoulay D, et al. Rescue surgery for unresectable colorectal liver metastases downstaged by chemotherapy: a model to predict long-term survival. Ann Surg. 2004;240:644–57. [PMID: 15383792]. https://doi.org/10.1097/01.sla.0000141198.92114.f6.
5. Chiba N, Shimazu M, Takano K, Oshima G, Tomita K, Sano T, et al. Predicting hepatic failure with a new diagnostic technique by preoperative liver scintigraphy and computed tomography: a pilot study in 123 patients undergoing liver resection. Patient Saf Surg. 2017;11:29. [PMID: 29270223]. https://doi.org/10.1186/s13037-017-0143-z.
6. Mann CD, Metcalfe MS, Leopardi LN, Maddern GJ. The clinical risk score: emerging as a reliable preoperative prognostic index in hepatectomy for colorectal metastases. Arch Surg. 2004;139:1168–72. [PMID: 15545561]. https://doi.org/10.1001/archsurg.139.11.1168.
7. Beppu T, Sakamoto Y, Hasegawa K, Honda G, Tanaka K, Kotera Y, et al. A nomogram predicting disease-free survival in patients with colorectal liver metastases treated with hepatic resection: multicenter data collection as a Project Study for Hepatic Surgery of the Japanese Society of Hepato-Biliary-Pancreatic Surgery. J Hepatobiliary Pancreat Sci. 2012;19:72–84. [PMID: 22020927]. https://doi.org/10.1007/s00534-011-0460-z.
8. Kim CW, Lee JL, Yoon YS, Park IJ, Lim SB, Yu CS, et al. Resection after preoperative chemotherapy versus synchronous liver resection of colorectal cancer liver metastases: a propensity score matching analysis. Medicine (Baltimore). 2017;96:e6174. [PMID: 28207557]. https://doi.org/10.1097/MD.0000000000006174.
9. Abbott DE, Cantor SB, Hu CY, Aloia TA, You YN, Nguyen S, et al. Optimizing clinical and economic outcomes of surgical therapy for patients with colorectal cancer and synchronous liver metastases. J Am Coll Surg. 2012;215:262–70. [PMID: 22560316]. https://doi.org/10.1016/j.jamcollsurg.2012.03.021.
10. Ono Y, Saiura A, Arita J, Takahashi Y, Takahashi M, Inoue Y. Short-term outcomes after simultaneous colorectal and major hepatic resection for synchronous colorectal liver metastases. Dig Surg. 2017;34:447–54. [PMID: 28319941]. https://doi.org/10.1159/000455295.
11. Tanaka K, Matuo K, Murakami T, Kawaguchi D, Hiroshima Y, Koda K, et al. Associating liver partition and portal vein ligation for staged hepatectomy (ALPPS): short-term outcome, functional changes in the future liver remnant, and tumor growth activity. EJSO. 2015;41:506–12. [PMID: 25704556]. https://doi.org/10.1016/j.ejso.2015.01.031.

Immunotherapy in the Management of Colorectal Cancer Liver Metastasis

21

Thuy B. Tran and Ajay V. Maker

Introduction

Colorectal cancer (CRC) is one of the most common malignancies in the United States, with approximately 134,490 new cases diagnosed per year, and it remains the second leading cause of cancer-related deaths in the United States [1]. The majority of patients will die of metastatic disease with the liver being the most common site of spread [2]. Currently, hepatic resection of isolated colorectal liver metastases (CRLM) remains the cornerstone of curative-intent treatment. While a combination of advancements in surgical and systemic therapies have increased survival of patients with resectable CRLM, recurrence rates remain as high as 70% in the liver.

Five-year survival after resection of CRLM ranges from 33% to 61% [3–5]; however, 34% of 5-year survivors will experience disease progression [4]. Furthermore, though it may enhance patient selection for surgery, perioperative chemotherapy in randomized controlled trials does not appear to improve survival in this patient population [5]. Thus, there is a need to better select patients who may benefit from both surgery and adjuvant treatment for CRLM and, perhaps more importantly, to develop more effective and durable targeted therapies. Perhaps what is most alarming for the future is that while patient selection for treatment has improved, treatment strategies have remained largely unchanged, and the majority of improvement in colon cancer mortality over the decades has been secondary solely to improved screening.

T. B. Tran · A. V. Maker (✉)
Department of Surgery, Division of Surgical Oncology, University of Illinois at Chicago, Chicago, IL, USA

Creticos Cancer Center, Advocate Illinois Masonic Medical Center, Chicago, IL, USA
e-mail: amaker@uic.edu

M. M. Correia et al. (eds.), *Colorectal Cancer Liver Metastases*,
https://doi.org/10.1007/978-3-030-25486-5_21

Based on checkpoint blockade trials that have shown unprecedented responses in other cancer histologies [6, 7], there has been growing excitement for the potential of immunotherapy in CRC, and there is a strong scientific premise for this contention. Patient survival can be accurately determined by the number and location of tumor-infiltrating lymphocytes (TIL) trafficking to primary CRC tumors [8–14]. In CRLM, a similar association has been demonstrated between increased TIL and improved survival [10, 11]. Furthermore, it has been identified through gene ontology analysis that recurrence after CRLM resection is mainly determined by the ability of the host to mount, and the tumor to support, lymphocyte proliferation, activation, and cytotoxicity [11]. Thus, there is a reason to believe that interventions that activate anti-tumor immunocytes above an immunoediting threshold, or that inhibit immunosuppressive signals, hold potential as new strategies to combat this disease process.

Unfortunately, the use of immunotherapy for gastrointestinal (GI) cancers, in general, has met significant challenges and is not part of the standard armamentarium to battle these diseases [15]. Checkpoint blockade has not resulted in clinically meaningful responses in microsatellite stable (>95%) colon cancer [16, 17]. Similarly, adoptive transfer of CEA-specific T cells resulted in dose-limiting toxicity resulting in termination of that trial [18]. Thus, current immunotherapy strategies successful in other histologies have not been successful in CRC. Until GI cancer-specific antigens are identified across patients, new strategies to enhance tumor-infiltrating lymphocyte activation in the tumor microenvironment are needed.

In this chapter, the emerging role and efficacy of immunotherapy in the management of CRLM is examined, recent advancements in immunotherapy are summarized, and pathways to overcome resistance to anti-tumor immunity are highlighted.

Emerging Immunotherapies

Increased understanding of the interaction between the immune system and the tumor microenvironment has led to a burgeoning interest in enhancing the anti-tumor immune response both within the tumor and systemically. We herein highlight approaches that have been used, are in trial, or are in development for the management of metastatic CRC (Table 21.1).

Table 21.1 Selected clinical trials of metastatic CRC treated with immunotherapy

Author/ year/study type	Regimen/strategy	Cohort	Survival	Complications
Foon (1997) [19] Phase Ib clinical trial	3H1 anti-idiotype monoclonal CEA antibody (anti-CEA vaccine)	$N = 24$ Metastatic CRC	Median OS 11.3 months Median time to progression 2.3 months	Local injection reaction – mild erythema and induration
Wong (2000) [20] Phase I clinical trial	^{90}Y-labeled DTPA-cT84.66 (anti-CEA vaccine)	$N = 22$ Metastatic CRC (18), lung (2), pseudomyxoma peritonei (1), 1 thyroid	Stable disease 3/22	Overall AE 19/22 Grade 1 AE (13/22) Grade 2 AE (4/22) Grade 3–4 AE (2/22) Transaminitis (2/22) Fatigue 4/22 Anemia 3/22 Rash 1/22
Posner (2007) [21] Phase II clinical trial	CeaVac TriAb (anti-idiotype monoclonal antibody vaccines)	$N = 52$ Post-hepatic resection for colorectal liver metastasis	Median time to recurrence 1.3 years Median RFS 16 months 2-year OS 94%	Grade 2 AE 22% Hematologic 6% Non-hematologic complications 24% Mortality 0%
Mazzaferro (2003) [22] Pilot study	HSPPC-gp96 (Oncophage) (autogenous tumor-derived heat-shock protein Gp96 vaccine)	$N = 29$ Patients who underwent resection of CRLM	2-year OS 100% 2-year DFS 46%	Grade 0–1 AE 9/29 (31%)
Harrop (2006) [23] Phase I/II clinical trial	TroVax (anti-5T4 vaccine)	$N = 17$ patients with metastatic CRC	Stable disease 5/17 patients (disease control ranging from 3 to 18 months)	Not reported
Elkord (2008) [24] Phase II clinical trial	TroVax (anti-5T4 vaccine)	$N = 15$ Patients who underwent complete resection and received at least 4 vaccinations	Patients who mount an above median 5TA-specific antibody and proliferative response had significantly increased survival ($P = 0.016$) compared to those with minimal or no 5T4 response after vaccination	Not reported

(continued)

Table 21.1 (continued)

Author/ year/study type	Regimen/strategy	Cohort	Survival	Complications
Harrop (2008) [25] Phase II clinical trial	TroVax + chemotherapy (anti-5T4 and 5-fluorouracil, leucovorin, and irinotecan)	*N* = 19 Metastatic CRC	Response rate 7/19 (58.3%) PR 6/19 (31%) SD 5/19 (26%) CR 1/19 (5%) Median survival 15.4 months	Not reported
Barth (2000) [26]	Autologous tumor lysate dendritic cell vaccine	*N* = 26 Resected CRLM	5-year RFS 63%	Not reported
Katz (2015) [27] Phase I clinical trial	Hepatic intra-arterial CAR-T therapy	*N* = 6 Unresectable CRC liver metastasis	Median OS 15 months Stable disease 1/6	Grade 1–3 AE 5/6 Grade 4–5 AE 0% Fever 4/6
Le (2015) [16] Phase II clinical trial	Pembrolizumab (PD-1 inhibitor)	*N* = 41 (11/41 patients with metastatic mismatch repair deficient CRC)	Response rate 40% PFS 78%	Overall morbidity 40/41 Grade 3–4 AE 17/41 Anemia 8/41 Lymphopenia 8/41 Diarrhea 24/41 Pancreatitis 6/41 Bowel obstruction 3/41
Overman (2017) [28] Phase II clinical trial	Nivolumab (PD-1 inhibitor)	*N* = 74 (dMMR and MSI-H CRC)	Response rate 31% Median PFS 14.3 months 12-month OS 73% 12-month PFS 50% Disease control rate > 12 weeks 69%	Grade 1–2 AE 29/74 (39%) Grade 3 AE 30/74 (30%) Grade 4 AE 10/74 (14%) Treatment-related mortality 0% Treatment-related AE 52/74 (70%) Treatment-related grade 3–4 AE 15/74 (20%)

(continued)

Table 21.1 (continued)

Author/year/study type	Regimen/strategy	Cohort	Survival	Complications
Overman (2018) [29]	Nivolumab + ipilimumab for 4 weeks, followed by nivolumab every 2 weeks (combination PD-1 inhibitor and CTLA-4 antibody)	*N* = 119 (dMMR and MSI-H metastatic CRC)	Response rate 55% Disease control rate > 12 weeks 80% 12-month PFS 71% 12-month OS 85%	Overall morbidity 73% Diarrhea 26/119 (22%) Fatigue 21/119 (18%) Pruritis 20/119 (17%) Grade 1–2 AE 49/119 (41%) Grade 3 AE 32/119 (27%) Grade 4 AE 6/119 (5%) Treatment-related mortality 0%

Abbreviation: *CRC* colorectal cancer, *CRLM* colorectal liver metastasis, *PFS* progression-free survival, *PD-1* programmed death-1, *CTLA-4* cytotoxic T-cell lymphocyte antigen-4, *AE* adverse events, *RFS* recurrence-free survival, *CR* complete response, *SD* stable disease, *PR* partial response, *CAR-T* chimeric antigen receptor-modified T cell

Peptide-Based Vaccines and Oncoviruses

Cancer vaccines are designed with the goal of sensitizing patients with tumor-specific antigens to generate anti-tumor lymphocyte responses and long-term memory. Colorectal cancers are a reasonable target for vaccines because they are known to express tumor-related antigens such as CEA, melanoma antigen gene family (MAGE), p53, and MUC-1 [30, 31]. In the last few decades, several vaccines have been developed to treat metastatic CRC, though few have resulted in clinically relevant tumor regressions [32–34]. Peptide vaccines, in general, have demonstrated the ability to increase antigen-specific circulating T cells; however, tumor regressions are rare. Anti-CEA monoclonal antibody was one of the earliest vaccines developed, but failed to gain traction due to no improvement in long-term recurrence or overall survival after surgical resection of CRLM. In a phase II multi-institutional study consisting 52 patients who underwent curative resection of CRLM followed by adjuvant anti-idiotype monoclonal antibody vaccines with tumor-associated antigens carcinoembryonic antigen (CeaVac) and human milk fat globule (TriAb), a 2-year recurrence-free survival was comparable to hepatectomy alone [24].

The therapeutic vaccine, TroVax (MVA-5TA), was developed as a potential treatment for solid tumors by utilizing the oncofetal antigen 5T4. 5T4 is known to be associated with poor survival [35–38], and increased tumor expression is associated with cancer progression and metastasis [24, 39]. The antigen is presented by a highly attenuated vaccinia virus (modified vaccinia Ankara (MVA)) that harbors the gene for 5TA. In early studies, the vaccine was safe and effective in inducing anti-5T4 cellular and humoral immune responses. A phase I/II trial consisting of 17 patients with metastatic colorectal cancer who received TroVax revealed the magnitude of anti-5T4 immunologic response was an independent predictor of improved survival within 5T4 antibody responders [23]. A subsequent phase II study in patients with resected CRLM demonstrated that 7/8 (88%) patients who mounted a response to 5T4 after vaccination were long-term survivors [24]. Further, combining TroVax with systemic chemotherapy resulted in decreases in serum CEA levels and partial responses in 31% of patients and complete responses in 5% [25]. While there was a positive association between the development of 5TA antibody response and patient survival or time to progression, these trials did not show a correlation between survival and 5T4 antibody level.

Few studies have evaluated the use of vaccines in the adjuvant setting after resection of colon cancer. Phase III trials of an adjuvant tumor vaccine of irradiated tumor cells administered with Bacillus Calmette-Guerin (BCG) after resection of primary colon cancer did not enhance overall survival in the entire cohort, but those who developed an immune response demonstrated improved survival compared to those who did not mount a response [40, 41]. Another vaccination strategy, that of arming dendritic cells (DCs) with tumor antigens, has generated anti-tumor immune responses measured by quantification of antigen-specific cytotoxic T lymphocytes (CTL) in the circulation or tumor marker responses. This has been accomplished with DCs loaded with CEA peptides, WT1, MAGE, MUC1, HER2, and whole tumor mRNA, cells, or lysate. In a randomized trial of 26 resected CRLM patients who received tumor lysate-pulsed DC, it was reported that patients with early tumor-specific T-cell proliferation or cytokine responses had a significantly higher 5-year RFS compared with patients who did not mount an anti-tumor immune response following vaccination [26]. These vaccine strategies have supported the ability to generate tumor antigen-specific circulating CTL; however, improved design, combinations, and identification of novel neoantigens are likely necessary to improve clinical tumor responses and the utility of this approach.

Oncolytic viruses are replication-competent viruses that are targeted to tumor tissues where they can selectively replicate and cause tumor lysis. They can also function to simultaneously deliver genes for immunostimulatory cytokines. Oncolysis has been shown to generate damage-associated molecular patterns, which have the added effect of inducing immunogenic cell death. This process exposes tumor antigens and activates anti-tumor immune responses that can enhance clinical responses and potentially work synergistically with combination immunotherapy. A handful of viruses have been evaluated clinically in CRLM. The genetically engineered, replication-selective adenovirus d11520 (ONYX-015) was administered through the hepatic artery in phase I/II dose-escalation trials combined with 5-fluorouracil. This virus was well-tolerated and resulted in partial responses and stabilization of disease in select patients [42]. In addition, the genetically engineered herpes simplex virus, NV1020, infused arterially in the liver has been shown to be safe without significant systemic adverse events or liver dysfunction in patients with CRLM refractory to first-line chemotherapy, [43] and resulted in stable disease in 50% of patients with a 1-year survival of 47.2% [44]. Pexa-Vec (pexastimogene devacirepvec, JX-594) is a thymidine kinase gene-inactivated oncolytic vaccinia virus engineered to selectively target cancer cells and to stimulate anti-tumor immunity through delivery of granulocyte-macrophage colony-stimulating factor (GM-CSF) and β-galactosidase [45]. While Pexa-Vec improved survival in patients with hepatocellular carcinoma [46], a recent phase Ib trial in CRLM demonstrated no serious adverse events and stable disease in 67% of patients on the study [47]. Studies on the efficacy of newer oncolytic immunotherapeutic vaccines for CRLM, including the FDA-approved for melanoma HSV talimogene laherparepvec (T-VEC), are currently under investigation (NCT02509507). As a group, there is evidence of clinical efficacy using oncolytic viruses in CRLM both through direct tumor lysis and as a vehicle to deliver immunostimulatory cytokines into the tumor microenvironment. Challenges that remain to be overcome to improve success rates with these viruses include techniques to enhance viral delivery into the tumors and tumor selectivity and to decrease viral clearance by the host immune system. That oncolytic cell death exposes tumor antigens and generates immunogenic cell death does imply a future for oncolytic immunotherapy in combination with other strategies, e.g., checkpoint blockade, to inhibit suppressive immune signals in the tumor microenvironment.

Chimeric Antigen Receptor-Modified T-Cell (CAR-T) Therapy

In recent years, there has been considerable interest in engineering T cells for adoptive transfer with chimeric antigen receptors (CAR) to recognize overexpressed or specific tumor antigens, particularly in hematologic malignancies [48, 49]. These reprogrammed T cells, or CAR-T, can theoretically target tumor antigens and result in T-cell proliferation and cytotoxic lysis of tumor cells. The first set of CAR-T utilized in metastatic CRC targeted the tumor-associated glycoprotein (TAG)-72, and though the infusions were well-tolerated and resulted in a decrease in serum TAG-72 levels, there were not any clinical responses. In the absence of other known CRC antigens, the most studied target has been CEA. In the initial clinical trial adoptively transferring anti-CEA T cells to three patients, all experienced decreased CEA, and one had a tumor regression; however, severe dose-limiting colitis resulted in termination of that trial [18]. Since that time, next-generation CEA+ CAR-T have been shown to be well-tolerated in patients with metastatic CRC [50, 51], but with limited efficacy. In an attempt to limit administration to the liver using hepatic artery infusion of anti-CEA CAR-T, local delivery was well-tolerated, but five out of the six patients with CRLM died from disease progression with a median survival of 15 months [27]. Thus, the premise of CAR-T cell therapy and potential for enhanced anti-tumor immune responses depends on identification of novel CRC tumor antigens and, likely, increased expression of engineered co-stimulatory molecules in next-generation CAR-Ts.

Blockade of Immunoinhibitory Signals

It is well-established that immunosuppressive cytokines, e.g., TGFb and IL10, in the tumor microenvironment, and increased intra-tumoral T-regulatory cells are associated with poor outcomes [10]. Thus, strategies to block immunosuppressive cells and signals may have the potential to "release the brakes" on the immune system and to free tumor antigen-specific T cells. Preliminary research has implicated support of tumor-associated macrophages, inhibition of myeloid-derived suppressor cells, Treg inhibition, and engagement of checkpoint blockade molecules to potentially enhance anti-tumor immune responses in CRLM [52]. It has become increasingly evident that the more unique mutated neoantigens expressed by tumors, the more effective an immune response can be generated through these strategies. As the vast majority, >95%, of CRCs are microsatellite stable, the frequency of mutated antigens available for presentation is few; however, emerging data in microsatellite instable disease has provided proof of principle for the clinical utility of these strategies. The most effective strategy to date that highlights this approach in CRC has been to block the PD-1/PD-L1 interaction.

The PD-1 pathway is a negative feedback system that suppresses cytotoxic T cells and is thus often upregulated in many tumors. Blockade of the PD-1 pathway has been shown to hinder the disease progression of various cancers [53, 54]. Previous studies demonstrated an approximately 25% response rate in patients treated with PD-1 blockade for non-small cell lung cancer, melanoma, or renal cell cancer [7]. Recent studies have hypothesized that deficient mismatch repair (dMMR) CRC have a greater immune response to PD-1 blockade [55]. In the recent phase II clinical trial evaluating the impact of the PD-1 inhibitor pembrolizumab in patients with treatment-refractory metastatic CRC, there was a 40% response rate and 78% progression-free survival (PFS) rate in patients with dMMR, while MMR-proficient CRC patients experienced a 0% response rate and 11% PFS rate [16].

Nivolumab is a PD-1 inhibitor that has been shown to provide durable immunologic response and disease control in metastatic CRC with dMMR or high microsatellite instability (MSI-H). In the CheckMate-142 open-label multicenter phase II trial, patients experienced a response rate of 31% ($n = 23/74$) with a median PFS 14.3 months. The 12-month overall survival (OS) and PFS were 86% and 50%, respectively [28]. A follow-up study consisting of 119 patients with dMMR/MSI-H metastatic CRC evaluating the efficacy of combination immunotherapy with nivolumab and ipilimumab (CTLA-4 inhibitor) revealed a higher response rate compared to the previous published study with nivolumab alone [29]. CTLA-4 inhibits T-cell activation when it binds to CD28 during T-cell priming, and it is thought to augment the anti-tumor immunity response of PD-1 inhibitors; however, CTLA-4 blockade as monotherapy was found not to be effective in advanced colorectal cancer [17, 56]. The higher efficacy and anti-tumor responses observed in the studies using nivolumab plus ipilimumab combination therapy underscore the benefits of multidrug immunotherapy as a potential strategy to improve survival in patients with metastatic CRC compared to anti-PD-1 or anti-CTLA-4 monotherapy alone. The ongoing challenges for the future are to better understand the limitations of checkpoint blockade in dMMR tumors and to improve response rates in these, the majority, of CRLM patients.

Radioimmunotherapy

Given the activity of radiation therapy against CRC, a potential approach to treat CRLM is targeted delivery of radiation to the tumor using monoclonal antibodies against tumor antigens [57–61]. In a study treating patients with metastatic cancer using ^{90}Y-labeled DTPA-cT84.66, which consists of human/murine T84.66 chimeric IgG with a high affinity to the carcinoembryonic antigen (CEA), there was no tumor response in patients with liver metastases due to rapid clearance of the antibody in patients [20]. As newer CRC-specific tumor antigens are identified and techniques to limit their clearance are utilized, radiolabeled antibodies may become more effective. Several studies are evaluating the combination of liver-directed stereotactic radiotherapy, external beam radiation, or radiofrequency ablation with PD-1 inhibitors (NCT02437071, NCT02888743) [62]. Combining immunogenic cell death and abscopal effects secondary to radiation with other immune modulators and checkpoint blockade remains an avenue of active research with great potential.

Immune Modulators

Neutrophil Extracellular Traps

In patients undergoing curative-intent CRLM resection, increased postoperative neutrophil extracellular trap (NET) formation was associated with a significant reduction in disease-free survival [63]. These snares, formed by expelled neutrophil chromatin, are considered to promote metastasis in preclinical models; therefore, interventions that decrease NET formation may improve outcomes in these patients. One such intervention, hydroxychloroquine, is currently under investigation for this purpose for gastrointestinal cancers (NCT01128296).

LIGHT

LIGHT is a tumor necrosis factor superfamily member (TNFSF14) that is naturally expressed on immature dendritic cells and activated T cells [64–66]. Stimulation leads to augmentation of T-cell responses at tumor sites and induction of strong antitumor immunity.

It promotes priming of T cells and overcomes immunological tolerance by acting as a strong co-stimulatory molecule for T-cell activation and expansion. Recent experiments suggest that LIGHT expression facilitates T-cell recruitment and activation, thereby enhancing antigen recognition and rejection of tumors [67–69]. Moreover, LIGHT stimulation amplifies DC activity for T-cell mediated anti-tumor immunity [70], promotes apoptosis of tumor cells, and inhibits tumor growth [71, 72].

In CRLM, increased LIGHT expression is significantly associated with improved outcomes. Studies of resected CRLM have demonstrated that increased expression of LIGHT and LIGHT + lymphocytes in tumors was associated with improved OS and recurrence-free survival [11]. In preclinical models of CRLM, the number of T cells infiltrating CRLM and expressing LIGHT is very low, leading to rapid tumor progression and death [24]. However, increasing expression of LIGHT within CRLM amplified T-cell infiltration and activation, leading to anti-tumor immune responses and clinical regressions [73]. Thus, there is potential for LIGHT alone or in combination with checkpoint blockade to be developed for clinical use.

Conclusion

Improved understanding of the complex interplay of immunostimulatory and regulatory signals in the tumor microenvironment, combined with new technologies and targeted checkpoint blockade antibodies, has resulted in a shift in focus from traditional chemotherapy toward immunotherapeutics in the battle against metastatic gastrointestinal cancers. Evidence supports that strategies to increase tumor-infiltrating lymphocytes in the tumor microenvironment, combined with inhibition of suppressive signals, have great promise specifically for the treatment of CRLM. Further investigation is warranted to establish durability and long-term survival benefits with immunotherapy in these patients; however, the preclinical models and human clinical trials reviewed in this chapter suggest that a combination of immunotherapeutic strategies holds great promise for the near future.

References

1. Miller KD, Siegel RL, Lin CC, Mariotto AB, Kramer JL, Rowland JH, et al. Cancer treatment and survivorship statistics, 2016. CA Cancer J Clin. 2016;66(4):271–89.
2. Siegel RL, Miller KD, Jemal A. Cancer statistics, 2015. CA Cancer J Clin. 2015;65(1):5–29.
3. House MG, Kemeny NE, Gonen M, Fong Y, Allen PJ, Paty PB, et al. Comparison of adjuvant systemic chemotherapy with or without hepatic arterial infusional chemotherapy after hepatic resection for metastatic colorectal cancer. Ann Surg. 2011;254(6):851–6.
4. Tomlinson JS, Jarnagin WR, DeMatteo RP, Fong Y, Kornprat P, Gonen M, et al. Actual 10-year survival after resection of colorectal liver metastases defines cure. J Clin Oncol. 2007;25(29):4575–80.
5. Nordlinger B, Sorbye H, Glimelius B, Poston GJ, Schlag PM, Rougier P, et al. Perioperative FOLFOX4 chemotherapy and surgery versus surgery alone for resectable liver metastases from colorectal cancer (EORTC 40983): long-term results of a randomised, controlled, phase 3 trial. Lancet Oncol. 2013;14(12):1208–15.
6. Maker AV, Phan GQ, Attia P, Yang JC, Sherry RM, Topalian SL, et al. Tumor regression and autoimmunity in patients treated with cytotoxic T lymphocyte-associated antigen 4 blockade and interleukin 2: a phase I/II study. Ann Surg Oncol. 2005;12(12):1005–16.

7. Topalian SL, Hodi FS, Brahmer JR, Gettinger SN, Smith DC, McDermott DF, et al. Safety, activity, and immune correlates of anti-PD-1 antibody in cancer. N Engl J Med. 2012;366(26):2443–54.
8. Chiba T, Ohtani H, Mizoi T, Naito Y, Sato E, Nagura H, et al. Intraepithelial CD8+ T-cell-count becomes a prognostic factor after a longer follow-up period in human colorectal carcinoma: possible association with suppression of micrometastasis. Br J Cancer. 2004;91(9):1711–7.
9. Galon J, Costes A, Sanchez-Cabo F, Kirilovsky A, Mlecnik B, Lagorce-Pages C, et al. Type, density, and location of immune cells within human colorectal tumors predict clinical outcome. Science. 2006;313(5795):1960–4.
10. Katz SC, Bamboat ZM, Maker AV, Shia J, Pillarisetty VG, Yopp AC, et al. Regulatory T cell infiltration predicts outcome following resection of colorectal cancer liver metastases. Ann Surg Oncol. 2013;20(3):946–55.
11. Maker AV, Ito H, Mo Q, Weisenberg E, Qin LX, Turcotte S, et al. Genetic evidence that intratumoral T-cell proliferation and activation are associated with recurrence and survival in patients with resected colorectal liver metastases. Cancer Immunol Res. 2015;3(4):380–8.
12. Naito Y, Saito K, Shiiba K, Ohuchi A, Saigenji K, Nagura H, et al. CD8+ T cells infiltrated within cancer cell nests as a prognostic factor in human colorectal cancer. Cancer Res. 1998;58(16):3491–4.
13. Pages F, Berger A, Camus M, Sanchez-Cabo F, Costes A, Molidor R, et al. Effector memory T cells, early metastasis, and survival in colorectal cancer. N Engl J Med. 2005;353(25):2654–66.
14. Prall F, Duhrkop T, Weirich V, Ostwald C, Lenz P, Nizze H, et al. Prognostic role of CD8+ tumor-infiltrating lymphocytes in stage III colorectal cancer with and without microsatellite instability. Hum Pathol. 2004;35(7):808–16.
15. Rosenberg SA, Yang JC, Restifo NP. Cancer immunotherapy: moving beyond current vaccines. Nat Med. 2004;10(9):909–15.
16. Le DT, Uram JN, Wang H, Bartlett BR, Kemberling H, Eyring AD, et al. PD-1 blockade in tumors with mismatch-repair deficiency. N Engl J Med. 2015;372(26):2509–20.
17. Chung KY, Gore I, Fong L, Venook A, Beck SB, Dorazio P, et al. Phase II study of the anti-cytotoxic T-lymphocyte-associated antigen 4 monoclonal antibody, tremelimumab, in patients with refractory metastatic colorectal cancer. J Clin Oncol. 2010;28(21):3485–90.
18. Parkhurst MR, Yang JC, Langan RC, Dudley ME, Nathan DA, Feldman SA, et al. T cells targeting carcinoembryonic antigen can mediate regression of metastatic colorectal cancer but induce severe transient colitis. Mol Ther. 2011;19(3):620–6.
19. Foon KA, John WJ, Chakraborty M, Sherratt A, Garrison J, Flett M, Bhattacharya-Chatterjee M. Clinical and immune responses in advanced colorectal cancer patients treated with anti-idiotype monoclonal antibody vaccine that mimics the carcinoembryonic antigen. Clin Cancer Res. 1997;3(8):1267–76.
20. Wong JYC, Chu DZ, Yamauchi DM, Williams LE, Liu A, Wilczynski S, et al. A phase I radioimmunotherapy trial evaluating 90yttrium-labeled anti-carcinoembryonic antigen (CEA) chimeric T84.66 in patients with metastatic CEA-producing malignancies. Clin Cancer Res. 2000;6(10):3855–63.
21. Posner MC, Niedzwiecki D, Venook AP, Hollis DR, Kindler HL, Martin EW, et al. A phase II prospective multi-institutional trial of adjuvant active specific immunotherapy following curative resection of colorectal cancer hepatic metastases: cancer and leukemia group B study 89903. Ann Surg Oncol. 2008;15(1):158–64.
22. Mazzaferro V, Coppa J, Carrabba MG, Rivoltini L, Schiavo M, Regalia E, et al. Vaccination with autologous tumor-derived heat-shock protein gp96 after liver resection for metastatic colorectal cancer. Clin Cancer Res. 2003;9(9):3235–45.
23. Harrop R, Connolly N, Redchenko I, Valle J, Saunders M, Ryan MG, et al. Vaccination of colorectal cancer patients with modified vaccinia Ankara delivering the tumor antigen 5T4 (TroVax) induces immune responses which correlate with disease control: a phase I/II trial. Clin Cancer Res. 2006;12(11 Pt 1):3416–24.
24. Elkord E, Dangoor A, Drury NL, Harrop R, Burt DJ, Drijfhout JW, et al. An MVA-based vaccine targeting the oncofetal antigen 5T4 in patients undergoing surgical resection of colorectal cancer liver metastases. J Immunother. 2008;31(9):820–9.

25. Harrop R, Drury N, Shingler W, Chikoti P, Redchenko I, Carroll MW, et al. Vaccination of colorectal cancer patients with TroVax given alongside chemotherapy (5-fluorouracil, leukovorin and irinotecan) is safe and induces potent immune responses. Cancer Immunol Immunother. 2008;57(7):977–86.
26. Barth RJ Jr, Fisher DA, Wallace PK, Channon JY, Noelle RJ, Gui J, et al. A randomized trial of ex vivo CD40L activation of a dendritic cell vaccine in colorectal cancer patients: tumor-specific immune responses are associated with improved survival. Clin Cancer Res. 2010;16(22):5548–56.
27. Katz SC, Burga RA, McCormack E, Wang LJ, Mooring W, Point GR, et al. Phase I hepatic immunotherapy for metastases study of intra-arterial chimeric antigen receptor-modified T-cell therapy for CEA+ liver metastases. Clin Cancer Res. 2015;21(14):3149–59.
28. Overman MJ, McDermott R, Leach JL, Lonardi S, Lenz HJ, Morse MA, et al. Nivolumab in patients with metastatic DNA mismatch repair-deficient or microsatellite instability-high colorectal cancer (CheckMate 142): an open-label, multicentre, phase 2 study. Lancet Oncol. 2017;18(9):1182–91.
29. Overman MJ, Lonardi S, Wong KYM, Lenz HJ, Gelsomino F, Aglietta M, et al. Durable clinical benefit with nivolumab plus ipilimumab in DNA mismatch repair-deficient/microsatellite instability-high metastatic colorectal cancer. J Clin Oncol. 2018;36(8):773–9.
30. Lou E, Marshall J, Aklilu M, Cole D, Chang D, Morse M. A phase II study of active immunotherapy with PANVAC or autologous, cultured dendritic cells infected with PANVAC after complete resection of hepatic metastases of colorectal carcinoma. Clin Colorectal Cancer. 2006;5(5):368–71.
31. Nagorsen D, Scheibenbogen C, Marincola FM, Letsch A, Keilholz U. Natural T cell immunity against cancer. Clin Cancer Res. 2003;9(12):4296–303.
32. Grenier JM, Yeung ST, Khanna KM. Combination immunotherapy: taking cancer vaccines to the next level. Front Immunol. 2018;9:610.
33. Klebanoff CA, Acquavella N, Yu Z, Restifo NP. Therapeutic cancer vaccines: are we there yet? Immunol Rev. 2011;239(1):27–44.
34. Melero I, Gaudernack G, Gerritsen W, Huber C, Parmiani G, Scholl S, et al. Therapeutic vaccines for cancer: an overview of clinical trials. Nat Rev Clin Oncol. 2014;11(9):509–24.
35. Naganuma H, Kono K, Mori Y, Takayoshi S, Stern PL, Tasaka K, et al. Oncofetal antigen 5T4 expression as a prognostic factor in patients with gastric cancer. Anticancer Res. 2002;22(2B):1033–8.
36. Starzynska T, Marsh PJ, Schofield PF, Roberts SA, Myers KA, Stern PL. Prognostic significance of 5T4 oncofetal antigen expression in colorectal carcinoma. Br J Cancer. 1994;69(5):899–902.
37. Starzynska T, Wiechowska-Kozlowska A, Marlicz K, Bromley M, Roberts SA, Lawniczak M, et al. 5T4 oncofetal antigen in gastric carcinoma and its clinical significance. Eur J Gastroenterol Hepatol. 1998;10(6):479–84.
38. Wrigley E, McGown AT, Rennison J, Swindell R, Crowther D, Starzynska T, et al. 5T4 oncofetal antigen expression in ovarian carcinoma. Int J Gynecol Cancer. 1995;5(4):269–74.
39. Cavallaro U, Christofori G. Cell adhesion and signalling by cadherins and Ig-CAMs in cancer. Nat Rev Cancer. 2004;4(2):118–32.
40. Harris JE, Ryan L, Hoover HC Jr, Stuart RK, Oken MM, Benson AB 3rd, et al. Adjuvant active specific immunotherapy for stage II and III colon cancer with an autologous tumor cell vaccine: Eastern Cooperative Oncology Group Study E5283. J Clin Oncol. 2000;18(1):148–57.
41. Vermorken JB, Claessen AM, van Tinteren H, Gall HE, Ezinga R, Meijer S, et al. Active specific immunotherapy for stage II and stage III human colon cancer: a randomised trial. Lancet. 1999;353(9150):345–50.
42. Reid TR, Freeman S, Post L, McCormick F, Sze DY. Effects of Onyx-015 among metastatic colorectal cancer patients that have failed prior treatment with 5-FU/leucovorin. Cancer Gene Ther. 2005;12(8):673–81.
43. Kemeny N, Brown K, Covey A, Kim T, Bhargava A, Brody L, et al. Phase I, open-label, dose-escalating study of a genetically engineered herpes simplex virus, NV1020, in subjects with metastatic colorectal carcinoma to the liver. Hum Gene Ther. 2006;17(12):1214–24.

44. Geevarghese SK, Geller DA, de Haan HA, Horer M, Knoll AE, Mescheder A, et al. Phase I/II study of oncolytic herpes simplex virus NV1020 in patients with extensively pretreated refractory colorectal cancer metastatic to the liver. Hum Gene Ther. 2010;21(9):1119–28.
45. Breitbach CJ, Bell JC, Hwang TH, Kirn DH, Burke J. The emerging therapeutic potential of the oncolytic immunotherapeutic Pexa-Vec (JX-594). Oncolytic Virother. 2015;4:25–31.
46. Heo J, Reid T, Ruo L, Breitbach CJ, Rose S, Bloomston M, et al. Randomized dose-finding clinical trial of oncolytic immunotherapeutic vaccinia JX-594 in liver cancer. Nat Med. 2013;19(3):329–36.
47. Park SH, Breitbach CJ, Lee J, Park JO, Lim HY, Kang WK, et al. Phase 1b trial of biweekly intravenous Pexa-Vec (JX-594), an oncolytic and immunotherapeutic vaccinia virus in colorectal cancer. Mol Ther. 2015;23(9):1532–40.
48. Grupp SA, Kalos M, Barrett D, Aplenc R, Porter DL, Rheingold SR, et al. Chimeric antigen receptor-modified T cells for acute lymphoid leukemia. N Engl J Med. 2013;368(16):1509–18.
49. Porter DL, Levine BL, Kalos M, Bagg A, June CH. Chimeric antigen receptor-modified T cells in chronic lymphoid leukemia. N Engl J Med. 2011;365(8):725–33.
50. Hege KM, Bergsland EK, Fisher GA, Nemunaitis JJ, Warren RS, McArthur JG, et al. Safety, tumor trafficking and immunogenicity of chimeric antigen receptor (CAR)-T cells specific for TAG-72 in colorectal cancer. J Immunother Cancer. 2017;5:22.
51. Zhang C, Wang Z, Yang Z, Wang M, Li S, Li Y, et al. Phase I escalating-dose trial of CAR-T therapy targeting CEA(+) metastatic colorectal cancers. Mol Ther. 2017;25(5):1248–58.
52. Thorn M, Guha P, Cunetta M, Espat NJ, Miller G, Junghans RP, et al. Tumor-associated GM-CSF overexpression induces immunoinhibitory molecules via STAT3 in myeloid-suppressor cells infiltrating liver metastases. Cancer Gene Ther. 2016;23(6):188–98.
53. Hamid O, Robert C, Daud A, Hodi FS, Hwu WJ, Kefford R, et al. Safety and tumor responses with lambrolizumab (anti-PD-1) in melanoma. N Engl J Med. 2013;369(2):134–44.
54. Powles T, Eder JP, Fine GD, Braiteh FS, Loriot Y, Cruz C, et al. MPDL3280A (anti-PD-L1) treatment leads to clinical activity in metastatic bladder cancer. Nature. 2014;515(7528):558–62.
55. Bodmer W, Bishop T, Karran P. Genetic steps in colorectal cancer. Nat Genet. 1994;6(3):217–9.
56. Sharma P, Allison JP. The future of immune checkpoint therapy. Science. 2015;348(6230):56–61.
57. Abdel-Nabi HH, Schwartz AN, Higano CS, Wechter DG, Unger MW. Colorectal carcinoma: detection with indium-111 anticarcinoembryonic-antigen monoclonal antibody ZCE-025. Radiology. 1987;164(3):617–21.
58. Divgi CR, McDermott K, Griffin TW, Johnson DK, Schnobrich KE, Fallone PS, et al. Lesion-by-lesion comparison of computerized tomography and indium-111-labeled monoclonal antibody C110 radioimmunoscintigraphy in colorectal carcinoma: a multicenter trial. J Nucl Med. 1993;34(10):1656–61.
59. Lind P. Application of radioimmunodetection with a radiolabeled monoclonal antibody to CEA (BW 431/26) in colorectal and breast cancer. Pathol Biol (Paris). 1993;41(1):39.
60. Riva P, Moscatelli G, Paganelli G, Benini S, Siccardi A. Antibody-guided diagnosis: an Italian experience on CEA-expressing tumours. Int J Cancer Suppl. 1988;2:114–20.
61. Stillwagon GB, Order SE, Haulk T, Herpst J, Ettinger DS, Fishman EK, et al. Variable low dose rate irradiation (131I-anti-CEA) and integrated low dose chemotherapy in the treatment of nonresectable primary intrahepatic cholangiocarcinoma. Int J Radiat Oncol Biol Phys. 1991;21(6):1601–5.
62. Duffy AG, Makarova-Rusher OV, Ulahannan SV, Rahma OE, Fioravanti S, Walker M, et al. Modulation of tumor eIF4E by antisense inhibition: a phase I/II translational clinical trial of ISIS 183750-an antisense oligonucleotide against eIF4E-in combination with irinotecan in solid tumors and irinotecan-refractory colorectal cancer. Int J Cancer. 2016;139(7):1648–57.
63. Tohme S, Yazdani HO, Al-Khafaji AB, Chidi AP, Loughran P, Mowen K, et al. Neutrophil extracellular traps promote the development and progression of liver metastases after surgical stress. Cancer Res. 2016;76(6):1367–80.
64. Mauri DN, Ebner R, Montgomery RI, Kochel KD, Cheung TC, Yu GL, et al. LIGHT, a new member of the TNF superfamily, and lymphotoxin alpha are ligands for herpesvirus entry mediator. Immunity. 1998;8(1):21–30.

65. Tamada K, Shimozaki K, Chapoval AI, Zhu G, Sica G, Flies D, et al. Modulation of T-cell-mediated immunity in tumor and graft-versus-host disease models through the LIGHT co-stimulatory pathway. Nat Med. 2000;6(3):283–9.
66. Yu P, Fu YX. Targeting tumors with LIGHT to generate metastasis-clearing immunity. Cytokine Growth Factor Rev. 2008;19(3–4):285–94.
67. Yu P, Lee Y, Liu W, Chin RK, Wang J, Wang Y, et al. Priming of naive T cells inside tumors leads to eradication of established tumors. Nat Immunol. 2004;5(2):141–9.
68. Yu P, Spiotto MT, Lee Y, Schreiber H, Fu YX. Complementary role of CD4+ T cells and secondary lymphoid tissues for cross-presentation of tumor antigen to CD8+ T cells. J Exp Med. 2003;197(8):985–95.
69. Mortarini R, Scarito A, Nonaka D, Zanon M, Bersani I, Montaldi E, et al. Constitutive expression and costimulatory function of LIGHT/TNFSF14 on human melanoma cells and melanoma-derived microvesicles. Cancer Res. 2005;65(8):3428–36.
70. Morel Y, Truneh A, Sweet RW, Olive D, Costello RT. The TNF superfamily members LIGHT and CD154 (CD40 ligand) costimulate induction of dendritic cell maturation and elicit specific CTL activity. J Immunol. 2001;167(5):2479–86.
71. Browning JL, Miatkowski K, Sizing I, Griffiths D, Zafari M, Benjamin CD, et al. Signaling through the lymphotoxin beta receptor induces the death of some adenocarcinoma tumor lines. J Exp Med. 1996;183(3):867–78.
72. Zhai Y, Guo R, Hsu TL, Yu GL, Ni J, Kwon BS, et al. LIGHT, a novel ligand for lymphotoxin beta receptor and TR2/HVEM induces apoptosis and suppresses in vivo tumor formation via gene transfer. J Clin Invest. 1998;102(6):1142–51.
73. Qin JZ, Upadhyay V, Prabhakar B, Maker AV. Shedding LIGHT (TNFSF14) on the tumor microenvironment of colorectal cancer liver metastases. J Transl Med. 2013;11:70.

Adjuvant Hepatic Arterial Infusion Therapy

22

Vitor Moutinho, Louise C. Connell, and Nancy Kemeny

Introduction

Colorectal cancer represents a significant global health burden, with over one million new cases diagnosed worldwide each year. In the United States alone, it is estimated that 140,250 new colorectal cancer cases will be diagnosed in 2018, with an anticipated 50,630 deaths attributable to this disease [1]. The most common organ that harbors metastases from colorectal cancer is the liver. Hepatic metastatic disease is the main prognostic driver, accounting for approximately 50% of colorectal cancer deaths [2]. Twenty to twenty-five percent of patients will have synchronous hepatic metastases at diagnosis. De novo liver metastases occur in approximately 15% of colorectal cancer patients, while 60% of people who develop metastatic disease will have liver metastases [3].

Traditionally, patients with liver metastatic disease were treated in a very conservative and palliative manner. More recently, however, there has been a shift in thinking of colorectal cancer patients with liver metastases as untreatable to potentially curable. Surgery confers the best survival advantage and for a long time was the only therapeutic option, which was offered to just a very small proportion of patients. Early studies demonstrated 5-year survival rates of ~30% in patients with low-volume liver metastatic disease who successfully underwent hepatic resection [4]. However, curative surgery such as this was only feasible in a small minority of patients, approximately 10%, given the strict criteria implied for resectability [5].

The portal vein drainage from the colon and rectum to the liver is one of the reasons why the liver is a preferred site for malignant cells from colorectal cancer to

V. Moutinho
AMV Medical Associates, São Paulo, Brazil
e-mail: vitormoutinho@mail.harvard.edu

L. C. Connell · N. Kemeny (✉)
Memorial Sloan Kettering Cancer Center, New York, NY, USA
e-mail: connelll@mskcc.org; kemenyn@mskcc.org

M. M. Correia et al. (eds.), *Colorectal Cancer Liver Metastases*,
https://doi.org/10.1007/978-3-030-25486-5_22

settle, and then the rich blood supply to the liver allows growth. With increasing knowledge and understanding of this background, the concept of metastatic colorectal cancer and its subsequent treatment has evolved. Metastatic colorectal cancer is no longer identified as a single group of patients with a systemic disease, but as various subgroups of patients with a systemic disease, which, in the context of liver metastases, has a very attainable treatment target in the liver to increase disease control.

Hepatic arterial infusion (HAI) chemotherapy as a liver-directed therapy in colorectal cancer was developed more than 50 years ago. Over the past few decades, this technique has been continually refined, with more liberal use of various chemotherapeutic agents. The combination of systemic therapy and regional HAI has been associated with improved locoregional responses in the treatment of liver metastases and in a number of studies with an increased overall survival. Additionally, several studies of hepatic arterial infusion therapies report increased rates of conversion to resection. Many patients who were initially considered unresectable were later offered the opportunity for liver resection after a treatment with hepatic arterial infusion.

Other concurrent types of arterial therapies such as radioembolization with yttrium-90 and chemoembolization with spheres have subsequently ensued in the ongoing effort to adequately and successfully control liver metastatic progression. These other types of treatments will be approached in different sections of this book, leaving this specific chapter to the description and discussion specifically of hepatic arterial infusion chemotherapy.

Hepatic arterial infusion (HAI) was initially described back in the 1960s. A study by Sullivan et al. in 1964 reported 10 objective responses with clinical benefit when 16 patients with gastrointestinal cancers metastatic to the liver were treated with continuous HAI [6].

During the following decades, the treatment has evolved with better systemic chemotherapy to be coupled with the arterial infusion chemotherapy. Initially the main drug used for hepatic arterial infusion was fluorouracil (5-FU); now a prodrug with a higher liver extraction rate, floxuridine (FUDR), is most often used in the United States.

Rationale for Hepatic Arterial Infusion and Choice of Drug

The rationale behind the use of a regional chemotherapy to treat liver metastases via hepatic arterial infusion is based on several principles. Liver metastases, once above 2–3 mm in size, from colorectal and other gastrointestinal tumors are supplied and maintained by the hepatic artery. The normal liver parenchyma, on the other hand, receives its blood supply from another source, the portal vein [7]. Consequently, infusion of chemotherapeutic drugs via the hepatic artery will lead to toxic levels within the tumor cells, with relative sparing of normal liver tissue. Drug extraction from the hepatic arterial circulation via first-pass metabolism results in high local drug concentration with minimal systemic toxicity. The ideal drugs for hepatic arterial infusion are those with a rapid total body clearance and a short plasma half-life, which in turn allows for the delivery of high chemotherapy concentrations directly to liver metastases while minimizing toxicity to the remaining liver and body [8, 9].

The liver is the first site of metastases from colorectal tumors in the majority of cases due to the hematogenous spread of tumor cells via the portal circulation [10]. Direct treatment of hepatic metastases therefore may lead to arrest of further metastatic spread to other organs. Following numerous studies of multiple drugs, FUDR, a prodrug of fluorouracil (5-FU), is now considered the ideal agent for administration via HAI, being the most effective and least toxic drug. During first-pass metabolism, up to 99% of FUDR is extracted by the liver which results in a hepatic/systemic ratio of 100–400, compared to a liver extraction rate of 19–55% for 5-FU resulting in a hepatic/systemic ratio around 10 [8].

Biliary toxicity and gastric ulceration are the predominant toxicities associated with FUDR HAI chemotherapy. Management of patients undergoing FUDR HAI treatment includes standard use of proton pump inhibitors and frequent liver function monitoring. Elevation of aspartate transaminase, alkaline phosphatase, and bilirubin require decreasing or holding the dose of FUDR [11]. If diarrhea is pronounced, shunting of HAI therapy to the bowel should be considered. Primary tumor obstruction versus a surgical stricture should always be ruled out first in a clinically jaundiced patient, before one assumes that it is due to FUDR HAI toxicity.

The use of steroids in conjunction with standard FUDR HAI therapy has been shown to improve hyperbilirubinemia. In a randomized study of patients with metastatic colorectal cancer liver metastases, the addition of dexamethasone to HAI FUDR therapy reduced the incidence of hyperbilirubinemia from 30% to 9%. The response rate was also increased in those patients who received FUDR plus dexamethasone compared to FUDR HAI alone [12].

FUDR has two main drawbacks, the associated biliary toxicity and also the fact that the drug is not available in many countries worldwide. Over the years, several other chemotherapeutic drugs have been trialed as possible alternatives for HAI therapy, including 5-FU, mitomycin, oxaliplatin, and irinotecan, either as single agents or in combination. Most of these agents were tested in a small number of patients in either a phase I or phase II clinical trial as demonstrated in Table 22.1.

Until now, there has been no prospective randomized trial comparing the various chemotherapeutic agents administered via HAI to determine the optimal drug choice. FUDR and oxaliplatin are both acceptable choices based on the available studies to date. Perhaps as important, if not even more important than the specific drug chosen for HAI treatment, one should prioritize the particular institution to oversee this highly specialized treatment, with a dedicated and experienced multidisciplinary team of surgeons, medical oncologists, radiologists, and nurses acquainted with this method and with knowledge and experience to deliver the best care possible.

Regional therapies are increasing as a whole, with an increased understanding that oligometastatic disease may be treated in a more aggressive manner than traditionally thought. Hyperthermic intraperitoneal chemotherapy (HIPEC),

Table 22.1 Retrospective cohorts and clinical trials

Author	Study design	Sample size	Investigational arm	Control arm	Adjuvant HAI vs treatment of unresectable CRLM	Progression-free survival – median (95% CI)	Overall survival – median (95% CI)
Kemeny et al. (1999) [16]	Phase II	156	HAI FUDR/Dex + IV 5-FU/LV	5-FU/LV	Adjuvant	37 vs 17	72 vs 59
Kern et al. (2001) [47]	Phase I	21	Oxaliplatin + 5-FU/ leucovorin HAI	–		Median PFS not reached	Median OS not reached
Mancuso et al. (2003) [48]	Phase I	15	Oxaliplatin HAI	–		10	19
Fiorentini et al. (2004) [49]	Phase II	76	5-FU/leucovorin IV + FUDR HAI	FUDR HAI		12 vs 8	20 vs 14
Boige et al. (2008) [50]	Phase II	44	5-FU/leucovorin IV + oxaliplatin HAI	–		7.0	16
Ducreux et al. (2005) [39]	Phase II	28	(5-FU/leucovorin + oxaliplatin) HAI	–		27.0	27.0
Del Freo et al. (2006) [51]	Phase II	21	(5-FU/leucovorin + oxaliplatin) HAI	–		5.9	36.1
Kemeny et al. (2006) [34]	Phase II	135	HAI FUDR/Dex	5-FU/LV	Unresectable	7.3 vs 9.8	24 vs 20
Lorenz et al. (1998) [19]	Phase II	226	HAI 5-FU/LV	Surgery only	Adjuvant	14.2 vs 13.7	34.5 vs 40.8
Bouchahda et al. (2009) [52]	Retrospective cohort	29	(Oxaliplatin + irinotecan + 5-FU) HAI	–		4.5 (2.4–6.5)	18 (5.8–30.2)
Guan et al. (2012) [53]	Phase II	27	(Oxaliplatin, 5-FU/ leucovorin) HAI + FOLFOX4 IV	–		11	24
Levi et al. (2016) [42]	Phase II	64	(Oxaliplatin + irinotecan + 5-FU) HAI + cetuximab IV	–		9.3 (7.8–10.9)	25.5 (18.8–32.1)

Lim et al. (2017) [54]	Retrospective cohort	61	Oxaliplatin HAI 5-FU/LV IV Monoclonal AB IV	–		9	Median not reached (80% in 2 years)
NCT02316028	Phase I/II	11	Decitabine HAI	–		NA	NA
NCT00268463	Phase III	22	FUDR + oxaliplatin + capecitabine	Oxaliplatin + capecitabine		NA	NA
Ongoing trials							
NCT01312857	Phase II	Recruiting	HAI + irinotecan, 5-FU, leucovorin, panitumumab	HAI + irinotecan, 5-FU, leucovorin		NA March 2018	NA
NCT02529774	Phase II/ III – parallel	Recruiting	Floxuridine (FUDR), dexamethasone (Dex), heparin	1. Oxaliplatin and capecitabine (CAPOX) 2. Oxaliplatin and leucovorin and 5-FU (mFOLFOX6)		NA September 2021	NA
NCT02494973	Phase II/III	Recruiting	Adjuvant HAI oxaliplatin and systemic LV5FU2	Adjuvant systemic chemotherapy with mFOLFOX6		NA May 2026	NA
NCT03069950	Phase II	Recruiting	HAI FUDR/Dex in addition to panitumumab plus FOLFIRI	Panitumumab plus FOLFIRI		NA February 2020	NA
NCT02102789	Phase III	Recruiting	mFOLFOX6 + HAI	mFOLFOX6		NA August 2020	NA
NCT01348412	Phase II	Recruiting	HAI (raltitrexed + oxaliplatin)	Standard chemotherapy		NA May 2019	NA

Abbreviations: *CRLM* colorectal liver metastases; *HAI* hepatic arterial infusion therapy; *5-FU* fluorouracil; *FUDR* floxuridine; *Dex* dexamethasone; *FOLFIRI* bolus and infusional 5-fluorouracil, leucovorin, and irinotecan; *NCT* national clinical trial; *FOLFOX* bolus and infusional 5-fluorouracil, leucovorin, and oxaliplatin; *CAPOX* capecitabine and oxaliplatin radioembolization, chemoembolization, and hepatic arterial infusion are all locoregional treatment modalities that may be used to control locally metastatic colorectal cancer. HAI specifically is increasingly recognized as a valuable locoregional treatment for the management of colorectal liver metastases, with more and more cancer centers worldwide developing specialist expertise in this technique [13, 14].

Over the past few decades, there have been multiple ways to refer to the treatment of colorectal liver metastases. Nonetheless there is a paramount need to standardize the nomenclature of such treatments to benchmark results so that they are comparable across studies.

In order to standardize the terms used for the purpose of this book chapter, and as a suggestion for the oncology community going forward, we will solely use the terminology "adjuvant hepatic arterial infusion" (ADJ-HAI) and "treatment of unresectable liver metastases" with hepatic arterial infusion (TULM-HAI). The first (ADJ-HAI) will refer to treatment given to reduce the risk of developing further colorectal liver metastases, as the term "adjuvant" implies, when hepatic arterial infusion follows a complete resection of liver metastases. The second modality of treatment, addressing unresectable liver metastases (TULM-HAI), is probably the most common application of hepatic arterial infusion to date. It has been used in many different clinical trials and retrospective cohorts (Table 22.1), and its most important feature is the possibility to offer surgical resection to patients previously deemed incurable (conversion to resection).

It is important to state that a few studies addressed the treatment of liver metastases after resection of the primary colorectal cancer (prophylactic HAI). This modality of treatment is an exception and will be considered as one, preventing the use of cross-reference and mixed terms in this text. Only three studies from Asia were conducted in this setting, and an applicability to Western countries has not been performed.

Adjuvant HAI Therapy After Liver Resection (ADJ-HAI)

The liver is the most frequent site for colorectal cancer metastases, with greater than 60% chance of recurrence [15]. In order to mitigate this risk, four randomized controlled trials were conducted comparing HAI treatment versus standard adjuvant systemic regimens or a control arm, and at least another six trials are currently being performed with results expected by 2020. Increased hepatic disease-free survival (DFS) and overall disease-free survival were demonstrated in three out of the four completed adjuvant studies with the use of HAI [11, 16–19].

One of these studies, performed as a single-institution study at Memorial Sloan Kettering Cancer Center, enrolled 156 patients. The trial reported a significantly higher 2-year survival (which was the chosen endpoint of this study) for the HAI FUDR plus systemic chemotherapy group compared with systemic chemotherapy alone (5-FU/LV). The overall survival at 2 years was 86% and 72%, respectively, at $p = 0.03$. The same group published a long-term follow-up of these patients, with a median follow-up of 10.3 years, reaffirming the benefit of HAI treatment, with a median overall survival of 72.2 months for combined therapy of HAI plus systemic chemotherapy versus 59.3 months for the systemic chemotherapy-alone arm. The progression-free survival (PFS) again favored the combination arm, with a median PFS of 31 versus 17 months for the combined therapy group versus the systemic therapy-alone arm, respectively ($p = 0.02$) [16, 17].

Another randomized controlled trial was conducted by the Eastern Cooperative Oncology Group (ECOG) and Southwest Oncology Group (SWOG), which had a slightly different trial design, with the intervention arm consisting of adjuvant HAI (FUDR) plus infusional intravenous 5-FU compared to no further therapy as the control arm. Of note, only 75 patients were eligible for adjuvant therapy post liver resection. The study was powered to assess for improvement in both recurrence-free survival and hepatic disease-free survival, but not overall survival. The study detected a significant improvement in recurrence-free survival at 4 years of follow-up, with a recurrence-free survival of 46% versus 25% in the chemotherapy- and surgery-alone arms, respectively ($p = 0.04$). The 4-year hepatic disease-free survival was also significantly improved in the treatment arm compared to the control arm, 67% versus 43% ($p = 0.03$) [11].

Two hundred and twenty-six patients from a German multicenter prospective trial were randomized to receive either adjuvant HAI therapy with 5-FU and LV versus surveillance. One important limitation of this study is that only 77% of the patients randomized to the intervention arm actually received treatment. The study was a negative study. When subgroup analysis was conducted, comparing those patients in the intervention arm that actually received treatment versus the observation group, improvements in both progression-free survival and hepatic progression-free survival were detected in favor of adjuvant HAI treatment. The median time to hepatic PFS and PFS for adjuvant HAI 5-FU/LV compared to observation was 44.8 versus 23.3 months and 20 versus 12.6 months, respectively [19].

Another prospective, European trial randomized resected patients intraoperatively to receive locoregional immunochemotherapy plus systemic chemotherapy with mitomycin, FU, and IL-2 compared to systemic chemotherapy alone. The 5-year survival favored combination therapy, with a 5-year survival of 73% in the HAI plus systemic group versus 60% in the systemic chemotherapy group [18].

A French retrospective comparative study published in 2013 by Goere et al. compared patients with colorectal liver metastases post liver resection who were treated adjuvantly with either HAI oxaliplatin therapy plus systemic 5-FU versus systemic chemotherapy alone. A total of 98 patients with resected colorectal liver metastases were included in this study, of whom 44 underwent HAI therapy with oxaliplatin plus systemic 5-FU and 54 patients underwent modern chemotherapy regimens as the control arm. After 3 years of follow-up, a slight benefit was seen in overall survival for the intervention group (HAI), but this did not reach statistical significance (75% vs 62%, $p = 0.17$). The 3-year disease-free survival was significantly better in favor of HAI therapy (33% vs 5%, $p < 0.001$). This study reports both HAI adjuvant therapy and R0 resection as independent predictive factors for prolonged disease-free survival in multivariate analysis [20].

Upon entering a new phase of modern chemotherapy with increased use of oxaliplatin and irinotecan in addition to 5-FU, it was crucial to study HAI in conjunction with these new agents for safety and efficacy mainly through phase II studies. The first phase I/II study published in 2003 showed a maximum tolerated FUDR dose of 0.12 mg/kg and as a secondary endpoint a 2-year survival rate of 89% for 96 patients who underwent systemic chemotherapy with irinotecan and 5-FU and HAI FUDR [21]. A second phase I trial of 35 patients tested systemic chemotherapy with oxaliplatin, 5-FU, and LV in combination with HAI FUDR and demonstrated a maximum tolerated dose of 85 mg/m^2 and as a secondary outcome a 4-year survival of 88% and progression-free survival of 50% [22]. A phase II study from the Mayo Clinic also investigated the efficacy of HAI FUDR therapy in alternation with CAPOX (systemic capecitabine plus oxaliplatin) in 55 patients. A caveat of this study is that both patients who had undergone resection or cryoablation were eligible to enter the study. Overall survival of this study at 2 years was 85% with a disease-free survival of 59.7% [23].

Evaluating the use of monoclonal antibodies (namely, bevacizumab) was the next logical step in clinical trial work which combined adjuvant systemic therapy and HAI treatment. A randomized phase II trial enrolled a total of 73 patients who were randomized to either HAI (FUDR-DEX) plus FOLFOX or FOLFIRI with bevacizumab as the intervention arm or without the VEGF antibody as the control arm. Thirty-five patients were randomized to the bevacizumab group and thirty-eight patients to the control arm. This was a negative trial. The addition of bevacizumab did not improve either overall survival or disease-free survival and actually increased biliary toxicity in the intervention arm. With a median follow-up of 30 months, the 4-year survival for the no bevacizumab and bevacizumab arms were 85% and 81%, respectively ($P = 0.5$), and 4-year recurrence-free survival (RFS) was 46% versus 37% [24].

Other studies also demonstrated high toxicity rates with the combination of bevacizumab and HAI therapy. An analysis including 203 patients from 3 separate prospective studies evaluating HAI FUDR plus bevacizumab demonstrated a consistent increase in the incidence of hyperbilirubinemia and biliary toxicity with increased stent placement required across all 3 studies. Also, the addition of bevacizumab did not seem to be associated with improved progression-free or overall survival in any of these three studies [25].

A large historical retrospective study from Memorial Sloan Kettering analyzed HAI in the adjuvant setting comparing patients treated on four separate treatment adjuvant protocols between 1991 and 2009. The study group was subdivided into those patients treated prior to the year 2003 versus those treated after 2003, mirroring the changes in the modern systemic chemotherapy employed. Results showed a significant increase in overall survival with 10-year survivals of 61% for the post 2003 group versus 40% for the group resected between 1991 and 2003, respectively. This study depicts more clearly the benefit of modern chemotherapy as well as improvements in surgical technique, with a statistical difference both in 3-year and 5-year survival analyses. The difference in the 3-year and 5-year overall survival between the two patient groups (before 2003 or after 2003) was 73% and 92% versus 56% and 78% ($p < 0.01$), respectively [26].

A recently published propensity score analysis of 2368 patients who had undergone liver resection for colorectal metastases was also performed at Memorial Sloan Kettering. Patients were treated with adjuvant hepatic arterial infusion or systemic chemotherapy. Patients were matched for seven prognostic factors in order to assure comparability between groups. Despite having a higher disease burden, the HAI group had a longer median survival of 67 months versus 44 months for those treated with HAI post liver resection versus systemic chemotherapy alone. The overall survival hazard ratio for patients who underwent HAI compared to those who did not receive was 0.67 (95% CI 0.59–0.76, $p > 0.01$) [27].

Treatment of Unresectable Liver Metastases (TULM) and Resectability Conversion Rates

In a scenario where colorectal liver metastases are considered unresectable, multiple studies have demonstrated that hepatic arterial infusion is a feasible, safe, and effective treatment. This strategy coupled with systemic chemotherapy makes it possible to convert patients to resectability in 3.3–37% of cases [28–32].

With improvements in modern systemic chemotherapy, coupled with contemporary use of novel biological and immunological agents, the prognosis of patients with metastatic colorectal cancer has dramatically improved. A recent systematic review including 10 observational studies with a total of 1886 patients showed that in patients who were initially deemed unresectable, an objective response was observed in 64% (range 43–79%) of patients and 14.4% of cases were converted to resectability following a course of systemic chemotherapy. The median overall survival was 45 months (range 36–60), with 19% of patients alive and recurrence-free [33].

The use of hepatic arterial infusion in this context might increase the ability to get to resection. When patients are treated with HAI FUDR as a first-line intervention, several randomized studies have shown that patients with unresectable colorectal liver metastases have two- to fourfold higher response rates compared to systemic 5-FU [34–36]. Ensuing phase I/II studies have shown response rates greater than 64% in chemotherapy-naive patients who were treated with combined HAI and modern systemic chemotherapy and response rates of 74–85% for previously treated patients with liver metastatic colorectal cancer.

A phase I study from the Memorial Sloan Kettering Cancer Center enrolled 49 patients with unresectable colorectal liver metastases to receive HAI FUDR/dexamethasone plus systemic chemotherapy with oxaliplatin and irinotecan. Fifty-three percent of patients had been previously treated with chemotherapy. The study indicated a high response rate of 92% with a 47% conversion to resectability. These results were especially more pronounced in chemo-naive patients, with a 57% rate of conversion. Median survival for patients who had previously undergone chemotherapy was 35 months versus 50.8 months for chemo-naive group [37].

A French retrospective study assessed 87 patients with unresectable colorectal liver metastases, 79% of whom had received prior systemic chemotherapy, who were then treated with HAI -oxaliplatin plus systemic 5-FU. Twenty-four percent of patients were converted to resectability. Five-year overall survival was 56% in the converted group, while none of the non-operated patients actually survived 5 years ($p < 0.001$). Median overall survival for the operated cohort was 41.9 months [38].

A second multicentric study from France also assessed this combination of HAI oxaliplatin with systemic 5-FU chemotherapy, with an objective response rate of 64% (95% CI 44–81%; 18 of 28 patients) and a conversion rate of 18% in patients with initially unresectable colorectal liver metastases [39].

A retrospective study evaluated the efficacy and toxicity of HAI oxaliplatin compared to intravenous oxaliplatin in patients with initially unresectable colorectal liver metastases who subsequently were converted to liver resection. In this study, the hepatic arterial route of administration was associated with significantly higher rates of complete pathological response and increased overall survival compared to intravenous oxaliplatin. However, there was increased toxicity with severe oxaliplatin-related pathologic lesions within the normal noncancerous liver parenchyma. Biliary sinusoidal obstruction and regenerative nodular hyperplasia were both seen in a greater percentage of patients undergoing HAI therapy. Patients in this study who underwent HAI oxaliplatin were observed to have a threefold increase in lesions related to the drug use. Despite the increased toxicity, data from this study did not indicate a lower overall survival attributable to oxaliplatin-related adverse events [40].

A single-institution phase II study of HAI FUDR plus systemic therapy enrolled 49 patients with unresectable colorectal liver metastases with conversion to resection as its primary outcome. An important characteristic of this study was the fact that 65% of the patient population were heavily pretreated. The trial initially also includes treatment with bevacizumab. A high biliary toxicity rate was found, in the first 24 patients whose treatment included bevacizumab. The remaining 25 patients were treated without bevacizumab. Around 10% of patients had complete responses, and the overall response rate was 76%. Conversion to resection was reached in 47% of study population, at a median of 6 months from treatment initiation. Secondary outcomes reported a median overall survival of 38 months and median progression-free survival of 13 months. Bevacizumab administration did not impact outcome. On multivariate analysis, results showed that the only variable of the regression model that could significantly predict prolonged overall survival and progression-free survival was conversion to resection [41].

The use of HAI plus systemic chemotherapy in relation to a patient's KRAS mutational status has also been reported. A phase II multicenter European study enrolled wild-type KRAS patients with unresectable colorectal liver metastases, who had previously progressed on 1–3 lines of systemic chemotherapy. Extrahepatic disease was documented in 40.6% of the patients. The primary endpoint of this study was R0–R1 hepatectomy, posttreatment with one to three HAI and systemic chemotherapy protocols. Systemic cetuximab was used in conjunction with a triplet HAI treatment regimen including a combination of 5-FU, oxaliplatin, and irinotecan. The rate of liver resection was 29.7%. Median overall survival was 25.7 months, and progression-free survival was 9.3 months. Those with R0–R1 hepatectomy had a median OS of 35.2 months (32.6–37.8), with 37.4% (23.6–51.2) alive at 4 years [42].

Conclusion

Approximately 50% of colorectal cancer deaths are due to liver metastases. Surgery remains the optimal therapeutic approach for colorectal liver metastases and confers the best outcomes. However, nearly 70% of these patients develop recurrent disease after hepatic resection, usually within 2 years, and 30–50% develop isolated liver metastases [43, 44].

Adjuvant locoregional therapy with HAI can target any residual micrometastatic hepatic disease, in conjunction with systemic therapy to reduce systemic recurrence. Several randomized studies as outlined above have compared HAI plus systemic therapy versus systemic therapy alone and show that this is a safe and effective treatment option, with a clear survival advantage. Three of four randomized trials comparing HAI and systemic chemotherapy versus systemic chemotherapy alone or control showed a significant increase in disease-free survival and hepatic disease-free survival [11, 16–18].

Large retrospective series of HAI therapy have also confirmed a benefit for adjuvant treatment [45, 46]. A new review of data from the Memorial Sloan Kettering Cancer Center experience demonstrated a 5-year overall survival rate of 78% for this combination approach of HAI and systemic therapy when used in the adjuvant setting following liver resection in patients treated after 2003 [26].

Floxuridine (FUDR) is not available worldwide. Many European-based studies offer compelling data to employ oxaliplatin as an alternative to FUDR. The potential benefit of adding systemic, anti-EGFR-based monoclonal antibodies for those with KRAS wild-type disease to HAI and combination systemic chemotherapy remains unanswered.

Hepatic arterial infusion therapy has been studied for decades, with significant evidence supporting its role in the management of colorectal liver metastases, but yet has not been universally embraced to date. It requires specialized expertise across the multidisciplinary team to facilitate HAI pump insertion, administration of therapy, and careful patient monitoring and management of side effects.

The management of colorectal cancer liver metastases continues to evolve with a number of liver-directed therapeutic options now existing beyond systemic chemotherapy as adjunctive therapy to surgery. The evidence to date indicates that HAI with systemic chemotherapy is a reasonable treatment option in select patients with oligometastatic disease to the liver in order to achieve improved outcomes.

References

1. Siegel RL, Miller KD, Jemal A. Cancer statistics, 2018. CA Cancer J Clin. 2018;68(1):7–30.
2. Helling TS, Martin M. Cause of death from liver metastases in colorectal cancer. Ann Surg Oncol. 2014;21(2):501–6.
3. Al-Asfoor A, Fedorowicz Z, Lodge M. Resection versus no intervention or other surgical interventions for colorectal cancer liver metastases. Cochrane Database Syst Rev. 2008;(2):CD006039.

4. Fong Y, Fortner J, Sun RL, Brennan MF, Blumgart LH. Clinical score for predicting recurrence after hepatic resection for metastatic colorectal cancer: analysis of 1001 consecutive cases. Ann Surg. 1999;230:309–18; discussion 18–21.
5. Poston GJ, Figueras J, Giuliante F, et al. Urgent need for a new staging system in advanced colorectal cancer. J Clin Oncol. 2008;26:4828–33.
6. Sullivan RD, Norcross JW, Watkins E Jr. Chemotherapy of metastatic liver cancer by prolonged hepatic-artery infusion. N Engl J Med. 1964;270:321–7.
7. Breedis C, Young G. The blood supply of neoplasms in the liver. Am J Pathol. 1954;30(5):969–77.
8. Ensminger WD, Rosowsky A, Raso V, et al. A clinical-pharmacological evaluation of hepatic arterial infusions of 5-fluoro-2′-deoxyuridine and 5-fluorouracil. Cancer Res. 1978;38:3784–92.
9. Ensminger WD, Gyves JW. Clinical pharmacology of hepatic arterial chemotherapy. Semin Oncol. 1983;10:176–82.
10. Weiss L, Grundmann E, Torhorst J, et al. Haematogenous metastatic patterns in colonic carcinoma: an analysis of 1541 necropsies. J Pathol. 1986;150(3):195–203.
11. Kemeny MM, Adak S, Gray B, et al. Combined-modality treatment for resectable metastatic colorectal carcinoma to the liver: surgical resection of hepatic metastases in combination with continuous infusion of chemotherapy--an intergroup study. J Clin Oncol. 2002;20:1499–505.
12. Kemeny N, Seiter K, Niedzwiecki D, et al. A randomized trial of intrahepatic infusion of fluorodeoxyuridine with dexamethasone versus fluorodeoxyuridine alone in the treatment of metastatic colorectal cancer. Cancer. 1992;69:327–34.
13. Karanicolas PJ, Ko YJ. Hepatic arterial infusion for unresectable liver metastases from colorectal cancer: the dawn of a new era? Ann Surg Oncol. 2017;24:6–7.
14. Dhir M, Jones HL, Shuai Y, et al. Hepatic arterial infusion in combination with modern systemic chemotherapy is associated with improved survival compared with modern systemic chemotherapy alone in patients with isolated unresectable colorectal liver metastases: a case-control study. Ann Surg Oncol. 2017;24:150–8.
15. Ye LC, Liu TS, Ren L, et al. Randomized controlled trial of cetuximab plus chemotherapy for patients with KRAS wild-type unresectable colorectal liver limited metastases. J Clin Oncol. 2013;31:1931–8.
16. Kemeny N, Huang Y, Cohen AM, et al. Hepatic arterial infusion of chemotherapy after resection of hepatic metastases from colorectal cancer. N Engl J Med. 1999;341:2039–48.
17. Kemeny NE, Gonen M. Hepatic arterial infusion after liver resection. N Engl J Med. 2005;352:734–5.
18. Lygidakis NJ, Sgourakis G, Vlachos L, et al. Metastatic liver disease of colorectal origin: the value of locoregional immunochemotherapy combined with systemic chemotherapy following liver resection. Results of a prospective randomized study. Hepato-Gastroenterology. 2001;48:1685–91.
19. Lorenz M, Muller HH, Schramm H, et al. Randomized trial of surgery versus surgery followed by adjuvant hepatic arterial infusion with 5-fluorouracil and folinic acid for liver metastases of colorectal cancer. German Cooperative on Liver Metastases (Arbeitsgruppe Lebermetastasen). Ann Surg. 1998;228:756–62.
20. Goere D, Benhaim L, Bonnet S, et al. Adjuvant chemotherapy after resection of colorectal liver metastases in patients at high risk of hepatic recurrence: a comparative study between hepatic arterial infusion of oxaliplatin and modern systemic chemotherapy. Ann Surg. 2013;257:114–20.
21. Kemeny N, Jarnagin W, Gonen M, et al. Phase I/II study of hepatic arterial therapy with floxuridine and dexamethasone in combination with intravenous irinotecan as adjuvant treatment after resection of hepatic metastases from colorectal cancer. J Clin Oncol. 2003;21:3303–9.
22. Kemeny N, Capanu M, D'Angelica M, et al. Phase I trial of adjuvant hepatic arterial infusion (HAI) with floxuridine (FUDR) and dexamethasone plus systemic oxaliplatin, 5-fluorouracil and leucovorin in patients with resected liver metastases from colorectal cancer. Ann Oncol. 2009;20:1236–41.

23. Alberts SR, Roh MS, Mahoney MR, et al. Alternating systemic and hepatic artery infusion therapy for resected liver metastases from colorectal cancer: a North Central Cancer Treatment Group (NCCTG)/National Surgical Adjuvant Breast and Bowel Project (NSABP) phase II intergroup trial, N9945/CI-66. J Clin Oncol. 2010;28:853–8.
24. Kemeny NE, Jarnagin WR, Capanu M, et al. Randomized phase II trial of adjuvant hepatic arterial infusion and systemic chemotherapy with or without bevacizumab in patients with resected hepatic metastases from colorectal cancer. J Clin Oncol. 2011;29:884–9.
25. Cercek A, D'Angelica M, Power D, et al. Floxuridine hepatic arterial infusion associated biliary toxicity is increased by concurrent administration of systemic bevacizumab. Ann Surg Oncol. 2014;21:479–86.
26. Kemeny NE, Chou JF, Boucher TM, et al. Updated long-term survival for patients with metastatic colorectal cancer treated with liver resection followed by hepatic arterial infusion and systemic chemotherapy. J Surg Oncol. 2016;113:477–84.
27. Groot Koerkamp B, Sadot E, Kemeny NE, et al. Perioperative hepatic arterial infusion pump chemotherapy is associated with longer survival after resection of colorectal liver metastases: a propensity score analysis. J Clin Oncol. 2017;35(17):1938–44.
28. Beppu T, Hayashi N, Masuda T, et al. FOLFOX enables high resectability and excellent prognosis for initially unresectable colorectal liver metastases. Anticancer Res. 2010;30:1015–20.
29. Adam R, Delvart V, Pascal G, et al. Rescue surgery for unresectable colorectal liver metastases downstaged by chemotherapy: a model to predict long-term survival. Ann Surg. 2004;240:644–57; discussion 57–8.
30. Delaunoit T, Alberts SR, Sargent DJ, et al. Chemotherapy permits resection of metastatic colorectal cancer: experience from Intergroup N9741. Ann Oncol. 2005;16:425–9.
31. Pozzo C, Basso M, Cassano A, et al. Neoadjuvant treatment of unresectable liver disease with irinotecan and 5-fluorouracil plus folinic acid in colorectal cancer patients. Ann Oncol. 2004;15:933–9.
32. Falcone A, Ricci S, Brunetti I, et al. Phase III trial of infusional fluorouracil, leucovorin, oxaliplatin, and irinotecan (FOLFOXIRI) compared with infusional fluorouracil, leucovorin, and irinotecan (FOLFIRI) as first-line treatment for metastatic colorectal cancer: the Gruppo Oncologico Nord Ovest. J Clin Oncol. 2007;25:1670–6.
33. Lam VW, Spiro C, Laurence JM, et al. A systematic review of clinical response and survival outcomes of downsizing systemic chemotherapy and rescue liver surgery in patients with initially unresectable colorectal liver metastases. Ann Surg Oncol. 2012;19:1292–301.
34. Kemeny NE, Niedzwiecki D, Hollis DR, et al. Hepatic arterial infusion versus systemic therapy for hepatic metastases from colorectal cancer: a randomized trial of efficacy, quality of life, and molecular markers (CALGB 9481). J Clin Oncol. 2006;24:1395–403.
35. Rougier P, Laplanche A, Huguier M, et al. Hepatic arterial infusion of floxuridine in patients with liver metastases from colorectal carcinoma: long term results of a prospective randomized trial. J Clin Oncol. 1992;10:1112–8.
36. Hohn DC, Stagg RJ, Friedman MA, et al. A randomized trial of continuous intravenous versus hepatic intraarterial floxuridine in patients with colorectal cancer metastatic to the liver: the Northern California Oncology Group trial. J Clin Oncol. 1989;7:1646–54.
37. Kemeny NE, Melendez FD, Capanu M, et al. Conversion to resectability using hepatic artery infusion plus systemic chemotherapy for the treatment of unresectable liver metastases from colorectal carcinoma. J Clin Oncol. 2009;27:3465–71.
38. Goere D, Deshaies I, de Baere T, et al. Prolonged survival of initially unresectable hepatic colorectal cancer patients treated with hepatic arterial infusion of oxaliplatin followed by radical surgery of metastases. Ann Surg. 2010;251:686–91.
39. Ducreux M, Ychou M, Laplanche A, et al. Hepatic arterial oxaliplatin infusion plus intravenous chemotherapy in colorectal cancer with inoperable hepatic metastases: a trial of the gastrointestinal group of the Federation Nationale des Centres de Lutte Contre le Cancer. J Clin Oncol. 2005;23:4881–7.

40. Allard MA, Sebagh M, Baillie G, et al. Comparison of complete pathologic response and hepatic injuries between hepatic arterial infusion and systemic administration of oxaliplatin in patients with colorectal liver metastases. Ann Surg Oncol. 2015;22(6):1925–32.
41. D'Angelica MI, Correa-Gallego C, Paty PB, et al. Phase II trial of hepatic artery infusional and systemic chemotherapy for patients with unresectable hepatic metastases from colorectal cancer: conversion to resection and long term outcomes. Ann Surg. 2015;261:353–60.
42. Levi FA, Boige V, Hebbar M, et al. Conversion to resection of liver metastases from colorectal cancer with hepatic artery infusion of combined chemotherapy and systemic cetuximab in multicenter trial OPTILIV. Ann Oncol. 2016;27:267–74.
43. Muratore A, Polastri R, Bouzari H, et al. Repeat hepatectomy for colorectal liver metastases: a worthwhile operation? J Surg Oncol. 2001;76(2):127–32.
44. Topal B, Kaufman L, Aerts R, et al. Patterns of failure following curative resection of colorectal liver metastases. Eur J Surg Oncol. 2003;29(3):248–53.
45. Tomlinson JS, Jarnagin WR, DeMatteo RP, et al. Actual 10-year survival after resection of colorectal liver metastases defines cure. J Clin Oncol. 2007;25:4575–80.
46. Ito H, Are C, Gonen M, et al. Effect of postoperative morbidity on long-term survival after hepatic resection for metastatic colorectal cancer. Ann Surg. 2008;247:994–1002.
47. Kern W, Beckert B, Lang N, et al. Phase I and pharmacokinetic study of hepatic arterial infusion with oxaliplatin in combination with folinic acid and 5-fluorouracil in patients with hepatic metastases from colorectal cancer. Ann Oncol. 2001;12:599–603.
48. Mancuso A, Giuliani R, Accettura C, et al. Hepatic arterial continuous infusion (HACI) of oxaliplatin in patients with unresectable liver metastases from colorectal cancer. Anticancer Res. 2003;23:1917–22.
49. Fiorentini G, Rossi S, Dentico P, et al. Oxaliplatin hepatic arterial infusion chemotherapy for hepatic metastases from colorectal cancer: a phase I–II clinical study. Anticancer Res. 2004;24:2093–6.
50. Boige V, Malka D, Elias D, et al. Hepatic arterial infusion of oxaliplatin and intravenous LV5FU2 in unresectable liver metastases from colorectal cancer after systemic chemotherapy failure. Ann Surg Oncol. 2008;15:219–26.
51. Del Freo A, Fiorentini G, Sanguinetti F, et al. Hepatic arterial chemotherapy with oxaliplatin, folinic acid and 5-fluorouracil in pre-treated patients with liver metastases from colorectal cancer. In Vivo. 2006;20:743–6.
52. Bouchahda M, Adam R, Giacchetti S, et al. Rescue chemotherapy using multidrug chronomodulated hepatic arterial infusion for patients with heavily pretreated metastatic colorectal cancer. Cancer. 2009;115:4990–9.
53. Guan M, Chen S-C, Ying H-Y, et al. Folfox4 regimen administered through combined hepatic arterial and systemic infusion for treatment of colorectal cancer with unresectable liver metastases. Chin Med J. 2012;125:3640–5.
54. Lim A, Le Sourd S, Senellart H, et al. Hepatic arterial infusion chemotherapy for unresectable liver metastases of colorectal cancer: a multicenter retrospective study. Clin Colorectal Cancer. 2017;16(4):308–15.

Sequencing of Systemic Chemotherapy for Unresectable CRLM

23

Marc T. Roth and Laura W. Goff

First-Line Chemotherapy

Four main cytotoxic agents are available to serve as backbones or in combination with one another. Fluoropyridines are the most common backbone and typically used with another agent as described later. Fluorouracil (5-FU) [1] has been used in gastrointestinal malignancies for many years, dating back to the 1950s. Common side effects include mucositis, anorexia, cytopenias, alopecia, and dermatologic reactions. Capecitabine [2] is an oral prodrug of 5-FU that is converted to the active antimetabolite and was made available in the 1990s. The most common side effects include gastrointestinal upset, cytopenias, and dermatologic reactions. Both 5-FU and capecitabine are pyrimidine analogs that work through inhibition of thymidylate synthetase. Oxaliplatin [3] is a platinum-based drug that inhibits cell division by cross-linking DNA. Side effects include neuropathy, gastrointestinal upset, and cytopenias. Finally, irinotecan [4] is a topoisomerase inhibitor that works through inhibition of DNA replication. Common side effects include gastrointestinal upset, alopecia, fever, and cytopenias. First-line treatment heavily influences the sequence of latter lines, and for this reason, more emphasis will be placed on this section.

Cytotoxic Regimens

The four drugs described above first showed promise as monotherapy but, in the modern era, most often are used in combination with other agents to increase the resection rate or, in our case, prolong survival, response rate, and quality of life. Choice of first-line regimen is dependent on patient characteristics, and those with

M. T. Roth · L. W. Goff (✉)
Vanderbilt University Medical Center, Nashville, TN, USA
e-mail: marc.roth@vumc.org; laura.goff@vumc.org

M. M. Correia et al. (eds.), *Colorectal Cancer Liver Metastases*,
https://doi.org/10.1007/978-3-030-25486-5_23

a good performance status and few limiting comorbidities should be considered for intensive upfront therapy. A number of drug pairs have been studied.

FOLFOX (folinic acid (LV) [5], 5-FU, oxaliplatin) was shown to offer improved progression-free survival (PFS) over 5-FU alone [6, 7]. The combination resulted in higher toxicities, but importantly, quality of life was not found to be impaired. Around the same time, FOLFIRI (folinic acid, 5-FU, irinotecan) was being investigated, and both OS and PFS were significantly improved compared to 5-FU alone [8, 9]. Once capecitabine was introduced and had shown acceptable safety and efficacy [10], it was used in combination with oxaliplatin in the regimen XELOX (Xeloda® [capecitabine], oxaliplatin).[1]

In pursuit of a superior cytotoxic doublet, these regimens were compared head to head in several large, randomized controlled trials (RCTs). FOLFIRI and FOLFOX were shown to have generally similar effects on response rate, time to progression, and overall survival, only differing in their toxicity profiles. Irinotecan caused a higher incidence of alopecia and gastrointestinal toxicity, whereas oxaliplatin caused more neuropathy and thrombocytopenia, as expected [11, 12]. XELOX and FOLFOX were also compared in a non-inferiority trial and were similar in outcomes [13].

The push for better resection and survival rates resulted in the comparison of FOLFIRI with the combination of all available agents in an upfront regimen called FOLFOXIRI (folinic acid, 5-FU, oxaliplatin, irinotecan). This high-intensity regimen is, in theory, the only way to guarantee exposure of all available cytotoxic agents during the disease course. FOLFOXIRI failed to demonstrate a statistically significant difference in overall survival [14] (although it resulted in one of the longest reported in literature), but did show a higher response rate and R0 resection rate in the neoadjuvant setting [15]. The additional cytotoxic agent did come with increased toxicities with a higher incidence of alopecia, diarrhea, and neuropathy. This regimen is typically used in patients with a good performance status when the goal is to downstage to resection in pursuit of cure.

All regimens discussed above are generally regarded as equivalent in efficacy, and choice of backbone agent and intensity depends on toxicity profile and patient comorbidities. For example, oxaliplatin should be used with caution in those with baseline neuropathy or those in whom it develops during treatment. Similarly, an elevated bilirubin and patients with inherited disorders of bilirubin metabolism may require a dose reduction with irinotecan or an alternative agent altogether. If neither irinotecan nor oxaliplatin can be used, fluoropyrimidine monotherapy is an acceptable treatment alternative with the understanding that it is not as intensive. These patients should be evaluated for additional agent candidacy should their comorbidities improve if it aligns with their goals of care.

[1] Other combinations were investigated (IROX, IFL), but are not as commonly used as first line and therefore will not be covered in this chapter. Of note, capecitabine combinations with irinotecan have led to excessive toxicity and are not recommended.

Duration and Sequence

Many derivations of regimen length and order have been investigated and are worthy of mention as they represent core concepts in the treatment of neoplasias.

Continuous vs Intermittent The MRC COIN trial [16] compared continuous fluoropyrimidine and oxaliplatin regimens to an intermittent schedule. Patients in the latter group were given a pre-planned treatment holiday if no progressive disease (PD) was discovered after 12 weeks, but once it occurred, the same first-line regimen was resumed. Median overall survival did not appear to be different between the two groups, and the intermittent cohort saw a decrease in side effects and improved quality of life (results supported by the GISCAD study [17]). It is important to note, however, that this trial did not demonstrate non-inferiority and that maintenance therapy is recommended by most major guidelines (see section "Maintenance Therapy").

Combination vs Sequential Two large, well-known trials (MRC FOCUS [18] and CAIRO [19]) investigated whether overall survival was influenced by the order and timing of drugs received. Both trials included a single-agent fluoropyrimidine arm that transitioned to irinotecan after PD (sequential arm). The other cohort started with either a fluoropyrimidine + oxaliplatin or a fluoropyrimidine + irinotecan and transitioned to the alternate doublet (combination arm) after disease progression. Generally, neither study found that the upfront combination improved OS significantly over the sequential arm. In addition, toxicity was unsurprisingly higher in the combination group. However, although there are many analyses of these studies and others with similar aims, they do suggest that survival improves when all available cytotoxic agents are made available.

To investigate this, one meta-analysis of phase III trials calculated the survival of patients based on the number of agents they received over the course of their disease [20]. Overall survival was shown to improve significantly if all three classes of cytotoxic agents were received and if combination protocols over monotherapy were provided in the first-line setting. For this reason, it is imperative that all agents are offered to the patient provided there are no contraindications.

Biologic Agents in the First-Line Setting

The addition of antibody therapy to the armamentarium of systemic agents has revolutionized the treatment of neoplasia and allowed for more personalized treatment based on specific molecular characteristics of a given tumor. Bevacizumab [21] is a monoclonal antibody that inhibits vascular endothelial growth factor A (VEGF-A), slowing the growth of new blood vessels. It was the first inhibitor of angiogenesis available in the USA. Side effects include hypertension, cytopenias, dermatologic manifestations, venous thromboembolism, increased infection risk, and impaired wound healing, which thus must be timed appropriately in those who may undergo resection. Cetuximab [22] is a chimeric monoclonal antibody that inhibits epidermal growth factor receptor (EGFR). Panitumumab [23] is similar to cetuximab in that it targets EGFR but differs in that it is an IgG2 fully human monoclonal antibody. Both EGFR inhibitors can cause severe dermatologic manifestations, gastrointestinal upset, and decreased magnesium levels. Of note, development of skin toxicity is associated with an improvement in PFS and OS [24].

Intensive Treatment with Bevacizumab

Bevacizumab has shown safety and efficacy in combination with all first-line chemotherapy doublets [25, 26]. In a recent meta-analysis of 9 trials and nearly 4000 patients, the addition of VEGF inhibition to standard first-line cytotoxic chemotherapy resulted in a statistically significant increase in response rate, progression-free survival, and overall survival [27]. Of note, adverse events in the bevacizumab group included higher rates of hypertension, proteinuria, gastrointestinal perforation, bleeding, and thromboembolic events. Comparisons have been made between standard first-line doublets in search of a superior regimen, but survival statistics appear similar [28, 29].

FOLFOXIRI plus bevacizumab has been investigated with increasing frequency in recent years due to its potential for downstaging unresectable disease in liver-only metastases. The OLIVIA trial provided safety and efficacy data for the regimen and saw an increase in resection rates and progression-free survival [30], with only modest increases in grade 3–5 adverse events compared to the triplet alone. It should be noted that although FOLFOXIRI + bevacizumab is a first-line option for untreated metastatic colorectal cancer, there is limited data from large, phase III RCTs for the combination, although some trials are currently underway [31]. Pooled results from a systematic review, however, report that the regimen is associated with improved overall response rate and a resection rate of nearly 40% for disease initially considered unresectable at diagnosis [32].

Intensive Treatment with EGFR Inhibitors

Use of the EGFR inhibitors corresponded to an era of increased utilization of molecular testing of tumor tissue, and many studies evaluating their use underwent subgroup analyses based on *KRAS* (an oncogene) mutation status given the significant correlations found. For this reason, information provided in this section will focus on utilization based on *KRAS* subtype.

The use of cetuximab with all first-line doublet regimens has demonstrated safety and efficacy [33, 34] and shown a promise with increased resection rates in synchronous disease [35]. Early studies found an increase in progression-free survival and response rate in combination with oxaliplatin- and irinotecan-containing regimens, but failed to show overall survival benefit [36, 37]. After separation of *KRAS* wild-type (wt) and mutant genotypes, wild-type disease did exhibit an improvement in survival over cytotoxic therapy alone [38]. Panitumumab was shown to be safe [39] and demonstrated similar results in phase III trials with first-line doublet regimens [40].

Importantly, a subgroup analysis of the OPUS trial comparing FOLFOX with and without cetuximab regardless of *KRAS* status saw no benefit and potentially detrimental effects in *RAS* mutants (both *KRAS* and *NRAS*) [41]. Similarly, panitumumab was associated with decreased progression-free and overall survival in this population [42]. For this reason, anti-EGFR antibody therapy is only recommended for *RAS* wt patients by major published guidelines [43, 44].

FOLFOXIRI and cetuximab have been investigated in a recent phase II trial and resulted in a high surgical resection rate similar to triplet therapy plus bevacizumab [45], but data from large, phase III trials is yet to be published on its use in this setting.

Comparing Biologic Agents

Many initial studies suggested a benefit to early EGFR inhibition in patients whose tumor was *KRAS* wt [48, 49]. A meta-analysis of major head-to-head trials evaluating EGFR and VEGF inhibitors combined with chemotherapy in the first-line setting favored EGFR inhibition in terms of overall survival and response rate [46]. Subsequently, however, data from the large, prospective phase III trial CALGB/SWOG 80405 comparing first-line bevacizumab to cetuximab when added to combination chemotherapy in *KRAS* wt patients did not demonstrate a difference in overall survival [47].

Combining Biologic Agents

The drive for improvement in outcomes led to the combination of bevacizumab and EGFR inhibitors (both cetuximab and panitumumab) [50, 51]. Surprisingly, the combination was associated with a significant decrease in PFS, and quality of life scores were lower. Given the increased incidence in adverse outcomes, combination biologic treatment is not recommended [43, 44].

Non-intensive Treatment

In the elderly and those unsuitable for irinotecan or oxaliplatin, treatment with fluoropyrimidine monotherapy may be appropriate. Addition of VEGF and EGFR inhibition was shown to be safe in this population [52, 53], and an improvement in progression-free survival was seen with bevacizumab [54]. As the population grows older, accurately evaluating patients for therapy candidacy has become crucial. New screening tools and risk assessments are being studied to assist in the decision-making process [55] but are beyond the scope of this chapter.

Given the lesser side effect profile of these biologic agents compared to traditional cytotoxic chemotherapy, they have found use in the elderly population as monotherapy when candidacy for a more intensive regimen is lacking [56].

Special Considerations

As we acquire more information about tumor biology, it has become apparent that an individualized approach must be used to treat patients effectively. Tumor genetics and sidedness are being heavily studied insofar as how they relate to prognosis and response to available therapies.

Role of Extended Mutational Testing

As described above, *KRAS* mutation status influences the efficacy of anti-EGFR therapy. *KRAS* mutations in exon 2 have been well described, but further studies have shown that even if this gene is wild type, mutations in other *KRAS* and *NRAS* genes are common and can be detected with extended *RAS* testing [57]. A systematic review and meta-analysis of 9 RCTs and nearly 6000 patients revealed that there was no progression-free or overall survival benefit in patients with any *RAS* mutation with EGFR inhibition [58], and as such, the American Society of Clinical Oncology (ASCO) released a provisional clinical opinion update recommending anti-EGFR therapy only after extended *RAS* testing has demonstrated wild-type disease [59].

An emerging marker with prognostic and potential therapeutic implications is *BRAF V600E*. Studies have consistently demonstrated its negative impact on prognosis [42], but its implication in treatment is less clear. *BRAF*-mutant inhibitors have been developed, and clinical trials are currently underway.

Microsatellite instability (MSI) and mismatch repair deficiency (dMMR) are hallmarks of cancer and seen in colorectal malignancies. Pembrolizumab [60] is a humanized antibody that targets the programmed cell death-1 (PD-1) receptor and was initially approved to treat melanomas but has found clinical success in other malignancies. Its use has been described in colorectal cancer, with impressive response rates and progression-free survival in tumors where MSI burden is high and dMMR is present [61]. Nivolumab [62] is a human monoclonal antibody that targets PD-1 and is currently under investigation in the same setting [63]. These treatments are only recommended in the first-line setting when patients are not appropriate for intensive therapy, but are appropriate for later lines after failure of standard induction regimens [43].

Sidedness

Much attention has been paid to tumor "sidedness" in recent trials, referring to the side of origin of the primary tumor. The colon originates from different embryologic tissue: right side from the midgut and left side from the hindgut. Additionally, bacterial flora is variable throughout the length of the colon [64]. These and other variants yield tumors of differing molecular composition depending on the location. Right-sided tumors tend to be MSI-high and have higher rates of *BRAF* and *PI3KCA* mutations, as well as a higher mutational burden overall when compared to tumors originating on the left side [65].

Many large RCTs have performed retrospective subgroup analyses with primary tumor location (PTL) in mind, and systemic reviews have merged this data. One such review found that right-sided malignancies fared worse than left-sided [66]. Left-sided *RAS* wt tumors saw increased response rates and overall survival benefit (but not PFS) with anti-EGFR therapy compared to the same with bevacizumab. Right-sided tumors, on the other hand, saw a significant increase in progression-free survival with VEGF inhibition when added to standard of care, although survival was worse overall. Other reviews have shown comparable results of EGFR and VEGF inhibition regardless of PTL [67], making clear associations from clinical trials more difficult. Although the data are intriguing, little is available from prospective trials taking primary tumor location in account, and guidelines have not yet recommended making treatment decisions based on this tumor characteristic.

Maintenance Therapy

Maintenance therapy refers to less intensive treatment, usually a single agent of the initial regimen with or without a biologic agent, after standard induction chemotherapy is completed in an effort to delay disease progression and lower treatment-associated toxicity. Study results are mixed, and the determination of appropriate candidates for de-escalation therapy is not well-established, but major guidelines suggest that maintenance therapy in metastatic colorectal cancer after the appropriate induction regimen can be considered [43, 44]. The *OPTIMOX* trials yielded some of the earliest data on this strategy. In their first study [68], FOLFOX was administered continuously until PD or development of toxicity versus FOLFOX for six cycles followed by 5-FU maintenance. Survival statistics did not differ between the two groups and found that oxaliplatin could be stopped prior to PD to limit accrual of treatment toxicity. In *OPTIMOX2*, maintenance 5-FU was compared with observation alone after FOLFOX induction, but duration of disease control (and PFS, OS) was significantly shorter, favoring maintenance therapy [69].

Bevacizumab has been explored in this setting, exhibiting improvements in progression-free survival after standard induction in a meta-analysis of three major trials investigating its use, but large, prospective trials have had conflicting results, and we do not recommend single-agent bevacizumab as a maintenance strategy at this time.

Second-Line Therapy

Second-line chemotherapy refers to the treatment regimen after the first-line chemotherapy backbone is changed, usually initiated upon disease progression or unacceptable toxicity with first-line agents. Fit patients with good performance status and organ function should receive second-line treatment if it is within their goals. Additional agents are available for second and subsequent lines, but with so many options, it can seem overwhelming. In general, if first-line treatment consisted of an oxaliplatin backbone, irinotecan should be considered, either as FOLFIRI or monotherapy. Alternatively, if treatment was initiated with an irinotecan backbone, FOLFOX should be trialed. Depending on the first-line regimen and performance status, addition of VEGF or EGFR inhibition, or their use alone, may be appropriate.

Intensive Treatment

Support for alternating backbones was derived from phase III RCT data [70], and use of a cytotoxic doublet was superior in this setting over monotherapy with either 5-FU or oxaliplatin [71]. No specific doublet was shown to be superior in the second-line setting in regard to sequence, although toxicity profiles varied as expected.

Patients who were treated with less intensive 5-FU monotherapy until progression should be evaluated for addition of irinotecan or oxaliplatin, if appropriate [72]. If neither oxaliplatin nor irinotecan were used in first-line, the combination (IROX) may be used in the appropriate patient as it has been shown to be superior over irinotecan alone [73].

Both VEGF and EGFR inhibitions have shown improvement in overall survival, progression-free survival, and response rate beyond first-line treatment in a meta-analysis of large RCTs [74], and one has not been shown to be consistently superior to the other [75]. Bevacizumab has exhibited these effects when added to an alternate backbone after failure of a first-line cytotoxic doublet [76, 77] and when continued with second-line chemotherapy even if given during induction [78, 79]. Cetuximab and panitumumab have been shown to improve progression-free survival when added to FOLFIRI in the second-line setting [80]. In general, guidelines do not recommend one EGFR inhibitor over the other, and there is no data for alternating from cetuximab to panitumumab (or vice versa) after progression on one.

Two additional VEGF inhibitors are available for the treatment of metastatic colorectal cancer in the second-line setting. Ziv-aflibercept [81] is a recombinant fusion protein of the VEGF-binding portions of VEGFR (1 and 2) fused to an IgG1 Fc region. Overall survival and progression-free survival both improved over chemotherapy alone when the agent was added to FOLFIRI after failure of an oxaliplatin-based first-line regimen, even if bevacizumab was given [82]. Of note, a greater benefit was seen in those with liver-isolated metastatic disease in a subgroup analysis [83]. Ramucirumab [84] is a monoclonal antibody that inhibits angiogenesis through binding to VEGFR2 and blocking VEGF. Similarly, when added to FOLFIRI in second-line treatment, overall survival improved, even if bevacizumab was used for induction [85]. Side effects of these agents are similar to that of bevacizumab.

Non-intensive Treatment

Optimal treatment strategy in the non-intensive setting after disease progression should be based on previous lines, side effect profile, mutation status, and performance status. If patients are not appropriate candidates for a trial of doublet chemotherapy upon progression, irinotecan monotherapy may be considered [86]. VEGF and EGFR inhibitors described previously should also be evaluated for use, either in combination with cytotoxic chemotherapy [87, 88] or as single agents.

Subsequent Lines and Refractory Setting

Decisions regarding treatment in later lines are similar to those for preceding therapies and must take multiple previously discussed factors into consideration. As discussed above, improved survival statistics have been demonstrated when all available cytotoxic agents are made available. If the patient has other tumor characteristics with specific drug implications (i.e., *RAS* mutation status, sidedness, MSI-H/dMMR, other targetable mutations, etc.), the applicable agents should be trialed in appropriate candidates.

Bevacizumab, cetuximab, and panitumumab have all been evaluated in later lines with chemotherapy or alone and have been shown to have some efficacy compared to best supportive care (BSC) [89–91].

Additionally, two oral drugs have been approved in this setting. Trifluridine/tipiracil [92] is a combination drug that works by incorporating the nucleoside analog portion into DNA and preventing further synthesis. Side effects include fatigue, gastrointestinal upset, and cytopenias. A large RCT showed a statistically improved overall survival compared to BSC in the refractory setting [93]. Regorafenib [94] is a multi-kinase inhibitor (including VEGFR) that has been shown to improve overall survival in heavily pretreated metastatic colorectal cancer [95]. These agents are approved for use after failure of all available cytotoxic chemotherapies, bevacizumab, and an EGFR inhibitor.

Early involvement of palliative care is important for these complex patients.

Conclusions

The systemic treatment of metastatic colorectal cancer can be complex due to the number of agents and their potential combinations. As discussed, the administration of all available cytotoxic agents during disease course and the addition of VEGF and EGFR inhibition (in *KRAS* wt patients) have shown the most success in terms of survival statistics. Mutational profiling of the tumor is increasingly important in regard to prognosis and treatment availability, which influences decisions in first and later lines. Although intensive treatment regimens tend to exhibit better response, this may not be appropriate for patients based on their performance status, and less intensive treatment has still demonstrated efficacy.

Systemic treatment of unresectable, metastatic colorectal cancer is an active area of research with the goal of continuing to extend survival for patients with this disease.

References

1. Adrucil (5-fluorouracil) [package insert]. North Wales PTPU, Inc.; 2016.
2. Xeloda (capecitabine) [packet insert]. South San Francisco CGU, Inc.; 2016.
3. Eloxatin (oxaliplatin) [package insert]. Bridgewater NS-AUSL.
4. Camptosar (irinotecan) [package insert]. New York NPUCDoP, Inc.); 2014.
5. Leucovorin (folinic acid) [package insert]. Bedford OBL.
6. de Gramont A, Figer A, Seymour M, Homerin M, Hmissi A, Cassidy J, et al. Leucovorin and fluorouracil with or without oxaliplatin as first-line treatment in advanced colorectal cancer. J Clin Oncol. 2000;18(16):2938–47. https://doi.org/10.1200/JCO.2000.18.16.2938.
7. Giacchetti S, Perpoint B, Zidani R, Le Bail N, Faggiuolo R, Focan C, et al. Phase III multicenter randomized trial of oxaliplatin added to chronomodulated fluorouracil-leucovorin as first-line treatment of metastatic colorectal cancer. J Clin Oncol. 2000;18(1):136–47. https://doi.org/10.1200/JCO.2000.18.1.136.
8. Douillard JY, Cunningham D, Roth AD, Navarro M, James RD, Karasek P, et al. Irinotecan combined with fluorouracil compared with fluorouracil alone as first-line treatment for metastatic colorectal cancer: a multicentre randomised trial. Lancet. 2000;355(9209):1041–7.
9. Saltz LB, Cox JV, Blanke C, Rosen LS, Fehrenbacher L, Moore MJ, et al. Irinotecan plus fluorouracil and leucovorin for metastatic colorectal cancer. Irinotecan Study Group. N Engl J Med. 2000;343(13):905–14. https://doi.org/10.1056/NEJM200009283431302.
10. Van Cutsem E, Hoff PM, Harper P, Bukowski RM, Cunningham D, Dufour P, et al. Oral capecitabine vs intravenous 5-fluorouracil and leucovorin: integrated efficacy data and novel analyses from two large, randomised, phase III trials. Br J Cancer. 2004;90(6):1190–7. https://doi.org/10.1038/sj.bjc.6601676.
11. Colucci G, Gebbia V, Paoletti G, Giuliani F, Caruso M, Gebbia N, et al. Phase III randomized trial of FOLFIRI versus FOLFOX4 in the treatment of advanced colorectal cancer: a multicenter study of the Gruppo Oncologico Dell'Italia Meridionale. J Clin Oncol. 2005;23(22):4866–75. https://doi.org/10.1200/JCO.2005.07.113.
12. Madi A, Fisher D, Wilson RH, Adams RA, Meade AM, Kenny SL, et al. Oxaliplatin/capecitabine vs oxaliplatin/infusional 5-FU in advanced colorectal cancer: the MRC COIN trial. Br J Cancer. 2012;107(7):1037–43. https://doi.org/10.1038/bjc.2012.384.
13. Cassidy J, Clarke S, Diaz-Rubio E, Scheithauer W, Figer A, Wong R, et al. Randomized phase III study of capecitabine plus oxaliplatin compared with fluorouracil/folinic acid plus oxaliplatin as first-line therapy for metastatic colorectal cancer. J Clin Oncol. 2008;26(12):2006–12. https://doi.org/10.1200/JCO.2007.14.9898.
14. Souglakos J, Androulakis N, Syrigos K, Polyzos A, Ziras N, Athanasiadis A, et al. FOLFOXIRI (folinic acid, 5-fluorouracil, oxaliplatin and irinotecan) vs FOLFIRI (folinic acid, 5-fluorouracil and irinotecan) as first-line treatment in metastatic colorectal cancer (MCC): a multicentre randomised phase III trial from the Hellenic Oncology Research Group (HORG). Br J Cancer. 2006;94(6):798–805. https://doi.org/10.1038/sj.bjc.6603011.
15. Falcone A, Ricci S, Brunetti I, Pfanner E, Allegrini G, Barbara C, et al. Phase III trial of infusional fluorouracil, leucovorin, oxaliplatin, and irinotecan (FOLFOXIRI) compared with infusional fluorouracil, leucovorin, and irinotecan (FOLFIRI) as first-line treatment for metastatic colorectal cancer: the Gruppo Oncologico Nord Ovest. J Clin Oncol. 2007;25(13):1670–6. https://doi.org/10.1200/JCO.2006.09.0928.
16. Adams RA, Meade AM, Seymour MT, Wilson RH, Madi A, Fisher D, et al. Intermittent versus continuous oxaliplatin and fluoropyrimidine combination chemotherapy for first-line

treatment of advanced colorectal cancer: results of the randomised phase 3 MRC COIN trial. Lancet Oncol. 2011;12(7):642–53. https://doi.org/10.1016/S1470-2045(11)70102-4.
17. Labianca R, Sobrero A, Isa L, Cortesi E, Barni S, Nicolella D, et al. Intermittent versus continuous chemotherapy in advanced colorectal cancer: a randomised 'GISCAD' trial. Ann Oncol. 2011;22(5):1236–42. https://doi.org/10.1093/annonc/mdq580.
18. Seymour MT, Maughan TS, Ledermann JA, Topham C, James R, Gwyther SJ, et al. Different strategies of sequential and combination chemotherapy for patients with poor prognosis advanced colorectal cancer (MRC FOCUS): a randomised controlled trial. Lancet. 2007;370(9582):143–52. https://doi.org/10.1016/S0140-6736(07)61087-3.
19. Koopman M, Antonini NF, Douma J, Wals J, Honkoop AH, Erdkamp FL, et al. Sequential versus combination chemotherapy with capecitabine, irinotecan, and oxaliplatin in advanced colorectal cancer (CAIRO): a phase III randomised controlled trial. Lancet. 2007;370(9582):135–42. https://doi.org/10.1016/S0140-6736(07)61086-1.
20. Grothey A, Sargent D, Goldberg RM, Schmoll HJ. Survival of patients with advanced colorectal cancer improves with the availability of fluorouracil-leucovorin, irinotecan, and oxaliplatin in the course of treatment. J Clin Oncol. 2004;22(7):1209–14. https://doi.org/10.1200/JCO.2004.11.037.
21. AVASTIN (bevacizumab) [package insert]. South San Francisco CG, Inc.; 2015.
22. Erbitux (cetuximab) [package insert]. Branchburg NISI.
23. Vectibix (panitumumab) [package insert]. Thousand Oaks CAI.
24. Petrelli F, Borgonovo K, Barni S. The predictive role of skin rash with cetuximab and panitumumab in colorectal cancer patients: a systematic review and meta-analysis of published trials. Target Oncol. 2013;8(3):173–81. https://doi.org/10.1007/s11523-013-0257-x.
25. Kozloff M, Yood MU, Berlin J, Flynn PJ, Kabbinavar FF, Purdie DM, et al. Clinical outcomes associated with bevacizumab-containing treatment of metastatic colorectal cancer: the BRiTE observational cohort study. Oncologist. 2009;14(9):862–70. https://doi.org/10.1634/theoncologist.2009-0071.
26. Van Cutsem E, Rivera F, Berry S, Kretzschmar A, Michael M, DiBartolomeo M, et al. Safety and efficacy of first-line bevacizumab with FOLFOX, XELOX, FOLFIRI and fluoropyrimidines in metastatic colorectal cancer: the BEAT study. Ann Oncol. 2009;20(11):1842–7. https://doi.org/10.1093/annonc/mdp233.
27. Botrel TEA, Clark LGO, Paladini L, Clark OAC. Efficacy and safety of bevacizumab plus chemotherapy compared to chemotherapy alone in previously untreated advanced or metastatic colorectal cancer: a systematic review and meta-analysis. BMC Cancer. 2016;16:677. https://doi.org/10.1186/s12885-016-2734-y.
28. Saltz LB, Clarke S, Diaz-Rubio E, Scheithauer W, Figer A, Wong R, et al. Bevacizumab in combination with oxaliplatin-based chemotherapy as first-line therapy in metastatic colorectal cancer: a randomized phase III study. J Clin Oncol. 2008;26(12):2013–9. https://doi.org/10.1200/JCO.2007.14.9930.
29. Passardi A, Nanni O, Tassinari D, Turci D, Cavanna L, Fontana A, et al. Effectiveness of bevacizumab added to standard chemotherapy in metastatic colorectal cancer: final results for first-line treatment from the ITACa randomized clinical trial. Ann Oncol. 2015;26(6):1201–7. https://doi.org/10.1093/annonc/mdv130.
30. Gruenberger T, Bridgewater J, Chau I, Garcia Alfonso P, Rivoire M, Mudan S, et al. Bevacizumab plus mFOLFOX-6 or FOLFOXIRI in patients with initially unresectable liver metastases from colorectal cancer: the OLIVIA multinational randomised phase II trial. Ann Oncol. 2015;26(4):702–8. https://doi.org/10.1093/annonc/mdu580.
31. Cremolini C, Marmorino F, Loupakis F, Masi G, Antoniotti C, Salvatore L, et al. TRIBE-2: a phase III, randomized, open-label, strategy trial in unresectable metastatic colorectal cancer patients by the GONO group. BMC Cancer. 2017;17(1):408. https://doi.org/10.1186/s12885-017-3360-z.
32. Tomasello G, Petrelli F, Ghidini M, Russo A, Passalacqua R, Barni S. FOLFOXIRI Plus Bevacizumab as conversion therapy for patients with initially unresectable metastatic

colorectal cancer: a systematic review and pooled analysis. JAMA Oncol. 2017;3(7):e170278. https://doi.org/10.1001/jamaoncol.2017.0278.
33. Hazama S, Maeda H, Iwamoto S, Kim HM, Takemoto H, Kobayashi K, et al. A phase II study of XELOX and Cetuximab as first-line therapy in patients with KRAS wild type metastatic colorectal cancer (FLEET2 study). Clin Colorectal Cancer. 2016;15(4):329–36. https://doi.org/10.1016/j.clcc.2016.07.003.
34. Colucci G, Giuliani F, Garufi C, Mattioli R, Manzione L, Russo A, et al. Cetuximab plus FOLFOX-4 in untreated patients with advanced colorectal cancer: a Gruppo Oncologico dell'Italia Meridionale multicenter phase II study. Oncology. 2010;79(5–6):415–22. https://doi.org/10.1159/000323279.
35. Ye LC, Liu TS, Ren L, Wei Y, Zhu DX, Zai SY, et al. Randomized controlled trial of cetuximab plus chemotherapy for patients with KRAS wild-type unresectable colorectal liver-limited metastases. J Clin Oncol. 2013;31(16):1931–8. https://doi.org/10.1200/JCO.2012.44.8308.
36. Van Cutsem E, Kohne CH, Hitre E, Zaluski J, Chang Chien CR, Makhson A, et al. Cetuximab and chemotherapy as initial treatment for metastatic colorectal cancer. N Engl J Med. 2009;360(14):1408–17. https://doi.org/10.1056/NEJMoa0805019.
37. Maughan TS, Adams RA, Smith CG, Meade AM, Seymour MT, Wilson RH, et al. Addition of cetuximab to oxaliplatin-based first-line combination chemotherapy for treatment of advanced colorectal cancer: results of the randomised phase 3 MRC COIN trial. Lancet. 2011;377(9783):2103–14. https://doi.org/10.1016/S0140-6736(11)60613-2.
38. Van Cutsem E, Bajetta E, Valle J, Kohne CH, Hecht JR, Moore M, et al. Randomized, placebo-controlled, phase III study of oxaliplatin, fluorouracil, and leucovorin with or without PTK787/ZK 222584 in patients with previously treated metastatic colorectal adenocarcinoma. J Clin Oncol. 2011;29(15):2004–10. https://doi.org/10.1200/JCO.2010.29.5436.
39. Berlin J, Posey J, Tchekmedyian S, Hu E, Chan D, Malik I, et al. Panitumumab with irinotecan/leucovorin/5-fluorouracil for first-line treatment of metastatic colorectal cancer. Clin Colorectal Cancer. 2007;6(6):427–32. https://doi.org/10.3816/CCC.2007.n.011.
40. Douillard JY, Siena S, Cassidy J, Tabernero J, Burkes R, Barugel M, et al. Final results from PRIME: randomized phase III study of panitumumab with FOLFOX4 for first-line treatment of metastatic colorectal cancer. Ann Oncol. 2014;25(7):1346–55. https://doi.org/10.1093/annonc/mdu141.
41. Bokemeyer C, Kohne CH, Ciardiello F, Lenz HJ, Heinemann V, Klinkhardt U, et al. FOLFOX4 plus cetuximab treatment and RAS mutations in colorectal cancer. Eur J Cancer. 2015;51(10):1243–52. https://doi.org/10.1016/j.ejca.2015.04.007.
42. Douillard JY, Oliner KS, Siena S, Tabernero J, Burkes R, Barugel M, et al. Panitumumab-FOLFOX4 treatment and RAS mutations in colorectal cancer. N Engl J Med. 2013;369(11):1023–34. https://doi.org/10.1056/NEJMoa1305275.
43. Benson AB 3rd, Venook AP, Cederquist L, Chan E, Chen YJ, Cooper HS, et al. Colon Cancer, version 1.2017, NCCN clinical practice guidelines in oncology. J Natl Compr Cancer Netw. 2017;15(3):370–98.
44. Van Cutsem E, Cervantes A, Adam R, Sobrero A, Van Krieken JH, Aderka D, et al. ESMO consensus guidelines for the management of patients with metastatic colorectal cancer. Ann Oncol. 2016;27(8):1386–422. https://doi.org/10.1093/annonc/mdw235.
45. Cremolini C, Antoniotti C, Lonardi S, Aprile G, Bergamo F, Masi G, et al. Activity and safety of cetuximab plus modified FOLFOXIRI followed by maintenance with Cetuximab or Bevacizumab for RAS and BRAF wild-type metastatic colorectal cancer: a randomized phase 2 clinical trial. JAMA Oncol. 2018;4(4):529–36. https://doi.org/10.1001/jamaoncol.2017.5314.
46. Heinemann V, Rivera F, O'Neil BH, Stintzing S, Koukakis R, Terwey JH, et al. A study-level meta-analysis of efficacy data from head-to-head first-line trials of epidermal growth factor receptor inhibitors versus bevacizumab in patients with RAS wild-type metastatic colorectal cancer. Eur J Cancer. 2016;67:11–20. https://doi.org/10.1016/j.ejca.2016.07.019.
47. Venook AP, Niedzwiecki D, Lenz HJ, Innocenti F, Fruth B, Meyerhardt JA, et al. Effect of first-line chemotherapy combined with Cetuximab or Bevacizumab on overall survival in patients

with KRAS wild-type advanced or metastatic colorectal cancer: a randomized clinical trial. JAMA. 2017;317(23):2392–401. https://doi.org/10.1001/jama.2017.7105.
48. Rivera F, Karthaus M, Hecht JR, Sevilla I, Forget F, Fasola G, et al. Final analysis of the randomised PEAK trial: overall survival and tumour responses during first-line treatment with mFOLFOX6 plus either panitumumab or bevacizumab in patients with metastatic colorectal carcinoma. Int J Color Dis. 2017;32(8):1179–90. https://doi.org/10.1007/s00384-017-2800-1.
49. Heinemann V, von Weikersthal LF, Decker T, Kiani A, Vehling-Kaiser U, Al-Batran SE, et al. FOLFIRI plus cetuximab versus FOLFIRI plus bevacizumab as first-line treatment for patients with metastatic colorectal cancer (FIRE-3): a randomised, open-label, phase 3 trial. Lancet Oncol. 2014;15(10):1065–75. https://doi.org/10.1016/S1470-2045(14)70330-4.
50. Hecht JR, Mitchell E, Chidiac T, Scroggin C, Hagenstad C, Spigel D, et al. A randomized phase IIIB trial of chemotherapy, bevacizumab, and panitumumab compared with chemotherapy and bevacizumab alone for metastatic colorectal cancer. J Clin Oncol. 2009;27(5):672–80. https://doi.org/10.1200/JCO.2008.19.8135.
51. Tol J, Koopman M, Cats A, Rodenburg CJ, Creemers GJ, Schrama JG, et al. Chemotherapy, bevacizumab, and cetuximab in metastatic colorectal cancer. N Engl J Med. 2009;360(6):563–72. https://doi.org/10.1056/NEJMoa0808268.
52. Feliu J, Safont MJ, Salud A, Losa F, Garcia-Giron C, Bosch C, et al. Capecitabine and bevacizumab as first-line treatment in elderly patients with metastatic colorectal cancer. Br J Cancer. 2010;102(10):1468–73. https://doi.org/10.1038/sj.bjc.6605663.
53. Munemoto Y, Kanda M, Oba K, Kim HM, Takemoto H, Denda T, et al. A phase II trial to evaluate the efficacy of panitumumab combined with fluorouracil-based chemotherapy for metastatic colorectal cancer: the PF trial. Cancer Chemother Pharmacol. 2018;81(5):829–38. https://doi.org/10.1007/s00280-018-3556-1.
54. Kabbinavar FF, Schulz J, McCleod M, Patel T, Hamm JT, Hecht JR, et al. Addition of bevacizumab to bolus fluorouracil and leucovorin in first-line metastatic colorectal cancer: results of a randomized phase II trial. J Clin Oncol. 2005;23(16):3697–705. https://doi.org/10.1200/JCO.2005.05.112.
55. Battaglin F, Schirripa M, Buggin F, Pietrantonio F, Morano F, Boscolo G, et al. The PANDA study: a randomized phase II study of first-line FOLFOX plus panitumumab versus 5FU plus panitumumab in RAS and BRAF wild-type elderly metastatic colorectal cancer patients. BMC Cancer. 2018;18(1):98. https://doi.org/10.1186/s12885-018-4001-x.
56. Pietrantonio F, Cremolini C, Aprile G, Lonardi S, Orlandi A, Mennitto A, et al. Single-agent Panitumumab in frail elderly patients with advanced RAS and BRAF wild-type colorectal cancer: challenging drug label to light up new hope. Oncologist. 2015;20(11):1261–5. https://doi.org/10.1634/theoncologist.2015-0171.
57. Douillard JY, Rong A, Sidhu R. RAS mutations in colorectal cancer. N Engl J Med. 2013;369(22):2159–60. https://doi.org/10.1056/NEJMc1312697.
58. Sorich MJ, Wiese MD, Rowland A, Kichenadasse G, McKinnon RA, Karapetis CS. Extended RAS mutations and anti-EGFR monoclonal antibody survival benefit in metastatic colorectal cancer: a meta-analysis of randomized, controlled trials. Ann Oncol. 2015;26(1):13–21. https://doi.org/10.1093/annonc/mdu378.
59. Allegra CJ, Rumble RB, Hamilton SR, Mangu PB, Roach N, Hantel A, et al. Extended RAS gene mutation testing in metastatic colorectal carcinoma to predict response to anti-epidermal growth factor receptor monoclonal antibody therapy: American Society of Clinical Oncology provisional clinical opinion update 2015. J Clin Oncol. 2016;34(2):179–85. https://doi.org/10.1200/JCO.2015.63.9674.
60. KEYTRUDA (pembrolizumab) [package insert]. Whitehouse Station NMC, Inc.; 2016.
61. Le DT, Uram JN, Wang H, Bartlett BR, Kemberling H, Eyring AD, et al. PD-1 blockade in tumors with mismatch-repair deficiency. N Engl J Med. 2015;372(26):2509–20. https://doi.org/10.1056/NEJMoa1500596.
62. OPDIVO (nivolumab) [package insert]. Princeton NB-MSC.
63. Overman MJ, McDermott R, Leach JL, Lonardi S, Lenz HJ, Morse MA, et al. Nivolumab in patients with metastatic DNA mismatch repair-deficient or microsatellite instability-high

colorectal cancer (CheckMate 142): an open-label, multicentre, phase 2 study. Lancet Oncol. 2017;18(9):1182–91. https://doi.org/10.1016/S1470-2045(17)30422-9.
64. Raskov H, Burcharth J, Pommergaard HC. Linking gut microbiota to colorectal cancer. J Cancer. 2017;8(17):3378–95. https://doi.org/10.7150/jca.20497.
65. Salem ME, Weinberg BA, Xiu J, El-Deiry WS, Hwang JJ, Gatalica Z, et al. Comparative molecular analyses of left-sided colon, right-sided colon, and rectal cancers. Oncotarget. 2017;8(49):86356–68. https://doi.org/10.18632/oncotarget.21169.
66. Holch JW, Ricard I, Stintzing S, Modest DP, Heinemann V. The relevance of primary tumour location in patients with metastatic colorectal cancer: a meta-analysis of first-line clinical trials. Eur J Cancer. 2017;70:87–98. https://doi.org/10.1016/j.ejca.2016.10.007.
67. Snyder M, Bottiglieri S, Almhanna K. Impact of primary tumor location on first-line Bevacizumab or Cetuximab in metastatic colorectal cancer. Rev Recent Clin Trials. 2018; https://doi.org/10.2174/1574887113666180328104109.
68. Tournigand C, Cervantes A, Figer A, Lledo G, Flesch M, Buyse M, et al. OPTIMOX1: a randomized study of FOLFOX4 or FOLFOX7 with oxaliplatin in a stop-and-go fashion in advanced colorectal cancer--a GERCOR study. J Clin Oncol. 2006;24(3):394–400. https://doi.org/10.1200/JCO.2005.03.0106.
69. Chibaudel B, Maindrault-Goebel F, Lledo G, Mineur L, Andre T, Bennamoun M, et al. Can chemotherapy be discontinued in unresectable metastatic colorectal cancer? The GERCOR OPTIMOX2 Study. J Clin Oncol. 2009;27(34):5727–33. https://doi.org/10.1200/JCO.2009.23.4344.
70. Tournigand C, Andre T, Achille E, Lledo G, Flesh M, Mery-Mignard D, et al. FOLFIRI followed by FOLFOX6 or the reverse sequence in advanced colorectal cancer: a randomized GERCOR study. J Clin Oncol. 2004;22(2):229–37. https://doi.org/10.1200/JCO.2004.05.113.
71. Rothenberg ML, Oza AM, Bigelow RH, Berlin JD, Marshall JL, Ramanathan RK, et al. Superiority of oxaliplatin and fluorouracil-leucovorin compared with either therapy alone in patients with progressive colorectal cancer after irinotecan and fluorouracil-leucovorin: interim results of a phase III trial. J Clin Oncol. 2003;21(11):2059–69. https://doi.org/10.1200/JCO.2003.11.126.
72. Andre T, Louvet C, Maindrault-Goebel F, Couteau C, Mabro M, Lotz JP, et al. CPT-11 (irinotecan) addition to bimonthly, high-dose leucovorin and bolus and continuous-infusion 5-fluorouracil (FOLFIRI) for pretreated metastatic colorectal cancer. GERCOR. Eur J Cancer. 1999;35(9):1343–7.
73. Haller DG, Rothenberg ML, Wong AO, Koralewski PM, Miller WH Jr, Bodoky G, et al. Oxaliplatin plus irinotecan compared with irinotecan alone as second-line treatment after single-agent fluoropyrimidine therapy for metastatic colorectal carcinoma. J Clin Oncol. 2008;26(28):4544–50. https://doi.org/10.1200/JCO.2008.17.1249.
74. Segelov E, Chan D, Shapiro J, Price TJ, Karapetis CS, Tebbutt NC, et al. The role of biological therapy in metastatic colorectal cancer after first-line treatment: a meta-analysis of randomised trials. Br J Cancer. 2014;111(6):1122–31. https://doi.org/10.1038/bjc.2014.404.
75. Hecht JR, Cohn A, Dakhil S, Saleh M, Piperdi B, Cline-Burkhardt M, et al. SPIRITT: a randomized, multicenter, phase II study of Panitumumab with FOLFIRI and Bevacizumab with FOLFIRI as second-line treatment in patients with unresectable wild type KRAS metastatic colorectal cancer. Clin Colorectal Cancer. 2015;14(2):72–80. https://doi.org/10.1016/j.clcc.2014.12.009.
76. Giantonio BJ, Catalano PJ, Meropol NJ, O'Dwyer PJ, Mitchell EP, Alberts SR, et al. Bevacizumab in combination with oxaliplatin, fluorouracil, and leucovorin (FOLFOX4) for previously treated metastatic colorectal cancer: results from the Eastern Cooperative Oncology Group Study E3200. J Clin Oncol. 2007;25(12):1539–44. https://doi.org/10.1200/JCO.2006.09.6305.
77. Beretta GD, Petrelli F, Stinco S, Cabiddu M, Ghilardi M, Squadroni M, et al. FOLFIRI + bevacizumab as second-line therapy for metastatic colorectal cancer pretreated with oxaliplatin: a pooled analysis of published trials. Med Oncol. 2013;30(1):486. https://doi.org/10.1007/s12032-013-0486-y.

78. Masi G, Salvatore L, Boni L, Loupakis F, Cremolini C, Fornaro L, et al. Continuation or reintroduction of bevacizumab beyond progression to first-line therapy in metastatic colorectal cancer: final results of the randomized BEBYP trial. Ann Oncol. 2015;26(4):724–30. https://doi.org/10.1093/annonc/mdv012.
79. Bennouna J, Sastre J, Arnold D, Osterlund P, Greil R, Van Cutsem E, et al. Continuation of bevacizumab after first progression in metastatic colorectal cancer (ML18147): a randomised phase 3 trial. Lancet Oncol. 2013;14(1):29–37. https://doi.org/10.1016/S1470-2045(12)70477-1.
80. Peeters M, Price TJ, Cervantes A, Sobrero AF, Ducreux M, Hotko Y, et al. Randomized phase III study of panitumumab with fluorouracil, leucovorin, and irinotecan (FOLFIRI) compared with FOLFIRI alone as second-line treatment in patients with metastatic colorectal cancer. J Clin Oncol. 2010;28(31):4706–13. https://doi.org/10.1200/JCO.2009.27.6055.
81. ZALTRAP (ziv-aflibercept) [package insert]. Bridgewater NRP, Inc./sanofi-aventis U.S. LLC; 2016. .
82. Van Cutsem E, Tabernero J, Lakomy R, Prenen H, Prausova J, Macarulla T, et al. Addition of aflibercept to fluorouracil, leucovorin, and irinotecan improves survival in a phase III randomized trial in patients with metastatic colorectal cancer previously treated with an oxaliplatin-based regimen. J Clin Oncol. 2012;30(28):3499–506. https://doi.org/10.1200/JCO.2012.42.8201.
83. Tabernero J, Van Cutsem E, Lakomy R, Prausova J, Ruff P, van Hazel GA, et al. Aflibercept versus placebo in combination with fluorouracil, leucovorin and irinotecan in the treatment of previously treated metastatic colorectal cancer: prespecified subgroup analyses from the VELOUR trial. Eur J Cancer. 2014;50(2):320–31. https://doi.org/10.1016/j.ejca.2013.09.013.
84. CYRAMZA (ramucirumab) [package insert]. Indianapolis IELaC.
85. Tabernero J, Yoshino T, Cohn AL, Obermannova R, Bodoky G, Garcia-Carbonero R, et al. Ramucirumab versus placebo in combination with second-line FOLFIRI in patients with metastatic colorectal carcinoma that progressed during or after first-line therapy with bevacizumab, oxaliplatin, and a fluoropyrimidine (RAISE): a randomised, double-blind, multicentre, phase 3 study. Lancet Oncol. 2015;16(5):499–508. https://doi.org/10.1016/S1470-2045(15)70127-0.
86. Cunningham D, Pyrhonen S, James RD, Punt CJ, Hickish TF, Heikkila R, et al. Randomised trial of irinotecan plus supportive care versus supportive care alone after fluorouracil failure for patients with metastatic colorectal cancer. Lancet. 1998;352(9138):1413–8. https://doi.org/10.1016/S0140-6736(98)02309-5.
87. Seymour MT, Brown SR, Middleton G, Maughan T, Richman S, Gwyther S, et al. Panitumumab and irinotecan versus irinotecan alone for patients with KRAS wild-type, fluorouracil-resistant advanced colorectal cancer (PICCOLO): a prospectively stratified randomised trial. Lancet Oncol. 2013;14(8):749–59. https://doi.org/10.1016/S1470-2045(13)70163-3.
88. Sobrero AF, Maurel J, Fehrenbacher L, Scheithauer W, Abubakr YA, Lutz MP, et al. EPIC: phase III trial of cetuximab plus irinotecan after fluoropyrimidine and oxaliplatin failure in patients with metastatic colorectal cancer. J Clin Oncol. 2008;26(14):2311–9. https://doi.org/10.1200/JCO.2007.13.1193.
89. Geva R, Vecchione L, Tejpar S, Piessevaux H, Van Cutsem E, Prenen H. Bevacizumab plus chemotherapy as salvage treatment in chemorefractory patients with metastatic colorectal cancer. Onco Targets Ther. 2013;6:53–8. https://doi.org/10.2147/OTT.S41383.
90. Van Cutsem E, Peeters M, Siena S, Humblet Y, Hendlisz A, Neyns B, et al. Open-label phase III trial of panitumumab plus best supportive care compared with best supportive care alone in patients with chemotherapy-refractory metastatic colorectal cancer. J Clin Oncol. 2007;25(13):1658–64. https://doi.org/10.1200/JCO.2006.08.1620.
91. Price TJ, Peeters M, Kim TW, Li J, Cascinu S, Ruff P, et al. Panitumumab versus cetuximab in patients with chemotherapy-refractory wild-type KRAS exon 2 metastatic colorectal cancer (ASPECCT): a randomised, multicentre, open-label, non-inferiority phase 3 study. Lancet Oncol. 2014;15(6):569–79. https://doi.org/10.1016/S1470-2045(14)70118-4.
92. LONSURF (trifluridine and tipiracil) [package insert]. Tokyo JTPC, Ltd.; 2015.

93. Mayer RJ, Van Cutsem E, Falcone A, Yoshino T, Garcia-Carbonero R, Mizunuma N, et al. Randomized trial of TAS-102 for refractory metastatic colorectal cancer. N Engl J Med. 2015;372(20):1909–19. https://doi.org/10.1056/NEJMoa1414325.
94. STIVARGA (regorafenib) [package insert]. Whippany NBHPI.
95. Grothey A, Van Cutsem E, Sobrero A, Siena S, Falcone A, Ychou M, et al. Regorafenib monotherapy for previously treated metastatic colorectal cancer (CORRECT): an international, multicentre, randomised, placebo-controlled, phase 3 trial. Lancet. 2013;381(9863):303–12. https://doi.org/10.1016/S0140-6736(12)61900-X.

Role of Hepatic Artery Infusion Pump Chemotherapy for Unresectable Colorectal Cancer Liver Metastases

24

Jashodeep Datta and Michael I. D'Angelica

Abbreviations

FOLFIRI	5-FU, leucovorin, irinotecan
FOLFOX	5-FU, leucovorin, oxaliplatin
FOLFOXIRI	5-FU, leucovorin, oxaliplatin, irinotecan

Introduction

Despite the declining incidence of colorectal cancer (CRC) in patients 50 years or older, CRC remains the third most common cancer in the United States, accounting for an estimated 140,000 new cases and 50,000 deaths in 2017 [1]. Liver metastasis, either synchronous or metachronous, develops in over half of patients [2]. Complete resection in selected patients with limited colorectal liver metastasis (CRLM) is associated with 5-year overall survival (OS) exceeding 50% in select series [3]. Although most patients recur after hepatectomy, approximately 20% are cured after resection at long-term follow-up [3].

J. Datta
Hepatopancreatobiliary Service, Department of Surgery,
Memorial Sloan Kettering Cancer Center, New York, NY, USA

The Dewitt Daughtry Family Department of Surgery, Sylvester Comprehensive Cancer Center, University of Miami Miller School of Medicine, Miami, FL, USA

Memorial Sloan Kettering Cancer Center, Weill Cornell Unviersity School of Medicine, Miami, FL, USA

M. I. D'Angelica (✉)
Hepatopancreatobiliary Service, Department of Surgery,
Memorial Sloan Kettering Cancer Center, New York, NY, USA
e-mail: dangelim@mskcc.org

M. M. Correia et al. (eds.), *Colorectal Cancer Liver Metastases*,
https://doi.org/10.1007/978-3-030-25486-5_24

Unfortunately, only 15–20% of CRLM patients are deemed resectable at presentation [4]. Given that resection is a dominant contributor to long-term survival, major efforts have focused on expanding the pool of resectable patients. The advent of effective systemic chemotherapeutics (e.g., irinotecan [5], oxaliplatin [6]) and modern combination regimens (e.g., FOLFOX, FOLFIRI [7], and FOLFOXIRI) with or without targeted molecular therapies (e.g., anti-EGFR [for KRAS wild-type tumors] and anti-VEGF agents [8–10]) has been transformative in this regard. As such, several series/trials have demonstrated downstaging of CRLM patients from initially inoperable to potentially resectable, with similar 5-year survival compared with initially resectable patients [4, 11–13]. However, inconsistent reporting of resectability criteria and/or responses required for conversion to resection (CTR) in such studies has made interpretation of these data difficult [14, 15]. Moreover, modern chemotherapy rarely results in long-term cure in unresectable CRLM patients or those with extrahepatic disease (EHD), with median survival of 22–24 months [16], progression-free survival (PFS) averaging 10 months, and response rates (RR) in the second-line setting of 10–30% [16, 17].

Hepatic arterial infusion chemotherapy (HAIC) has evolved as an attractive strategy to expand resectability and/or control disease progression in unresectable CRLM patients with liver-only or liver-dominant disease. The hepatic artery is the predominant blood supply to liver metastases >3 mm in diameter, while normal hepatocytes are perfused predominantly by the portal circulation. Consequently, administration of chemotherapy into the hepatic artery allows selective drug delivery to the tumor with relative sparing of normal parenchyma [18]. This anatomic phenomenon, along with pharmacologic factors discussed below, provides much of the rationale for liver-directed HAIC in the management of CRLM. HAIC is typically administered via the gastroduodenal artery by a surgically implanted pump, hepatic arterial port, or percutaneously placed catheter connected to an external pump. Intra-arterial delivery of agents with high first-pass hepatic extraction (e.g., floxuridine [FUDR]) limits systemic toxicity and allows for concomitant administration of systemic chemotherapy at near-full doses [19]. Modern chemotherapeutic agents with lower first-pass extraction (e.g., irinotecan and oxaliplatin) have also been used for intra-arterial delivery, mostly in Europe and Asia [20, 21]. The most common adverse event from HAI-FUDR is biliary toxicity, which can be mitigated by concurrent administration of dexamethasone via pump and judicious dose cessations or adjustments [22].

Some of the evidence of the benefit of HAIC can be discerned from its use in the adjuvant setting. In an Eastern Cooperative Oncology Group (ECOG) trial randomizing completely resected CRLM patients to HAI-FUDR and intravenous 5-FU versus surgery alone, adjuvant HAIC/5-FU improved 4-year disease-free (46 vs. 25%) and hepatic recurrence-free (67 vs. 43%) survival [23]. A trial conducted at Memorial Sloan Kettering Cancer Center (MSKCC), randomizing resected patients to adjuvant HAI-FUDR plus 5-FU/leucovorin versus 5-FU/leucovorin alone, demonstrated improved overall, disease-free, and hepatic disease-free survival [24]. While these results cannot directly be extrapolated to unresectable CRLM, they provide level I evidence for HAIC efficacy.

Lingering questions remain regarding utilization of HAIC for unresectable CRLM patients and are explored in the following sections.

What Is the Role for HAIC Alone Versus Systemic Chemotherapy Alone in Unresectable CRLM?

Prospective trials published in the 1990s comparing HAIC alone to systemic chemotherapy alone demonstrated superior RRs (40–60%) in favor of HAIC but failed to consistently demonstrate an improvement in OS [25–27]. A meta-analysis by Mocellin et al. summarizing these data was cast as a moratorium on the use of HAIC alone for unresectable CRLM: "Evidence does not support the clinical or investigational use of fluoropyrimidine-based HAI alone for the treatment of patients with unresectable CRLM as first-line therapy" [28].

Meta-analyses such as this, however, failed to account for the inherent heterogeneity and the following critical methodologic limitations of summarized studies: (i) relatively small numbers of patients in individual trials; (ii) majority of studies conducted at single institutions; (iii) variations in technique of HAI delivery (e.g., use of port vs. pump); (iv) utilization of HAI-5-FU—known to have reduced efficacy compared with its prodrug FUDR—in at least two of the larger trials included; (v) even HAI-FUDR trials did not employ modern HAIC regimens, which include concomitant administration of leucovorin (LV) and DEX; and (vi) acceptance of crossover to HAIC for patients who experienced disease progression after receiving systemic therapy in eight included trials, confounding the assessment of the independent impact of HAIC on survival [29].

In an effort to overcome these limitations, a multi-institutional prospective randomized trial Cancer and Leukemia Group B (CALGB) 9481 was designed to compare HAI-FUDR/LV/DEX versus systemic bolus 5-FU/LV; notably, crossover between treatments was disallowed. Median OS was significantly longer for HAI-FUDR ($n = 68$) versus systemic 5-FU/LV treatment ($n = 67$; 24.4 vs. 20 months; $P = 0.003$), as were RRs (47% vs. 24%; $P = 0.012$) and time to hepatic progression (9.8 vs. 7.3 months; $P = 0.034$). Conversely, time to extrahepatic progression (7.7 vs. 14.8 months; $P = 0.029$) was significantly shorter in the HAIC cohort. The OS advantage conferred by HAI-FUDR persisted in multivariable modeling, despite inclusion of post-progression systemic treatment with newer chemotherapeutics (e.g., irinotecan, oxaliplatin) in both arms [30].

While results of this trial stimulated lively debate in oncology circles regarding the relevance of HAIC *alone* in unresectable CRLM patients, most institutions had already abandoned the HAIC-alone paradigm in favor of combinations with modern systemic chemotherapy in this setting. Indeed, several phase I/II trials investigating the efficacy of such combinations were underway at the time of its publication.

Does Combination HAIC and Systemic Chemotherapy Offer Improvement in Outcomes in Unresectable CRLM?

The competing tensions between improved hepatic disease control and EHD progression observed in unresectable CRLM patients receiving HAIC alone prompted exploration of HAIC with concurrent administration of systemic chemotherapy. A small randomized trial performed by Fiorentini and colleagues demonstrated superiority of HAI-FUDR plus systemic bolus 5-FU/LV over *HAI-FUDR alone* (median OS 20 vs. 14 months, respectively; $P = 0.003$) in patients with unresectable CRLM [31].

The approval of more effective systemic agents (e.g., oxaliplatin and irinotecan) in the late 1990s spurred the next generation of HAI-related trials, focusing on safety/efficacy of HAIC combined with these modern agents and/or combinations (Table 24.1). One of the earliest reported phase I trials examined HAI-FUDR/DEX combined with systemic irinotecan in 46 pretreated patients. In addition to establishing the maximum tolerated dose of irinotecan and impact of HAI-FUDR on irinotecan metabolism, a promising 74% RR was observed; median time to progression and OS were 8.1 and 20 months, respectively [32]. A subsequent phase I trial performed at MSKCC reported combination of HAI-FUDR/DEX with two separate

Table 24.1 Select trials of initially unresectable colorectal liver metastases treated with combination hepatic artery infusion and systemic chemotherapy

Author (year)	No. of pts	Treatment	RR (%)	Conversion to resection (%)	Median overall survival (months)
Allen-Mersh (2000) [57]	84	HAI-FUDR and SYS 5-FU/LV vs. SYS alone	45 vs. 23	NR	NR
Fallik (2003) [58]	75	HAI-pirarubicin and SYS 5-FU/LV	34.4	NR	20
Mancini (2003) [59]	123	HAI-cisplatin and SYS 5-FU	52	NR	18
Ducreux (2005) [20]	26	HAI-OX and SYS 5-FU/LV	64	17.8	27
Shimonov (2005) [21]	23	HAI-IRI and SYS 5-FU/LV+CARBO	40	NR	NR
Fiorentini (2006) [31]	76	HAI-5-FU/LV and SYS 5-FU/LV vs. HAI alone	47.5 vs. 41.7	NR[a]	20 vs. 14
Tsutsumi (2008) [60]	16	HAI-5-FU/LV and SYS UFT/LV	87.5	NR	22
Idelevich (2009) [61]	21	HAI-IRI+5-FU/LV and SYS UFT/LV	65	NR	36
Kemeny (2009) [35]	49	HAI-FUDR/DEX and SYS IRI+OX	92[b]	47	51 (chemo naive) 35 (prior chemo)
Goere (2010) [50]	87	HAI-OX and SYS 5-FU/LV	55	26	NR[c]
D'Angelica (2015) [48]	49	HAI-FUDR/DEX and best systemic therapy	76	47	38
Pak (2017) [49]	64	HAI-FUDR/DEX and best systemic therapy[d]	73	52	81

RR Response rate, *HAI* Hepatic artery infusion, *FUDR* Floxuridine, *SYS* Systemic, *5-FU* 5-Fluorouracil, *LV* Leucovorin, *NR* Not reported, *OX* Oxaliplatin, *IRI* Irinotecan, *CARBO* Carboplatin, *UFT* Uracil-tegafur, *DEX* Dexamethasone

[a]RFA performed in 33%

[b]Complete response observed in 8%

[c]5-yr survival 56%

[d]Expanded phase II study included 49 pts from D'Angelica et al. (2015)

oxaliplatin-based regimens (i.e., with irinotecan [group A] or infusional 5-FU/LV [FOLFOX; group B]) in 36 patients progressing on prior lines of chemotherapy. RRs (partial or complete) were nearly 90% in both groups; median OS was 36 and 22 months for groups A and B, respectively [33]. Li and colleagues reported combinations of HAI-FUDR with m-FOLFOX6 in 35 Chinese patients; RR was 69% for patients without EHD, and median PFS and OS were 8.2 and 25 months, respectively [34]. In a separate phase I trial from MSKCC, 49 patients received HAI-FUDR/DEX with oxaliplatin and irinotecan; RR was 92% in this heavily pretreated population, while median OS was 50.8 months and 35 months for chemotherapy-naive and previously treated patients [35].

In unresectable CRLM patients who progress on *all* standard chemotherapies, systemic options are essentially limited to investigational agents (e.g., regorafenib [36], TAS-102 [37], etc.). In this setting, HAIC represents a viable salvage approach for hepatic disease control. In 110 unresectable CRLM patients refractory to 5-FU/LV, irinotecan, oxaliplatin, ±bevacizumab, and anti-EGFR therapy (for RAS wild-type tumors) treated at MSKCC between 2003 and 2014, RRs of 35% were observed following treatment with HAI-FUDR and best systemic therapy [38]. Although nuanced clinical judgment is undoubtedly a factor when selecting patients that will tolerate HAIC in the setting of a heavily pretreated liver, the magnitude of tumor response observed with salvage HAIC in this treatment-refractory setting is extremely rare with investigational systemic chemotherapy alone.

While there is no randomized evidence comparing the *survival* impact of HAI-FUDR and modern systemic chemotherapy with systemic chemotherapy alone in unresectable CRLM, a retrospective analysis reported by the University of Pittsburgh group suggested that the addition of HAI-FUDR to systemic chemotherapy was associated with improved OS (32.8 vs. 15.3 months, $P < 0.0001$). Multivariable modeling revealed that HAIC plus systemic chemotherapy, ECOG status, and complexity of systemic chemotherapy receipt were independently associated with OS [39]. While the two groups appeared relatively well matched in terms of tumor burden and treatment-related characteristics, this study has been criticized for its low rates of CTR in either cohort, as well as the surprisingly poor survival statistics in the chemotherapy-alone cohort (most patients received therapy at community cancer centers) [40], thereby limiting applicability of these data to the broader group of patients treated with modern systemic regimens.

The efficacy of *non-FUDR* HAI with systemic chemotherapy combinations has also been established in several phase I/II studies. A German phase II trial evaluating HAI with oxaliplatin (HAI-OX) plus systemic 5-FU/LV in 26 patients demonstrated an RR of 64% and median OS of 27 months [20]. A group from Israel reported HAI-irinotecan with chronomodulated systemic 5-FU/folinic acid and carboplatin, yielding RR of 40% [21]. Taken together, these studies assessing combinatorial treatment with FUDR or non-FUDR HAIC and modern systemic chemotherapy suggested that, in general, this strategy was safe and generated a signal for effectiveness.

With increasing understanding of therapeutically actionable molecular alterations in metastatic colorectal cancer (e.g., anti-EGFR for KRAS wild type, anti-VEGF), combinations of systemic chemotherapy ± targeted agents with HAIC have been investigated. Despite some level I evidence supporting addition of anti-VEGF bevacizumab (BEV) to systemic chemotherapy, utilization of HAI-BEV with systemic regimens in a phase II trial from MSKCC increased the risk of biliary toxicity, precluding its use [41]. Use of cetuximab—an anti-EGFR antibody—in combination with an HAI infusate comprising 5-FU, oxaliplatin, and irinotecan in 64 KRAS wild-type patients revealed modest RRs, median PFS, and median OS outcomes (40.6%, 9.3 months, 25.5 months, respectively) [42]. Interestingly, there is preclinical evidence that suggests hepatic arterial infusion, but not systemic delivery, of cetuximab reduced outgrowth of CRLM in a murine model by inhibiting angiogenesis and inducing tumor cell apoptosis [43]. This paradigm is yet to be explored in the clinical setting.

Efforts at molecular/biologic prognostication of outcomes in the subset of unresectable CRLM receiving liver-directed therapies remain in their infancy. Connell and colleagues evaluated the interaction between KRAS-mutant status and serum biomarkers (i.e., CEA and LDH) in 193 unresectable CRLM patients receiving HAI-FUDR/DEX and systemic chemotherapy. Two distinct patterns of survival emerged. In patients with liver-restricted disease (n = 121), mutant-KRAS and serum LDH were negatively associated with survival, whereas in patients with extrahepatic disease (n = 72), only elevated LDH, but not mutant-KRAS, negatively impacted survival [44]. As knowledge of the genomic landscape of CRC expands, molecular-driven selection of patients as well as investigation of novel combinations of HAI/systemic agents is eagerly anticipated in these patients.

How Effective Is HAIC in Converting Initially Unresectable CRLM to Resectable and/or Abatable Disease?

One critically important endpoint to consider in the multimodality management of CRLM patients is complete resection. As such, determination of resectability is a complex biological and technical decision. Definitions of *upfront* resectability vary greatly between centers and are contingent on technical expertise, operative volume, institutional experience, and multidisciplinary oncologic care delivery. Similar factors limit interpretability in retrospective studies and clinical trials evaluating rates of CTR in initially unresectable patients. Notwithstanding, the data are clear in that initially unresectable CRLM patients who *do* convert to resection have similar long-term oncologic outcomes compared with those who were resectable upfront [4, 13]. Moreover, studies evaluating neoadjuvant chemotherapy in unresectable CRLM have demonstrated a reproducible correlation between RRs and resectability; this correlation was strongest in CRLM patients with liver-dominant disease ($r = 0.96$, $P = 0.002$) [45].

Arguably, the predominant goal of multimodality therapy in unresectable CRLM is to optimize RRs to facilitate resection; indeed, resectability has been proposed as a novel endpoint for trials evaluating neoadjuvant chemotherapy for metastatic liver disease. A substantial body of literature documents the impact of modern systemic chemotherapy *alone* on radiographic RRs and ensures CTR in initially unresectable

CRLM patients. Lam and colleagues systematically reviewed ten such observational studies examining 1886 patients with initially unresectable CRLM treated with systemic chemotherapy. Albeit quite heterogeneous in their design, prespecified definitions of irresectability, and systemic agents/regimens utilized, median objective RR of 64% (range 43–79%) was observed with first-line chemotherapy in initially unresectable patients [14]. When juxtaposing these results with responses seen in patients receiving HAIC *and* systemic chemotherapy, it appears that addition of liver-directed therapy augments RRs to 74–85% in pretreated, and up to 92% in chemotherapy-naive, patients with liver-dominant CRLM [46]. Therefore, if we were to accept that HAIC plus systemic chemotherapy generates improved RRs compared with systemic therapy alone, and that hepatic response is reliably predictive of ultimate resectability, it should logically follow that combination HAIC and systemic chemotherapy might enhance CTR in initially unresectable CRLM. The data appear to bear this out, with the caveat that there are no randomized trials directly comparing conversion rates from systemic chemotherapy alone to HAIC plus systemic chemotherapy.

In a retrospective analysis of 373 unresectable CRLM patients receiving HAI-FUDR/DEX and systemic chemotherapy (on and off clinical protocols) at MSKCC from 2000 to 2009, 93 patients (25%) subsequently underwent complete resection or ablation. Factors associated with CTR on multivariable analysis were contemporary treatment protocols (2004–2009), naivete to previous chemotherapy, clinical risk score (composite of 5 preoperative criteria: lymph node-positive primary, disease-free interval <12 months, ≥1 hepatic metastasis, largest metastasis ≥5 cm, and preoperative CEA level ≥ 200 ng/ml^2) ≥3, and younger age. Notwithstanding the likely biologic selection inherent in the subset achieving resection/ablation, median (59 vs. 16 months) and predicted 5-year OS (47% vs. 6%) was significantly improved in converted compared with non-converted patients [47]. Given the limitations of this retrospective study—nonstandardized definitions of irresectability, evolution of systemic and surgical treatment over time, and inclusion of patients on and off clinical protocols—it became clear that prospective trials would better define the role of HAIC in this setting (Table 24.1).

One of the first prospective studies to address the question of CTR with combination liver-directed and systemic chemotherapy was a phase I trial at MSKCC; 49 patients received HAI-FUDR/DEX and systemic oxaliplatin and irinotecan. This study retrospectively documented the rationale for initial irresectability: 24% of patients with all vessels involved, 73% with >5 liver lesions, 98% with bilobar disease, and 86% with ≥6 segments involved. In this cohort, the overall RR was 92% (complete: 8%; partial: 84%). CTR was achieved in 47%, reaching as high as 57% in chemotherapy-naive patients. Median OS from initiation of HAIC was 50.8 months in chemotherapy-naive, and 35 months in previously treated, patients, respectively [35].

A prospective phase II study from MSKCC (2007–2010) evaluated HAI-FUDR/DEX with best systemic therapy, in 49 patients with a strictly *prespecified* definition of irresectability. This included technical (i.e., margin-negative resection would require resection of 3 hepatic veins, both portal veins, or retrohepatic vena cava; or a resection that leaves <2 adequately perfused and drained segments) or biological (i.e., >6 metastases in a single lobe, with one lesion ≥5 cm; or ≥ 6 bilobar metastases) considerations. Despite a substantial burden of hepatic disease (i.e., median number of tumors was 14) in heavily pretreated (i.e., 65% received prior chemotherapy) patients, overall RR was 76%. Moreover, 47% of patients achieved CTR; in fact, CTR was the only factor independently associated with prolonged OS and PFS. A landmark analysis confirmed a higher 3-year OS among patients who underwent hepatectomy compared with those remaining unresectable (80% vs. 26%, $P = 0.005$) [48].

Results from this phase II trial were recently updated with longitudinal follow-up in an expanded cohort of 64 patients (2007–2012). At a median follow-up of *86 months* from initiation of HAI-FUDR and systemic chemotherapy, 52% had achieved CTR; as such, this study reached its primary endpoint with a CTR rate well over double the anticipated historical rate. Median PFS and OS were 13 and 38 months, respectively, with 5-year OS of 36%. RRs differed between chemotherapy-naive (86%) and previously treated (61%) patients; importantly, significant differences in PFS (19.7 vs. 10 months, $P = 0.021$) as well as OS (median 76.6 vs. 29.7 months, $P = 0.022$) were observed between chemotherapy-naive and previously treated patients, respectively. When controlling for appropriate demographic and high-risk clinical/anatomic characteristics, only CTR remained significantly associated with OS on multivariate analysis. Lastly, the curative potential of this therapeutic strategy was underscored by the fact that 9 of 64 patients (14%) were alive without evidence of disease at last follow-up [49].

CTR has also been investigated with *non-FUDR* HAI regimens. Goéré and colleagues retrospectively reviewed 87 French patients treated with HAI-OX and systemic 5-FU/LV for unresectable CRLM; 86% were deemed to have insufficient estimated functional liver remnant [FLR] precluding surgery. Objective RR was 55%, despite 79% of patients having previously received either systemic oxaliplatin or irinotecan. Following treatment, 26% of patients were submitted for curative-intent resection. CTR was significantly higher in patients who received HAI-OX as first line compared with patients receiving HAI-OX after failure of prior chemotherapy (53% vs. 19%) [50]. Levi and colleagues reported results from the prospective multicenter European phase II OPTILIV trial investigating CTR with triplet HAIC (5-FU, oxaliplatin, and irinotecan) and intravenous cetuximab in 64 patients with unresectable KRAS wild-type CRLM who had progressed on 1–3 lines of chemotherapy. RRs and disease control rates were 40.6% and 84.4%, respectively. CTR was achieved in 33.3% of patients (per protocol); when this therapeutic strategy was delivered in the second-line setting, CTR was achieved in 46.4% of patients compared with 16.7% when utilized in the third-line setting and beyond ($P = 0.014$). Median OS was significantly longer among patients completing therapeutic strategy as second versus third/fourth line (31.8 vs. 15.7 months, $P = 0.001$) [42]. Taken together, these data suggest that liver-directed approaches incorporating FUDR or non-FUDR HAIC, in conjunction with systemic chemotherapy, are associated with dramatic responses in the liver, far exceeding that expected with non-first-line chemotherapy regimens alone. In turn, these responses translate into encouraging rates of CTR in initially unresectable patients. One such dramatic example is provided in Fig. 24.1.

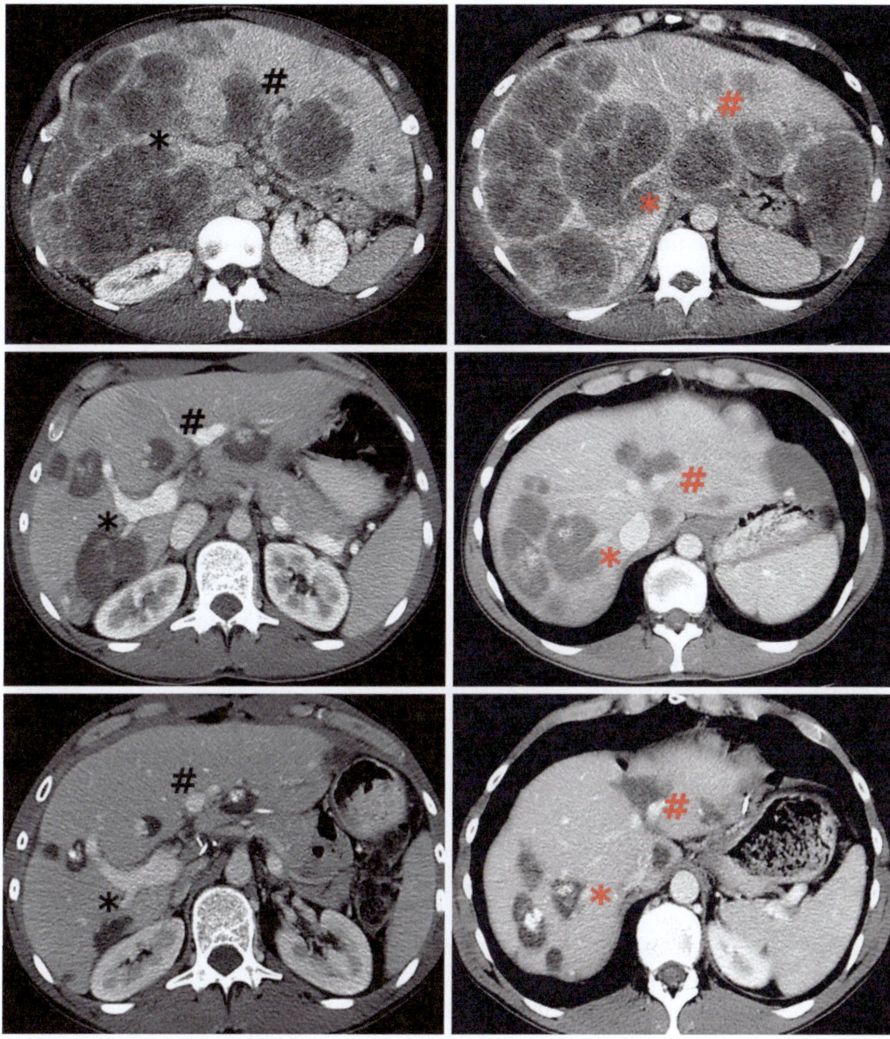

Fig. 24.1 Dramatic hepatic response in a patient treated with HAI-FUDR and systemic FOLFIRI, following initial progression on FOLFOX. Extensive bilobar unresectable disease involving both right (black ∗) and left (black #) portal pedicles, as well as right hepatic vein (red ∗) and middle/left hepatic veins (red #), is shown. Descending images demonstrate progressive response and clearance of inflow/outflow, and the patient was ultimately able to undergo a combination of curative-intent resection and ablation/irreversible electroporation. Patient remains recurrence-free 2 years after resection

Juxtaposition of Conversion to Resection Rates Using Systemic Chemotherapy Alone with Conversion Rates Achieved with Combination HAIC and Systemic Chemotherapy

The logical next questions that might inform decision-making in this setting are as follows: How do these aforementioned data compare with rates of CTR with *systemic chemotherapy alone*? And is it worth the additional toxicity? While the latter question will be addressed in section "Morbidity and Toxicity of HAIC" below, it is worthwhile to explore the former question. The largest study to date on this topic was a retrospective review of 1104 patients with initially unresectable CRLM treated at Hospital Paul-Brousse in France; patients received FOLFOX (70%), FOLFIRI (7%), or both (4%), and criteria for irresectability included inability to preserve >30% of non-tumoral liver parenchyma or presence of concomitant EHD. One hundred thirty-eight (12.5%) of patients had tumor downsizing allowing surgical resection; in this subset of patients, DFS and OS were 17% and 23% at 10 years, respectively [4]. These outcomes were mirrored in a meta-analysis summarizing the aggregate impact of CTR with modern chemotherapy ± anti-EGFR/VEGF regimens in 1886 unresectable CRLM patients; complete resection was achieved in 23.1% of patients [14].

Several other retrospective series and prospective trials have reported CTR rates between 7 and 60% in initially unresectable CRLM patients following modern chemotherapy alone [15]. Closer inspection of the methodology in these studies, however, reveals likely underreporting of the true denominator of unresectable patients, inconsistent definitions of irresectability, and variability in prescribed chemotherapy regimens and degree of pretreatment. For instance, an Italian prospective phase II trial evaluating irinotecan and 5-FU/LV in 40 unresectable CRLM patients reported conversion in 33%; however, pretreated patients were excluded [51]. Furthermore, *conservative* definitions of resectability in studies reporting the highest resectability rates likely overestimate the benefit of conversion chemotherapy. Giachetti and colleagues reported CTR rate of 38% with FOLFOX but deemed patients with tumors >5 cm initially unresectable [52]. Folprecht et al. reported an impressive CTR rate of 46% in 111 initially unresectable CRLM patients randomized to receive FOLFOX or FOLFIRI plus cetuximab in the CELIM trial; although this prospective study had prespecified criteria for irresectability, post hoc central review by a blinded committee comprising 7 hepatobiliary surgeons adjudicated nearly a third of enrolled patients to be *resectable* at initial presentation [53].

In general, rates of CTR with combination HAI and systemic chemotherapy, higher than those historically reported with systemic chemotherapy alone, remain the most compelling indication for liver-directed chemotherapy in this subset of patients. Based on the aforementioned data, an argument can be made for both earlier initiation/referral for consideration of HAIC in *chemotherapy-naive* patients with unresectable CRLM and utilization of HAIC to augment resectability rates in patients who have failed first-line systemic chemotherapy *before* proceeding to second-/third-line regimens. It will be increasingly important to identify which patients with initially unresectable CRLM might benefit from earlier initiation of liver-directed chemotherapy to improve CTR rates; indeed, at our institution, the molecular underpinnings of such conversion are being actively investigated.

Morbidity and Toxicity of HAIC

The enthusiasm for liver-directed therapy must be balanced with procedure-related morbidity and drug-related toxicity. Allen and colleagues reported on complications in 544 patients receiving HAIC at MSKCC (1986–2001). Overall complication rate was 22% (arterial thrombosis [6%], extrahepatic perfusion [3%], incomplete hepatic perfusion [2%], and hemorrhage [2%]); the incidence of complications improved with surgical experience. A majority of complications were salvageable, with 80% of pumps functioning for a minimum of 2 years [54].

A review of drug-related toxicity from HAI in 4580 cases found gastrointestinal symptoms in 22%, hepatic toxicity in 19%, and myelosuppression in 8%; HAI-FUDR was primarily associated with biliary sclerosis [55]. In 475 patients undergoing HAI-FUDR at MSKCC, 4.6% developed biliary sclerosis requiring a stent. Notably, no difference in survival was found between those with biliary sclerosis salvaged with stenting/dilation and those without biliary complications [56]. Several mitigating strategies can counteract the sclerosing effects of HAI-FUDR. A randomized trial of 50 patients found greater dose tolerance of FUDR at 5 months ($P = 0.05$) and increased RR ($P = 0.03$) when administered with HAI-DEX [22].

Conclusion

Hepatic disease control and CTR are important considerations in unresectable CRLM patients with liver-dominant disease. The role of combination HAIC and systemic chemotherapy in these patients is now well established by numerous retrospective and prospective studies. Administration of HAIC can be complex, and the importance of a dedicated multidisciplinary infrastructure that incorporates the surgical, medical, radiologic, and nursing aspects of HAIC management cannot be overemphasized and remains critical to the ultimate success of an HAIC "program."

While HAIC is certainly not a modern innovation per se, having been around for over three decades now, its potential is being increasingly acknowledged by the broader oncologic community. This is exemplified by the initiation of new HAIC programs in several centers across North America, Europe, and Asia. Moreover, it is heartening to see active recruitment of patients into phase II/III clinical trials examining the comparative effectiveness of HAIC plus systemic chemotherapy versus chemotherapy alone—a yet unanswered question. These include a phase III Chinese trial comparing HAI-FUDR/DEX plus mFOLFOX6 versus FOLFOX6 alone in unresectable CRLM, with margin-negative resection as primary outcome (NCT02102789), as well as a multi-institutional North American phase II trial randomizing patients with KRAS wild-type CRLM to either HAI-FUDR/DEX with FOLFIRI plus panitumumab or FOLFIRI plus panitumumab alone as second-line therapy, with CTR as primary outcome (NCT03069950).

Future directions in the field will entail refinements in the patient selection process—including investigation of the genetic determinants of response and outcome—for HAIC in the unresectable setting, incorporation of rapidly growing knowledge of molecularly driven systemic therapies into rational trial design, and development of prospective multi-institutional registries comparing combination HAI regimens not only to systemic chemotherapy alone but also to alternative liver-directed treatment approaches (e.g., Yttrium-90 radioembolization, transarterial chemoembolization, etc.) increasingly utilized in unresectable CRLM. Such efforts promise to further improve contemporary survival outcomes, already at a previously unimaginable level, in this difficult-to-treat subset of patients.

References

1. American Cancer Society: Key Statistics for Colorectal Cancer. 2017; Available from: www.cancer.org/cancer/colonandrectumcancer/detailedguide/colorectal-cancer-key-statistics.
2. Siegel R, Naishadham D, Jemal A. Cancer statistics, 2012. CA Cancer J Clin. 2012;62(1):10–29.
3. Tomlinson JS, et al. Actual 10-year survival after resection of colorectal liver metastases defines cure. J Clin Oncol. 2007;25(29):4575–80.
4. Adam R, et al. Patients with initially unresectable colorectal liver metastases: is there a possibility of cure? J Clin Oncol. 2009;27(11):1829–35.
5. Saltz LB, et al. Irinotecan plus fluorouracil and leucovorin for metastatic colorectal cancer. Irinotecan Study Group. N Engl J Med. 2000;343(13):905–14.
6. de Gramont A, et al. Leucovorin and fluorouracil with or without oxaliplatin as first-line treatment in advanced colorectal cancer. J Clin Oncol. 2000;18(16):2938–47.
7. Tournigand C, et al. FOLFIRI followed by FOLFOX6 or the reverse sequence in advanced colorectal cancer: a randomized GERCOR study. J Clin Oncol. 2004;22(2):229–37.
8. Cunningham D, et al. Cetuximab monotherapy and cetuximab plus irinotecan in irinotecan-refractory metastatic colorectal cancer. N Engl J Med. 2004;351(4):337–45.
9. Hurwitz HI, et al. Bevacizumab in combination with fluorouracil and leucovorin: an active regimen for first-line metastatic colorectal cancer. J Clin Oncol. 2005;23(15):3502–8.
10. Amado RG, et al. Wild-type KRAS is required for panitumumab efficacy in patients with metastatic colorectal cancer. J Clin Oncol. 2008;26(10):1626–34.
11. Alberts SR, et al. Oxaliplatin, fluorouracil, and leucovorin for patients with unresectable liver-only metastases from colorectal cancer: a North Central Cancer Treatment Group phase II study. J Clin Oncol. 2005;23(36):9243–9.
12. Folprecht G, et al. Survival of patients with initially unresectable colorectal liver metastases treated with FOLFOX/cetuximab or FOLFIRI/cetuximab in a multidisciplinary concept (CELIM study). Ann Oncol. 2014;25(5):1018–25.
13. Masi G, et al. Long-term outcome of initially unresectable metastatic colorectal cancer patients treated with 5-fluorouracil/leucovorin, oxaliplatin, and irinotecan (FOLFOXIRI) followed by radical surgery of metastases. Ann Surg. 2009;249(3):420–5.
14. Lam VW, et al. A systematic review of clinical response and survival outcomes of downsizing systemic chemotherapy and rescue liver surgery in patients with initially unresectable colorectal liver metastases. Ann Surg Oncol. 2012;19(4):1292–301.
15. Mokdad A, Choti MA, Yopp AC. Conversion chemotherapy for unresectable colorectal liver metastases: are we making a difference? Curr Colorectal Cancer Rep. 2015;11(4):160–7.

16. Sanoff HK, et al. Five-year data and prognostic factor analysis of oxaliplatin and irinotecan combinations for advanced colorectal cancer: N9741. J Clin Oncol. 2008;26(35):5721–7.
17. Peeters M, et al. Final results from a randomized phase 3 study of FOLFIRI {+/−} panitumumab for second-line treatment of metastatic colorectal cancer. Ann Oncol. 2014;25(1):107–16.
18. Breedis C, Young G. The blood supply of neoplasms in the liver. Am J Pathol. 1954;30(5):969–77.
19. Ensminger WD, Gyves JW. Clinical pharmacology of hepatic arterial chemotherapy. Semin Oncol. 1983;10(2):176–82.
20. Ducreux M, et al. Hepatic arterial oxaliplatin infusion plus intravenous chemotherapy in colorectal cancer with inoperable hepatic metastases: a trial of the gastrointestinal group of the Federation Nationale des Centres de Lutte Contre le Cancer. J Clin Oncol. 2005;23(22):4881–7.
21. Shimonov M, et al. Combined systemic chronotherapy and hepatic artery infusion for the treatment of metastatic colorectal cancer confined to the liver. Chemotherapy. 2005;51(2–3):111–5.
22. Kemeny N, et al. A randomized trial of intrahepatic infusion of fluorodeoxyuridine with dexamethasone versus fluorodeoxyuridine alone in the treatment of metastatic colorectal cancer. Cancer. 1992;69(2):327–34.
23. Kemeny MM, et al. Combined-modality treatment for resectable metastatic colorectal carcinoma to the liver: surgical resection of hepatic metastases in combination with continuous infusion of chemotherapy--an intergroup study. J Clin Oncol. 2002;20(6):1499–505.
24. Kemeny N, et al. Hepatic arterial infusion of chemotherapy after resection of hepatic metastases from colorectal cancer. N Engl J Med. 1999;341(27):2039–48.
25. Kemeny N, et al. Intrahepatic or systemic infusion of fluorodeoxyuridine in patients with liver metastases from colorectal carcinoma. A randomized trial. Ann Intern Med. 1987;107(4):459–65.
26. Kerr DJ, et al. Intrahepatic arterial versus intravenous fluorouracil and folinic acid for colorectal cancer liver metastases: a multicentre randomised trial. Lancet. 2003;361(9355):368–73.
27. Rougier P, et al. Hepatic arterial infusion of floxuridine in patients with liver metastases from colorectal carcinoma: long-term results of a prospective randomized trial. J Clin Oncol. 1992;10(7):1112–8.
28. Mocellin S, et al. Meta-analysis of hepatic arterial infusion for unresectable liver metastases from colorectal cancer: the end of an era? J Clin Oncol. 2007;25(35):5649–54.
29. D'Angelica M, et al. Hepatic arterial infusion chemotherapy for metastases from colorectal cancer: is it really the end of an era? J Clin Oncol. 2008;26(16):2788–9; author reply 2789-90.
30. Kemeny NE, et al. Hepatic arterial infusion versus systemic therapy for hepatic metastases from colorectal cancer: a randomized trial of efficacy, quality of life, and molecular markers (CALGB 9481). J Clin Oncol. 2006;24(9):1395–403.
31. Fiorentini G, et al. Hepatic arterial chemotherapy in combination with systemic chemotherapy compared with hepatic arterial chemotherapy alone for liver metastases from colorectal cancer: results of a multi-centric randomized study. In Vivo. 2006;20(6A):707–9.
32. Kemeny N, et al. Phase I study of hepatic arterial infusion of floxuridine and dexamethasone with systemic irinotecan for unresectable hepatic metastases from colorectal cancer. J Clin Oncol. 2001;19(10):2687–95.
33. Kemeny N, et al. Phase I trial of systemic oxaliplatin combination chemotherapy with hepatic arterial infusion in patients with unresectable liver metastases from colorectal cancer. J Clin Oncol. 2005;23(22):4888–96.
34. Li C, et al. Phase I trial of hepatic arterial infusion (HAI) of floxuridine with modified oxaliplatin, 5-fluorouracil and leucovorin (m-FOLFOX6) in Chinese patients with unresectable liver metastases from colorectal cancer. Cancer Chemother Pharmacol. 2014;74(5):1079–87.
35. Kemeny NE, et al. Conversion to resectability using hepatic artery infusion plus systemic chemotherapy for the treatment of unresectable liver metastases from colorectal carcinoma. J Clin Oncol. 2009;27(21):3465–71.
36. Grothey A, et al. Regorafenib monotherapy for previously treated metastatic colorectal cancer (CORRECT): an international, multicentre, randomised, placebo-controlled, phase 3 trial. Lancet. 2013;381(9863):303–12.

37. Mayer RJ, et al. Randomized trial of TAS-102 for refractory metastatic colorectal cancer. N Engl J Med. 2015;372(20):1909–19.
38. Cercek A, et al. Response rates of hepatic arterial infusion pump therapy in patients with metastatic colorectal cancer liver metastases refractory to all standard chemotherapies. J Surg Oncol. 2016;114(6):655–63.
39. Dhir M, et al. Hepatic arterial infusion in combination with modern systemic chemotherapy is associated with improved survival compared with modern systemic chemotherapy alone in patients with isolated unresectable colorectal liver metastases: a case-control study. Ann Surg Oncol. 2017;24(1):150–8.
40. Karanicolas PJ, Ko YJ. Hepatic arterial infusion for unresectable liver metastases from colorectal cancer: the dawn of a new era? Ann Surg Oncol. 2017;24(1):6–7.
41. Kemeny NE, et al. Randomized phase II trial of adjuvant hepatic arterial infusion and systemic chemotherapy with or without bevacizumab in patients with resected hepatic metastases from colorectal cancer. J Clin Oncol. 2011;29(7):884–9.
42. Levi FA, et al. Conversion to resection of liver metastases from colorectal cancer with hepatic artery infusion of combined chemotherapy and systemic cetuximab in multicenter trial OPTILIV. Ann Oncol. 2016;27(2):267–74.
43. Sperling J, et al. Hepatic arterial infusion but not systemic application of cetuximab in combination with oxaliplatin significantly reduces growth of CC531 colorectal rat liver metastases. Int J Color Dis. 2013;28(4):555–62.
44. Connell LC, et al. Relevance of CEA and LDH in relation to KRAS status in patients with unresectable colorectal liver metastases. J Surg Oncol. 2017;115(4):480–7.
45. Folprecht G, et al. Neoadjuvant treatment of unresectable colorectal liver metastases: correlation between tumour response and resection rates. Ann Oncol. 2005;16(8):1311–9.
46. Kelly CM, Kemeny NE. Liver-directed therapy in metastatic colorectal cancer. Expert Rev Anticancer Ther. 2017;17(8):745–58.
47. Ammori JB, et al. Conversion to complete resection and/or ablation using hepatic artery infusional chemotherapy in patients with unresectable liver metastases from colorectal cancer: a decade of experience at a single institution. Ann Surg Oncol. 2013;20(9):2901–7.
48. D'Angelica MI, et al. Phase II trial of hepatic artery infusional and systemic chemotherapy for patients with unresectable hepatic metastases from colorectal cancer: conversion to resection and long-term outcomes. Ann Surg. 2015;261(2):353–60.
49. Pak LM, et al. Prospective phase II trial of combination hepatic artery infusion and systemic chemotherapy for unresectable colorectal liver metastases: long term results and curative potential. J Surg Oncol. 2018;117(4):634–43.
50. Goere D, et al. Prolonged survival of initially unresectable hepatic colorectal cancer patients treated with hepatic arterial infusion of oxaliplatin followed by radical surgery of metastases. Ann Surg. 2010;251(4):686–91.
51. Barone C, et al. Final analysis of colorectal cancer patients treated with irinotecan and 5-fluorouracil plus folinic acid neoadjuvant chemotherapy for unresectable liver metastases. Br J Cancer. 2007;97(8):1035–9.
52. Giacchetti S, et al. Long-term survival of patients with unresectable colorectal cancer liver metastases following infusional chemotherapy with 5-fluorouracil, leucovorin, oxaliplatin and surgery. Ann Oncol. 1999;10(6):663–9.
53. Folprecht G, et al. Tumour response and secondary resectability of colorectal liver metastases following neoadjuvant chemotherapy with cetuximab: the CELIM randomised phase 2 trial. Lancet Oncol. 2010;11(1):38–47.
54. Allen PJ, et al. Technical complications and durability of hepatic artery infusion pumps for unresectable colorectal liver metastases: an institutional experience of 544 consecutive cases. J Am Coll Surg. 2005;201(1):57–65.
55. Kanat O, Gewirtz A, Kemeny N. What is the potential role of hepatic arterial infusion chemo-therapy in the current armamentorium against colorectal cancer. J Gastrointest Oncol. 2012;3(2):130–8.

56. Ito K, et al. Biliary sclerosis after hepatic arterial infusion pump chemotherapy for patients with colorectal cancer liver metastasis: incidence, clinical features, and risk factors. Ann Surg Oncol. 2012;19(5):1609–17.
57. Allen-Mersh TG, et al. Randomized trial of regional plus systemic fluorinated pyrimidine compared with systemic fluorinated pyrimidine in treatment of colorectal liver metastases. Eur J Surg Oncol. 2000;26(5):468–73.
58. Fallik D, et al. Hepatic arterial infusion using pirarubicin combined with systemic chemotherapy: a phase II study in patients with nonresectable liver metastases from colorectal cancer. Ann Oncol. 2003;14(6):856–63.
59. Mancini R, et al. Hepatic arterial infusion (HAI) of cisplatin and systemic fluorouracil in the treatment of unresectable colorectal liver metastases. Anticancer Res. 2003;23(2C):1837–41.
60. Tsutsumi S, et al. Hepatic arterial infusion combined with oral UFT/UZEL systemic chemotherapy for unresectable liver metastasis of colorectal cancer. Hepato-Gastroenterology. 2008;55(85):1419–22.
61. Idelevich E, et al. Phase II study of UFT with leucovorin plus hepatic arterial infusion with irinotecan, 5-fluorouracil and leucovorin for non-resectable liver metastases of colorectal cancer. Chemotherapy. 2009;55(2):76–82.

Enhanced Recovery After Liver Surgery

25

Eve Simoneau, Thomas A. Aloia, and Ching-Wei D. Tzeng

Introduction

The first postoperative fast-track protocols, also called "enhanced recovery after surgery" (ERAS), were instituted by colorectal surgeons almost three decades ago in order to modulate surgical stress and hasten recovery [1]. Since then, the implementation of enhanced recovery programs has had an exponential expansion across most surgical specialties, including gynecology, urology, breast, vascular, and orthopedic surgery [2–6]. "Enhanced recovery after liver surgery" (ERLS) was first introduced in 2008 [7] and has incrementally gained acceptance as being an integral part of perioperative care for hepatectomy patients. Several outcome metrics have shown to be improved with the adoption of a multimodal evidence-based strategy in liver surgery, many of which are also shared by other surgical specialties practicing in an enhanced recovery framework. Improved clinical outcomes such as length of stay, morbidity rates, and hospital costs tend to support implementation of fast-track programs in general, but other metrics specific to liver surgery and to patients with colorectal liver metastases (CLM) further endorse this strategy when managing CLM.

The implementation of an ERLS program represents a collaborative approach in which the different team players, including anesthesia, surgery, nutrition, pharmacy, nursing, and most importantly the patient and his/her family, engage actively in the perioperative pathway, in an evidence-based, patient-centered approach [8]. The

E. Simoneau
Division of Hepatobiliary Surgery and Liver Transplantation, Department of Surgery, University of Montreal, Montreal, Quebec, Canada
e-mail: evesimoneau@me.com

T. A. Aloia · C.-W. D. Tzeng (✉)
Department of Surgical Oncology, The University of Texas MD Anderson Cancer Center, Houston, TX, USA
e-mail: taaloia@mdanderson.org; cdtzeng@mdanderson.org

M. M. Correia et al. (eds.), *Colorectal Cancer Liver Metastases*,
https://doi.org/10.1007/978-3-030-25486-5_25

development of such programs also requires dedicated continuing education for the team members, flexibility in terms of perioperative management and decision-making by the health-care providers, support from the hospital administration, and systematic quality control measures to ensure implementation and accurate reporting. We will review here the different core elements of ERLS and discuss different outcomes associated with this system-based approach, with an emphasis on oncological patients.

Enhanced Recovery Core Elements

Although certain elements of ERLS programs share significant overlap with colorectal surgery, several core elements specific to liver surgery have been integrated into ERLS pathways (Table 25.1) and will be reviewed in this section.

Table 25.1 Summary of core items of enhanced recovery after liver surgery

	Recommendations	References
Preoperative instructions	Overnight fasting is only recommended for solid food Patients should be drinking high-carbohydrates clear liquids until 2 hours prior to surgery No "bowel prep" or laxatives for clearance of colon the day before surgery	[91, 92]
Perioperative analgesia	Opioid-sparing approach Epidural analgesia can be associated with a reduced need for intravenous opiates Transversus abdominis plane block is a promising strategy that can be used with multimodal analgesia	[17, 21, 22]
Perioperative antimicrobial prophylaxis	Preoperative antibiotics should be administered within an hour before surgical incision	[11, 26]
Venous thromboembolism prophylaxis	Preoperative single-dose chemoprophylaxis (heparin) can be administered without risk of hemorrhage, although the evidence currently lacks to show a clear benefit Postoperative VTE chemoprophylaxis should be given for 28 days, starting immediately on the day of surgery	[33–37]
Fluid therapy	A low CVP should be maintained during surgery Transfusions should be avoided or limited if needed A strategy of judicious goal-directed fluid therapy should be utilized in the postoperative period (i.e., BNP-driven fluid therapy)	[38–44, 51]
Early gastrointestinal function	Early oral diet should be initiated Promotility agents allowed but not required Early mobilization is required	[54]
Surgical drain management	The placement of routine prophylactic drains is not recommended Nasogastric tubes are not recommended	[56–58, 68, 69]
Surgical approach	When feasible, a minimally invasive approach is favored	[70–72, 74, 93]

Preoperative Instructions

Although there is no strong evidence to support a nutritional strategy specifically for liver surgery in the immediate preoperative period, several recommendations have been adopted from abdominal/intestinal surgical literature. In fact, complete overnight fasting is not recommended, and patients are allowed solid food until midnight but also advised to have carbohydrate-rich drinks until 2 hours before anesthesia induction [9]. This was shown to be safe and to reduce risks of insulin resistance, which in turn can be beneficial for hepatic surgery in the context of liver regeneration requirements [10–12]. Specific agents such as immunonutrition failed to have a significant impact on postoperative outcomes after liver surgery and are therefore not required [13].

Perioperative Analgesia

One of the pillars of ERLS is adequate and opiate-sparing perioperative analgesia. The integration of multimodal analgesia starts in the preoperative period, with patient evaluation, assessment of prior narcotic usage, patient education, and discussions on expectations related to pain management in the perioperative period [8]. Engaging patients early in the process of perioperative pain control has been shown to improve surgical recovery [14, 15]. In fact, a randomized controlled trial of 652 surgical patients ≥65 years of age showed that preoperative patient education and empowerment through patient booklets and diaries had significant positive impact with regard to short-term quality of life and postoperative pain [15]. In terms of type of perioperative analgesia, studies have evaluated the benefits of various modalities, which include epidural anesthesia (EA), transversus abdominis plane (TAP) blocks, quadratus lumborum (QL) blocks, and intravenous patient-controlled analgesia (IV-PCA). Regarding EA, a recent analysis of the national utilization patterns was done using the National Inpatient Sample (NIS) database and demonstrated that for over 53,000 patients who underwent hepatobiliary operations, for which the majority (94.7%) were open procedures, only 7.4% received EA. This low utilization rate may partially be explained by controversies around EA for hepatobiliary surgeries. For example, it was hypothesized that epidural-induced hemodynamic changes could result in reflexive boluses of excess IV fluid with subsequent compromise of enteric anastomoses and gastrointestinal recovery including ascites formation, due to the extra fluid shifts [16]. This concept has been challenged as several advantages of thoracic EA after major hepatobiliary surgery have been demonstrated [17]. A recent randomized controlled trial comparing 106 patients with thoracic EA to 34 patients who received IV-PCA alone for hepatobiliary operations showed superior pain control (as measured by pain scores in the first 48 hours postoperatively), less narcotic requirements, and improved patient satisfaction for the EA group [17]. In addition to the opioid-sparing advantages of EA, there may be an oncological benefit for adequate pain control with EA, which has been shown in a series of 510 patients who underwent liver resection for colorectal liver metastasis and exhibited superior recurrence-free survival. This oncological benefit was thought to be due to the modulation of perioperative inflammatory and immune mechanisms [18–20]. On the other hand, prospective evidence favoring IV-PCA has suggested that this strategy could potentially be advantageous in terms of length of stay as another measure of immediate postoperative recovery [21]. In this trial, however, the investigators evaluated combination therapy (IV-PCA plus regional anesthesia) as the "PCA" group, compared to EA. That study showed pain scores favoring EA, consistent with the results reported by Aloia et al.; however, the time required to fulfill discharge criteria was longer in the EA group. Finally, the transversus abdominis plane block, or TAP block, which was first described in 2001 and consists of an ultrasound-guided regional nerve block [22], is one of several promising regional anesthetic block strategies that can be used as part of a multimodal analgesia regimen. However, there are currently no randomized data evaluating its benefits over other modalities such as IV-PCA alone or EA for hepatectomy. A recent randomized controlled trial showed superiority of TAP block over EA in terms of reduction of hypotension episodes and IV opioid usage, but the cohort was heterogenous with different types of abdominal surgeries and not specifically for patients undergoing hepatectomy [23]. At the time of the writing of this chapter, a trial comparing TAP block to EA was enrolling at the same institution that published the previous IV-PCA vs. EA study (clinicaltrial.gov, NCT03214510), hoping to clarify the more advantageous approach for patients undergoing liver resection.

The optimal analgesia multimodality plan for liver resection remains debatable and is likely a combination of regional anesthesia within the framework of non-opioid bundles. Several prospective randomized controlled studies are currently ongoing in the aim of determining the optimal strategy in the enhanced recovery framework, such as comparison of continuous wound infusion and PCA vs. epidural for hepatobiliary procedures [24]. Regardless of the modality used, which can be institution and/or surgeon dependent, favoring an opioid-sparing strategy remains at the forefront of the enhanced recovery approach.

Perioperative Antimicrobial Prophylaxis

Before liver surgery, antimicrobial prophylaxis is part of the routine preoperative management for hepatectomy patients. Liver resection is classified as a clean-contaminated surgery due to the planned violation of the biliary system. There is no evidence for systematic use of antimicrobial prophylaxis and a specific antimicrobial in liver surgery [25]; however, the current recommendations point out to administration of a single dose of antibiotics less than an hour before the incision as with other gastrointestinal surgery [11, 26].

Venous Thromboembolism Prophylaxis

Regarding antithrombotic prophylaxis, the incidence of clinically detected venous thromboembolism (VTE) after hepatectomy is approximately 2.9% based on national databases [27, 28]. Hepatectomy itself is considered an independent risk factor for pulmonary embolism (PE) [29], and the extent of liver resection has in fact been shown to have a correlation directly proportional to the incidence of VTE, [28] with partial hepatectomy and extended hepatectomy having associated VTE in 2.1 and 5.8% of cases, respectively. In terms of risk factors, the presence of previous thromboembolic event will further increase the odds of having a PE after liver resection (OR 8.8) [30]. Moreover, additional elements—some of which potentially modifiable—such as extended operative time, presence of organ space infection, return to the operating room, and prolonged length of hospital stay are risk factors for VTE [31, 32].

As in any major operative procedures, perioperative VTE prophylaxis is recommended for hepatectomy although the evidence is lacking for preoperative administration. In fact, given the lack of clear benefit, coupled with the unpredictable nature of the procedure with potential hemorrhage and need for transfusions, pre-incision VTE chemoprophylaxis (subcutaneous heparin 5000 units or enoxaparin 40 mg daily) is not a "required" guideline item, as recently stated by an expert panel [33]. While this expert panel did not require pre-incision VTE chemoprophylaxis, a large series of HPB operations with preoperative and postoperative thromboelastograms showed no increase in post-hepatectomy hemorrhage and/or transfusions with almost no VTE when chemoprophylaxis is used pre-incision and then again 6 hours after closure, in the recovery room [34]. The use of sequential pneumatic device is however supported by current evidence as an intraoperative measure of prophylaxis. In the postoperative period, VTE chemoprophylaxis should be administered with low-molecular-weight heparin (enoxaparin), or heparin if renal impairment, and should be initiated in the immediate postoperative period [33] and for a total of 28 days, given the high-risk profile of these patients [34–37]. Special considerations include postoperative liver insufficiency, with or without concomitant cirrhosis, during which the risk of VTE is paradoxically increased [28]. However, no evidence exists to justify withholding VTE chemoprophylaxis in the setting of cirrhosis, unless the baseline platelet count is less than 100,000 mm/m3 and/or INR more than 1.8, both implying portal hypertension and/or intrinsic liver dysfunction [33].

Fluid Therapy

Fluid management represents a major component of ERLS, both in intraoperative and postoperative settings. Utilization of a low central venous pressure (CVP) during liver resection to reduce hepatic venous congestion and facilitate parenchymal transection and caval dissection has been the cornerstone of intraoperative fluid management. This technique has been associated with a reduction in blood loss, subsequent need for perioperative transfusions, as well as overall morbidity and mortality [25, 38–44]. Of note, this does not require a CVP line but simply judicious fluid management and noninvasive monitors of stroke volume variance using just an arterial line. Reduction of blood loss is particularly important in patients with CLM given the known detrimental effects of perioperative blood transfusions on oncological outcomes [45]. A recent Cochrane review by Moggia et al. [46] also suggested that a strategy of normovolemic hemodilution plus low central venous pressure, as opposed to low central venous pressure only, was associated with less blood transfusions during hepatectomy (OR 3.19, 95% CI 1.56 to 6.95), although based on low-level evidence. The goal in this approach is to maintain euvolemia by immediate preoperative removal of a calculated volume of autologous blood and storage during the procedure. This volume is then replaced appropriately with crystalloid or colloid solutions [47, 48]. As the hematocrit decreases, the red blood cell count loss is reduced as well, contributing to reduced need for packed red blood cell transfusions while maintaining intravascular volume and cardiac output [49]. Still, the main strategy revolves around low CVP-assisted liver surgery and constant communication and collaboration between surgeons and anesthetists to optimize intraoperative management and outcomes. With attentive fluid restriction, hemodilution protocols are viewed by many as unnecessarily complicated protocols since a goal of zero allogeneic transfusion is possible even without autotransfusions [34, 50].

Immediately postoperatively, goal-directed fluid therapy should be continued in order to avoid potential morbidity associated with hyper- or hypovolemia. A recent study by Patel et al. [51] evaluated the impact of utilizing serum brain natriuretic peptide (BNP)-guided fluid therapy. The proposed algorithm suggests that fluid bolus should be given when BNP is <100 pg/mL, suggesting intravascular depletion, that a range of 100–200 pg/mL signifies euvolemia, and that a value of >200 pg/mL indicated the need for intravenous fluid reduction or diuresis. In this series of 460 patients, cardiopulmonary and renal complications were reduced from 4% to 0.9% using this hepatobiliary fluid protocol.

Early Gastrointestinal Function

Although evidence suggests that implementation of ERAS protocols is associated with a significant reduction in postoperative ileus [43, 52, 53], no specific medical intervention such as use of promotility agents and laxatives have been shown to effectively shorten the length of stay by accelerating gastrointestinal function recovery after liver surgery [54]. However, since they are relatively benign in nature, promotility agents and gentle laxatives are usual components of ERLS protocols as well as early oral diet on the day of surgery and advancement per the patient rather than waiting for flatus or a bowel movement. Early patient mobilization in the immediate postoperative period is also strongly encouraged, as immobilization is known to have detrimental effects as well as potentially increases the risk of ileus.

Surgical Drain Management

Depending on the reported series and the extent of resection, post-hepatectomy bile leak can occur in approximately 12% of patients undergoing liver resection without biliary reconstruction, which is the case for most CLM resections. Judicious use of intra-abdominal drains after liver surgery is a critical component of an ERLS approach. Although some authors suggested that prophylactic abdominal drainage after hepatectomy might reduce the incidence of subphrenic abscesses [55], overwhelming evidence suggests that restrictive use of operative drains is more favorable. A large analysis of 2583 patients using the National Surgical Quality Improvement Program (NSQIP) targeted procedure database for hepatectomies reported that routine operative drainage was associated with more adverse short-term outcomes and did not facilitate early diagnosis of biliary collections, advocating against the routine placement of drains [56]. These results were also corroborated in patients specifically undergoing major hepatectomy [57]. Although specific indications for operative drainage were not prospectively evaluated, active strategies exist in order to maximize the benefits of using operative drains after hepatectomy. The air leak test (ALT), which was first described by Zimmitti et al. in 2013, was shown to be effective in reducing the risk of bile leaks for patients undergoing major liver resection, with a rate decreasing to 1.9% with ALT compared to 10.8% without ALT ($p = 0.008$) [58].

Although this strategy is effective in reducing bile leaks as well as risks for organ space infections [58, 59], specific recommendations on drain placement if the test is initially positive are not clear, as the placement of operative drain was at the discretion of the surgeons in these studies. Given that routine drains have fallen out of favor, the use of operative drains when performing an air leak test should be reserved to situations when the leak test remains positive after multiple repair attempts. It is also important to differentiate that the air leak test is performed after any more evident or larger leak is seen and repaired using a white sponge applied on the transected parenchymal surface. Its use is reserved for detection of occult bile leaks that would not be obvious but would later develop into an intra-abdominal collection. A similar technique, the "white test," had been reported in the past where injection of 5% fat emulsion in the biliary system was described in order to facilitate detection of bile leaks. However, air injection might represent a more practical technique as opposed to using fat emulsion or other agents like methylene blue or indocyanine green, as previously reported [60–63]. Nevertheless, once an operative drain is placed based on the surgeon's clinical decision, early removal has been advocated as a strategy integral to an enhanced recovery strategy [64]. Although the optimal timing of removal remains debatable and not standardized, several investigators reported safe removal of the operative on postoperative day 3, as long as the drain bilirubin level remains less than 3 times the serum bilirubin [64–67]. Given the sum of evidence, prophylactic drains should be avoided since they seem to be associated with more bile leaks, and they go against a basic ERAS tenet of reducing tubes and drains. On the topic of tubes and drains, the same principle goes with the use of a nasogastric tube, for which there is strong evidence that its prophylactic use should be avoided, given the increase risks of pulmonary complications associated with it [68, 69].

Surgical Approach

Although minimally invasive hepatic surgery is beyond the scope of this chapter, minimizing incisions when technically feasible is in line with principles of enhanced surgical recovery. In a recent review reporting over 9000 cases, laparoscopic cases were associated with significant short-term advantages such as a reduced length of stay, complications, and mortality, which was shown for both minor and major liver resections [70]. Overall, evidence suggests not only safety of a minimally invasive approach but favorable short-term outcomes over open liver resection, provided that the procedures are performed by trained and experienced surgeons. The main reasons contributing for superiority of a minimally invasive approach are by reducing the complication rates and length of stay [71–74]. These core elements are summarized in Table 25.1.

ERLS-Associated Outcomes

Short-Term Surgical Outcomes

Several short-term metrics can be evaluated to measure the impact of ERLS. Pooled analyses of reported enhanced recovery programs after hepatectomy [75–77] suggested that ERLS programs significantly reduce the complication rate, reduce the median length of stay to 4–5 days from 7 to 11 days, and are safe with similar mortality. Specifically for CLM, Dunne et al. reported similar effect in terms of reduced length of stay, decreased rate of intensive care unit utilization, and no significant increase in terms of overall complications or mortality compared to the non-ERLS group [78]. Certainly for elderly patients considered for CLM resection, [79] a multimodal approach through an ERLS program has been shown to confer acceptable outcomes, facilitating the performance of hepatectomy in selected octogenarians.

Long-Term Oncological Outcomes

Given that ERLS promotes a multimodal approach that aims for reductions in perioperative inflammation, transfusions, and complication rates, along with overall efficient recovery, the benefits of implementing ERLS pathways in oncological patients are obvious. Several analyses [80, 81] demonstrated clear evidence that postoperative complications have a negative oncological impact in patients undergoing resection of colorectal liver metastasis, in terms of worse disease-free survival and overall survival. Postoperative complications can preclude or delay timely administration of adjuvant therapy. A novel mnemonic was recently proposed by Aloia et al. called "RIOT," which stands for "return to intended oncologic treatment" [82]. In one RIOT study, patients with CLM with delayed or omitted timely adjuvant therapy were more likely to have experienced postoperative complications ($p = 0.039$). As expected, this non-RIOT group exhibited significantly worse disease-free and overall survival. Further studies should aim to evaluate the exact impact of ERLS on RIOT. The long-term benefits were also highlighted in a study where ERLS patients had significantly superior survival after 2 years compared to traditional pathway, implying an advantage of this strategy that extends beyond the immediate postoperative period [83].

Cost-Effectiveness and Economic Benefit

In an era of increasing awareness of resource utilization, implementation of ERAS programs in general has also proven to have an economic benefit, mainly by reduced medical costs with less complications. Joliat et al. [84] investigated the economic impact of ERAS, and despite higher costs related to anesthesia and operating room expenses, encouraging results overall favored the ERAS approach. A benefit of ERLS protocols over traditional care was also indicated by cost-effectiveness analyses in patients undergoing laparoscopic hepatectomies, again mainly by the significant decrease in postoperative complications [71, 85], as well as length of stay [72].

Patient-Reported Outcomes

Interference with oncological treatment plans can negatively affect patients' long-term outcomes but can also be detrimental to quality of life and overall functional status. Patient-reported outcomes (PROs) attempt to capture the patients' perspective for a given intervention or treatment strategy, which are particularly important in oncological patients. Day et al. reported that the implementation of ERLS was beneficial for patients in terms of functional recovery, and although no significant differences were detected in terms of symptom burden, the impact of ERLS was shown to accelerate functional recovery by returning to baseline interference earlier. This positive effect from ERLS seems more pronounced in patients undergoing open hepatectomy over those already benefiting from minimally invasive surgery [86].

Challenges in Implementation

Despite the overwhelming evidence endorsing the implementation of fast-track protocols, several barriers exist that explain variability in implementation and adherence in clinical practice. Adherence to the items of enhanced recovery programs has been evaluated and has a direct correlation with postoperative outcomes [87]. Since it is known that perioperative management can sometimes be highly variable among individual practitioners and can deviate from evidence-based medicine [88, 89], it is not surprising that the implementation of a somewhat more rigid structure that guides perioperative management is challenging to implement and sustain. Another challenge is coming from the multidisciplinary aspect of enhanced recovery, which requires the different specialties to engage in the perioperative care of these patients in a more standardized way, which requires agreement a priori.

At another level, reproducibility of ERAS programs from one institution to the other could be improved and would facilitate the accurate measurement of ERAS impact and outcomes at a larger scale. One starting point consists of accurately reporting in detail the elements of ERAS programs, including their adherence, in order to facilitate not only reproducibility but to ensure quality improvement across institutions and over time. A study evaluated the extent of reporting as well as program compliance and in fact demonstrated a low level of completeness in terms of reporting the individual enhanced surgical recovery elements [90]. Common outcome measures of interest, like morbidity, mortality, and length of stay, seem to be consistently reported in studies, but describing the core elements and their adherence remains of low quality and warrants more attention in order to have these concepts adopted into surgical practice.

Conclusion

ERLS programs are safe and highly effective for patients undergoing hepatectomy. The advantages are particularly relevant for patients with CLM, who oftentimes have longitudinal treatment strategies during which optimal operative recovery has a positive impact on long-term oncological outcomes. Hence, the benefits for these patients extend beyond commonly reported short-term surgical outcomes, such as length of stay and morbidity. Although implementation of such programs is rapidly spreading in the surgical community, ongoing efforts are still needed to continuously improve reporting in studies, enhance protocol compliance, and ultimately optimize patient-centered outcomes and quality of life.

References

1. Kehlet H. Fast-track colorectal surgery. Lancet. 2008;371:791–3.
2. Muehling B, Schelzig H, Steffen P, Meierhenrich R, Sunder-Plassmann L, Orend K-H. A prospective randomized trial comparing traditional and fast-track patient care in elective open infrarenal aneurysm repair. World J Surg. 2009;33:577–85.
3. Arsalani-Zadeh R, ELFadl D, Yassin N, MacFie J. Evidence-based review of enhancing postoperative recovery after breast surgery. Br J Surg. 2010;98:181–96.
4. Magheli A, Knoll N, Lein M, Hinz S, Kempkensteffen C, Gralla O. Impact of fast-track postoperative care on intestinal function, pain, and length of hospital stay after laparoscopic radical prostatectomy. J Endourol. 2011;25:1143–7.
5. Owens K, Stovall DW. Use of Enhanced Recovery After Surgery (ERAS) in major gynecologic surgery [1R]. Obstet Gynecol. 2018;131:194S–5S.
6. Scott NB, McDonald D, Campbell J, Smith RD, Carey AK, Johnston IG, James KR, Breusch SJ. The use of enhanced recovery after surgery (ERAS) principles in Scottish orthopaedic units—an implementation and follow-up at 1 year, 2010–2011: a report from the Musculoskeletal Audit, Scotland. Arch Orthop Trauma Surg. 2012;133:117–24.

7. van Dam RM, Hendry PO, Coolsen MME, Bemelmans MHA, Lassen K, Revhaug A, Fearon KCH, Garden OJ, Dejong CHC, on behalf of the Enhanced Recovery After Surgery (ERAS) Group. Initial experience with a multimodal enhanced recovery programme in patients undergoing liver resection. Br J Surg. 2008;95:969–75.
8. Kim BJ, Aloia TA. What is "Enhanced Recovery," and how can i do it? J Gastrointest Surg. 2017;22:164–71.
9. Nygren J, Thacker J, Carli F, Fearon KCH, Norderval S, Lobo DN, Ljungqvist O, Soop M, Ramirez J, Enhanced Recovery After Surgery Society. Guidelines for perioperative care in elective rectal/pelvic surgery: Enhanced Recovery After Surgery (ERAS®) Society recommendations. Clin Nutr. 2012;31:801–16.
10. Hassanain M, Metrakos P, Fisette A, Doi SAR, Schricker T, Lattermann R, Carvalho G, Wykes L, Molla H, Cianflone K. Randomized clinical trial of the impact of insulin therapy on liver function in patients undergoing major liver resection. Br J Surg. 2013;100:610–8.
11. Melloul E, Hübner M, Scott M, et al. Guidelines for perioperative care for liver surgery: Enhanced Recovery After Surgery (ERAS) Society recommendations. World J Surg. 2016;40:2425–40.
12. Bilku DK, Dennison AR, Hall TC, Metcalfe MS, Garcea G. Role of preoperative carbohydrate loading: a systematic review. Ann R Coll Surg Engl. 2014;96:15–22.
13. Zacharias T, Ferreira N, Carin A-J. Preoperative immunonutrition in liver resection—a propensity score matched case-control analysis. Eur J Clin Nutr. 2014;68:964–9.
14. Chou R, Gordon DB, de Leon-Casasola OA, et al. Management of postoperative pain: a clinical practice guideline from the American Pain Society, the American Society of Regional Anesthesia and Pain Medicine, and the American Society of Anesthesiologists' Committee on Regional Anesthesia, Executive Committee, and Administrative Council. J Pain. 2016;17:131–57.
15. Schmidt M, Eckardt R, Scholtz K, Neuner B, von Dossow-Hanfstingl V, Sehouli J, Stief CG, Wernecke K-D, Spies CD, PERATECS Group. Patient empowerment improved perioperative quality of care in cancer patients aged ≥ 65 years - a randomized controlled trial. PLoS One. 2015;10:e0137824.
16. Pratt WB, Steinbrook RA, Maithel SK, Vanounou T, Callery MP, Vollmer CM Jr. Epidural analgesia for pancreatoduodenectomy: a critical appraisal. J Gastrointest Surg. 2008;12:1207–20.
17. Aloia TA, Kim BJ, Segraves-Chun YS, et al. A randomized controlled trial of postoperative thoracic epidural analgesia versus intravenous patient-controlled analgesia after major hepatopancreatobiliary surgery. Ann Surg. 2017;266:545–54.
18. Zimmitti G, Soliz J, Aloia TA, Gottumukkala V, Cata JP, Tzeng C-WD, Vauthey J-N. Positive impact of epidural analgesia on oncologic outcomes in patients undergoing resection of colorectal liver metastases. Ann Surg Oncol. 2015;23:1003–11.
19. Cummings KC III, Xu F, Cummings LC, Cooper GS. A comparison of epidural analgesia and traditional pain management effects on survival and cancer recurrence after colectomy. Surv Anesthesiol. 2013;57:153–4.
20. Wuethrich PY, Hsu Schmitz S-F, Kessler TM, Thalmann GN, Studer UE, Stueber F, Burkhard FC. Potential influence of the anesthetic technique used during open radical prostatectomy on prostate cancer-related outcome. Anesthesiology. 2010;113:1–576.
21. Revie EJ, McKeown DW, Wilson JA, Garden OJ, Wigmore SJ. Randomized clinical trial of local infiltration plus patient-controlled opiate analgesia vs. epidural analgesia following liver resection surgery. HPB. 2012;14:611–8.
22. Lissauer J, Mancuso K, Merritt C, Prabhakar A, Kaye AD, Urman RD. Evolution of the transversus abdominis plane block and its role in postoperative analgesia. Best Pract Res Clin Anaesthesiol. 2014;28:117–26.
23. Shaker TM, Carroll JT, Chung MH, Koehler TJ, Lane BR, Wolf AM, Wright GP. Efficacy and safety of transversus abdominis plane blocks versus thoracic epidural anesthesia in patients undergoing major abdominal oncologic resections: a prospective, randomized controlled trial. Am J Surg. 2018;215:498–501.

24. Mungroop TH, Veelo DP, Busch OR, et al. Continuous wound infiltration or epidural analgesia for pain prevention after hepato-pancreato-biliary surgery within an enhanced recovery program (POP-UP trial): study protocol for a randomized controlled trial. Trials. 2015;16:562.
25. Gurusamy KS, Naik P, Davidson BR. Methods of decreasing infection to improve outcomes after liver resections. Cochrane Database Syst Rev. 2011;383:CD006933.
26. Bratzler DW, Houck PM. Antimicrobial prophylaxis for surgery: an advisory statement from the National Surgical Infection Prevention Project. Am J Surg. 2005;189:395–404.
27. Turley RS, Reddy SK, Shortell CK, Clary BM, Scarborough JE. Venous thromboembolism after hepatic resection: analysis of 5,706 patients. J Gastrointest Surg. 2012;16:1705–14.
28. Tzeng C-WD, Katz MHG, Fleming JB, Pisters PWT, Lee JE, Abdalla EK, Curley SA, Vauthey J-N, Aloia TA. Risk of venous thromboembolism outweighs post-hepatectomy bleeding complications: analysis of 5651 National Surgical Quality Improvement Program patients. HPB. 2012;14:506–13.
29. Melloul E, Dondéro F, Vilgrain V, Raptis DA, Paugam-Burtz C, Belghiti J. Pulmonary embolism after elective liver resection: a prospective analysis of risk factors. J Hepatol. 2012;57:1268–75.
30. Nobili C, Marzano E, Oussoultzoglou E, Rosso E, Addeo P, Bachellier P, Jaeck D, Pessaux P. Multivariate analysis of risk factors for pulmonary complications after hepatic resection. Ann Surg. 2012;255:540–50.
31. Ejaz A, Spolverato G, Kim Y, et al. Defining incidence and risk factors of venous thromboembolism after hepatectomy. J Gastrointest Surg. 2013;18:1116–24.
32. Tzeng C-WD, Curley SA, Vauthey J-N, Aloia TA. Distinct predictors of pre- versus post-discharge venous thromboembolism after hepatectomy: analysis of 7621 NSQIP patients. HPB. 2013;15:773–80.
33. Aloia TA, Geerts WH, Clary BM, Day RW, Hemming AW, D'Albuquerque LC, Vollmer CM, Vauthey J-N, Toogood GJ. Venous thromboembolism prophylaxis in liver surgery. J Gastrointest Surg. 2015;20:221–9.
34. Le A-T, Harris JW, Maynard E, Dineen SP, Tzeng C-WD. Thromboelastography demonstrates perioperative hypercoagulability in hepato-pancreato-biliary patients and supports routine administration of preoperative and early postoperative venous thromboembolism chemoprophylaxis. HPB. 2017;19:154–61.
35. Fagarasanu A, Alotaibi GS, Hrimiuc R, Lee AYY, Wu C. Role of extended thromboprophylaxis after abdominal and pelvic surgery in cancer patients: a systematic review and meta-analysis. Ann Surg Oncol. 2016;23:1422–30.
36. Rasmussen MS, Jørgensen LN, Wille-Jørgensen P. Prolonged thromboprophylaxis with low molecular weight heparin for abdominal or pelvic surgery. Cochrane Database Syst Rev. 2009;346:975.
37. Akl EA, Kahale LA, Schünemann HJ. Association between perioperative low-molecular-weight heparin vs unfractionated heparin and clinical outcomes in patients with cancer undergoing surgery. JAMA. 2015;313:1364.
38. Correa Gallego C, Berman A, Denis SC, et al. Renal function after low central venous pressure-assisted liver resection: assessment of 2116 cases. HPB. 2015;17:258–64.
39. Melendez JA, Arslan V, Fischer ME, Wuest D, Jarnagin WR, Fong Y, Blumgart LH. Perioperative outcomes of major hepatic resections under low central venous pressure anesthesia: blood loss, blood transfusion, and the risk of postoperative renal dysfunction. J Am Coll Surg. 1998;187:620–5.
40. Chen H. Hepatic resection using intermittent vascular inflow occlusion and low central venous pressure anesthesia improves morbidity and mortality. J Gastrointest Surg. 2000;4:162–7.
41. Jones, Moulton, Hardy. Central venous pressure and its effect on blood loss during liver resection. Br J Surg. 1998;85:1058–60.
42. Li Z. Controlled low central venous pressure reduces blood loss and transfusion requirements in hepatectomy. World J Gastroenterol. 2014;20:303–9.
43. Hughes MJ, Ventham NT, Harrison EM, Wigmore SJ. Central venous pressure and liver resection: a systematic review and meta analysis. HPB. 2015;17:863–71.

44. Gurusamy KS, Li J, Vaughan J, Sharma D, Davidson BR. Cardiopulmonary interventions to decrease blood loss and blood transfusion requirements for liver resection. Cochrane Database Syst Rev. 2012;20:369.
45. Hallet JI, Tsang M, Cheng E, Kulyk IB, Hanna S, Law C, Coburn NG, Karanicolas PJ. The impact of perioperative red blood cell transfusion on long-term survival after hepatectomy for colorectal liver metastases. J Clin Oncol. 2015;33:725.
46. Moggia E, Rouse B, Simillis C, Li T, Vaughan J, Davidson BR, Gurusamy KS. Methods to decrease blood loss during liver resection: a network meta-analysis. Cochrane Database Syst Rev. 2016;92:954.
47. Guo J-R, Shen H-C, Liu Y, Xu F, Zhang Y-W, Shao Y, Su Y-J. Effect of acute Normovolemic Hemodilution combined with controlled low central venous pressure on blood coagulation function and blood loss in patients undergoing resection of liver cancer operation. Hepato-Gastroenterology. 2015;62:992–6.
48. Jarnagin WR, Gönen M, Maithel SK, et al. A prospective randomized trial of acute Normovolemic Hemodilution compared to standard intraoperative management in patients undergoing major hepatic resection. Trans Meet Am Surg Assoc. 2008;126:10–9.
49. Huntington JT, Royall NA, Schmidt CR. Minimizing blood loss during hepatectomy: a literature review. J Surg Oncol. 2013;109:81–8.
50. Day RW, Brudvik KW, Vauthey J-N, Conrad C, Gottumukkala V, Chun YS, Katz MH, Fleming JB, Lee JE, Aloia TA. Advances in hepatectomy technique: toward zero transfusions in the modern era of liver surgery. Surgery. 2016;159:793–801.
51. Patel SH, Kim BJ, Tzeng C-WD, Chun YS, Conrad C, Vauthey J-N, Aloia TA. Reduction of cardiopulmonary/renal complications with serum BNP-guided volume status management in posthepatectomy patients. J Gastrointest Surg. 2018;22:467–76.
52. Jones C, Kelliher L, Dickinson M, Riga A, Worthington T, Scott MJ, Vandrevala T, Fry CH, Karanjia N, Quiney N. Randomized clinical trial on enhanced recovery versus standard care following open liver resection. Br J Surg. 2013;100:1015–24.
53. Ni CY, Yang Y, Chang YQ, Cai H, Xu B, Yang F, Lau WY, Wang ZH, Zhou WP. Fast-track surgery improves postoperative recovery in patients undergoing partial hepatectomy for primary liver cancer: a prospective randomized controlled trial. Eur J Surg Oncol. 2013;39: 542–7.
54. Hendry PO, van Dam RM, Bukkems SFFW, McKeown DW, Parks RW, Preston T, Dejong CHC, Garden OJ, Fearon KCH. Randomized clinical trial of laxatives and oral nutritional supplements within an enhanced recovery after surgery protocol following liver resection. Br J Surg. 2010;97:1198–206.
55. Kyoden Y, Imamura H, Sano K, Beck Y, Sugawara Y, Kokudo N, Makuuchi M. Value of prophylactic abdominal drainage in 1269 consecutive cases of elective liver resection. J Hepatobiliary Pancreat Sci. 2009;17:186–92.
56. Brauer DG, Nywening TM, Jaques DP, Doyle MBM, Chapman WC, Fields RC, Hawkins WG. Operative site drainage after hepatectomy: a propensity score matched analysis using the American College of Surgeons NSQIP targeted hepatectomy database. J Am Coll Surg. 2016;223:774–783.e2.
57. Squires MH III, Lad NL, Fisher SB, et al. Value of primary operative drain placement after major hepatectomy: a multi-institutional analysis of 1,041 patients. J Am Coll Surg. 2015;220:396–402.
58. Zimmitti G, Vauthey J-N, Shindoh J, Tzeng C-WD, Roses RE, Ribero D, Capussotti L, Giuliante F, Nuzzo G, Aloia TA. Systematic use of an intraoperative air leak test at the time of major liver resection reduces the rate of postoperative biliary complications. J Am Coll Surg. 2013;217:1028–37.
59. Tran Cao HS, Phuoc V, Ismael H, Denbo JW, Passot G, Yamashita S, Conrad C, Aloia TA, Vauthey JN. Rate of organ space infection is reduced with the use of an air leak test during major hepatectomies. J Gastrointest Surg. 2016;21:85–93.
60. McFadden DW. The white test: a new dye test for intraoperative detection of bile leakage during major liver resection--invited critique. Arch Surg. 2008;143:404.

61. Li J, Malagó M, Sotiropoulos GC, Lang H, Schaffer R, Paul A, Broelsch CE, Nadalin S. Intraoperative application of "white test" to reduce postoperative bile leak after major liver resection: results of a prospective cohort study in 137 patients. Langenbeck's Arch Surg. 2008;394:1019–24.
62. Lam C-M, Lo C-M, Liu C-L, Fan S-T. Biliary complications during liver resection. World J Surg. 2014;25:1273–6.
63. Yamashita Y-I, Hamatsu T, Rikimaru T, Tanaka S, Shirabe K, Shimada M, Sugimachi K. Bile leakage after hepatic resection. Ann Surg. 2001;233:45–50.
64. Hokuto D, Nomi T, Yasuda S, Kawaguchi C, Yoshikawa T, Ishioka K, Obara S, Yamada T, Kanehiro H. The safety of the early removal of prophylactic drainage after liver resection based solely on predetermined criteria: a propensity score analysis. HPB. 2017;19:359–64.
65. Yamazaki S, Takayama T, Moriguchi M, Mitsuka Y, Okada S, Midorikawa Y, Nakayama H, Higaki T. Criteria for drain removal following liver resection. Br J Surg. 2012;99:1584–90.
66. Tanaka K, Kumamoto T, Nojiri K, Takeda K, Endo I. The effectiveness and appropriate management of abdominal drains in patients undergoing elective liver resection: a retrospective analysis and prospective case series. Surg Today. 2012;43:372–80.
67. Torzilli G, Nagino M, Tzeng C-WD, et al. SSAT State-of-the-Art Conference: new frontiers in liver surgery. J Gastrointest Surg. 2016;21:175–85.
68. Verma R, Nelson RL. Prophylactic nasogastric decompression after abdominal surgery. Cochrane Database Syst Rev. 2007;8:85.
69. Pessaux P, Regimbeau JM, Dondéro F, Plasse M, Mantz J, Belghiti J. Randomized clinical trial evaluating the need for routine nasogastric decompression after elective hepatic resection. Br J Surg. 2007;94:297–303.
70. Ciria R, Cherqui D, Geller DA, Briceno J, Wakabayashi G. Comparative short-term benefits of laparoscopic liver resection. Ann Surg. 2016;263:761–77.
71. Mirnezami R, Mirnezami AH, Chandrakumaran K, Abu Hilal M, Pearce NW, Primrose JN, Sutcliffe RP. Short- and long-term outcomes after laparoscopic and open hepatic resection: systematic review and meta-analysis. HPB. 2011;13:295–308.
72. Cleary SP, Han H-S, Yamamoto M, Wakabayashi G, Asbun HJ. The comparative costs of laparoscopic and open liver resection: a report for the 2nd international consensus conference on laparoscopic liver resection. Surg Endosc. 2016;30:4691–6.
73. Nguyen KT. Comparative benefits of laparoscopic vs open hepatic resection. Arch Surg. 2011;146:348.
74. Cherqui D. Evolution of laparoscopic liver resection. Br J Surg. 2016;103:1405–7.
75. Coolsen MME, Wong-Lun-Hing EM, van Dam RM, van der Wilt AA, Slim K, Lassen K, Dejong CHC. A systematic review of outcomes in patients undergoing liver surgery in an enhanced recovery after surgery pathways. HPB. 2013;15:245–51.
76. Hughes MJ, McNally S, Wigmore SJ. Enhanced recovery following liver surgery: a systematic review and meta-analysis. HPB. 2014;16:699–706.
77. Ni T-G. Enhanced recovery after surgery programs in patients undergoing hepatectomy: a meta-analysis. World J Gastroenterol. 2015;21:9209–16.
78. Dunne DFJ, Yip VS, Jones RP, et al. Enhanced recovery in the resection of colorectal liver metastases. J Surg Oncol. 2014;110:197–202.
79. Tufo A, Dunne DFJ, Manu N, Joshi H, Lacasia C, Jones L, Malik HZ, Poston GJ, Fenwick SW. Hepatectomy for octogenarians with colorectal liver metastasis in the era of enhanced recovery. Eur J Surg Oncol. 2018; https://doi.org/10.1016/j.ejso.2018.01.089.
80. Matsuda A, Matsumoto S, Seya T, Matsutani T, Kishi T, Yokoi K, Wang P, Uchida E. Does postoperative complication have a negative impact on long-term outcomes following hepatic resection for colorectal liver metastasis?: a meta-analysis. Ann Surg Oncol. 2013;20:2485–92.
81. Yin Z, Huang X, Ma T, Jin H, Lin Y, Yu M, Jian Z. Postoperative complications affect long-term survival outcomes following hepatic resection for colorectal liver metastasis. World J Surg. 2015;39:1818–27.

82. Aloia TA, Zimmitti G, Conrad C, Gottumukalla V, Kopetz S, Vauthey J-N. Return to intended oncologic treatment (RIOT): a novel metric for evaluating the quality of oncosurgical therapy for malignancy. J Surg Oncol. 2014;110:107–14.
83. Morrison B, Jones C, Kelliher L, Scott M, Dickinson M, Karanjia N, Quiney N. ERAS for open liver resection surgery improves two-year survival but not five-year survival. Clin Nutr ESPEN. 2017;19:78.
84. Joliat G-R, Labgaa I, Hübner M, Blanc C, Griesser A-C, Schäfer M, Demartines N. Cost–benefit analysis of the implementation of an enhanced recovery program in liver surgery. World J Surg. 2016;40:2441–50.
85. Wang C, Zheng G, Zhang W, Zhang F, Lv S, Wang A, Fang Z. Enhanced recovery after surgery programs for liver resection: a meta-analysis. J Gastrointest Surg. 2017;21:472–86.
86. Day RW, Cleeland CS, Wang XS, Fielder S, Calhoun J, Conrad C, Vauthey J-N, Gottumukkala V, Aloia TA. Patient-reported outcomes accurately measure the value of an enhanced recovery program in liver surgery. J Am Coll Surg. 2015;221:1023–1030.e2.
87. Feroci F, Lenzi E, Baraghini M, Garzi A, Vannucchi A, Cantafio S, Scatizzi M. Fast-track colorectal surgery: protocol adherence influences postoperative outcomes. Int J Color Dis. 2012;28:103–9.
88. Fearon KCH, Ljungqvist O, Meyenfeldt Von M, et al. Enhanced recovery after surgery: a consensus review of clinical care for patients undergoing colonic resection. Clin Nutr. 2005;24:466–77.
89. Lassen K, Hannemann P, Ljungqvist O, Fearon K, Dejong CHC, von Meyenfeldt MF, Hausel J, Nygren J, Andersen J, Revhaug A. Patterns in current perioperative practice: survey of colorectal surgeons in five northern European countries. BMJ. 2005;330:1420–1.
90. Day RW, Fielder S, Calhoun J, Kehlet H, Gottumukkala V, Aloia TA. Incomplete reporting of enhanced recovery elements and its impact on achieving quality improvement. Br J Surg. 2015;102:1594–602.
91. Gustafsson UO, Scott MJ, Schwenk W, et al. Guidelines for perioperative care in elective colonic surgery: Enhanced Recovery After Surgery (ERAS®) Society Recommendations. World J Surg. 2012;37:259–84.
92. Practice guidelines for preoperative fasting and the use of pharmacologic agents to reduce the risk of pulmonary aspiration. Anesthesiology. 2017;126:376–93.
93. Nguyen KT, Laurent A, Dagher I, et al. Minimally invasive liver resection for metastatic colorectal cancer: a multi-institutional, international report of safety, feasibility, and early outcomes. Ann Surg. 2009;250:842–8.

Surgical Results for Synchronous Colorectal Cancer Liver Metastases

26

Rinaldo Gonçalves, Marcus Valadão, and Rodrigo Araújo

Colorectal cancer (CRC) is the third most commonly diagnosed malignancy and the fourth leading cause of cancer death in the world, accounting for about 1.4 million new cases and almost 700,000 deaths in 2012 and projected 1.1 million cancer deaths by 2030 [1]. The most common metastatic site is the liver, with 15–25% of patients presenting colorectal liver metastases (CRLM) at the time of diagnosis [2, 3].

The presence of (CRLM) is the main prognostic factor, conferring a median survival of 6–12 months in untreated patients [4]. Surgical treatment is the best chance for long-term survival, with 5-year survival of patients who underwent complete surgical resection for (CRLM) reaching 40–58% [5–7]. The optimal surgical management of patients with colorectal cancer and synchronous liver metastasis is a matter of debate. To date, there have been no randomized controlled trials on surgical approach of colorectal synchronous hepatic metastases. The information available are based on retrospective series with biases inherent to these types of studies [4].

Three strategies are possible when managing synchronous colorectal liver metastasis: the traditional approach, starting with the resection of the primary tumor followed by chemotherapy and liver resection at a later stage (colorectal-first approach); a combined approach, where both the primary tumor and metastatic liver disease are resected on a same procedure; and a reverse approach (liver-first approach), starting with chemotherapy and then going to the liver surgery followed by the colorectal surgery [8].

Traditionally, patients with synchronic liver metastases would undergo staged resection of their colorectal and hepatic tumors. Due to concerns about the progression of the primary tumor resulting in complications such as tumor bleeding, obstruction, and intestinal perforation, in the classical strategy, colorectal tumors would usually be resected at first, followed by chemotherapy, and liver metastases

R. Gonçalves (✉) · M. Valadão · R. Araújo
Department of Abdomino-Pelvic Surgery, Instituto Nacional de Câncer (INCA), Rio de Janeiro, Brazil
e-mail: rinaldo.silva@inca.gov.br; mvaladao@inca.gov.br; raraujo@inca.gov.br

M. M. Correia et al. (eds.), *Colorectal Cancer Liver Metastases*,
https://doi.org/10.1007/978-3-030-25486-5_26

resected at a later time. This would provide initial control of the primary tumor, eliminating the source of future metastases and the risk of urgent surgery related to tumor complications during the course of chemotherapy.

In addition, it would allow a better selection of patients so that patients who present disease progression after resection of the primary could be spared from unnecessary liver surgeries.

Recent advances in systemic chemotherapy, like infusional fluorouracil/leucovorin with oxaliplatin or irinotecan, and the addition of targeted therapeutic agents such as bevacizumab or cetuximab to the above combinations have provided response rates of up to 82% and disease control rates of 85% in prospective clinical trials, both in hepatic metastases and in the primary tumor, resulting in a relative infrequency of complications from unresected primary tumors [9–12].

Poultsides et al. analyzed the frequency of interventions necessary to palliate the primary tumor in patients who present with synchronous, stage IV colorectal cancer (CRC) and who receive up-front chemotherapy. Of 233 patients, 217 (93%) never required surgical palliation of their primary tumor. Sixteen patients (7%) required emergent surgery for primary tumor obstruction or perforation, 10 patients (4%) required nonoperative intervention (i.e., stent or radiotherapy), and 213 (89%) never required any direct symptomatic management for their intact primary tumor [13].

A multicenter phase II trial involving asymptomatic primary tumor and unresectable CRLMs analyzed the need for surgical resection due to symptoms related to the primary tumor in patients receiving oxaliplatin (mFOLFOX6) combined with bevacizumab. Among 86 eligible cases, there were 12 patients (14%) with major morbidity related to the primary tumor: 10 required surgery (eight, obstruction; one, perforation; and one, abdominal pain), and two patients died. The 24-month cumulative incidence of major morbidity was 16.3% [14]. On the other hand, a randomized study comparing open versus laparoscopic colectomy in 1082 patients with colon cancer found overall complication rate of 21%, anastomotic failure in 3%, and reintervention in 7% of the patients [15]. Similarly, a multicenter trial assessed the rate of symptomatic anastomotic leakage in patients operated on with low anterior resection for rectal cancer and who were intraoperatively randomized to a defunctioning stoma or not. The overall rate of symptomatic leakage was 19.2% (45 of 234). The need for urgent abdominal reoperation was 8.6% (10 of 116) in those randomized to stoma and 25.4% (30 of 118) in those without ($P < 0.001$) [16].

Thus, the initial surgical approach of the colorectal primary can determine a postoperative complication rate higher than the rate of complications related to the presence of the primary tumor left in situ and treated initially with chemotherapy. These possible surgical complications associated with postoperative immunodeficiency status may prevent or significantly delay the onset of chemotherapy, resulting in progression and loss of the possibility of a curative surgical approach to the liver metastases.

Tevis et al. reported the surgical results of 355 patients that underwent proctectomy with total mesorectal excision. Overall complication rate was 30%. Postoperative complications and 30-day readmissions were associated with delays in chemotherapy ≥8 weeks after surgery. Patients who received chemotherapy

≥8 weeks postoperatively were found to have worse local and distant recurrence rates and worse overall survival as compared with patients who received chemotherapy within 8 weeks of surgery [17]. In the multi-institutional LiverMetSurvey study, only 30% of patients managed with the classical approach were able undergo both colorectal and liver resections, comparing to 80% of treatment completion when the liver was approached first [18].

Most patients with colorectal metastases will succumb due to their liver metastases, making the liver approach a priority. In this way, some centers recommend liver approach before the primary tumor resection, especially in patients with a large-volume liver disease, in order to prevent delay in liver-directed therapy or in systemic treatment. In this strategy, the "liver-first" or reverse approach, a highly effective neoadjuvant chemotherapy is given first in order to control the CRLM at the same time as the colorectal primary, optimizing the chances of a curative liver resection and allowing an unhurried later resection of the primary tumor, especially in rectal cancer when chemoradiation is needed.

Mentha and colleagues first described this approach [19]. On their study, twenty consecutive patients with nonobstructive colonic (nine patients) or rectal (11 patients) cancer and advanced synchronous liver metastases were treated according to this strategy. Patients received between two and six cycles of 5-fluorouracil-, oxaliplatin-, and irinotecan-based chemotherapy before liver resection. Surgery of the colorectal primary was planned within 3–8 weeks after liver surgery or after completion of radiotherapy. Sixteen patients (80%) responded to treatment and underwent liver surgery with posterior removal of the colorectal primary. Overall actuarial survival rates at 1, 2, 3, and 4 years for the 16 patients whose tumors were resected were 100, 93, 81, and 61%.

The authors concluded that "This strategy produced resectability and survival rates better than those expected from the published data on patients with disease of similar severity. It allows initial control and downstaging of liver metastases, and delivery of preoperative radiotherapy for rectal cancer without the fear that liver metastases will meanwhile progress beyond the possibility of cure "[19].

De Rosa et al. analyzed thirty-seven patients with synchronous CRLM considered for this same strategy. After induction chemotherapy, thirty patients underwent hepatic resections with no postoperative deaths. Following liver resection, five patients failed to proceed to colorectal resection, and one patient had complete response to chemoradiotherapy. The overall 1- and 3-year survival rates were 65.9% and 30.4%, respectively [20].

Some groups have proposed simultaneous resection of both the primary and metastatic liver disease. This strategy would eliminate the need for two surgical procedures, resulting in less surgical and anesthetic trauma, with a consequent shorter period of postsurgical immunosuppression and overall reduction in the total hospital length of stay and costs. Despite the possible benefits of this strategy, the greater complexity involved in performing two surgical procedures at a single opportunity would invariably lead to greater complexity and safety and long-term survival issues, necessitating appropriate patient selection for this strategy as well as surgical teams trained to approach the primary tumor and liver lesions.

In spite of the theoretical benefits inherent in each of the approaches, there is no prospective randomized study comparing simultaneous or delayed approach. Retrospective studies comparing these strategies generally involve referral bias, institutional bias, and patient bias (different clinical profiles, different degrees of hepatic involvement, and nonhomogeneous localization of primary tumors—colon vs. rectum), making the data difficult to interpret [21–32, 34, 35].

Some series found similar perioperative and long-term results with both delayed and simultaneous strategies, but with overall less severe liver involvement and less major hepatectomies in the simultaneous group [21–32, 34–36]. One author reported worse disease-free survival in simultaneously treated patients [33]. Others reported no difference in morbidity and mortality even in patients who underwent major hepatic resections and more complex colorectal surgeries but with shorter length of hospital stay [28–31]. These inhomogeneous results reinforce the need for an individualized approach for each patient.

Weber et al. analyzed 97 patients presented with synchronous colorectal liver metastases. Thirty-five patients (36%) underwent a simultaneous resection, and 62 patients (64%) had a delayed resection. The morbidity (23% after simultaneous resection and 32% after delayed resection) and the 5 years overall survival rate (21% simultaneous resection and 22% delayed resection) did not differ significantly. However, the incidence of more than four liver metastases and a bilobar distribution were significantly higher in the delayed resection group than in the simultaneous resection group (37 and 68% vs. 17 and 23%, respectively), as well as the rate of major hepatectomies [21].

Martin et al. reported 134 patients who underwent simultaneous resection of a colorectal primary and hepatic metastases and 106 patients who underwent staged operations. Length of hospital stay was shorter for the simultaneous group (10 days vs. 18 days, $p < 0.001$), as well as the complication rate ($p < 0.003$), with similar perioperative mortality. However, the simultaneous resections tended to be performed for right colon primaries ($p < 0.001$), smaller ($p < 0.01$) and fewer ($p < 0.001$) liver metastases, and less extensive liver resection ($p < 0.001$) [22].

In a retrospective multicenter study involving 610 patients with synchronous colorectal cancer and liver metastases, 135 patients (22.1%) underwent simultaneous primary colorectal tumor and hepatic resection. The simultaneous group more often had smaller and fewer hepatic metastases and was mainly treated with wedge resections, whereas staged patients had larger hepatic metastases and more often underwent major hepatic resections. Staged patients more often were treated with left colectomy and low anterior resection, whereas simultaneous patients had more right colectomies. In this series, simultaneous colorectal resection and minor hepatectomy presented no differences in mortality, severe morbidity, hepatic-related morbidity, intraoperative blood loss, or frequency of blood transfusion compared to minor hepatic resection alone. However, among patients who underwent major hepatectomy, intraoperative blood loss, frequency of microscopic positive hepatic resection margins (R1 resection), mortality, overall morbidity, severe morbidity, and length of hospital stay were all greater after simultaneous resections compared to hepatectomy alone. The simultaneous approach was associated with a more than threefold risk of severe morbidity [23].

The same trend in increased mortality and morbidity associated with major hepatectomies and synchronous colorectal resection was observed in other series. Bolton and Fuhrman reported a mortality rate of 12% after synchronous resection and of 24% in case of major hepatectomies [24]. Tanaka et al. analyzed 39 consecutive patients who underwent simultaneous hepatectomy and colorectal resection. The mean volume of the resected liver appeared as a risk factor for postoperative complications (350 g in patients with postoperative complications vs. 150 g in those without complications) [25]. Nordlinger reported an operative mortality of 7% for simultaneous resections, compared with 2% for staged resections [26].

Similarly, Thelen et al. reported 40 patients who underwent simultaneous resection of liver metastases and primary colorectal cancer and 179 who underwent staged resections. Although morbidity and survival did not differ significantly between groups, the mortality rate was significantly higher in patients with simultaneous liver resection (10% vs. 1.1%, $p = 0.012$), in spite of the less extensive liver surgery performed more frequently in this group. The mortality after simultaneous liver resection ($n = 4$) occurred only after major hepatectomies [27].

Differently from the previous series where a higher mortality rate was associated with major hepatectomy and simultaneous colorectal resection, some reports found similar results despite the extension of the hepatic resection. Chua et al. analyzed 96 consecutive patients who underwent concurrent (64 patients) or staged (32 patients) resections. The groups were similar in the characteristics of hepatic metastases and the type of colon and hepatic resection. The authors found overall shorter duration of hospitalization for simultaneous resection (mean, 11 vs. 22 days; $P <$ or $= 0.001$), with no differences in perioperative morbidity and overall survival from date of hepatectomy (median, 27 vs. 34 months; $P = 0.52$) [28].

Capussoti et al. described similar results of mortality and anastomotic leak rates in 31 patients who underwent synchronous major hepatectomies and colorectal surgery when compared to 48 patients who underwent delayed major liver resections. Considering both surgical procedures (colorectal and liver resection), in delayed hepatectomies, morbidity was higher (56.3% vs. 32.6%, $P = .0369$) and hospitalization was longer (20.5 vs. 13.9 days, $P = .00001$). Nine patients underwent major hepatectomy and concurrent anterior rectal resection with no mortality (morbidity 22.2%, mean hospitalization 12.4 days) [29].

Martin et al. also found similar results to those of Capusotti reporting 70 patients who underwent simultaneous resections compared with 160 patients who underwent staged resection. In his series, there was similar proportion of major hepatic resections (more than 3 segments) performed for both groups, as well as the same rate of patients requiring rectal resection. The overall complication rate for simultaneous resection (56%) was similar for staged resections (55%; $p < 0.90$), even when the analysis was restricted to the 97 patients who underwent major liver resection (lobectomy or greater), with the overall complications rate of simultaneous resections (17 of 33, 50%) being significantly less than for staged resections (38 of 64, 60%) and length of hospital stay significantly shorter for the simultaneous resections than for the combined hospitalizations of the staged colorectal and hepatic resections [30].

Slesser et al. reported surgical results of 112 patients with synchronous colorectal liver metastases. Thirty-six had a simultaneous resection and 76 had a sequential resection. The groups were homogenous regarding chemotherapy use, site of the primary tumor, nodal status, number and size of liver metastases, the presence of extrahepatic metastases, and the CEA level. The rate of major hepatic resections (64% and 79% of the patients in the simultaneous and sequential groups, respectively, *P*-value 0.089) was the same, with more patients in the simultaneous group underwent low anterior resection. The perioperative results were similar but with shorter length of hospital stay in the simultaneous group, 14 days compared to 18.5 days in the sequential group (*P*-value 0.03). No significant difference regarding three-year disease-free survival, three-year hepatic recurrence-free survival, and three-year overall survival was found [31].

Differently from the study of Slesser et al., de Haas et al. reported worse recurrence-free survival for patients who underwent simultaneous resections. In this report, 228 patients underwent limited hepatectomy (less than three segments) for synchronous CLMs. Fifty-five (24·1%) had a simultaneous colorectal resection and 173 (75.9%) had delayed hepatectomy. The authors founded similar mortality rate in the two groups (0% vs. 0.6%, respectively; $P = 0{\cdot}557$), but cumulative morbidity was significantly lower in the simultaneous group (11% vs. 25.4% in the delayed group; $P = 0{\cdot}015$). The 3-year overall survival rate was 74% in the simultaneous group versus 70.3% in the delayed group ($P = 0{\cdot}871$). Despite the fact that the simultaneous strategy group had more patients with less extensive liver disease, significantly more recurrences were observed in this population at 3 years (85% vs. 63.6%; $P = 0{\cdot}002$). In this series, preoperative chemotherapy was used in only 24% of the patients in the simultaneous group compared with 95% in the delayed group. This difference in the use of chemotherapy could explain the higher recurrence rate in the simultaneous group [32]. In fact, a randomized controlled trial assessed the combination of perioperative chemotherapy and surgery compared with surgery alone for patients with initially resectable liver metastases from colorectal cancer. The authors found an increase in the rate of progression-free survival at 3 years from 28.1% to 35.4%, as well as an increase of the median progression-free survival from 11.7 months to 18.7 months with chemotherapy [33]. However, on the series of de Hass et al., in multivariable analysis, preoperative chemotherapy was not a predictor of recurrence [31]. This worse recurrence-free survival was not found in other more recent series or review articles [4, 34–37].

Brouquet et al. analyzed 72 patients who underwent classic, 43 combined, and 27 reverse strategies. Although the number of CLMs were higher in the reverse group (1 in the combined, 3 in the classic, and 4 in the reverse strategy group [$p < 0.01$ classic vs. reverse; $p < 0.001$ reverse vs. combined]), as well as the proportion of rectal tumor and major liver resection (24 patients [89%] vs. 63 [55%] in the 2 other groups, $p < 0.001$), postoperative mortality and postoperative cumulative morbidity rates were similar. Three-year and 5-year overall survival rates were, respectively, 65% and 55% in the combined, 58% and 48% in the classic, and 79% and 39% in the reverse strategy (NS). On multivariate analysis, liver tumor size >3 cm and cumulative postoperative morbidity were independently associated with overall survival after surgery [34].

A multi-institutional study involving 1004 patients treated for synchronous colorectal liver metastases compared staged approach (further divided as colorectal-first and liver-first approach) and simultaneous resection. Simultaneous CRC and liver resection was performed in 329 (33%) patients. Patients with bilateral hepatic disease (64.8% vs. 35.3% in unilateral disease; $p < 0.001$) and presenting higher number of CRLM ($p < 0.001$) were managing predominantly by a combined approach. Of these 675 patients (67.2%) managed in a staged fashion, 647 (64.4%) had the CRC primary treated initially and 28 (2.8%) underwent liver-first resections. Patients managed with the liver-first approach had more hepatic lesions and were more likely to have bilateral disease than those in the other 2 groups ($p < 0.05$). Moreover, patients undergoing this approach were more likely to have a rectal primary tumor ($n = 15$; 53.6%) compared with patients undergoing either a colorectal-first or a simultaneous resection. Patients in the simultaneous resection group were more likely to undergo a minor hepatic resection ($n = 251$; 76.2%) compared with patients in either the classic ($n = 397$; 61.4%) or liver-first ($n = 18$; 64.2%) groups ($p < 0.001$). A major resection (>3 segments) was more common with a staged approach (39% vs. 24%; $p < 0.001$). Similarly, extended hepatectomy was more commonly performed in the staged setting (colorectal first, 16.2% and liver first, 17.9% vs. simultaneous, 7.6%; $p < 0.001$). The authors found no difference in morbidity and 90 days mortality between staged and simultaneous hepatectomies, even when considering patients who underwent a major hepatic resection ($p > 0.05$). Recurrence rate, overall median, and 5-year survivals were similar when comparing the colorectal-first, liver-first, or simultaneous approaches ($p = 0.526$) [35].

Silberhumer et al. reported the Memorial Sloan Kettering Cancer Center experience on this subject. In this series, the safety of simultaneous rectal and liver metastasis resection was studied. One hundred ninety-eight patients underwent surgical treatment for stage IV rectal cancer. In 145 (73%) patients, a simultaneous procedure was performed. The simultaneous treatment resulted in a shorter hospital stay (10 ± 5 vs. 18 ± 7 days; $P < .01$) with similar complication rates compared to staged resections. The authors stressed the importance of a careful patient selection in order to achieve good results. In this series, rectal tumors requiring abdominoperineal resections were more likely to be chosen for a staged approach ($P < .01$), and larger liver lesions requiring major liver procedures (3 or more segments) were performed in 73.6% staged hepatic resections compared with only 20.7% in the simultaneous groups [36].

Kelly and colleagues published a review where eighteen studies were included, reporting on 3605 patients comparing the three different surgical strategies, of which 2439 (67.7%) had classical colorectal-first resection, 133 (3.7%) had liver-first resection, and 1033 (28.6%) had combined resections. Colorectal-first approach had 71.2% colonic primaries and 23.8% rectal primaries. Liver-first approach had less colonic primaries at 50.4% and more rectal primaries at 49.6%. Combined approach had 67.8% colonic primaries and 32.2% rectal tumors. The colorectal-first approach had 48.3% unilobar and 51.7% bilobar CLM. The liver-first approach had 33.9% unilobar and 66.1% bilobar CLM. The combined approach had 64.7% unilobar and 35.3% bilobar CLM. Network meta-analysis did not find significant difference among the three groups regarding overall survival, 30-day mortality, or the mean number of complication events of the three surgical approaches. For the colorectal-first group, the complication rate was 29.3% (n.489), within which respiratory events (sepsis and pleural effusions, 12.2%, n.60), bile leak (7.9%, n.39), and intra-abdominal collection/abscess (5.9%, n.29) were the most common. The complication rate of the combined group was 30.7% (n.294) with the most common types of complications being intra-abdominal collection/abscess (9.8%, n.29), wound infection (7.8%, n.23), and respiratory sepsis/pleural effusions (6.8%, n.20) [4].

A more recent systematic review and meta-analysis yielded similar results. There were no statistically significant differences relating to safety and efficacy between the simultaneous and delayed hepatectomy groups, with similar trend to more bilobar disease or major hepatectomy in the delayed group and similar long-term survival. The average length of hospital stay was six days shorter with simultaneous approach [37].

A Canadian study compared the simultaneous and the staged strategy (cost for the two operations and hospital admissions) with regard to cost, defined as the absolute dollars spent by the institution admissions. Fifty-three cases were identified; 27 patients underwent staged resections and 26 simultaneous surgeries. There were no differences with respect to laparoscopic versus open surgical approach for either the colorectal or liver resection. There was no difference with respect to type of hepatectomy or extent of liver resection; however, the staged cohort had a higher proportion of patients undergoing rectal surgery compared to the simultaneous group (44.4% vs. 26.9%). Median length hospital stay (LOS) was significantly longer for the staged group, with a median LOS of 19 days compared to 10 days for the simultaneous group ($P < 0.01$). Total cost ($20297 vs. $27522), operating room ($6830 vs. $10376), postanesthetic care unit ($675 vs. $1182), ward ($7586 vs. $11603), and pharmacy costs ($728 vs. $1075) were all significantly less for the simultaneous group ($P < 0.05$). The adjusted rate ratio for total cost of care in the staged group compared to simultaneous group was 1.51 (95%CI: 1.16–1.97, $P < 0.05$) [38].

In conclusion, although there are no available data based on prospective trials, information from retrospective studies indicates that there is no strategy clearly superior to the others, allowing a unique approach for patients with colorectal tumors and synchronic metastases. Patients presenting synchronous liver metastases and a colorectal primary tumor should have their cases discussed at multidisciplinary meeting and the treatment planned according to their clinical characteristics, such as age, ECOG performance status, and comorbidities, in addition to tumor characteristics such as location (colon vs. rectum), characteristics of liver metastases, resectability, and need for neoadjuvant therapy.

Patients with unresectable liver disease with no conversion potential are managed with palliative chemotherapy. Primary tumors are evaluated for resection according to the criteria described in the chapter: Resection of the Primary in Unresectable Colorectal Liver Metastases: Is It Worth?

Patients with easily resectable primary and metastatic disease are initially treated with chemotherapy and considered for synchronous resection.

Patients with extensive liver disease requiring major hepatectomies are initially treated with chemotherapy and then undergo the liver resection, leaving the primary tumor as the last procedure, preceded by chemoradiation when indicated.

Patients with locally advanced rectal tumor and easily resectable liver metastases are treated with chemoradiation first and then concomitant surgical resection.

References

1. Ferlay J, Soerjomataram I, Ervik M et al. GLOBOCAN 2012 v1.1, Cancer Incidence and Mortality Worldwide: IARC CancerBase No. 11 [Internet].
2. McMillan DC, McArdle CS. Epidemiology of colorectal liver metastases. Surg Oncol. 2007;16:3–5.
3. Van Cutsem E, Nordlinger B, Adam R, et al. Towards a paneuropean consensus on the treatment of patients with colorectal liver metastases. Eur J Cancer. 2006;42:2212–21.
4. Kelly ME, Spolverato G, Lê GN, et al. Synchronous colorectal liver metastasis: a network meta-analysis review comparing classical, combined, and liver-first surgical strategies. J Surg Oncol. 2015;111(3):341–51.
5. deJong MC, Pulitano C, Ribero D, et al. Rates and patterns of recurrence following curative intent surgery for colorectal liver metastasis: an international multi-institutional analysis of 1669 patients. Ann Surg. 2009;250:440–8.
6. Abdalla EK, Vauthey JN, Ellis LM, et al. Recurrence and outcomes following hepatic resection, radiofrequency ablation and combined resection/ablation for colorectal liver metastasis. Ann Surg. 2004;239:818–25.
7. Mavros MN, de Jong M, Dogeas E, et al. Impact of complications on long-term survival after resection of colorectal liver metastases. Br J Surg. 2013;100:711–8.
8. Mentha G, Roth AD, Terraz S, et al. 'Liver First' approach in the treatment of colorectal cancer with synchronous liver metastases. Dig Surg. 2008;25:430–5.
9. Tournigand C, Andre T, Achille E, et al. FOLFIRI followed by FOLFOX6 or the reverse sequence in advanced colorectal cancer: a randomized GERCOR study. J Clin Oncol. 2004;22(2):229–37.
10. Goldberg RM, Sargent DJ, Morton RF, et al. A randomized controlled trial of fluorouracil plus leucovorin, irinotecan, and oxaliplatin combinations in patients with previously untreated metastatic colorectal cancer. J Clin Oncol. 2004;22(1):23–30.
11. Garufi C, Torsello A, Tumolo S, et al. Cetuximab plus chronomodulated irinotecan, 5-fluorouracil, leucovorin and oxaliplatin as neoadjuvant chemotherapy in colorectal liver metastases: POCHER trial. Br J Cancer. 2010;103(10):1542–7.
12. Cai S, et al. Abstracts of the 37th ESMO (European Society for Medical Oncology) congress. September 28-October 2, 2012. Vienna, Austria. Ann Oncol. 2012;23(Suppl 9):Abstract 643.
13. Poultsides GA, Servais EL, Saltz LB, et al. Outcome of primary tumor in patients with synchronous stage IV colorectal cancer receiving combination chemotherapy without surgery as initial treatment. J Clin Oncol. 2009;27(20):3379–84.
14. McCahill LE, Yothers G, et al. Primary mFOLFOX6 Plus Bevacizumab without resection of the primary tumor for patients presenting with surgically unresectable metastatic colon cancer and an intact asymptomatic colon cancer: definitive analysis of NSABP trial C-10. J Clin Oncol. 2012;30(26):3223–8.
15. Veldkamp R, Kuhry E, Hop WC, et al. Laparoscopic surgery versus open surgery for colon cancer: short-term outcomes of a randomised trial. Lancet Oncol. 2005;6(7):477–84.
16. Matthiessen P, Hallböök O, Rutegård J, et al. Defunctioning stoma reduces symptomatic anastomotic leakage after low anterior resection of the rectum for cancer. A randomized multicenter trial. Ann Surg. 2007;246(2):207–14.

17. Tevis SE, Kohlnhofer BM, Stringfield S, et al. Postoperative complications in patients with rectal cancer are associated with delays in chemotherapy that lead to worse disease-free and overall survival. Dis Colon Rectum. 2013;56(12):1339–48.
18. Andres A, Toso C, Adam R, et al. A survival analysis of the liver-first reversed management of advanced simultaneous colorectal liver metastases: a LiverMetSurvey-based study. Ann Surg. 2012;256(5):772–8.
19. Mentha G, Majno PE, Andres A, et al. Neoadjuvant chemotherapy and resection of advanced synchronous liver metastases before treatment of the colorectal primary. Br J Surg. 2006;93(7):872–8.
20. de Rosa A, Gomez D, Hossaini S, et al. Stage IV colorectal cancer: outcomes following the liver-first approach. J Surg Oncol. 2013;108(7):444–9.
21. Weber JC, Bachellier P, Oussoultzoglou E, et al. Simultaneous resection of colorectal primary tumour and synchronous liver metastases. Br J Surg. 2003;90(8):956–62.
22. Martin R, Paty P, Fong Y, et al. Simultaneous liver and colorectal resections are safe for synchronous colorectal liver metastasis. J Am Coll Surg. 2003;197(2):233–41.
23. Reddy SK, Pawlik TM, Zorzi D, et al. Simultaneous resections of colorectal cancer and synchronous liver metastases: a multi-institutional analysis. Ann Surg Oncol. 2007;14(12):3481–91.
24. Bolton JS, Fuhrman GM. Survival after resection of multiple bilobar hepatic metastases from colorectal carcinoma. Ann Surg. 2000;231:743–51.
25. Tanaka K, Shimada H, Matsuo K, et al. Outcome after simultaneous colorectal and hepatic resection for colorectal cancer with synchronous metastases. Surgery. 2004;136(3):650–9.
26. Nordlinger B, Guiguet M, Vaillant JC, et al. Surgical resection of colorectal carcinoma metastases to the liver. A prognostic scoring system to improve case selection, based on 1568 patients. Association Francaise de Chirurgie. Cancer. 1996;77:1254–62.
27. Thelen A, Jonas S, Benckert C, et al. Simultaneous versus staged liver resection of synchronous liver metastases from colorectal cancer. Int J Color Dis. 2007;22:1269–76.
28. Chua HK, Sondenaa K, Tsiotos GG, et al. Concurrent vs. staged colectomy and hepatectomy for primary colorectal cancer with synchronous hepatic metastases. Dis Colon Rectum. 2004;47(8):1310–6.
29. Capussotti L, Ferrero A, Viganò L, et al. Major liver resections synchronous with colorectal surgery. Ann Surg Oncol. 2007;14(1):195–201.
30. Martin RC 2nd, Augenstein V, Reuter NP, et al. Simultaneous versus staged resection for synchronous colorectal cancer liver metastases. J Am Coll Surg. 2009;208(5):842–50.
31. Slesser AA, Chand M, Goldin R, et al. Outcomes of simultaneous resections for patients with synchronous colorectal liver metastases. Eur J Surg Oncol. 2013;39(12):1384–93.
32. de Haas RJ, Adam R, Wicherts DA, et al. Comparison of simultaneous or delayed liver surgery for limited synchronous colorectal metastases. Br J Surg. 2010;97(8):1279–89.
33. Nordlinger B, Sorbye H, Glimelius B, et al. Perioperative chemotherapy with FOLFOX4 and surgery versus surgery alone for resectable liver metastases from colorectal cancer (EORTC Intergroup trial 40983): a randomised controlled trial. Lancet. 2008;371(9617):1007–16.
34. Brouquet A, Mortenson MM, Vauthey JN, et al. Surgical strategies for synchronous colorectal liver metastases in 156 consecutive patients: classic, combined or reverse strategy? J Am Coll Surg. 2010;210(6):934–41.
35. Mayo SC, Pulitano C, Marques H, et al. Surgical management of patients with synchronous colorectal liver metastasis: a multicenter international analysis. J Am Coll Surg. 2013;216:707–16.
36. Silberhumer GR, Paty PB, Temple LK, Araujo RL, et al. Simultaneous resection for rectal cancer with synchronous liver metastasis is a safe procedure. Am J Surg. 2015;209(6):935–42.
37. Gavriilidis P, Sutcliffe RP, Hodson J, et al. Simultaneous versus delayed hepatectomy for synchronous colorectal liver metastases: a systematic review and meta-analysis. HPB (Oxford). 2018;20(1):11–9.
38. Le Souder EB, Azin A, Hirpara DH, et al. Considering the cost of a simultaneous versus staged approach to resection of colorectal cancer with synchronous liver metastases in a publicly funded healthcare model. J Surg Oncol. 2018;117:1376.

Resection of Metachronous Colorectal Cancer Liver Metastases: Surgical Outcomes

27

Fábio Luiz Waechter, Uirá Fernandes Teixeira, Pablo Duarte Rodrigues, Marcio Boff, Rinaldo Danesi, and Mauro Monteiro Correia

Introduction

Colorectal cancer (CRC) is the third most common cancer affecting both men and women in the United States and the third leading cause of cancer-related deaths in that country. For 2018, 140,250 new CRC cases and 50,630 deaths have been estimated in the United States [1]. Despite the improvements in diagnosis and treatment of patients with CRC, which have led to a decline in mortality in some populations, global projections indicate a marked increase in the burden of CRC in the coming years, reaching 2.4 million new cases and 1.1 million deaths in 2030 [2, 3].

In CRC, the liver is the most common site of metastasis [3]. Metastatic disease to the liver is observed in approximately 50% of CRC patients during the course of the disease. Thus, adequate treatment of colorectal liver metastases (CRLM) is essential for the long-term survival of patients [4, 5].

F. L. Waechter (✉) · U. F. Teixeira · P. D. Rodrigues
Digestive Surgery Division, Universidade Federal de Ciências da Saúde de Porto Alegre, UFCSPA, Centro de Cirurgia Digestiva – CAD, Porto Alegre, RS, Brazil
e-mail: waechter@jaschter.com.br; https://www.centrodecirurgiadigestiva.com.br

M. Boff
Head of Surgical Oncology Mãe de Deus Cancer Center, Mãe de Deus Hospital, Porto Alegre, RS, Brazil

R. Danesi
Hepato-Pancreato-Biliary Surgical Division, Universidade de Blumenau, Santa Catarina Hospital, Blumenau, SC, Brazil

M. M. Correia
National Cancer Institute, Rio de Janeiro, Brazil

Department of Surgery, UNIVERSIDADE DO GRANDE RIO, Duque de Caxias, Brazil

M. M. Correia et al. (eds.), *Colorectal Cancer Liver Metastases*,
https://doi.org/10.1007/978-3-030-25486-5_27

Defining Terminology

Although, in principle, all CRLM are synchronous (occult or detectable at diagnosis), they are classified as synchronous or metachronous according to the timing of diagnosis in relation to the primary tumor. It is estimated that 30% of patients develop metastases that are metachronous in presentation [3, 5]. Nevertheless, the definition of metachronous metastasis varies: some authors consider as metachronous those metastases appearing 3 months after resection of the primary tumor, while others establish a disease-free interval of 4 to 6 months [6, 7].

In 1986, Ekberg et al. had already inferred that synchronous lesions show a more aggressive biological behavior and, consequently, a worse prognosis [8]. This view is supported by data from the LiverMetSurvey, an international registry of patients undergoing resection for CRLM [9], which showed significantly lower survival rates for patients with CRLM detected at the time of diagnosis or in the month preceding diagnosis as compared to those whose metastases were discovered 12 months after diagnosis. Analysis of these data indicates that detection of CRLM more than 1 month after diagnosis is associated with a statistical trend toward a poor prognosis [10].

In an attempt to standardize this definition, in 2015, Adam et al. presented the recommendations developed by an international panel of multidisciplinary experts. Based on the findings of the LiverMetSurvey [9, 10], the panel defined metachronous metastases as those arising after diagnosis or treatment of the primary tumor, regardless of timing. The panel then proposed a subdivision into early and late metachronous metastases – those detected within 12 months or >12 months after surgery, respectively [10].

In general, despite extensive research, the natural history of CRLM has not yet been completely elucidated, and understanding is still evolving. However, definitions such as those relating to metachronous metastases allow an adequate assessment regarding the best timing for therapeutic intervention and shed light on postoperative outcomes.

Tumor Biology of Metachronous Metastases

One of the central issues in the discussion of metastatic lesions is why some tumors develop synchronous while others develop metachronous metastases. Although metachronous lesions theoretically already exist initially, they have been shown to differ biologically in relation not only to synchronous lesions but also to the primary tumor [11]. It is believed that in their "metastasization process," primary lesions form a subpopulation of cells that develop the ability to metastasize [12–14]. For that, the primary tumor must undergo genetic alterations to ensure the survival of tumor cells throughout the metastatic cascade as well as a receptive microenvironment in the liver for the implant of cells [12, 15]. The main alterations with respect to this early process are related to the expression of molecular markers such as p27 [16, 17], cyclin E [18], thymidylate synthase [19, 20], ERCC1 [19], CCR6, CCR20,

CXCR4 [21–24], vascular endothelial growth factor (VEGF) [24, 25], insulin receptor substrate 1 (Irs1) [26, 27], and focal adhesion kinase (FAK) [28].

Conversely, the differences in biomarkers between synchronous and metachronous metastases are less noticeable, with discrepant results in the literature pointing to heterogeneities. Among the markers that have been studied, differences have been reported in cyclooxygenase-2 (COX-2) [29–33], epidermal growth factor receptor (EGFR) [32, 34], tumor growth factor [TGF]-α [34], number of dendritic cells [35], and Ang 1–2 [36].

Overall, there is increasing evidence showing that biological alterations determine greater or lesser tumor aggressiveness. In the near future, the identification of these factors will provide information regarding the type of follow-up needed by patients undergoing primary tumor resection, the basis of adjuvant treatment, and disease prognosis [11].

Survival after Resection of Metachronous Metastases of Colorectal Cancer

As a rule, metachronous metastases are surgically treated if there is a possibility of resection with free margins and adequate liver remnant. In general, the prognosis of this group of patients tends to be more favorable than that of patients with synchronous metastases, in whom curative resection is performed less frequently due to the more aggressive biological behavior of these lesions. Results from the main series of patients indicate a 5-year overall survival ranging from 25 to 58.5% in those subjected to resection of metachronous metastases with curative intent (Table 27.1). The comparatively worse prognosis of synchronous lesions has been described in several retrospective series from centers specialized in CRC [37–42], and also supported by epidemiological data from the French region of Burgundy, where 5-year survival was significantly better for metachronous metastases vs. synchronous metastases (17.6% vs. 7.2%) [43, 44]. However, the lack of consensus in the literature regarding the temporal cutoff point for the definition of metachronous metastases should be considered, as well as biases relating to diagnostic selection, when the data were obtained, types of surgical treatment, chemotherapy used, and also chemoresistance of the patient series [45].

Due to these possible biases, the literature is not unanimous with regard to these results. Van der Pool et al., in a study published in 2010, did not observe differences in overall and disease-free survival among patients undergoing hepatectomy for synchronous and metachronous LM (median survival of 44 months and 38% in 5 years) [46]. Jeong et al., in a recent series published in 2017 [6], did not report any difference in long-term survival between patients with synchronous and metachronous liver and pulmonary metastases. Survival at 5 years after surgery for resection of colorectal tumor was 77.8% in the synchronous group, similar to that of the metachronous group (73.1%). In addition, 5-year survival in the two groups after the first liver metastasectomy was 74.1% (synchronous) and 73.2% (metachronous), with no statistical difference. One possibility is that in studies reporting less

Table 27.1 Published series describing overall survival (OS) after surgical treatment of metachronous metastasis of colorectal cancer

Reference	Year	No. patients	Series type	5-year OS	Definition of metachronous lesion
Scheele et al. [52]	1995	434	Single center	43%	After colorectal tumor diagnosis
Fong et al. [54]	1999	1001	Single center	41%	12 months after colorectal tumor resection
Weber et al. [59]	2001	221	Single center	38%	Not specified
Manfredi et al. [43]	2006	3655	Population-based	29%	After colorectal tumor resection
Wang et al. [51]	2007	923	Population-based	25%	6 months after colorectal tumor diagnosis
Figueras et al. [58]	2007	501	Single center	43%	After colorectal tumor diagnosis
Tsai et al. [42]	2007	155	Single center	54.6%	12 months after colorectal tumor resection
Rees et al. [56]	2008	929	Single center	37.1%	3 months after colorectal tumor diagnosis
Beppu et al. [75]	2012	727	Multicentric	51.2%	Not specified
Sadot et al. [55]	2015	2368	Single center	44%	After colorectal tumor resection
Angelsen et al. [7]	2017	538	Population-based	28.1% (<12 months) 25.4% (12 months)[a]	After colorectal tumor diagnosis
Wang et al. [38]	2017	300	Single center	58.5%	Not specified

[a]3-year overall survival

favorable results with synchronous tumors, this difference is explained by the inclusion of patients who did not undergo the "test of time," that is, the interval between the diagnosis and evaluation was not sufficient for extrahepatic or biologically unfavorable disease to become evident [46].

Population-based series analyzing patients with a focus on the moment of CRC diagnosis showed a higher resection rate in the presence of metachronous metastases compared to synchronous disease, with greater survival in those with metastases developing at a later point in time [7, 43, 47]. One possible explanation for this difference is that patients with metachronous disease had fewer metastases and a higher rate of unilobar distribution [47–49], well-known favorable prognostic factors for resection [47, 48]. Meanwhile, in studies including only patients undergoing resection, the timing of metastases appearance was not associated with worse survival outcomes [7, 48–51]. Angelsen et al. [7] reported that among all patients diagnosed with LM, survival rate at 3 years was higher in the group with metachronous lesions (28.1 vs. 15%); however, when only patients with resection were selected, this difference was not significant.

The starting point of survival analysis is also important. In a study by Swan et al. [49], a survival advantage was observed in patients with hepatic resection 3 years after colorectal surgery as compared to patients with synchronous metastases (94.1 and 46.3%, respectively, at 5 years) only when the starting point of analysis was the date of colectomy; statistical significance was lost when the date of liver surgery was used.

In studies that did not rely on population-based data, the results can be evaluated, taking into account the year of patient inclusion. Findings from patients treated mostly in the 1990s and including a large number of cases, such as those by Scheele et al. (1995) [52], Nordlinger et al. (1996) [53], and Fong et al. (1999) [54], demonstrated that late-onset metastases were associated with better results in terms of survival. Conversely, more recent studies, such as those by Sadot et al. (2015) [55], Rees et al. (2008) [56], and Malik et al. (2007) [57], have failed to demonstrate an association between late metastases and survival. In the studies by Figueras et al. [58] and Tsai et al. [42], which included patients treated between 1990 and 2004, later timing in disease progression was not a risk factor for poor outcomes in terms of overall survival, but disease-free interval less than 12 months was a risk factor for shorter disease-free survival. In studies that demonstrated worse results in patients with synchronous disease, there was a decrease in overall survival, from 8 to 18% [43, 54, 59–61].

Such differences in the findings of these studies may be explained by (1) more frequent use of perioperative chemotherapy, (2) new drugs with more pronounced response rates, and (3) in more recent studies, more aggressive and standardized management of synchronous tumors. Supporting this association, Vigano et al. [60] demonstrated that patients with synchronous metastases are at increased risk of early recurrence (before 6 months after hepatic resection), which, in turn, is associated with worse overall survival; however, this association was not observed when only patients who received preoperative chemotherapy were included. Similarly, Ng et al. [61] evaluated the association of chemotherapy with post-hepatectomy results. In that study, synchronous tumors were associated with worse overall survival in patients without neoadjuvant treatment and in patients who received it but showed a poor response (no response or disease progression) (19.3 vs. 47.4 months). Survival was not less favorable in patients with response to chemotherapy.

Overall, when evaluating all patients with CRLM, prognostic factors associated with poor overall survival outcomes are advanced age (75 or 60 years) [47, 53, 62], multiple lesions (2, 3, or 4) [50, 53, 55, 56, 58, 62, 63], extrahepatic disease [7, 47, 49, 55, 56, 58], presence of lesion >5 cm [47, 48, 52, 53, 55, 56, 62, 63], positive lymph nodes close to the primary tumor [49, 52, 53, 55, 56, 64], high levels of carcinoembryonic antigen (CEA) (>60 or >200 ng/mL) [49, 55, 56], absence of adjuvant treatment [58, 64], resection with positive margins [49, 55, 56, 62], and palliative treatment [7, 48, 50].

Some series have evaluated factors related to overall survival in patients with metachronous liver disease. Positive lymph nodes in the resection of the primary tumor, tumors >5 cm, extrahepatic disease, and presence of four or more lesions were associated with a worse prognosis [49, 65]. Female sex, treatment at a specialized hospital (more than 29 surgeries per year), adjuvant chemotherapy after resection of primary tumor, and age <75 years were associated with better overall survival [43, 51].

Finally, it is clear that in highly selected patients with metachronous metastases, surgical treatment may lead to excellent results in terms of overall survival, with a 5-year survival rate of 58.5%. This group of patients has less aggressive tumors and better prognosis in the long term.

Disease-Free Survival in Patients with Metachronous Metastases of Colorectal Cancer

Although prognostic factors for CRLM have been identified in recent years and long-term survival outcomes have improved greatly, 40 to 81% of these patients will develop recurrence, mostly in the first 2 years after surgery [52, 53, 58, 60, 66–74]. Synchronous metastases and disease-free intervals of 12, 24, and up to 30 months from resection of the primary tumor to detection of liver disease have been reported as independent risk factors for recurrence or poor disease-free survival [42, 53, 58, 60, 67, 69, 72, 75].

In patients with metachronous metastases, 5-year disease-free survival after hepatic resection ranges from 21 to 36% [42, 52, 58, 59, 72]. The time interval between CRLM resection and recurrence is of extreme importance and has been reported to range from 9 to 23 months [52, 67, 68, 72, 73]. Patients with late recurrence show a tendency for better results. Takahashi et al. [74] demonstrated that early relapse (defined by these authors as relapse after 6 months) is directly correlated with a poor prognosis in terms of long-term survival, an observation that was confirmed by other series [60, 73]. Differently from patients who show early recurrence after hepatectomy (inferring a greater biological aggressiveness), those with late recurrence have higher resectability rates, as well as repeated resections, which would help explain the better results in the latter group [73, 74]. Vigano et al. [60] found that the presence of synchronous metastases was independently related to the occurrence of early recurrences after surgical treatment.

Other risk factors associated with these outcomes demonstrated in the main series published to date are positive lymph nodes close to the primary tumor [52, 54, 62, 68, 71, 75, 76], degree of primary invasion (T3 or T4) [42, 52, 53], multiple (2, 3, 4, or 5) nodules [53, 58, 62, 68, 69, 71, 75, 76], metastasis size (4, 5, or 8 cm) [52–54, 62, 68, 69, 71, 75, 76], high levels of CEA or carbohydrate antigen (CA) 19-9 prior to hepatectomy [54, 68, 75], no chemotherapy [58, 71, 72], positive resection margins [54, 58, 71, 75, 76], and extrahepatic disease [54, 58, 75, 76]. More specifically, elevated serum levels of CEA and CA 19-9 are related to greater lesion volume and number, which ultimately are markers of greater tumor aggressiveness [77, 78]. Regarding the assessment of surgical margins, Pawlik et al. [63] demonstrated that patients with resection margins <1 mm had increased risk of recurrence vs. those with negative margins (51.1 vs. 38%, respectively); this was the only factor associated with recurrence at the liver resection margin. Vigano et al. [79] further demonstrated that when the resection margin was positive along major intrahepatic vessels (vascular R1), recurrence and overall survival were similar as compared to R0 patients; in turn, standard R1 resections with parenchymal margin were associated with worse results. Several series have demonstrated the role of chemotherapy in improving postoperative outcomes. The EORTC Intergroup trial 40,983 [80] showed improvement in progression-free survival in patients undergoing perioperative chemotherapy (FOLFOX4) compared to patients undergoing surgery alone (36.2 vs. 28.1%, respectively, in patients eligible for treatment).

Recurrence after CRLM resection usually affects a single site, especially the liver [58, 68, 72–74]. Extrahepatic recurrences, in descending order of frequency, develop in the lungs, lymph nodes, and peritoneum [72–74]. In general, 20 to 58% of patients who develop recurrence undergo new resections [52, 58, 60, 67, 70, 71, 73, 74]. The positive impact of additional resections was demonstrated in a meta-analysis by Wurster et al. [81], which showed that survival in patients undergoing repeated hepatic resection with curative intent was similar to that of patients undergoing a first hepatectomy. In turn, when this group of patients is submitted to palliative treatment, the overall 5-year survival rate was extremely low (15.4 vs. 59.7%) [73].

Thus, the available evidence shows an association between the timing of CRLM and post-resection recurrence of CRLM. This should always be considered when making therapeutic decisions for these patients. Recurrence after hepatectomy is frequent, and the time interval between liver surgery and recurrence is an important prognostic marker. To achieve the best possible long-term results, treatment with curative intent should be the rule, even in patients with recurrent disease.

Curability of Patients with Metachronous Metastases of Colorectal Cancer

The main studies that focus on this topic define cure as actual 10-year survival after resection of the metastasis. Tomlinson et al. [82] were the first to show a plateau in the survival curve 10 years after CRLM resection. After that time, only a minority of patients will die from the disease. In their series with 612 patients undergoing hepatectomy, 17% survived more than 10 years, and of these, only one died due to cancer. This finding is supported by other studies [83, 84], which also highlighted the need for prolonged follow-up, since recurrence was found in 12–15% of patients after a 5-year disease-free interval following hepatectomy [83, 84].

Adam et al. [85] defined cure as a disease-free interval 5 years from last hepatic or extrahepatic resection until the last follow-up. In their series with initially unresectable patients, 16% were considered cured and none showed recurrence during follow-up. In turn, among those who survived 10 years, about 14% had extensive recurrence that could not be treated surgically. Predictors of cure included lesions <3 cm, presence of three or fewer metastases, and complete pathological response. More recently, the same group found similar results in terms of postoperative cure in patients with CRLM associated with extrahepatic disease. These authors identified a cure rate of 13.1% in the overall cohort and 19% in patients undergoing curative resection of all metastases; in that series, the presence of metachronous liver lesions was associated with a higher probability of cure [86].

The use of markedly different definitions of cure – 5-year vs. 10-year survival – might be explained, at least in part, by the fact that studies that define cure as 10-year survival were performed before the 2000s. At that time, only a small number of patients received perioperative chemotherapy, usually with adjuvant 5-fluorouracil; the chemotherapy regimens routinely used today were not available then.

More recently, Cuchetti et al. [87] have proposed a "cure model" based on disease-free survival. In a multicenter study, the authors showed that being alive without tumor recurrence 5.84 to 7.31 years after hepatic resection entails 99% certainty of cure. In addition, the authors also pointed out the following prognostic factors associated with a higher probability of cure: single metachronous tumor, <3 cm, and no positive lymph nodes next to the primary tumor. These patients would have a cure probability of 40.9% in 5.84 years.

Therefore, irrespective of the criterion used, 13 to 23% [82–87] of patients considered as having systemic disease were deemed cured after surgical management of CRLM.

Prognostic Scores and Metachronous Metastases

Prognostic scores, developed with the aim of stratifying CRLM patients according to risk for various outcomes (recurrence, long-term survival), are useful when defining the best therapeutic options for these patients. A variety of prognostic scores have been described in the literature, most of which were based on data from patients treated at a single center [53, 56, 57, 69, 75, 88–94]. Of these, at least six considers late metastases as an independent factor related to more favorable outcomes [53, 54, 69, 75, 89, 92] (Table 27.2).

Although the statistical methods employed in these studies support the reliability of the proposed prognostic models, applicability becomes questionable due to possible biases including patient selection, the use of various diagnostic modalities and different surgical techniques, and differences in treatment times, among others. Thus, these prognostic scores should be submitted to external validation (that is, reproduced in other populations) before routine use.

One of the most tested prognostic tools is the clinical risk score (CRS) proposed by Fong et al. [54]. The CRS relies on five variables that were independently associated with recurrence: lymph node involvement by primary tumor, disease-free interval from primary to metastases <12 months, number of hepatic tumors >1, largest hepatic tumor >5 cm, and preoperative CEA >200 ng/mL. One point is assigned to each criterion, and the final score ranges from 0 to 5. In its original publication, the probability of 5-year survival for patients with a score of zero was 60% vs. 14% for those with a score of 5. In fact, however, none of the patients with a score of 5 survived 5 years [54].

Table 27.2 Prognostic scores in colorectal liver metastases

Score system	Year	No. patients	Series type	Outcome	Prognostic factors associated with worse outcomes included in the scoring system
Nordlinger et al. [53]	1996	1568	Multicentric	Overall survival	Age >60 years, resection <1 cm, extension into serosa of primary cancer, 4 lesions, size of largest metastasis >5 cm, lymphatic spread of primary cancer, **disease-free interval between colorectal surgery and metastasis diagnosis <2 years**
Fong et al. [54]	1999	1001	Single center	Recurrence Overall survival	Presence of 2 lesions, preoperative CEA level >200 ng/dL, size of the largest tumor >5 cm, lymph node involvement in primary cancer, **disease-free interval between colorectal surgery and metastasis diagnosis <1 year**
Konopke et al. [89]	2009	201	Single center	Recurrence Overall survival	CEA level at diagnosis of metastases >200 ng/dL, 4 lesions, and **synchronous metastases**
Iwatsuki et al. [69]	1999	305	Single center	Tumor-free survival Overall survival	Positive surgical margins, extrahepatic disease, 3 lesions, size of largest tumor >8 cm, bilobar distribution, **time interval between colorectal and liver resection <30 months**
Ueno et al. [92]	2000	85	Single center	Overall survival Disease-free survival Recurrence	Presence of tumor budding in colorectal cancer, N2 or N3, **disease-free survival <12 months**, 3 lesions, elevated post-hepatectomy CEA level
Beppu et al. [75]	2012	727	Multicentric	Disease-free survival	**Synchronous tumor**, 2 lesions, CA 19-9 level >100 U/mL before hepatectomy, extrahepatic disease, lymph node involvement in primary cancer, size of largest tumor >5 cm

Regarding external validation of the CRS, Mann et al. [95] and Mala et al. [96] have demonstrated good accuracy of the score to predict long-term survival in different populations. In the series by Pulitano et al. [84], CRS >2 was associated with poor survival. None of the patients with CRS >3 was alive at the end of 10 years. Zakaria et al. [90] evaluated the ability of three prognostic scores (described by Fong et al. [54], Nordlingler et al. [53], and Iwatsuki et al. [69]) to predict survival and recurrence in a population of patients undergoing CRLM resection at the Mayo Clinic. In the end, none of the scores was able to correctly stratify the population according to the outcomes. CRS showed the best capacity to predict overall survival.

Given this scenario, prognostic scores should be used with caution when making decisions regarding curative surgery, which could even benefit patients with a poor prognosis [85, 86]. Nevertheless, prognostic scores seem useful in daily practice to identify patients who may benefit from chemotherapy and also for counseling patients and families regarding prognosis.

References

1. Siegel RL, Miller KD, Jemal A. Cancer statistics, 2018. CA Cancer J Clin. 2018;68(1):7–30. https://doi.org/10.3322/caac.21442.
2. Ferlay J, Soerjomataram I, Ervik M, Dikshit R, Eser C, Mathers M et al. GLOBOCAN 2012 v1.0, Cancer Incidence and Mortality Worldwide: IARC CancerBase No. 11. International Agency for Research on Cancer, Lyon, France. 2013. http://globocan.iarc.fr.
3. Arnold M, Sierra MS, Laversanne M, Soerjomataram I, Jemal A, Bray F. Global patterns and trends in colorectal cancer incidence and mortality. Gut. 2017;66(4):683–91. https://doi.org/10.1136/gutjnl-2015-310912.
4. Maher B, Ryan E, Little M, Boardman P, Stedman B. The management of colorectal liver metastases. Clin Radiol. 2017;72(8):617–25. https://doi.org/10.1016/j.crad.2017.05.016.
5. Jones RP, Kokudo N, Folprecht G, Mise Y, Unno M, Malik HZ, et al. Colorectal liver metastases: a critical review of state of the art. Liver Cancer. 2016;6(1):66–71. https://doi.org/10.1159/000449348.
6. Jeong S, Heo JS, Park JY, Choi DW, Choi SH. Surgical resection of synchronous and metachronous lung and liver metastases of colorectal cancers. Ann Surg Treat Res. 2017;92(2):82–9. https://doi.org/10.4174/astr.2017.92.2.82.
7. Angelsen JH, Horn A, Sorbye H, Eide GE, Loes IM, Viste A. Population-based study on resection rates and survival in patients with colorectal liver metastasis in Norway. Br J Surg. 2017;104(5):580–9. https://doi.org/10.1002/bjs.10457.
8. Ekberg H, Tranberg KG, Andersson R, Lundstedt C, Hagerstrand I, Ranstam J, et al. Determinants of survival in liver resection for colorectal secondaries. Br J Surg. 1986;73(9):727–31.
9. Adam R, Frilling A, Elias D, Laurent C, Ramos E, Capussotti L, et al. Liver resection of colorectal metastases in elderly patients. Br J Surg. 2010;97(3):366–76. https://doi.org/10.1002/bjs.6889.
10. Adam R, de Gramont A, Figueras J, Kokudo N, Kunstlinger F, Loyer E, et al. Managing synchronous liver metastases from colorectal cancer: a multidisciplinary international consensus. Cancer Treat Rev. 2015;41(9):729–41. https://doi.org/10.1016/j.ctrv.2015.06.006.
11. Slesser AA, Georgiou P, Brown G, Mudan S, Goldin R, Tekkis P. The tumour biology of synchronous and metachronous colorectal liver metastases: a systematic review. Clin Exp Metastasis. 2013;30(4):457–70. https://doi.org/10.1007/s10585-012-9551-8.
12. Bird NC, Mangnall D, Majeed AW. Biology of colorectal liver metastases: a review. J Surg Oncol. 2006;94(1):68–80. https://doi.org/10.1002/jso.20558.
13. Wang SC, Lin JK, Wang HS, Yang SH, Li AF, Chang SC. Nuclear expression of CXCR4 is associated with advanced colorectal cancer. Int J Color Dis. 2010;25(10):1185–91. https://doi.org/10.1007/s00384-010-0999-1.
14. Rudmik LR, Magliocco AM. Molecular mechanisms of hepatic metastasis in colorectal cancer. J Surg Oncol. 2005;92(4):347–59. https://doi.org/10.1002/jso.20393.
15. Li JQ, Miki H, Wu F, Saoo K, Nishioka M, Ohmori M, et al. Cyclin a correlates with carcinogenesis and metastasis, and p27(kip1) correlates with lymphatic invasion, in colorectal neoplasms. Hum Pathol. 2002;33(10):1006–15.
16. Thomas GV, Szigeti K, Murphy M, Draetta G, Pagano M, Loda M. Down-regulation of p27 is associated with development of colorectal adenocarcinoma metastases. Am J Pathol. 1998;153(3):681–7. https://doi.org/10.1016/S0002-9440(10)65610-6.
17. Lloyd RV, Erickson LA, Jin L, Kulig E, Qian X, Cheville JC, et al. p27kip1: a multifunctional cyclin-dependent kinase inhibitor with prognostic significance in human cancers. Am J Pathol. 1999;154(2):313–23. https://doi.org/10.1016/S0002-9440(10)65277-7.

18. Li JQ, Miki H, Ohmori M, Wu F, Funamoto Y. Expression of cyclin E and cyclin-dependent kinase 2 correlates with metastasis and prognosis in colorectal carcinoma. Hum Pathol. 2001;32(9):945–53. https://doi.org/10.1053/hupa.2001.27116.
19. Kobayashi H, Sugihara K, Uetake H, Higuchi T, Yasuno M, Enomoto M, et al. Messenger RNA expression of TS and ERCC1 in colorectal cancer and matched liver metastasis. Int J Oncol. 2008;33(6):1257–62.
20. Inokuchi M, Uetake H, Shirota Y, Yamada H, Tajima M, Sugihara K. Gene expression of 5-fluorouracil metabolic enzymes in primary colorectal cancer and corresponding liver metastasis. Cancer Chemother Pharmacol. 2004;53(5):391–6. https://doi.org/10.1007/s00280-003-0747-0.
21. Ghadjar P, Coupland SE, Na IK, Noutsias M, Letsch A, Stroux A, et al. Chemokine receptor CCR6 expression level and liver metastases in colorectal cancer. J Clin Oncol. 2006;24(12):1910–6. https://doi.org/10.1200/JCO.2005.04.1822.
22. Kim J, Takeuchi H, Lam ST, Turner RR, Wang HJ, Kuo C, et al. Chemokine receptor CXCR4 expression in colorectal cancer patients increases the risk for recurrence and for poor survival. J Clin Oncol. 2005;23(12):2744–53. https://doi.org/10.1200/JCO.2005.07.078.
23. Ghadjar P, Rubie C, Aebersold DM, Keilholz U. The chemokine CCL20 and its receptor CCR6 in human malignancy with focus on colorectal cancer. Int J Cancer. 2009;125(4):741–5. https://doi.org/10.1002/ijc.24468.
24. Wu Y, Jin M, Xu H, Shimin Z, He S, Wang L, et al. Clinicopathologic significance of HIF-1alpha, CXCR4, and VEGF expression in colon cancer. Clin Dev Immunol. 2010;2010:1. https://doi.org/10.1155/2010/537531.
25. Kim YW, Ko YT, Kim NK, Chung HC, Min BS, Lee KY, et al. A comparative study of protein expression in primary colorectal cancer and synchronous hepatic metastases: the significance of matrix metalloproteinase-1 expression as a predictor of liver metastasis. Scand J Gastroenterol. 2010;45(2):217–25. https://doi.org/10.3109/00365520903453158.
26. Esposito DL, Aru F, Lattanzio R, Morgano A, Abbondanza M, Malekzadeh R, et al. The insulin receptor substrate 1 (IRS1) in intestinal epithelial differentiation and in colorectal cancer. PLoS One. 2012;7(4):e36190. https://doi.org/10.1371/journal.pone.0036190.
27. Bommer GT, Feng Y, Iura A, Giordano TJ, Kuick R, Kadikoy H, et al. IRS1 regulation by Wnt/beta-catenin signaling and varied contribution of IRS1 to the neoplastic phenotype. J Biol Chem. 2010;285(3):1928–38. https://doi.org/10.1074/jbc.M109.060319.
28. Ayaki M, Komatsu K, Mukai M, Murata K, Kameyama M, Ishiguro S, et al. Reduced expression of focal adhesion kinase in liver metastases compared with matched primary human colorectal adenocarcinomas. Clin Cancer Res. 2001;7(10):3106–12.
29. Yamauchi T, Watanabe M, Kubota T, Hasegawa H, Ishii Y, Endo T, et al. Cyclooxygenase-2 expression as a new marker for patients with colorectal cancer. Dis Colon Rectum. 2002;45(1):98–103.
30. Watanabe T, Kobunai T, Yamamoto Y, Kanazawa T, Konishi T, Tanaka T, et al. Prediction of liver metastasis after colorectal cancer using reverse transcription-polymerase chain reaction analysis of 10 genes. Eur J Cancer. 2010;46(11):2119–26. https://doi.org/10.1016/j.ejca.2010.04.019.
31. Nakamoto RH, Uetake H, Iida S, Kolev YV, Soumaoro LT, Takagi Y, et al. Correlations between cyclooxygenase-2 expression and angiogenic factors in primary tumors and liver metastases in colorectal cancer. Jpn J Clin Oncol. 2007;37(9):679–85. https://doi.org/10.1093/jjco/hym080.
32. Pantaleo MA, Astolfi A, Nannini M, Paterini P, Piazzi G, Ercolani G, et al. Gene expression profiling of liver metastases from colorectal cancer as potential basis for treatment choice. Br J Cancer. 2008;99(10):1729–34. https://doi.org/10.1038/sj.bjc.6604681.
33. Prabhudesai SG, Rekhraj S, Roberts G, Darzi AW, Ziprin P. Apoptosis and chemo-resistance in colorectal cancer. J Surg Oncol. 2007;96(1):77–88. https://doi.org/10.1002/jso.20785.
34. De Jong KP, Stellema R, Karrenbeld A, Koudstaal J, Gouw AS, Sluiter WJ, et al. Clinical relevance of transforming growth factor alpha, epidermal growth factor receptor, p53, and Ki67 in colorectal liver metastases and corresponding primary tumors. Hepatology. 1998;28(4):971–9. https://doi.org/10.1002/hep.510280411.

35. Miyagawa S, Soeda J, Takagi S, Miwa S, Ichikawa E, Noike T. Prognostic significance of mature dendritic cells and factors associated with their accumulation in metastatic liver tumors from colorectal cancer. Hum Pathol. 2004;35(11):1392–6. https://doi.org/10.1016/j.humpath.2004.07.018.
36. van der Wal GE, Gouw AS, Kamps JA, Moorlag HE, Bulthuis ML, Molema G, et al. Angiogenesis in synchronous and metachronous colorectal liver metastases: the liver as a permissive soil. Ann Surg. 2012;255(1):86–94. https://doi.org/10.1097/SLA.0b013e318238346a.
37. Venderbosch S, de Wilt JH, Teerenstra S, Loosveld OJ, van Bochove A, Sinnige HA, et al. Prognostic value of resection of primary tumor in patients with stage IV colorectal cancer: retrospective analysis of two randomized studies and a review of the literature. Ann Surg Oncol. 2011;18(12):3252–60. https://doi.org/10.1245/s10434-011-1951-5.
38. Wang K, Liu W, Yan XL, Li J, Xing BC. Long-term postoperative survival prediction in patients with colorectal liver metastasis. Oncotarget. 2017;8(45):79927–34. https://doi.org/10.18632/oncotarget.20322.
39. Graf W, Bergstrom R, Pahlman L, Glimelius B. Appraisal of a model for prediction of prognosis in advanced colorectal cancer. Eur J Cancer. 1994;30A(4):453–7.
40. Freyer G, Rougier P, Bugat R, Droz JP, Marty M, Bleiberg H, et al. Prognostic factors for tumour response, progression-free survival and toxicity in metastatic colorectal cancer patients given irinotecan (CPT-11) as second-line chemotherapy after 5FU failure. CPT-11 F205, F220, F221 and V222 study groups. Br J Cancer. 2000;83(4):431–7. https://doi.org/10.1054/bjoc.2000.1303.
41. Etienne-Grimaldi MC, Formento JL, Francoual M, Francois E, Formento P, Renee N, et al. K-Ras mutations and treatment outcome in colorectal cancer patients receiving exclusive fluoropyrimidine therapy. Clin Cancer Res. 2008;14(15):4830–5. https://doi.org/10.1158/1078-0432.CCR-07-4906.
42. Tsai MS, Su YH, Ho MC, Liang JT, Chen TP, Lai HS, et al. Clinicopathological features and prognosis in resectable synchronous and metachronous colorectal liver metastasis. Ann Surg Oncol. 2007;14(2):786–94. https://doi.org/10.1245/s10434-006-9215-5.
43. Manfredi S, Lepage C, Hatem C, Coatmeur O, Faivre J, Bouvier AM. Epidemiology and management of liver metastases from colorectal cancer. Ann Surg. 2006;244(2):254–9. https://doi.org/10.1097/01.sla.0000217629.94941.cf.
44. Ghiringhelli F, Hennequin A, Drouillard A, Lepage C, Faivre J, Bouvier AM. Epidemiology and prognosis of synchronous and metachronous colon cancer metastases: a French population-based study. Dig Liver Dis. 2014;46(9):854–8. https://doi.org/10.1016/j.dld.2014.05.011.
45. Mekenkamp LJ, Koopman M, Teerenstra S, van Krieken JH, Mol L, Nagtegaal ID, et al. Clinicopathological features and outcome in advanced colorectal cancer patients with synchronous vs metachronous metastases. Br J Cancer. 2010;103(2):159–64. https://doi.org/10.1038/sj.bjc.6605737.
46. van der Pool AE, Lalmahomed ZS, Ozbay Y, de Wilt JH, Eggermont AM, Jzermans JN, et al. 'Staged' liver resection in synchronous and metachronous colorectal hepatic metastases: differences in clinicopathological features and outcome. Colorectal Dis. 2010;12(10 Online):e229–35. https://doi.org/10.1111/j.1463-1318.2009.02135.x.
47. Leporrier J, Maurel J, Chiche L, Bara S, Segol P, Launoy G. A population-based study of the incidence, management and prognosis of hepatic metastases from colorectal cancer. Br J Surg. 2006;93(4):465–74. https://doi.org/10.1002/bjs.5278.
48. Engstrand J, Nilsson H, Stromberg C, Jonas E, Freedman J. Colorectal cancer liver metastases - a population-based study on incidence, management and survival. BMC Cancer. 2018;18(1):78. https://doi.org/10.1186/s12885-017-3925-x.
49. Swan PJ, Welsh FK, Chandrakumaran K, Rees M. Long-term survival following delayed presentation and resection of colorectal liver metastases. Br J Surg. 2011;98(9):1309–17. https://doi.org/10.1002/bjs.7527.
50. Hackl C, Neumann P, Gerken M, Loss M, Klinkhammer-Schalke M, Schlitt HJ. Treatment of colorectal liver metastases in Germany: a ten-year population-based analysis of 5772

cases of primary colorectal adenocarcinoma. BMC Cancer. 2014;14:810. https://doi.org/10.1186/1471-2407-14-810.

51. Wang X, Hershman DL, Abrams JA, Feingold D, Grann VR, Jacobson JS, et al. Predictors of survival after hepatic resection among patients with colorectal liver metastasis. Br J Cancer. 2007;97(12):1606–12. https://doi.org/10.1038/sj.bjc.6604093.
52. Scheele J, Stang R, Altendorf-Hofmann A, Paul M. Resection of colorectal liver metastases. World J Surg. 1995;19(1):59–71.
53. Nordlinger B, Guiguet M, Vaillant JC, Balladur P, Boudjema K, Bachellier P, et al. Surgical resection of colorectal carcinoma metastases to the liver. A prognostic scoring system to improve case selection, based on 1568 patients. Association Francaise de Chirurgie. Cancer. 1996;77(7):1254–62.
54. Fong Y, Fortner J, Sun RL, Brennan MF, Blumgart LH. Clinical score for predicting recurrence after hepatic resection for metastatic colorectal cancer: analysis of 1001 consecutive cases. Ann Surg. 1999;230(3):309–18; discussion 18–21.
55. Sadot E, Groot Koerkamp B, Leal JN, Shia J, Gonen M, Allen PJ, et al. Resection margin and survival in 2368 patients undergoing hepatic resection for metastatic colorectal cancer: surgical technique or biologic surrogate? Ann Surg. 2015;262(3):476–85.; ; discussion 83–5. https://doi.org/10.1097/SLA.0000000000001427.
56. Rees M, Tekkis PP, Welsh FK, O'Rourke T, John TG. Evaluation of long-term survival after hepatic resection for metastatic colorectal cancer: a multifactorial model of 929 patients. Ann Surg. 2008;247(1):125–35. https://doi.org/10.1097/SLA.0b013e31815aa2c2.
57. Malik HZ, Prasad KR, Halazun KJ, Aldoori A, Al-Mukhtar A, Gomez D, et al. Preoperative prognostic score for predicting survival after hepatic resection for colorectal liver metastases. Ann Surg. 2007;246(5):806–14. https://doi.org/10.1097/SLA.0b013e318142d964.
58. Figueras J, Torras J, Valls C, Llado L, Ramos E, Marti-Rague J, et al. Surgical resection of colorectal liver metastases in patients with expanded indications: a single-center experience with 501 patients. Dis Colon Rectum. 2007;50(4):478–88. https://doi.org/10.1007/s10350-006-0817-6.
59. Weber JC, Nakano H, Bachellier P, Oussoultzoglou E, Inoue K, Shimura H, et al. Is a proliferation index of cancer cells a reliable prognostic factor after hepatectomy in patients with colorectal liver metastases? Am J Surg. 2001;182(1):81–8.
60. Vigano L, Capussotti L, Lapointe R, Barroso E, Hubert C, Giuliante F, et al. Early recurrence after liver resection for colorectal metastases: risk factors, prognosis, and treatment. A LiverMetSurvey-based study of 6,025 patients. Ann Surg Oncol. 2014;21(4):1276–86. https://doi.org/10.1245/s10434-013-3421-8.
61. Ng WW, Cheung YS, Wong J, Lee KF, Lai PB. A preliminary analysis of combined liver resection with new chemotherapy for synchronous and metachronous colorectal liver metastasis. Asian J Surg. 2009;32(4):189–97. https://doi.org/10.1016/S1015-9584(09)60394-8.
62. Wei AC, Greig PD, Grant D, Taylor B, Langer B, Gallinger S. Survival after hepatic resection for colorectal metastases: a 10-year experience. Ann Surg Oncol. 2006;13(5):668–76. https://doi.org/10.1245/ASO.2006.05.039.
63. Pawlik TM, Scoggins CR, Zorzi D, Abdalla EK, Andres A, Eng C, et al. Effect of surgical margin status on survival and site of recurrence after hepatic resection for colorectal metastases. Ann Surg. 2005;241(5):715–22, discussion 22–4.
64. Nanji S, Cleary S, Ryan P, Guindi M, Selvarajah S, Al-Ali H, et al. Up-front hepatic resection for metastatic colorectal cancer results in favorable long-term survival. Ann Surg Oncol. 2013;20(1):295–304. https://doi.org/10.1245/s10434-012-2424-1.
65. de Jong MC, Pulitano C, Ribero D, Strub J, Mentha G, Schulick RD, et al. Rates and patterns of recurrence following curative intent surgery for colorectal liver metastasis: an international multi-institutional analysis of 1669 patients. Ann Surg. 2009;250(3):440–8. https://doi.org/10.1097/SLA.0b013e3181b4539b.
66. Sugawara Y, Yamamoto J, Yamasaki S, Shimada K, Kosuge T, Makuuchi M. Estimating the prognosis of hepatic resection in patients with metastatic liver tumors from colorectal cancer

with special concern for the timing of hepatectomy. Surgery. 2001;129(4):408–13. https://doi.org/10.1067/msy.2001.112001.
67. Adam R, Bismuth H, Castaing D, Waechter F, Navarro F, Abascal A, et al. Repeat hepatectomy for colorectal liver metastases. Ann Surg. 1997;225(1):51–60; discussion −2.
68. Hallet J, Sa Cunha A, Adam R, Goere D, Bachellier P, Azoulay D, et al. Factors influencing recurrence following initial hepatectomy for colorectal liver metastases. Br J Surg. 2016;103(10):1366–76. https://doi.org/10.1002/bjs.10191.
69. Iwatsuki S, Dvorchik I, Madariaga JR, Marsh JW, Dodson F, Bonham AC, et al. Hepatic resection for metastatic colorectal adenocarcinoma: a proposal of a prognostic scoring system. J Am Coll Surg. 1999;189(3):291–9.
70. Xu J, Wei Y, Zhong Y, Fan J, Zhou J, Qin L, et al. Hepatectomy for liver metastasis of colorectal cancer. Int J Color Dis. 2009;24(4):419–25. https://doi.org/10.1007/s00384-008-0619-5.
71. Ito H, Are C, Gonen M, D'Angelica M, Dematteo RP, Kemeny NE, et al. Effect of postoperative morbidity on long-term survival after hepatic resection for metastatic colorectal cancer. Ann Surg. 2008;247(6):994–1002. https://doi.org/10.1097/SLA.0b013e31816c405f.
72. Angelsen JH, Viste A, Loes IM, Eide GE, Hoem D, Sorbye H, et al. Predictive factors for time to recurrence, treatment and post-recurrence survival in patients with initially resected colorectal liver metastases. World J Surg Oncol. 2015;13:328. https://doi.org/10.1186/s12957-015-0738-8.
73. Imai K, Allard MA, Benitez CC, Vibert E, Sa Cunha A, Cherqui D, et al. Early recurrence after hepatectomy for colorectal liver metastases: what optimal definition and what predictive factors? Oncologist. 2016;21(7):887–94. https://doi.org/10.1634/theoncologist.2015-0468.
74. Takahashi S, Konishi M, Nakagohri T, Gotohda N, Saito N, Kinoshita T. Short time to recurrence after hepatic resection correlates with poor prognosis in colorectal hepatic metastasis. Jpn J Clin Oncol. 2006;36(6):368–75. https://doi.org/10.1093/jjco/hyl027.
75. Bozzetti F, Doci R, Bignami P, Morabito A, Gennari L. Patterns of failure following surgical resection of colorectal cancer liver metastases. Rationale for a multimodal approach. Ann Surg. 1987;205(3):264–70.
76. Beppu T, Sakamoto Y, Hasegawa K, Honda G, Tanaka K, Kotera Y, et al. A nomogram predicting disease-free survival in patients with colorectal liver metastases treated with hepatic resection: multicenter data collection as a project study for hepatic surgery of the Japanese society of Hepato-biliary-pancreatic surgery. J Hepatobiliary Pancreat Sci. 2012;19(1):72–84. https://doi.org/10.1007/s00534-011-0460-z.
77. Ishizuka D, Shirai Y, Sakai Y, Hatakeyama K. Colorectal carcinoma liver metastases: clinical significance of preoperative measurement of serum carcinoembryonic antigen and carbohydrate antigen 19-9 levels. Int J Color Dis. 2001;16(1):32–7.
78. Lu Z, Peng J, Wang Z, Pan Z, Yuan Y, Wan D, et al. High preoperative serum CA19-9 level is predictive of poor prognosis for patients with colorectal liver oligometastases undergoing hepatic resection. Med Oncol. 2016;33(11):121. https://doi.org/10.1007/s12032-016-0838-5.
79. Vigano L, Procopio F, Cimino MM, Donadon M, Gatti A, Costa G, et al. Is tumor detachment from vascular structures equivalent to R0 resection in surgery for colorectal liver metastases? An Observational Cohort. Ann Surg Oncol. 2016;23(4):1352–60. https://doi.org/10.1245/s10434-015-5009-y.
80. Nordlinger B, Sorbye H, Glimelius B, Poston GJ, Schlag PM, Rougier P, et al. Perioperative chemotherapy with FOLFOX4 and surgery versus surgery alone for resectable liver metastases from colorectal cancer (EORTC intergroup trial 40983): a randomised controlled trial. Lancet. 2008;371(9617):1007–16. https://doi.org/10.1016/S0140-6736(08)60455-9.
81. Wurster EF, Tenckhoff S, Probst P, Jensen K, Dolger E, Knebel P, et al. A systematic review and meta-analysis of the utility of repeated versus single hepatic resection for colorectal cancer liver metastases. HPB (Oxford). 2017;19(6):491–7. https://doi.org/10.1016/j.hpb.2017.02.440.
82. Tomlinson JS, Jarnagin WR, DeMatteo RP, Fong Y, Kornprat P, Gonen M, et al. Actual 10-year survival after resection of colorectal liver metastases defines cure. J Clin Oncol. 2007;25(29):4575–80. https://doi.org/10.1200/JCO.2007.11.0833.

83. Vigano L, Ferrero A, Lo Tesoriere R, Capussotti L. Liver surgery for colorectal metastases: results after 10 years of follow-up. Long-term survivors, late recurrences, and prognostic role of morbidity. Ann Surg Oncol. 2008;15(9):2458–64. https://doi.org/10.1245/s10434-008-9935-9.
84. Pulitano C, Castillo F, Aldrighetti L, Bodingbauer M, Parks RW, Ferla G, et al. What defines 'cure' after liver resection for colorectal metastases? Results after 10 years of follow-up. HPB (Oxford). 2010;12(4):244–9. https://doi.org/10.1111/j.1477-2574.2010.00155.x.
85. Adam R, Wicherts DA, de Haas RJ, Ciacio O, Levi F, Paule B, et al. Patients with initially unresectable colorectal liver metastases: is there a possibility of cure? J Clin Oncol. 2009;27(11):1829–35. https://doi.org/10.1200/JCO.2008.19.9273.
86. Imai K, Castro Benitez C, Allard MA, Vibert E, Sa Cunha A, Cherqui D, et al. Potential of a cure in patients with colorectal liver metastases and concomitant extrahepatic disease. J Surg Oncol. 2017;115(4):488–96. https://doi.org/10.1002/jso.24539.
87. Cucchetti A, Ferrero A, Cescon M, Donadon M, Russolillo N, Ercolani G, et al. Cure model survival analysis after hepatic resection for colorectal liver metastases. Ann Surg Oncol. 2015;22(6):1908–14. https://doi.org/10.1245/s10434-014-4234-0.
88. Nagashima I, Takada T, Nagawa H, Muto T, Okinaga K. Proposal of a new and simple staging system of colorectal liver metastasis. World J Gastroenterol. 2006;12(43):6961–5.
89. Konopke R, Kersting S, Distler M, Dietrich J, Gastmeier J, Heller A, et al. Prognostic factors and evaluation of a clinical score for predicting survival after resection of colorectal liver metastases. Liver Int. 2009;29(1):89–102. https://doi.org/10.1111/j.1478-3231.2008.01845.x.
90. Zakaria S, Donohue JH, Que FG, Farnell MB, Schleck CD, Ilstrup DM, et al. Hepatic resection for colorectal metastases: value for risk scoring systems? Ann Surg. 2007;246(2):183–91. https://doi.org/10.1097/SLA.0b013e3180603039.
91. Lise M, Bacchetti S, Da Pian P, Nitti D, Pilati P. Patterns of recurrence after resection of colorectal liver metastases: prediction by models of outcome analysis. World J Surg. 2001;25(5):638–44. https://doi.org/10.1007/s002680020138.
92. Ueno H, Mochizuki H, Hatsuse K, Hase K, Yamamoto T. Indicators for treatment strategies of colorectal liver metastases. Ann Surg. 2000;231(1):59–66.
93. Schindl M, Wigmore SJ, Currie EJ, Laengle F, Garden OJ. Prognostic scoring in colorectal cancer liver metastases: development and validation. Arch Surg. 2005;140(2):183–9. https://doi.org/10.1001/archsurg.140.2.183.
94. Kanemitsu Y, Kato T. Prognostic models for predicting death after hepatectomy in individuals with hepatic metastases from colorectal cancer. World J Surg. 2008;32(6):1097–107. https://doi.org/10.1007/s00268-007-9348-0.
95. Mann CD, Metcalfe MS, Leopardi LN, Maddern GJ. The clinical risk score: emerging as a reliable preoperative prognostic index in hepatectomy for colorectal metastases. Arch Surg. 2004;139(11):1168–72. https://doi.org/10.1001/archsurg.139.11.1168.
96. Mala T, Bohler G, Mathisen O, Bergan A, Soreide O. Hepatic resection for colorectal metastases: can preoperative scoring predict patient outcome? World J Surg. 2002;26(11):1348–53. https://doi.org/10.1007/s00268-002-6231-x.

Laparoscopic Resections for Colorectal Cancer Liver Metastases

28

Giammauro Berardi and Go Wakabayashi

Introduction

Minimally invasive procedures have deeply changed the surgical practice worldwide and have gained interest in the last decades, thanks to the improved outcomes in terms of postoperative complications, hospitalization, aesthetics, and overall cost-effectiveness compared to open surgery [1]. A fast-growing development affected different surgical specialties such as colorectal surgery, gynecology, urology, and thoracic surgery. [2–5] Conversely, the application of minimally invasive techniques to the hepatobiliary field was somehow slower likely because of the technical difficulties requiring experience in both hepatobiliary and complex laparoscopy, together with a specific long and demanding learning curve. [6] The first laparoscopic partial liver resection is dated back in 1991 [7], followed by anatomic and major hepatectomies in 1996 and 1997, respectively [8, 9]. Since then, the number of laparoscopic liver resections (LLR) grew exponentially with many case series and multicenter experiences being reported, leading to the first Consensus Conference in Louisville and 6 years later to the recommendations from the second World Consensus Conference in Morioka, which represent a landmark in minimally invasive surgery of the liver. [10–15] From the initial small case series of selected patients to the large multicenter experiences and randomized control trials, laparoscopy nowadays represents a common practice for liver surgery in many centers worldwide. To date, more than 9000 LLRs have been described for both benign and malignant lesions [16]. Despite initial

G. Berardi (✉) · G. Wakabayashi
Center for Advanced Treatment of HBP Diseases, Ageo Central General Hospital, Ageo Shi, Saitama, Japan

M. M. Correia et al. (eds.), *Colorectal Cancer Liver Metastases*,
https://doi.org/10.1007/978-3-030-25486-5_28

skepticism in fact, LLR is now accepted also for the treatment of primary and secondary liver malignancies. [17, 18] In the latest systematic review, over 60% of the total LLR were performed for malignancies, being hepatocellular carcinoma and colorectal liver metastases (CRLM) the most frequent indications [16]. In fact, despite the progress reached in the last decades in terms of screening programs, chemotherapy regimens, and surgical treatments, colorectal cancer still represents a major health issue affecting nearly one million people worldwide; as a further issue, around 65% of patients with colorectal cancer develop metastases being the liver the most common site either at the time of diagnosis (15–25%) or during follow-up (20–30%). [19]

The treatment of CRLM is based on a multimodal approach including systemic therapies and surgical resection; when these are deemed resectable, surgical approach in combination with chemotherapy represents the standard of care as it offers long-term survival, with rates of 22–55% at 5 years from resection [20]. Being one of the most frequent indications to liver surgery, laparoscopic approach for CRLM has been increasingly reported over time. Nguyen et al. described one of the first case series of 109 patients reporting good and safe results and low rates of morbidity and mortality [21]. Later, several studies with different level of evidence compared the postoperative short- and long-term outcomes of laparoscopic versus open liver resection (OLR) for CRLM (Fig. 28.1). [22–31]

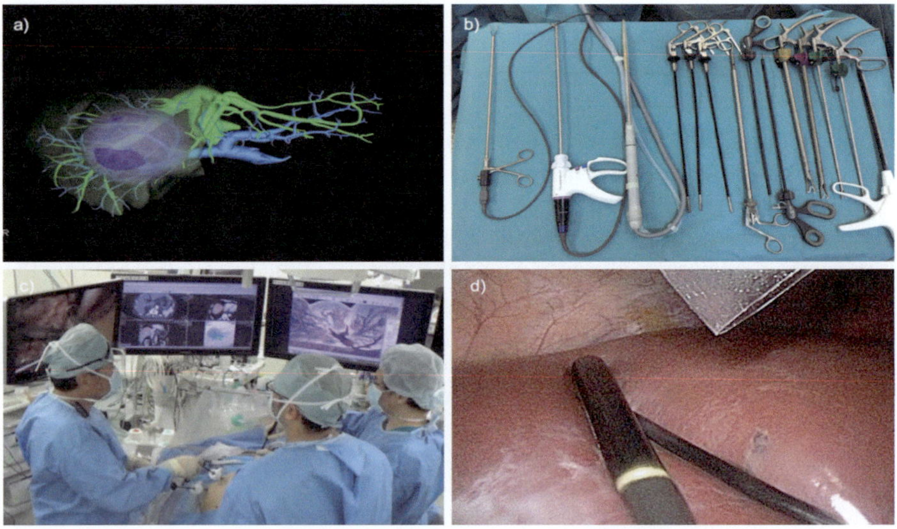

Fig. 28.1 Basics for laparoscopic liver resections. (**a**) Preoperative 3D reconstructions. (**b**) Surgical instruments. (**c**) Intraoperative position. (**d**) Intraoperative ultrasonography

Laparoscopic Versus Open resection for Colorectal Liver Metastases

To date, eight meta-analysis pooling studies that compared open and laparoscopic liver resections for CRLM have been reported, evaluating the results of more than four thousand patients. [17, 32–39] Moreover, a large amount of comparative and case-control studies, propensity score matchings, and even a randomized control trial focused on the role of laparoscopy in the treatment of CRLM, making the whole body of evidence large enough to draw reliable conclusions both in terms of postoperative and oncological outcomes.

In a well-designed 1:2 propensity score matching analysis, Beppu et al. showed that intraoperative blood loss (163 ml vs. 415 ml, $p < 0.001$) and transfusion rates (6.5% vs. 16.5%, $p = 0.004$) were significantly lower in LLR [40]. The buffer effect of the pneumoperitoneum and the magnification of vision are likely the major contributors, allowing for a detailed dissection with selective visualization of structures in a bloodless field during parenchymal transection. [32] It has too been mentioned that bleeding and transfusions have been claimed by some authors to negatively influence the oncological outcomes after liver resections and to prolong the time to adjuvant chemotherapy which might in turn improve long-term outcomes in LLR, despite no sufficient data is available to date. [32, 41]

Although some of the studies reported longer operative times during LLR, most of the available meta-analysis showed a comparable duration of surgery between the two approaches; the learning curve effect in this setting might play a major role, with improved intraoperative results in the later phases in which expertise is gained and standardization of procedures is reached.

Laparoscopic liver resection has comparable mortality rates to OLR and is associated with lower complications both in terms of overall morbidity and major morbidity (grade III or greater according to Clavien-Dindo classification). [16, 22, 23, 30] Furthermore, less requirement for analgesia and a shortened time to oral intake eventually result in reduced hospital stay. [24, 25, 40] The mini invasiveness of LLR reduces manipulation of the liver, electrolyte imbalance, postoperative ileus, and stress on the abdominal wall which in turn lead to a faster recovery and mobilization, reducing complications such as urinary tract infections, pneumonia, and wound infections, while it is possible that the magnified laparoscopic vision could significantly reduce major complications (i.e., bile leakage, bleeding) by allowing a more detailed revision of the transection line at the end of the procedure. Furthermore, two interesting randomized controlled studies showed a reduction in the inflammatory response after LLR for CRLM inducing a well-preserved immune function in the postoperative period, hence reducing the occurrence of complications. [42, 43]

Despite data is scant and severely biased by different healthcare systems, it is likely that laparoscopic approach is associated with overall cost-effectiveness compared to OLR. Indeed, despite the apparent intraoperative economic burden for the surgical equipment, the decrease in complications, the faster recovery, and the reduction in hospital stay eventually lead to an overall reduction in hospital costs. [32]

All the available studies and all the pooled meta-analysis reported comparable oncological outcomes between LLR and OLR in terms of surgical margins, recurrence rates, overall survival (OS), and disease-free survival (DFS). Furthermore, Beppu et al. observed no specific differences regarding recurrences' patterns when analyzing DFS from initial hepatecomy. [40] An interesting study by Montalti et al. showed a higher number of repeated hepatectomies for recurrence during follow-up, speculating that due to the reduced anatomical changes, LLR might be associated with higher resectability in case of recurrence [30]. Indeed, the rate of second hepatectomies in their study was 56% and 62% in OLR and LLR, while a third hepatectomy was possible in 14% versus 80% of cases who initially underwent laparotomy and laparoscopy, respectively ($p = 0.015$).

Therefore, the available evidence from retrospective comparisons highlights that LLR for CRLM is safe and feasible and associated with superior results in terms of intraoperative blood loss and postoperative outcomes, maintaining safety from the oncological point of view. Recently, the first randomized control trial, the OSLO-COMET trial, disclosed its results achieving the highest level of evidence currently available on the topic. [44] The enrollment of patients was dated between 2012 and 2016 and was limited to minor LLR for CRLM focusing on mortality, morbidity, and resection margins as principal outcomes: mortality was comparable between groups with only 1 reported event in the OLR, while morbidity was significantly lower in laparoscopy (31% in OLR and 19% in LLR $p = 0.02$) but comparable considering only major grade complications (11% in LLR and 14% in OLR). Hospital stay was shorter after LLR, and patients required less morphine-based analgesia. Resection margins were comparable between groups with 6% R1 resection rate in LLR and 7% in OLR. Quality of life was evaluated at baseline, 1- and 4-months, and LLR achieved superior results. Finally, a cost analysis showed that laparoscopy was cost-effective with a likelihood of 67%. The results from the OSLO-COMET trial confirm and further enhance the improved postoperative short-term outcomes of LLR compared to OLR; in the future, the secondary outcomes evaluating long-term survivals will be available for interpretation, finally achieving further evidence on the oncological value of LLR.

Selection Criteria for Laparoscopic Liver Resection for Colorectal Liver Metastases

According to the early experiences available in the literature, laparoscopic liver resection was strictly reserved to extremely selected cases as still considered as an innovative technique: small, single, peripheral lesions in the anterolateral segments were initially most commonly approached. [45] With the wider adoption and implementation of technique into practice, the number of patients increased, and the indications broadened with time, with more complex patients and demanding procedures being considered. [1] To date, around 20–50% of liver resections could be approached by laparoscopy depending on the referral and local expertise [46]. Similarly, over the past decades, the concept of tumor resectability in CRLM has significantly changed from a policy in which only patients with solitary liver lesions could benefit from operative treatment, to a concept in which surgery is considered regardless of the tumor's size and number, provided that negative margins and enough remnant liver are guaranteed. For the abovementioned reasons, laparoscopic liver surgeons are progressing and broadening the indications to LLR for CRLM, and selection criteria vary among the literature according to the learning curve and experience. Despite this, even in the most experienced centers, patient's and tumor's related factors still represent a limit in LLR selection. From a technical point of view, large lesions and bulky tumors infiltrating major structures requiring vascular and biliary reconstructions are still seen as a major hurdle. [38] Similarly, multiple and bilobar metastases should be cautiously approached as challenges during ultrasound evaluation, exposure, and maintenance of adequate margins are a matter of fact during laparoscopy.

Concerning type of procedures, according to the available evidence, laparoscopy is widely recognized as the gold standard approach for left lateral sectionectomy and for partial resections in the anterolateral segments [47]. Conversely, posterosuperior resections (Fig. 28.2), anatomical segmentectomies, major hepatectomies, central hepatectomy, and right anterior and posterior sectionectomies are certainly more demanding and should be approached after appropriate learning curve [48]. Indeed, learning curve might influence selection of candidates as surgeons gradually perform LLR in a stepwise manner with easier resections in the early phase likely broadening indications with proficiency.

During the recent Southampton Consensus Guidelines Meeting, LLR for colorectal liver metastases was recommended as a valid alternative to the open approach with shorter hospital stay and lower complication rates [49]. Advanced age and obesity were not considered as contraindications, while repeated hepatectomies, two-stage resections, proximity to major vessels, and lesions >10 cm were considered only in experienced hands as were major hepatectomies, difficult resections (i.e., posterosuperior segments), and anatomical segmentectomies. Therefore, selection of candidates for LLR should consider patients' characteristics, disease presentation, and expertise in order to minimize conversions, improve postoperative outcomes, and maintain safe survivals. [50]

Laparoscopic Parenchyma-Sparing Liver Resections

During the last decades, parenchyma-sparing liver resections have been demonstrated to be advantageous for the treatment of CRLM compared to more extensive resections. On one side, a radical resection of the tumor with clear margins sparing as much healthy parenchyma as possible is associated with lower rates of posthepatectomy liver failure, especially after neoadjuvant chemotherapy; on the other side, recurrence after resection for CRLM is frequent, and repeated hepatectomies have been reported to achieve satisfactory outcomes [40]; hence, preserving healthy parenchyma allows for re-resection in case of recurrence.

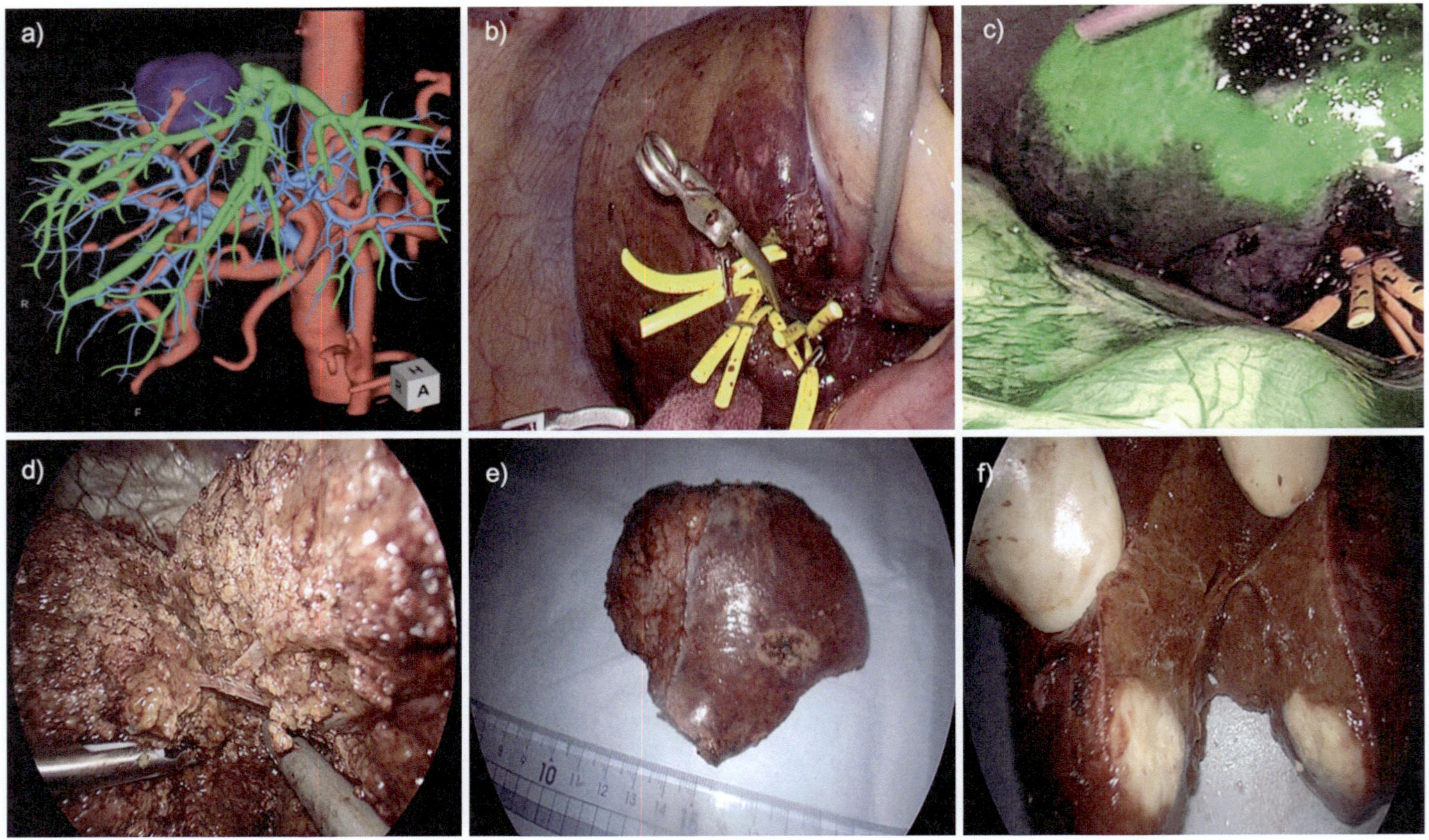

Fig. 28.2 Laparoscopic segment 7 resection for colorectal liver metastases. (**a**) Preoperative 3D reconstruction. (**b**) Glissonian approach to S7 pedicle. (**c**) Indocyanine green demarcation line. (**d**) Parenchymal transection. (**e**) S7 specimen. (**f**) Colorectal metastases

As far as negative margins and remnant liver are respected, parenchyma-sparing liver resections represent a milestone in the multimodal treatment of CRLM and are associated with less surgical stress and fewer complications. In this setting, multiple partial nonanatomical resections are performed in order to achieve complete removal of the tumor sparing as much healthy liver as possible.

Laparoscopic approach for parenchyma-sparing resections has been described as safe, with good short- and long-term outcomes; despite this, most of the studies reported the results of single lesions, while few focused on parenchyma-sparing resections for multiple metastases. In this setting, the number and the unfavorable localization of multiple tumors could represent a major challenge in laparoscopy due to the need of different patient position and port placement among right- and left-sided resections in bilobar lesions. Furthermore, the use of intraoperative ultrasonography is pivotal to locate the lesions and guide the resections in order to achieve safe margins. Aghayan et al. described a case series of 296 patients undergoing laparoscopic parenchymal-sparing resections for CRLM with a 5-year survival of 44% in 80 patients undergoing resections for multiple liver metastases. Furthermore, in case of deep and unfavorable locations, they reported the association of laparoscopic parenchyma-sparing resections with radiofrequency ablation, achieving a 39% survival at 5 years. [51]

Overall, the available results demonstrate that laparoscopic parenchyma-sparing resections are feasible and associated with low conversion rates and fewer complications, representing the preferred option over major resections; more studies should investigate the role of laparoscopic parenchyma sparing for multiple and bilobar colorectal liver metastases as the evidence is still scarce.

Laparoscopic Major Hepatectomies for Colorectal Liver Metastases

Laparoscopic major hepatectomies have been limited to tertiary referral centers and to experienced surgeons due to the associated technical demands (Fig. 28.3). [1] The percentages of left and right hepatectomies in the major LLR case series range between 0% and 55%, demonstrating wide variability depending on centers and expertise [33]. Good postoperative outcomes and safe oncological outcomes have been reported, and some studies even speculated shorter hospitalization, fewer complications, and decreased blood loss compared to the open approach. [52–56] Conversely, Topal et al. reported the results of 20 patients undergoing laparoscopic major hepatectomies for CRLM and compared the outcomes with the open approach [31]. In their study, no statistical differences in terms of blood loss, operative time, postoperative complications, and survival outcomes were observed. In a recent met-analysis of propensity score-matched studies comparing OLR and LLR for CRLM, a nice subgroup analysis of patients undergoing major hepatectomies was performed; in this manuscript, LLR was confirmed to have better short-term outcomes, maintaining safe and comparable survivals to the open approach, representing a potentially safe alternative for patients requiring major hepatectomies [33].

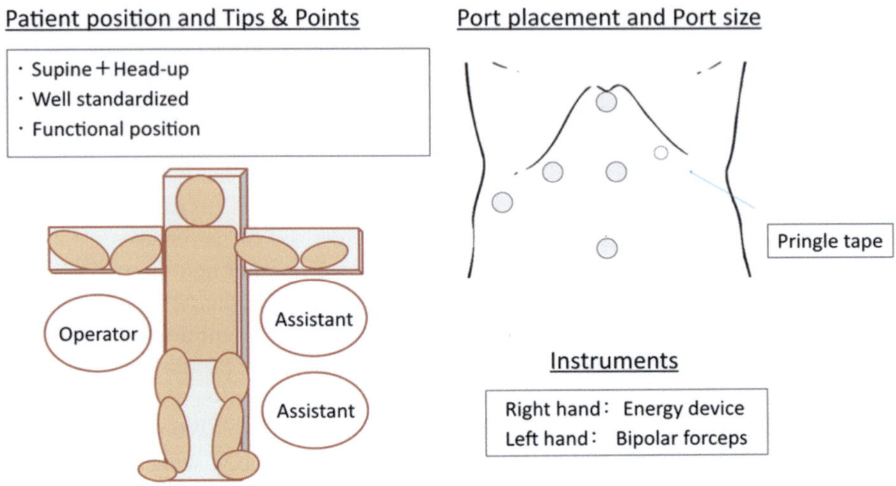

Fig. 28.3 Patients and port position for laparoscopic right and left hepatectomies

In another recent meta-analysis, laparoscopic major hepatectomies were associated with longer operative time, while blood loss, transfusion rates, and postoperative morbidity were significantly lower. Furthermore, oncological outcomes were comparable in terms of recurrence rates, OS, and DFS. LLR were associated with conversion rates ranging from 9% to 42% [53]: these rates are clearly higher than the average for minor hepatectomies and reasonably reflect the challenges of these procedures. The difficult mobilization, the large cut surface, and the numbers of potential intraoperative pitfalls certainly represent a challenge in this setting. Indeed, laparoscopic major hepatectomies should be performed in the final phases of the learning curve, after proficiency is achieved with minor and easier resections, in order to guarantee safety and improve postoperative outcomes.

All the studies currently available on the topic, including meta-analysis, suffer from selection bias as easier cases were likely selected for the laparoscopic approach. Furthermore, the referral policy and surgeon's experience and skills might hamper the reproducibility of results. The first randomized controlled trial comparing laparoscopic versus open major hepatectomies, the ORANGE-II plus trial (NCT01441856), has recently finished recruitment, and results will finally disclose the advantages of one or the other technique in terms of postoperative short-term outcomes.

Laparoscopic Two-Stage Hepatectomy for Bilobar Colorectal Liver Metastases

Only 20% of patients with bilobar CRLM are deemed resectable at the time of diagnosis. [57] One of the main limits in these patients is the future liver remnant (FLR) which must be adequate to avoid posthepatectomy liver failure. Two-stage

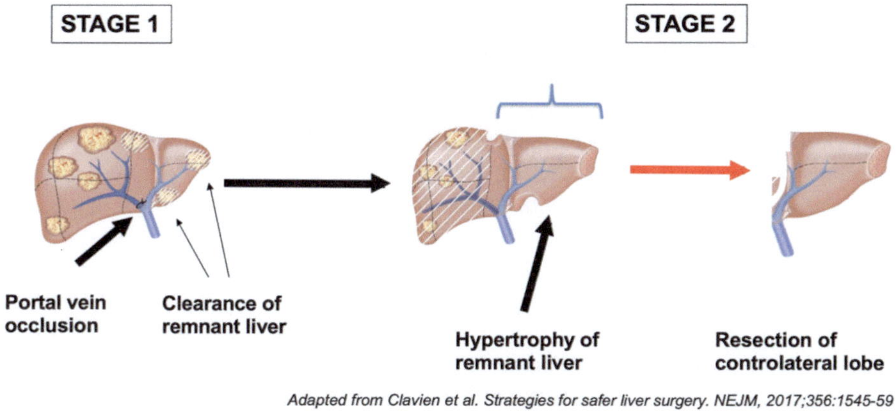

Fig. 28.4 Two-stage hepatectomy for bilobar colorectal liver metastases

hepatectomy has been proposed as a valid option for patients with bilobar CRLM and low FLR (Fig. 28.4). This consists of a first-stage operation in which the least diseased lobe is cleared from metastases and the contralateral portal vein is ligated, followed by a second stage in which after adequate FLR hypertrophy, the most diseased liver lobe is resected. This strategy has improved resectability rated by 10–50% in advanced patients.

Few studies have investigated the role of laparoscopy for two-stage hepatectomy [58–61]. Fuks et al. reported an overall feasibility of the procedure including both first and second stage, with 80% of patients completing the whole protocol. A low conversion rate was disclosed in this study (6% during first stage, 15% during second stage), and few major complications (11% during first stage, 26% during second stage) and posthepatectomy liver failures (0% during first stage, 7% during second stage) were observed. Furthermore, a 31% 5-year OS from first hepatectomy was reported. The first-stage laparoscopic hepatectomy, inducing fewer adhesions, less surgical stress, and rapid postoperative recovery, might play a positive role in the management of these patients, with fewer complications potentially reducing interstage dropout. On the other side, the second stage represents a challenge due to the technically demanding hilar dissection as a consequence of portal vein ligation and because of the changes in the anatomy due to the liver hypertrophy and should therefore be performed by expert laparoscopic hepatobiliary surgeons.

Laparoscopic Repeated Liver Resections for Recurrent Colorectal Metastases

Colorectal liver metastases have a 50–60% chance of recurrence during follow-up after liver resection, and in these cases, repeat hepatectomy has been shown to provide good oncological outcomes. [40, 62, 63] A recent worldwide survey reported that the long-term survival of patients undergoing a first liver resection was comparable to those who underwent up to four repeated liver resections. [63] However, adhesions and anatomical changes induced by previous resections and systemic treatments significantly increase the level of difficulty during repeated hepatecomy, and in the case of the laparoscopic approach, it may increase the rate of intraoperative conversions. [50] Despite this, some authors reported encouraging results from their experience with laparoscopy for recurrent CRLM. [64, 65] In a recent propensity score matching analysis, LLR was associated with shorter operative time (200 min vs. 256 min, $p < 0.001$) and shorter hospital stay (5 days vs. 6 days, $p = 0.02$); furthermore, a trend toward less blood loss was noted (200 ml vs. 300 ml, $p = 0.07$), while postoperative morbidity and mortality were comparable between groups. The laparoscopic caudal view and the need for minimum mobilization and adhesion takedown to achieve the target lesions may explain these better outcomes. However, the most noticeable finding was that LLR were more frequently preceded by laparoscopic liver resections compared to open [65]. This could be attributed to the fact that LLR is generally associated with less adhesion formation which could in turn improve accessibility to the abdomen in case of repeated abdominal procedures.

It still should be kept in mind that laparoscopic repeated liver resections are still challenging procedures as the liver anatomy may be changed by the previous resection, introducing a further issue on trocar placement and exposure. For these reasons, laparoscopic repeated resections should be avoided in the early phase of the learning curve and approached once proficiency is reached for easier resections.

Laparoscopic Combined Resection of Colorectal Cancer and Liver Metastases

Around 15–25% of patients with colorectal cancer present with synchronous liver metastases at the time of diagnosis. [66] Among patients with resectable synchronous liver disease, the optimal operative sequence for the management of the primary tumor and the metastases is still debated; "colorectal-first," "liver-first," and "combined" strategies have been described for this clinical scenario with different results and selection criteria. With the improvements in surgical techniques and perioperative care, an increasing number of patients are being treated with combined resection with acceptable morbidity, mortality, and long-term outcomes. [67–69] Furthermore, synchronous resection might offer potential benefits including shorter hospital stay and shorter time to systemic therapies, which could possibly affect long-term outcomes. Despite this, the available evidence is limited to few case series and comparative studies. In a recent systematic review, laparoscopic combined resections were reported in 199 patients over 12 studies [68]: fifty-eight percent of patients underwent a colon resection, and the vast majority underwent a minor hepatectomy (84%). In the studies comparing open versus laparoscopic combined resection, laparoscopy was associated with similar operative time and postoperative morbidity as well as shorter hospital stay. Importantly, the oncological long-term outcomes were comparable. Postoperative morbidity was 19.9% in laparoscopy and 32.8% in open, while mortality rate was similar.

Due to the limited evidence, conclusions and results should be interpreted with caution and laparoscopic combined resections should be performed in selected patients and in referral centers. Low-risk colorectal resections as well as minor hepatectomies should be preferred, and the availability of a laparoscopic colorectal surgeon as well as a laparoscopic liver surgeon is strongly suggested.

Conclusion

Laparoscopic liver resections represent a valid option for the treatment of colorectal liver metastases. In several settings, LLR has demonstrated superior short-term outcomes and similar survivals compared to open resections. Patients' characteristics and disease presentation as well as learning curve and experience play a major role in the selection of candidates. Difficult procedures such as major hepatectomies and posterosuperior resections as well as challenging clinical scenarios such as multiple bilobar lesions, recurrences, and synchronous metastases should be approached with caution in referral centers by experienced surgeons.

References

1. Berardi G, Van Cleven S, Fretland AA, et al. Evolution of laparoscopic liver surgery from innovation to implementation to mastery: perioperative and oncologic outcomes of 2,238 patients from 4 European specialized centers. J Am Coll Surg. 2017;225(5):639–49.
2. Ghezzi F, Cromi A, Ditto A, et al. Laparoscopic versus open radical hysterectomy for stage IB2-IIB cervical cancer in the setting of neoadjuvant chemotherapy: a multi-institutional cohort study. Ann Surg Oncol. 2013;20(6):2007–15.
3. Guillou PJ, Quirke P, Thorpe H, et al. Short-term endpoints of conventional versus laparoscopic-assisted surgery in patients with colorectal cancer (MRC CLASICC trial): multicentre, randomised controlled trial. Lancet. 2005;365(9472):1718–26.
4. Luketich JD, Pennathur A, Awais O, et al. Outcomes after minimally invasive esophagectomy: review of over 1000 patients. Ann Surg. 2012;256(1):95–103.
5. Trabulsi EJ, Guillonneau B. Laparoscopic radical prostatectomy. J Urol. 2005;173(4):1072–9.
6. Gagner M, Rogula T, Selzer D. Laparoscopic liver resection: benefits and controversies. Surg Clin North Am. 2004;84(2):451–62.
7. Reich H, McGlynn F, DeCaprio J, et al. Laparoscopic excision of benign liver lesions. Obstet Gynecol. 1991;78(5 Pt 2):956–8.
8. Azagra JS, Goergen M, Gilbart E, et al. Laparoscopic anatomical (hepatic) left lateral segmentectomy-technical aspects. Surg Endosc. 1996;10(7):758–61.
9. Huscher CG, Napolitano C, Chiodini S, et al. Hepatic resections through the laparoscopic approach. Ann Ital Chir. 1997;68(6):791–7.
10. Belli G, Limongelli P, Fantini C, et al. Laparoscopic and open treatment of hepatocellular carcinoma in patients with cirrhosis. Br J Surg. 2009;96(9):1041–8.
11. Wakabayashi G, Cherqui D, Geller DA, et al. Recommendations for laparoscopic liver resection: a report from the second international consensus conference held in Morioka. Ann Surg. 2015;261(4):619–29.
12. Buell JF, Cherqui D, Geller DA, et al. The international position on laparoscopic liver surgery: the Louisville statement, 2008. Ann Surg. 2009;250(5):825–30.

13. Cherqui D, Husson E, Hammoud R, et al. Laparoscopic liver resections: a feasibility study in 30 patients. Ann Surg. 2000;232(6):753–62.
14. Descottes B, Lachachi F, Sodji M, et al. Early experience with laparoscopic approach for solid liver tumors: initial 16 cases. Ann Surg. 2000;232(5):641–5.
15. Nguyen KT, Gamblin TC, Geller DA. World review of laparoscopic liver resection-2,804 patients. Ann Surg. 2009;250(5):831–41.
16. Ciria R, Cherqui D, Geller DA, et al. Comparative short-term benefits of laparoscopic liver resection: 9000 cases and climbing. Ann Surg. 2016;263(4):761–77.
17. Schiffman SC, Kim KH, Tsung A, et al. Laparoscopic versus open liver resection for metastatic colorectal cancer: a metaanalysis of 610 patients. Surgery. 2015;157(2):211–22.
18. Xiong JJ, Altaf K, Javed MA, et al. Meta-analysis of laparoscopic vs open liver resection for hepatocellular carcinoma. World J Gastroenterol. 2012;18(45):6657–68.
19. Sugihara K, Uetake H. Therapeutic strategies for hepatic metastasis of colorectal cancer: overview. J Hepatobiliary Pancreat Sci. 2012;19(5):523–7.
20. Simmonds PC, Primrose JN, Colquitt JL, et al. Surgical resection of hepatic metastases from colorectal cancer: a systematic review of published studies. Br J Cancer. 2006;94(7): 982–99.
21. Nguyen KT, Laurent A, Dagher I, et al. Minimally invasive liver resection for metastatic colorectal cancer: a multi-institutional, international report of safety, feasibility, and early outcomes. Ann Surg. 2009;250(5):842–8.
22. Cannon RM, Scoggins CR, Callender GG, et al. Laparoscopic versus open resection of hepatic colorectal metastases. Surgery. 2012;152(4):567–73; discussion 573-4.
23. Castaing D, Vibert E, Ricca L, et al. Oncologic results of laparoscopic versus open hepatectomy for colorectal liver metastases in two specialized centers. Ann Surg. 2009;250(5):849–55.
24. Cheung TT, Poon RT, Yuen WK, et al. Outcome of laparoscopic versus open hepatectomy for colorectal liver metastases. ANZ J Surg. 2013;83(11):847–52.
25. Guerron AD, Aliyev S, Agcaoglu O, et al. Laparoscopic versus open resection of colorectal liver metastasis. Surg Endosc. 2013;27(4):1138–43.
26. Hu MG, Ou-yang CG, Zhao GD, et al. Outcomes of open versus laparoscopic procedure for synchronous radical resection of liver metastatic colorectal cancer: a comparative study. Surg Laparosc Endosc Percutan Tech. 2012;22(4):364–9.
27. Huh JW, Koh YS, Kim HR, et al. Comparison of laparoscopic and open colorectal resections for patients undergoing simultaneous R0 resection for liver metastases. Surg Endosc. 2011;25(1):193–8.
28. Kazaryan AM, Marangos IP, Rosok BI, et al. Laparoscopic resection of colorectal liver metastases: surgical and long-term oncologic outcome. Ann Surg. 2010;252(6):1005–12.
29. Mala T, Edwin B, Gladhaug I, et al. A comparative study of the short-term outcome following open and laparoscopic liver resection of colorectal metastases. Surg Endosc. 2002;16(7):1059–63.
30. Montalti R, Berardi G, Laurent S, et al. Laparoscopic liver resection compared to open approach in patients with colorectal liver metastases improves further resectability: oncological outcomes of a case-control matched-pairs analysis. Eur J Surg Oncol. 2014;40(5):536–44.
31. Topal H, Tiek J, Aerts R, et al. Outcome of laparoscopic major liver resection for colorectal metastases. Surg Endosc. 2012;26(9):2451–5.
32. Cheng Y, Zhang L, Li H, et al. Laparoscopic versus open liver resection for colorectal liver metastases: a systematic review. J Surg Res. 2017;220:234–46.
33. Zhang XL, Liu RF, Zhang D, et al. Laparoscopic versus open liver resection for colorectal liver metastases: a systematic review and meta-analysis of studies with propensity score-based analysis. Int J Surg. 2017;44:191–203.
34. Hallet J, Beyfuss K, Memeo R, et al. Short and long-term outcomes of laparoscopic compared to open liver resection for colorectal liver metastases. Hepatobiliary Surg Nutr. 2016;5(4):300–10.
35. Luo LX, Yu ZY, Bai YN. Laparoscopic hepatectomy for liver metastases from colorectal cancer: a meta-analysis. J Laparoendosc Adv Surg Tech A. 2014;24(4):213–22.

36. Tian ZQ, Su XF, Lin ZY, et al. Meta-analysis of laparoscopic versus open liver resection for colorectal liver metastases. Oncotarget. 2016;7(51):84544–55.
37. Wei M, He Y, Wang J, et al. Laparoscopic versus open hepatectomy with or without synchronous colectomy for colorectal liver metastasis: a meta-analysis. PLoS One. 2014;9(1):e87461.
38. Xie SM, Xiong JJ, Liu XT, et al. Laparoscopic versus open liver resection for colorectal liver metastases: a comprehensive systematic review and meta-analysis. Sci Rep. 2017;7(1):1012.
39. Zhou Y, Xiao Y, Wu L, et al. Laparoscopic liver resection as a safe and efficacious alternative to open resection for colorectal liver metastasis: a meta-analysis. BMC Surg. 2013;13:44.
40. Beppu T, Wakabayashi G, Hasegawa K, et al. Long-term and perioperative outcomes of laparoscopic versus open liver resection for colorectal liver metastases with propensity score matching: a multi-institutional Japanese study. J Hepatobiliary Pancreat Sci. 2015;22(10):711–20.
41. Younes RN, Rogatko A, Brennan MF. The influence of intraoperative hypotension and perioperative blood transfusion on disease-free survival in patients with complete resection of colorectal liver metastases. Ann Surg. 1991;214(2):107–13.
42. Fretland AA, Sokolov A, Postriganova N, et al. Inflammatory response after laparoscopic versus open resection of colorectal liver metastases: data from the Oslo-CoMet trial. Medicine (Baltimore). 2015;94(42):e1786.
43. Kasai M, Van Damme N, Berardi G, et al. The inflammatory response to stress and angiogenesis in liver resection for colorectal liver metastases: a randomized controlled trial comparing open versus laparoscopic approach. Acta Chir Belg. 2018;118(3):172–80.
44. Fretland AA, Dagenborg VJ, Bjornelv GMW, et al. Laparoscopic versus open resection for colorectal liver metastases: the OSLO-COMET randomized controlled trial. Ann Surg. 2018;267(2):199–207.
45. Mala T, Edwin B. Role and limitations of laparoscopic liver resection of colorectal metastases. Dig Dis. 2005;23(2):142–50.
46. Cherqui D. Evolution of laparoscopic liver resection. Br J Surg. 2016;103(11):1405–7.
47. Chang S, Laurent A, Tayar C, et al. Laparoscopy as a routine approach for left lateral sectionectomy. Br J Surg. 2007;94(1):58–63.
48. Kawaguchi Y, Fuks D, Kokudo N, et al. Difficulty of laparoscopic liver resection: proposal for a new classification. Ann Surg. 2017.
49. Abu Hilal M, Aldrighetti L, Dagher I, et al. The Southampton consensus guidelines for laparoscopic liver surgery: from indication to implementation. Ann Surg. 2018;268(1):11–8.
50. Halls MC, Cipriani F, Berardi G, et al. Conversion for unfavorable intraoperative events results in significantly worse outcomes during laparoscopic liver resection: lessons learned from a multicenter review of 2861 cases. Ann Surg. 2018;268(6):1051–7.
51. Aghayan DL, Pelanis E, Avdem Fretland A, et al. Laparoscopic parenchyma-sparing liver resection for colorectal metastases. Radiol Oncol. 2018;52(1):36–41.
52. Dagher I, O'Rourke N, Geller DA, et al. Laparoscopic major hepatectomy: an evolution in standard of care. Ann Surg. 2009;250(5):856–60.
53. Kasai M, Cipriani F, Gayet B, et al. Laparoscopic versus open major hepatectomy: a systematic review and meta-analysis of individual patient data. Surgery. 2018;163(5):985–95.
54. Martin RC, Scoggins CR, McMasters KM. Laparoscopic hepatic lobectomy: advantages of a minimally invasive approach. J Am Coll Surg. 2010;210(5):627-34–634-6.
55. Ratti F, Cipriani F, Ariotti R, et al. Laparoscopic major hepatectomies: current trends and indications. A comparison with the open technique. Updat Surg. 2015;67(2):157–67.
56. Tozzi F, Berardi G, Vierstraete M, et al. Laparoscopic versus open approach for formal right and left hepatectomy: a propensity score matching analysis. World J Surg. 2018;42(8):2627–34.
57. Adam R. Chemotherapy and surgery: new perspectives on the treatment of unresectable liver metastases. Ann Oncol. 2003;14(Suppl 2):ii13–6.
58. Di Fabio F, Whistance R, Rahman S, et al. Exploring the role of laparoscopic surgery in two-stage hepatectomy for bilobar colorectal liver metastases. J Laparoendosc Adv Surg Tech A. 2012;22(7):647–50.
59. Fuks D, Nomi T, Ogiso S, et al. Laparoscopic two-stage hepatectomy for bilobar colorectal liver metastases. Br J Surg. 2015;102(13):1684–90.

60. Jain G, Parmar J, Mohammed MM, et al. "Stretching the limits of laparoscopic surgery": two-stage laparoscopic liver resection. J Laparoendosc Adv Surg Tech A. 2010;20(1):51–4.
61. Machado MA, Makdissi FF, Surjan RC, et al. Two-stage laparoscopic liver resection for bilateral colorectal liver metastasis. Surg Endosc. 2010;24(8):2044–7.
62. de Jong MC, Pulitano C, Ribero D, et al. Rates and patterns of recurrence following curative intent surgery for colorectal liver metastasis: an international multi-institutional analysis of 1669 patients. Ann Surg. 2009;250(3):440–8.
63. Wicherts DA, de Haas RJ, Salloum C, et al. Repeat hepatectomy for recurrent colorectal metastases. Br J Surg. 2013;100(6):808–18.
64. Nomi T, Fuks D, Ogiso S, et al. Second and third laparoscopic liver resection for patients with recurrent colorectal liver metastases. Ann Surg. 2016;263(5):e68–72.
65. van der Poel MJ, Barkhatov L, Fuks D, et al. Multicentre propensity score-matched study of laparoscopic versus open repeat liver resection for colorectal liver metastases. Br J Surg. 2019.
66. Siegel RL, Miller KD, Jemal A. Cancer statistics, 2019. CA Cancer J Clin. 2019;69(1):7–34.
67. Martin RC 2nd, Augenstein V, Reuter NP, et al. Simultaneous versus staged resection for synchronous colorectal cancer liver metastases. J Am Coll Surg. 2009;208(5):842–50. discussion 850-2
68. Moris D, Tsilimigras DI, Machairas N, et al. Laparoscopic synchronous resection of colorectal cancer and liver metastases: a systematic review. J Surg Oncol. 2019;119(1):30–9.
69. Reddy SK, Pawlik TM, Zorzi D, et al. Simultaneous resections of colorectal cancer and synchronous liver metastases: a multi-institutional analysis. Ann Surg Oncol. 2007;14(12):3481–91.

Robotic Partial Hepatectomy for Colorectal Cancer Liver Metastases

29

Eric C. H. Lai and Chung Ngai Tang

Introduction

Metastatic disease eventually develops in up to half of colorectal cancer patients after curative surgery and is present in about one-quarter of patients at initial presentation. Liver resection is the only potentially curative treatment for colorectal liver metastases (CRLM). With the introduction of improved patient selection, improved surgical techniques, and more effective systemic treatment, 5-year survival following curative intent surgery of CRLM now approaches 45% to 60% [1–4].

Minimally invasive surgical approach benefits patients in terms of aesthetics and early recovery and medical institutions in terms of the low cost associated with a short hospital stay. In recent years, laparoscopic hepatectomies of both benign and malignant liver tumors have been increasing in number. In addition, more complicated procedures, such as laparoscopic major hepatectomy or combined laparoscopic colonic and hepatectomy, have been gaining popularity. Two international expert consensus conferences on laparoscopic hepatectomy were held in Louisville, KY, USA, in 2008 and in Morioka, Japan, in 2014, respectively [5, 6]. The jury in the second consensus meeting concluded that minor laparoscopic hepatectomy had become standard practice and that major hepatectomies were still innovative procedures in the exploration phase. Continued cautious introduction of laparoscopic major hepatectomy was recommended. Technological advancement has resulted in exponential increase in the number of laparoscopic hepatectomies across the world in the past few years. In a review reported in 2009, 2804 cases of laparoscopic hepatectomies performed worldwide were analyzed [7]. Overall mortality was 0.3%, and morbidity was 10.5%, with no intraoperative deaths reported. In a recent review reported in 2016, 9527 cases of laparoscopic hepatectomies performed worldwide were analyzed, and 65% of cases were performed for malignant pathologies [8].

E. C. H. Lai (✉) · C. N. Tang
Department of Surgery, Pamela Youde Nethersole Eastern Hospital, Hong Kong, China
e-mail: tangcn@ha.org.hk

M. M. Correia et al. (eds.), *Colorectal Cancer Liver Metastases*,
https://doi.org/10.1007/978-3-030-25486-5_29

A total of 6190 laparoscopic hepatectomies have been reported for malignancies. As observed, hepatocellular carcinoma (HCC) and CRLM account for more than 75% of the cases reported worldwide. In minor resection series, results from the meta-analysis show that the number of overall complications, estimated blood loss, blood transfusion rate, and hospital stay favors laparoscopic approach. A trend toward a longer operative time in laparoscopic approach was seen compared with open approach, but this was not statistically significant. In major resection series, results from the meta-analysis show that the number of overall complications, estimated blood loss, and hospital stay favors laparoscopic approach. There were no significant differences in operative time and blood transfusion rate between the laparoscopic and open groups for major hepatectomy. Recent systematic review and meta-analyses also showed laparoscopic hepatectomy for CRLM is a beneficial alternative to open hepatectomy in selected patients, and it provides more favorable short-term outcomes such as less blood loss, lower blood transfusion rate, less overall morbidity, and shorter hospital stay [9, 10]. Simultaneously, laparoscopic hepatectomy does not compromise oncological outcomes including surgical margins R0, tumor recurrence, disease-free survival, and overall survival.

The recent introduction of robotic surgical system has revolutionized the field of minimally invasive surgery. The da Vinci surgical system is a sophisticated robotic platform designed to enable complex surgery in a minimally invasive approach. It consists of three main components: (1) patient cart, which holds the EndoWrist robotic instruments (Fig. 29.1), (2) vision cart (Fig. 29.2), and (3) surgeon console (Fig. 29.3). It was developed to overcome the disadvantages of conventional laparoscopic surgery. The surgeon sits comfortably and via hand manipulators controls the EndoWrist instrument's movements at the surgical site. The surgeon console operator sits outside of the sterile field and controls instruments and a 3-dimensional endoscope with his/her hands, using two master controllers, and with his/her feet, using foot pedals. The introduction of robotic system may lower the hurdle for entry for practice into minimally invasive hepatectomy. Well-known advantages of the robotic system included improved vision via 3-dimensional view, magnification, tremor suppression, and the dexterity of the instruments (Table 29.1). These features allow the surgeon to perform delicate tissue dissection and precise intracorporeal suturing (Fig. 29.4) [11, 12].

This chapter aimed at reviewing the current role and development of robotic hepatectomy for CRLM.

Robotic Versus Open Partial Hepatectomy

Five nonrandomized comparative studies compared robotic and open hepatectomy [13–17]. Patriti et al. showed no significant differences in postoperative outcomes as measured by blood loss, transfusion rate, overall complication rate, mortality, and hospital stay [13]. Kingham et al. showed a significant shorter operative time, lower estimated blood loss, and shorter hospital stay in robotic group [14]. The complication rate and mortality rate were similar in both groups. Daskalaki et al. showed less

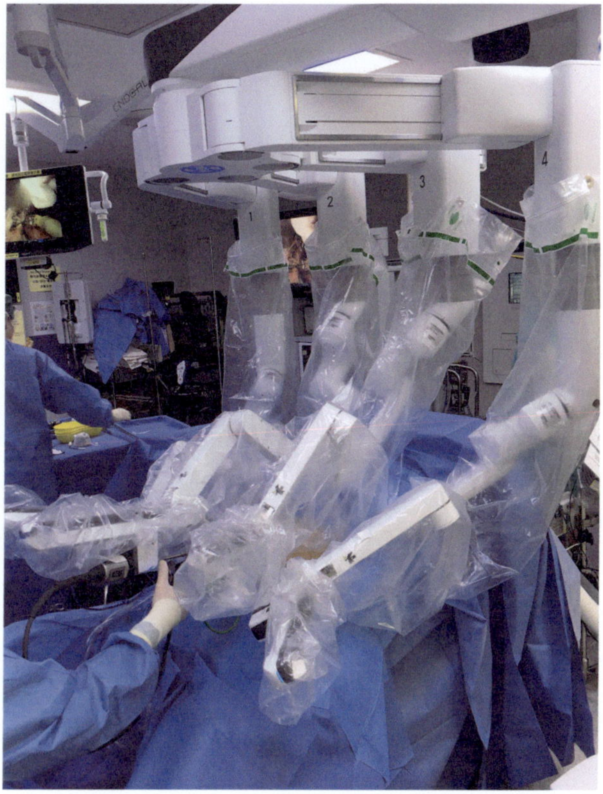

Fig. 29.1 Patient cart

overall complication rate, intensive care unit, and hospital stay in robotic group. This translates into decreased average costs for robotic surgery [15]. Chen et al. showed significantly longer operative time, shorter hospital stay, and lower dosages of postoperative patient-controlled analgesia in robotic group [16]. Wang et al. showed the robotic group had significantly longer operative time and shorter hospital stay [17]. The postoperative complication rate was slightly lower in the robotic group. All studies showed similar R0 resection rates, when compared to open approach. Based on current limited nonrandomized comparative studies, robotic approach has better perioperative outcomes, particularly blood loss and hospital stay, than open approach.

Robotic Versus Laparoscopic Partial Hepatectomy

Traditionally, laparoscopic hepatectomy can either be total laparoscopic or hand-assisted laparoscopic approach. Techniques of hand-assisted laparoscopic have been attempted to bridge the gap between open and conventional total laparoscopic approach. The benefits of hand-assisted laparoscopic approach in hepatectomy are as follows: [1] facilitation in manual retraction, which may be the best atraumatic

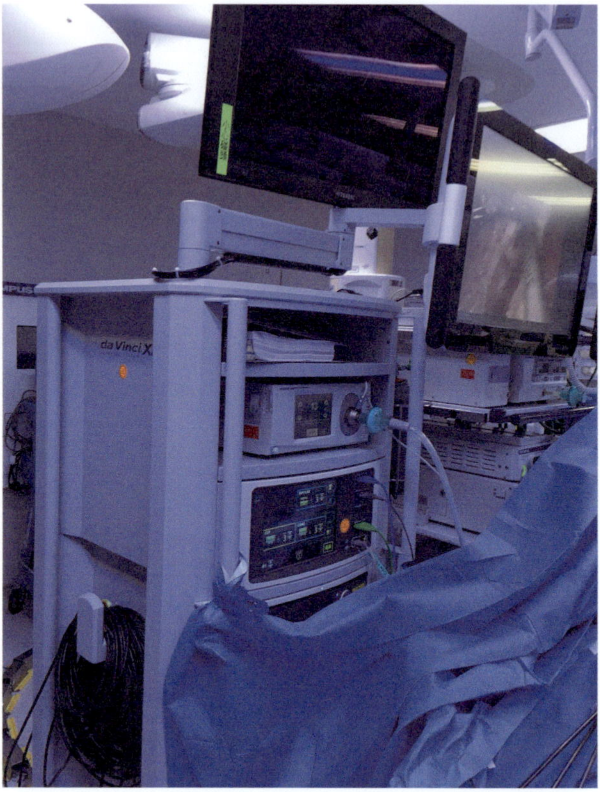

Fig. 29.2 Vision cart

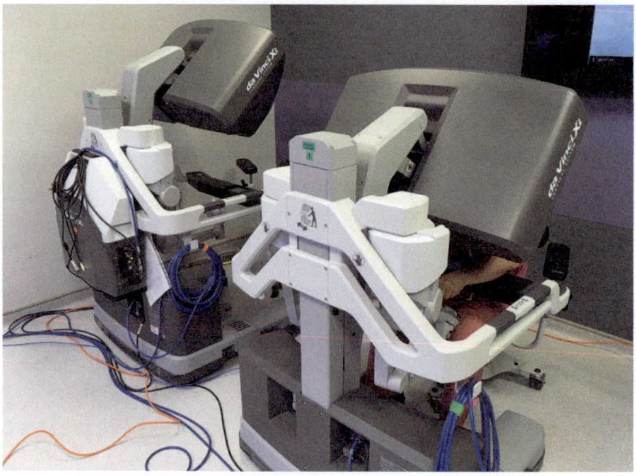

Fig. 29.3 Surgeon console

tool, [2] feasibility in assessing margins of resection with the use of tactile sensation, [3] safety in parenchymal dissection laparoscopically, and [4] possibility of immediate hemostasis and prevention of air embolism in case the hepatic vein is severed. Obviously, total laparoscopic procedure is superior to hand-assisted approach in terms of wound pain, and cosmetic outcome as hand-assisted

Table 29.1 Advantages and disadvantages of laparoscopic and robotic approaches

	Laparoscopic approach	Robotic approach
Advantages	Well-developed technology Less start-up cost Less maintenance cost	3-dimensional magnified view Good dexterity 7 degrees of freedom of motion Elimination of fulcrum effect Elimination of physiologic tremors Good in suturing Tele-surgery More ergonomic in working posture
Disadvantages	Compromised dexterity Limited degrees of motion Fulcrum effect Magnification of physiologic tremors loss of tactile feedback	New technology with limited evidence High start-up cost Expensive in maintenance Complete absence of tactile feedback

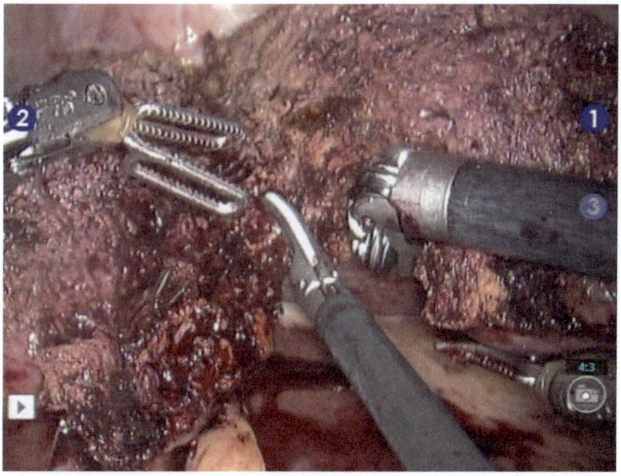

Fig. 29.4 Robotic liver parenchymal transection

laparoscopic hepatectomy usually required a 6–8 cm incision for the placement of the hand port. Another possible disadvantage of hand-assisted laparoscopic approach includes possible obstruction of the visual field by the surgeon's hand during the operation.

Based on the platform of the development and experiences of conventional laparoscopic hepatectomy, robotic surgical system was developed to overcome the limitations of conventional laparoscopic approach and hand-assisted laparoscopic approach, such as suturing of bleeding point, those resections of tumors located at difficult segments, or those tumors required major resections [18, 19]. Robotic hepatectomy was increasingly studied in recent years. Up till now, no randomized trials are available for robotic hepatectomy. All data have been reported as case series or case-control studies. Most data were obtained from prospectively maintained databases. Based on the current evidence, robotic surgical approach offers an alternative to conventional laparoscopic hepatectomy for minimally invasive hepatectomy. Tables 29.2 and 29.3 show the results of nonrandomized comparative studies comparing robotic and laparoscopic hepatectomy in patients with minor hepatectomies

Table 29.2 Nonrandomized comparative studies comparing robotic and laparoscopic minor hepatectomy (∗ <0.05)

Studies	*n*	Operating time (min)	Blood loss (ml)	Conversion (%)	Complication (%)	Mortality (%)	Hospital stay (days)	R0 resection (%)
Berber et al. [20]	9 vs. 23	258.5 vs. 233.6	136 vs. 155	11.1 vs. 0	11 vs. 17	\	\	\
Packiam et al. [21]	11 vs. 18	175 vs. 188	30 vs. 30	0 vs. 0	27 vs. 0∗	0 vs. 0	4 vs. 3∗	\
Lai et al. [22]	33 vs. 33	202.7 vs. 133.4∗	373.4 vs. 347.7	\	3 vs. 9	0 vs. 0	\	90.9 vs. 90.9
Tranchart et al. [23]	28 vs. 28	210 vs. 176 (median)	200 vs. 150	14.3 vs. 7.1	17.9 vs. 17.9	0 vs. 0	4.5 vs. 3	\
Yu et al. [24]	13 vs. 17	291.5 vs. 240.9∗	388.5 vs. 342.6	0 vs. 0	0 vs. 11.8	0 vs. 0	7.8 vs. 9.5	\
Kim et al. [25]	12 vs. 31	337.4 vs. 216.4∗	225 vs. 150 (median)	0 vs. 3.2	25 vs. 22.6	0 vs. 0	7 vs. 7	\
Montalti et al. [26]	36 vs. 72	306 vs. 295	415 vs. 437	13.9 vs. 9.7	19.4 vs. 19.4	2.8 vs. 0	6 vs. 4.9	88.9 vs. 87.5
Salloum et al. [27]	16 vs. 80	190 vs. 162	247 vs. 206	13 vs. 3	13 vs. 11	0 vs. 1	6 vs. 7	100 vs. 98

Table 29.3 Nonrandomized comparative studies comparing robotic and laparoscopic minor and major hepatectomy (∗ <0.05)

Studies	*n*	Operating time (min)	Blood loss (ml)	Conversion (%)	Complication (%)	Mortality (%)	Hospital stay (days)	R0 resection (%)	R1 resection (%)
Troisi et al. [28]	40 vs. 223	271 vs. 262	330 vs. 174∗	20 vs. 7.6∗	12.5 vs. 12.6	0 vs. 0	6.1 vs. 5.9	\	7.5 vs. 5.4
Tsung et al. [29]	57 vs. 114	253 vs. 198.5∗	200 vs. 100	7 vs. 8.8	19.3 vs. 26	0 vs. 1.8	4 vs. 4 (median)	\	\
Spampinato et al. [30]	25 vs. 25	430 vs. 360	250 vs. 400	4 vs. 4	16 vs. 36	0 vs. 4	8 vs. 7	100 vs. 91	\
Wu et al. [31]	38 vs. 41	380 vs. 227∗	325 vs. 173∗	5 vs. 12.2	8 vs. 10	0 vs. 0	7.9 vs. 7.2	\	\
Lee et al. [32]	70 vs. 66	251.5 vs. 215∗	100 vs. 100 (median)	5.7 vs. 12.1	11.4 vs. 4.5	0 vs. 0	5 vs. 5	\	\
Lai et al. [33]	100 vs. 35	207.4 vs. 134.2∗	334.6 vs. 336	4 vs. 5.7	14 vs. 20	0 vs. 0	7.3 vs. 7.1	96 vs. 91.4	\

and in patients with minor and major hepatectomies [20–33]. Although little data regarding robotic hepatectomy have been reported, robotic hepatectomy had similar to conventional laparoscopic hepatectomy in terms of operative time, estimated blood loss, morbidity, mortality rate, and hospital stay. However, robotic hepatectomy is more expensive than laparoscopic hepatectomy. The robotic approach tended to have longer operative time in these studies also. Robot-assisted laparoscopic hepatectomy may have longer operation time. However, the definition of operation time was variable. Some authors refer to a "total operation time" and specify an included "robot setup and docking time," whereas others refer to a "procedure time" with a separate "system time" (from positioning the robot over the patient to disconnection of the robot) and "dissection time" (surgeon's active time at the console); others calculate the time from "induction of anesthesia to incision" or from "incision to extubation."

The benefit of robotic hepatectomy was shown in four studies. Both Tsung et al. and Wu et al. showed that the robotic system facilitated the completion of partial hepatectomies by totally minimally invasive approach and allowed higher proportion of major hepatectomies. Tranchart et al. showed that the robotic system facilitated the resection of those tumors located over superior and posterior segments. Lai et al. showed that the robotic approach allowed higher proportion of major hepatectomies and resection of those tumors located over superior and posterior segments. Its future implementation will depend on the advantages that it can provide over conventional laparoscopy or open surgery. The indications for minimally invasive hepatectomy may be extended.

Oncological Outcomes After Robotic Hepatectomy for CRLM

At present, available survival data about robotic hepatectomy for CRLM in the literature are very limited still. Difficult learning curves, adequate resection margins, tumor seeding, and the long-term outcome are the major concerns in robotic surgery for malignancies. Technical feasibility and safety of one-stage or two-stage laparoscopic colectomy and robotic hepatectomy was reported [34–38].

In the cohort study of Giulianotti et al., 17 patients with malignant tumors (HCC, $n = 1$; CRLM, $n = 11$; non-colorectal liver metastases, $n = 4$; hepatoblastoma, $n = 1$) were reported. Among patients with CRLM, 9 of 11 were alive and disease free at a mean follow-up time of 36 months [39]. In the cohort study of Casciola et al., after mean follow-up time of 25.1 months, among 19 patients with malignant tumor (HCC, $n = 3$; CRLM, $n = 14$; clear cell renal metastasis, $n = 1$; gallbladder carcinoma metastasis, $n = 1$), 2 patients with CRLM died for tumor progression after discontinuation of adjuvant chemotherapy with hepatic, nodal, and peritoneal relapse [40]. Three patients with CRLM were alive with disease.

In the nonrandomized comparative study of Berber et al., patients with robotic resection for malignant liver tumors (HCC, $n = 3$; CRLM, $n = 4$; others, $n = 2$) and patients with laparoscopic resection for malignant liver tumors (HCC, $n = 7$; CRLM, $n = 14$; others, $n = 2$) had a similar overall and disease-free survival after a mean follow-up of 14 months. Eight patients (robotic group, $n = 2$; laparoscopic group, $n = 6$) developed tumor recurrence in the liver during follow-up. In the nonrandomized comparative study of Troisi et al., 40 patients underwent robotic hepatectomy and 223 patients underwent laparoscopic hepatectomy. Among the patients, 24 patients had CRLM in robotic group, while 108 patients had CRLM in laparoscopic group. The disease-free survivals at 1 and 3 years were 79% and 62% in robotic group for patients with colorectal metastasis after a median follow-up of 9.6 months and 81% and 41% in laparoscopic group after a median follow-up of 24 months, accounting for 37% and 44% total recurrence rate, respectively, for robotic group and laparoscopic group.

Based on the current limited evidence, the oncological outcomes of robotic approach for CRLM are still unclear. Controlled trials are needed to compare the long-term oncological results after robot-assisted laparoscopic hepatectomy with those of open surgery or laparoscopic surgery.

Conclusion

Although little data regarding robotic hepatectomy for CRLM have been reported, the robotic approach has similar perioperative outcomes to conventional laparoscopic approach in terms of estimated blood loss, complication rate, mortality rate, and hospital stay. The robotic system has allowed adopting the operating technique with more ease and extending the indications for minimally invasive hepatectomy. In light of the cost of robotic system and remaining uncertainties regarding oncological outcome, caution should be exercised in the assessment of the appropriateness of robotic approach for individual patients. Its future implementation and clinical value will depend on the advantages that it can provide over conventional laparoscopy or open surgery. It should be emphasized that considering robot-assisted laparoscopic partial hepatectomy requires 4 conditions: (1) appropriate selection of patients; (2) follow the principle of open liver surgery; (3) specific expertise and training, in both liver and laparoscopic surgeries; and (4) familiarization with the robotic machine and pay precaution of its potential dangers, such as visceral injury by robotic arm and total loss of tactile feedback. The approach to the patient with potentially resectable CRLM is getting more complicated and is ideally considered in a multidisciplinary tumor board to achieve the best possible outcome.

References

1. Lau WY, Lai EC. Hepatic resection for colorectal liver metastases. Singap Med J. 2007;48:635–9.
2. Nguyen KT, Laurent A, Dagher I, Geller DA, Steel J, Thomas MT, Marvin M, Ravindra KV, Mejia A, Lainas P, Franco D, Cherqui D, Buell JF, Gamblin TC. Minimally invasive liver resection for metastatic colorectal cancer: a multi-institutional, international report of safety, feasibility, and early outcomes. Ann Surg. 2009;250:842–8.
3. de Jong MC, Pulitano C, Ribero D, Strub J, Mentha G, Schulick RD, Choti MA, Aldrighetti L, Capussotti L, Pawlik TM. Rates and patterns of recurrence following curative intent surgery

for colorectal liver metastasis: an international multi-institutional analysis of 1669 patients. Ann Surg. 2009;250:440–8.
4. Beppu T, Wakabayashi G, Hasegawa K, et al. Long-term and perioperative outcomes of laparoscopic versus open liver resection for colorectal liver metastases with propensity score matching: a multi-institutional Japanese study. J Hepatobiliary Pancreat Sci. 2015;22:711–20.
5. Buell JF, Cherqui D, Geller DA, World Consensus Conference on Laparoscopic Surgery, et al. The international position on laparoscopic liver surgery: the Louisville statement, 2008. Ann Surg. 2009;250:825–30.
6. Wakabayashi G, Cherqui D, Geller DA, et al. Recommendations for laparoscopic liver resection: a report from the second international consensus conference held in Morioka. Ann Surg. 2015;261:619–29.
7. Nguyen KT, Gamblin TC, Geller DA. World review of laparoscopic liver resection-2,804 patients. Ann Surg. 2009;250:831–41.
8. Ciria R, Cherqui D, Geller DA, Briceno J, Wakabayashi G. Comparative short-term benefits of laparoscopic liver resection: 9000 cases and climbing. Ann Surg. 2016;263:761–77.
9. Zhang XL, Liu RF, Zhang D, Zhang YS, Wang T. Laparoscopic versus open liver resection for colorectal liver metastases: a systematic review and meta-analysis of studies with propensity score-based analysis. Int J Surg. 2017;44:191–203.
10. Cheng Y, Zhang L, Li H, Wang L, Huang Y, Wu L, Zhang Y. Laparoscopic versus open liver resection for colorectal liver metastases: a systematic review. J Surg Res. 2017;220:234–46.
11. Lai EC, Tang CN, Li MK. Conventional laparoscopic and robot-assisted laparoscopic liver resection for benign and malignant pathologies: a cohort study. J Robot Surg. 2012;6:295–300.
12. Lai EC, Tang CN, Yang GP, Li MK. Multimodality laparoscopic liver resection for hepatic malignancy--from conventional total laparoscopic approach to robot-assisted laparoscopic approach. Int J Surg. 2011;9:324–8.
13. Patriti A, Cipriani F, Ratti F, Bartoli A, Ceccarelli G, Casciola L, Aldrighetti L. Robot-assisted versus open liver resection in the right posterior section. JSLS. 2014;18:e2014.00040.
14. Kingham TP, Leung U, Kuk D, Gönen M, D'Angelica MI, Allen PJ, DeMatteo RP, Laudone VP, Jarnagin WR, Fong Y. Robotic liver resection: a case-matched comparison. World J Surg. 2016;40:1422–8.
15. Daskalaki D, Gonzalez-Heredia R, Brown M, Bianco FM, Tzvetanov I, Davis M, Kim J, Benedetti E, Giulianotti PC. Financial impact of the robotic approach in liver surgery: a comparative study of clinical outcomes and costs between the robotic and open technique in a single institution. J Laparoendosc Adv Surg Tech A. 2017;27:375–82.
16. Chen PD, Wu CY, Hu RH, Chou WH, Lai HS, Liang JT, Lee PH, Wu YM. Robotic versus open hepatectomy for hepatocellular carcinoma: a matched comparison. Ann Surg Oncol. 2017;24:1021–8.
17. Wang WH, Kuo KK, Wang SN, Lee KT. Oncological and surgical result of hepatoma after robot surgery. Surg Endosc. 2018;32:3918.
18. Lai ECH, Tang CN. Training robotic hepatectomy: the Hong Kong experience and perspective. Hepatobiliary Surg Nutr. 2017;6:222–9.
19. Lai EC, Tang CN, Li MK. Robot-assisted laparoscopic hemi-hepatectomy: technique and surgical outcomes. Int J Surg. 2012;10:11–5.
20. Berber E, Akyildiz HY, Aucejo F, Gunasekaran G, Chalikonda S, Fung J. Robotic versus laparoscopic resection of liver tumours. HPB (Oxford). 2010;12:583–6.
21. Packiam V, Bartlett DL, Tohme S, Reddy S, Marsh JW, Geller DA, Tsung A. Minimally invasive liver resection: robotic versus laparoscopic left lateral sectionectomy. J Gastrointest Surg. 2012;16:2233–8.
22. Lai EC, Yang GP, Tang CN. Robot-assisted laparoscopic liver resection for hepatocellular carcinoma: short-term outcome. Am J Surg. 2013 Jun;205(6):697–702.
23. Tranchart H, Ceribelli C, Ferretti S, Dagher I, Patriti A. Traditional versus robot-assisted full laparoscopic liver resection: a matched-pair comparative study. World J Surg. 2014;38:2904–9.
24. Yu YD, Kim KH, Jung DH, Namkoong JM, Yoon SY, Jung SW, Lee SK, Lee SG. Robotic versus laparoscopic liver resection: a comparative study from a single center. Langenbeck's Arch Surg. 2014;399:1039–45.

25. Kim JK, Park JS, Han DH, Choi GH, Kim KS, Choi JS, Yoon DS. Robotic versus laparoscopic left lateral sectionectomy of liver. Surg Endosc. 2016;30:4756–64.
26. Montalti R, Scuderi V, Patriti A, Vivarelli M, Troisi RI. Robotic versus laparoscopic resections of posterosuperior segments of the liver: a propensity score-matched comparison. Surg Endosc. 2016;30:1004–13.
27. Salloum C, Lim C, Lahat E, Gavara CG, Levesque E, Compagnon P, Azoulay D. Robotic-assisted versus laparoscopic left lateral sectionectomy: analysis of surgical outcomes and costs by a propensity score matched cohort study. World J Surg. 2017;41:516–24.
28. Troisi RI, Patriti A, Montalti R, Casciola L. Robot assistance in liver surgery: a real advantage over a fully laparoscopic approach? Results of a comparative bi-institutional analysis. Int J Med Robot. 2013;9:160–6.
29. Tsung A, Geller DA, Sukato DC, Sabbaghian S, Tohme S, Steel J, Marsh W, Reddy SK, Bartlett DL. Robotic versus laparoscopic hepatectomy: a matched comparison. Ann Surg. 2014;259:549–55.
30. Spampinato MG, Coratti A, Bianco L, Caniglia F, Laurenzi A, Puleo F, Ettorre GM, Boggi U. Perioperative outcomes of laparoscopic and robot-assisted major hepatectomies: an Italian multi-institutional comparative study. Surg Endosc. 2014;28:2973–9.
31. Wu YM, Hu RH, Lai HS, Lee PH. Robotic-assisted minimally invasive liver resection. Asian J Surg. 2014;37:53–7.
32. Lee KF, Cheung YS, Chong CC, Wong J, Fong AK, Lai PB. Laparoscopic and robotic hepatectomy: experience from a single centre. ANZ J Surg. 2016;86:122–6.
33. Lai EC, Tang CN. Robot-assisted laparoscopic partial caudate lobe resection for hepatocellular carcinoma in cirrhotic liver. Surg Laparosc Endosc Percutan Tech. 2014;24:e88–91.
34. Dwyer RH, Scheidt MJ, Marshall JS, Tsoraides SS. Safety and efficacy of synchronous robotic surgery for colorectal cancer with liver metastases. J Robot Surg. 2018;12(4):603–6.
35. Giulianotti PC, Giacomoni A, Coratti A, Addeo P, Bianco FM. Minimally invasive sequential treatment of synchronous colorectal liver metastases by laparoscopic colectomy and robotic right hepatectomy. Int J Color Dis. 2010;25:1507–11.
36. Patriti A, Ceccarelli G, Bartoli A, Spaziani A, Lapalorcia LM, Casciola L. Laparoscopic and robot-assisted one-stage resection of colorectal cancer with synchronous liver metastases: a pilot study. J Hepato-Biliary-Pancreat Surg. 2009;16:450–7.
37. Xu JM, Wei Y, Wang XY, Fan H, Chang WJ, Ren L, Jiang W, Fan J, Qin XY. Robot-assisted one-stage resection of rectal cancer with liver and lung metastases. World J Gastroenterol. 2015;21:2848–53.
38. Sunil S, Restrepo J, Azin A, Hirpara D, Cleary S, Cleghorn MC, Wei A, Quereshy FA. Robotic simultaneous resection of rectal cancer and liver metastases. Clin Case Rep. 2017;5:1913–8.
39. Giulianotti PC, Sbrana F, Coratti A, Bianco FM, Addeo P, Buchs NC, Ayloo SM, Benedetti E. Totally robotic right hepatectomy: surgical technique and outcomes. Arch Surg. 2011;146:844–50.
40. Casciola L, Patriti A, Ceccarelli G, Bartoli A, Ceribelli C, Spaziani A. Robot-assisted parenchymal-sparing liver surgery including lesions located in the posterosuperior segments. Surg Endosc. 2011;25:3815–24.

Navigation and Augmented Reality for Liver Surgery

30

Mauro Monteiro Correia

Abbreviations and Acronyms

3D	3-Dimensional
AR	Augmented reality
CT	Computer tomography
DICOM	Digital imaging and communications in medicine
EMTS	Electromagnetic tracking system
FIGS	Fluorescence image-guided surgery
IGLR	Image-guided liver resection
IGLS	Image-guided liver surgery
IOUS	Intraoperative ultrasound
MIS	Minimally invasive surgery
MRI	Magnetic resonance imaging
MWA	Microwave ablation
NS	Navigated surgery
RFA	Radiofrequency ablation
VLM	Vanished liver metastases

Introduction

In 1956, Claude Couinaud produced an extraordinary book entitled *The Liver – Anatomical Studies and Surgical Studies*. He showed in details, after studying casts of the liver, that according to the distribution of the portal and hepatic vein blood, the liver contains eight segments. This segmental division of the liver has

M. M. Correia (✉)
National Cancer Institute, Rio de Janeiro, Brazil

Department of Surgery, UNIVERSIDADE DO GRANDE RIO, Duque de Caxias, Brazil

M. M. Correia et al. (eds.), *Colorectal Cancer Liver Metastases*,
https://doi.org/10.1007/978-3-030-25486-5_30

been the basis of modern liver imaging interpretation, radiological intervention, and surgery [1, 2].

To define section planes in the liver, surgeons need to know the functional anatomy as defined by Couinaud. This plane recognition process depends on the mental ability of the surgeon to cognitively relate a few external landmarks of the liver with the portal fissures as defined by Couinaud. Then he needs to form a 3D mental image in which he will navigate during the resection. This mechanism does not provide real-time image guidance during surgery.

Even for experienced surgeons, this can be a difficult task sometimes, and, in spite of the introduction of IOUS, the heterogeneity of liver parenchyma, due to chemotherapy or steatosis, can make it hard to identify precisely tiny or disappearing metastases. Therefore, surgeons, mathematicians, and computer scientists have collaborated to develop new possibilities of a more precise liver surgery.

Computer-aided surgery, computer-assisted surgery planning, image-guided liver surgery, computer-assisted planning for navigated surgery, virtual reality, and enhanced or augmented reality in surgery are some terms with recent increasing referrals in the specialized medical literature.

They represent several computational applications that explore interfaces between 3D reconstruction and imaging software making detailed and delicate operations possible through the virtual identification of internal anatomical structures, estimation of volumes, and navigation of instruments during surgery, from point A to point B, accurately, and therefore making it a safer operation.

Cross-sectional imaging based on navigation and virtual reality planning tools are well stablished in the surgical routine in different medical specialties, such as interventional radiology, neurosurgery, head and neck surgery, urology, orthopedics, head and neck trauma surgery, and liver surgery since the twentieth century, but the first experiments to precisely localize anatomical structures inside the human body date back to the nineteenth century and in the area of neurosurgery [3, 4].

The present technology of navigated liver surgery, with or without augmented reality, took a long time to get to where it is now. It all began in 1889, when Zernov developed an “encephalometer” to target brain structures, based on surface landmarks of the skull and polar coordinates. It was used on at least three cases for anatomical operations on the human brain. This initiative gave birth to the stereotactic surgery, where coordinates are used for localizing inner areas of interest in the human body [5].

The subsequent efforts of neurosurgeons and mathematicians, in the first six decades of the twentieth century, made it possible to use frames based on Cartesian coordinate systems to perform psychosurgery, as a safer option to destructive frontal lobotomies. A number of breakthroughs in the field of stereotactic surgery that began in the 1970s–1980s with the introduction of computed tomography (CT), magnetic resonance imaging (MRI), the DICOM® (Digital Imaging and Communications in Medicine) standard, positron emission tomography (PET), and single photon emission computed tomography (SPECT) put the image-guided surgery into the modern era. One of the most significant computing evolutionary tools was the 3D volumetric reconstruction, and in 1986 David Roberts and John Strohbehn successfully accomplished a frameless stereotactic neurosurgery [6]. In

1987, potentiometers were used to track a surgical probe in real time, and in 1995 real-time instrument tracking was used combining acoustic tracking technology and computer vision system [7–9]. These initial advances in neurosurgery (brain and spine) have been transferred to oral and maxillofacial surgery and thoracic and abdominal surgery along these first decades of the twenty-first century.

Before the introduction of navigation systems, the liver surgeon would plan his surgery preoperatively based mostly on imaging findings (CT or MRI) and build a mental image. During the surgery, he would reassess the location and extent of disease based on intraoperative findings (inspection and palpation) and confirm or modify his primary surgical indication. Later on, with the introduction of intraoperative ultrasound (IOUS) for open and laparoscopic surgery, it became possible to check for new findings and limits, navigate along a planned resection line, and perform interventions.

It has been since the introduction of computer-based 3D image reconstruction software and different intraoperative navigation systems that virtual liver surgery planning has gained significant advances.

Marescaux and Diana have elegantly quoted Plato and his theory of the "World of the Ideas" to form a concept of virtual reality [10]. The Greek philosopher considered that "reality is a preconditioned phenomenon filtered by our senses"; therefore, the expansion of our senses through AR technology makes us more competent to recognize and immerse in the "real anatomy" of the patient.

Augmented reality is a technology similar to the virtual reality paradigm. It combines 3-dimensional (3D) computer-generated objects and text superimposed onto real images and video, all in real time. It allows the surgeon to visualize the 3D reconstructed structures of interest overlaid or projected to the patients' real liver image during a surgery [11].

Nevertheless, we still face significant technical obstacles in achieving a perfect intraoperative real-time navigation process in liver surgery, mostly because most systems do not adapt automatically to the liver deformation and dislocation that occur during surgery.

Navigation in surgery has become the standard of care for a variety of surgical specialties and is likely to become also for liver surgeons in the quest for safer, less invasive, and more cost-efficient surgery.

In the field of image-guided liver surgery (IGLS), navigated surgery (NS) and augmented reality (AR) things have evolved quickly. 3D reconstruction has been useful for preoperative surgery planning, definition of volumes, construction of risk maps, assurance of free margins, identification of individual vascular liver anatomy, and avoidance of futile hepatectomies by anticipating possible complications and increasing safety and (possibly) survival.

The cutting-edge strategy of integrating radiology, tele-transmission (Internet, infrared, electromagnetic), computer science, radio-immuno-scintigraphy, ultrasound, accelerometers, confocal laser endomicroscopy, and many other technologies has put forward the advances in the use of augmented reality in open, laparoscopic, and robotic surgery.

A proper understanding of the patient's real anatomy permits the liver team to analyze surgical and ablative possibilities, select technology, anticipate possible postoperative complications, and discuss the surgical plan with the patient based on sound visual information.

In this chapter, we expect to describe the latest significant advances in navigation and augmented reality for liver surgery. We would feel rewarded if we stimulate liver surgeons to adopt and develop a technology which has been growing at an unprecedented pace.

Very soon navigated and augmented reality will be a part of our surgical routines and later on integral parts of complete robotic autonomous surgical procedures.

Navigation Workflow

The workflow for IGLS usually comprises the following steps (Fig. 30.1):

1. Image acquisition (CT, MRI). In this process, special imaging protocols are necessary in order for proper image acquisition. Basically, a contrast-enhanced three-phase CT with 1 mm width slices.

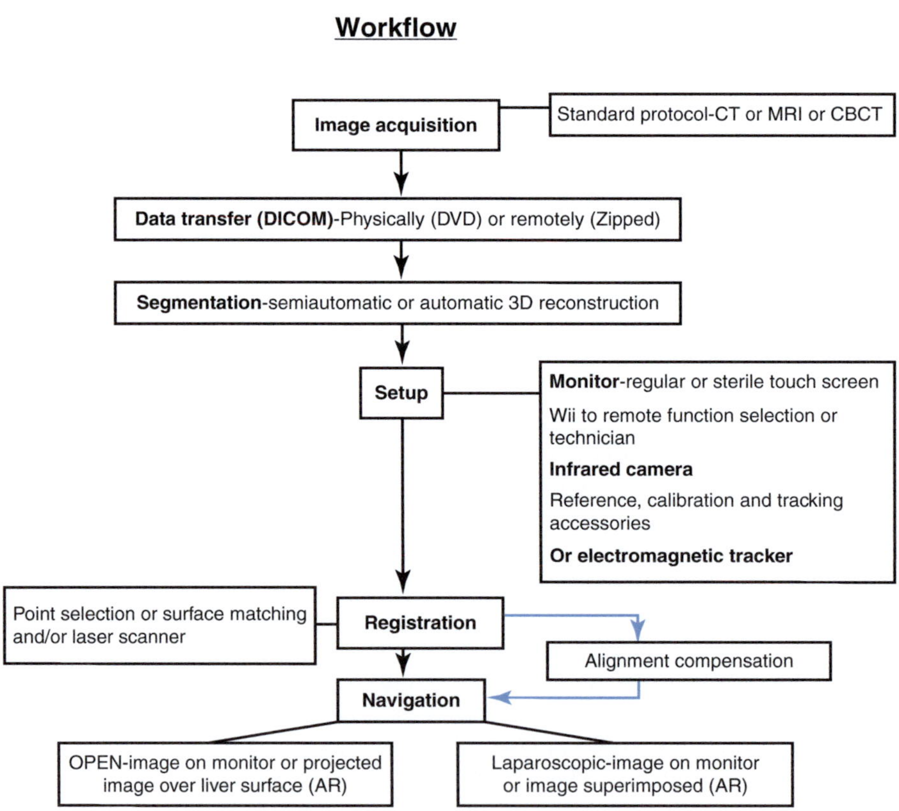

Fig. 30.1 Workflow for navigated liver surgery

2. 3D reconstruction and organs or structures selection (segmentation of the image of interest). Different public and private software and tools use the DICOM information for liver registration. Different semiautomatic and automatic methods are available for segmentation of liver vessels, parenchyma, and tumors for creating volumes (from pixels to voxels) of these structures. Different attributes such as control of transparency, zooming, rotations, translations, and volume calculations are ready for use.
3. Surgical planning. Definition of transection planes, construction of risk maps, simulation of ablation zones, and needle insertion trajectory are essential parts of a virtual hepatectomy plan.
4. Intraoperative registration of patient to 3D images. Different methods are used for this step. Infrared emitters and cameras or electromagnetic sensors and point selection and liver surface recognition with or without laser scanners will be used for matching external landmarks of the liver (base of the round ligament, gallbladder fossa, edges of the liver, suprahepatic vena cava, apparent tumors) to the virtual image of the liver.
5. Intraoperative instrument tracking (open/laparoscopic/robotic). Instruments are coupled with infrared reflective spheres or an electromagnetic wire that will make it possible to track them, according to the used method (Fig. 30.2).
6. Visualization and integration with other visual information. The final aspect of 3D reconstruction depends on the quality of the image acquisition and reconstruction. The display of the virtual liver can be shown in side-by-side monitors, overlaid/mixed images in a single monitor, projected with a beamer in the operative field or through AR glasses, depending on the system available. Integration with other images from fluorescence methods, real-time 3D ultrasound, real-time CT, or MRI, with or without elastic registration, is already under development.

Products

An image-guided surgery platform comprises several integrated tools:

- A high-definition monitor (in some cases with touch-screen properties)
- An optical tracking system (infrared camera) or an electromagnetic tracking system (EMTS) – a sensor coil and field generator
- Optional: handheld laser scanner, 2D or 3D ultrasound, real-time CT or MRI, a Wiimote pointing device (to be used for remotely active functions in the screen), seen through optical display – semitransparent mirror or eyewear, and beamer for video projection
- A navigation computer and planning workstation
- Accessories for registration of the patient anatomy to the 3D liver and instrument navigation (reflective spheres, holders, recognizable frames for spatial registration)

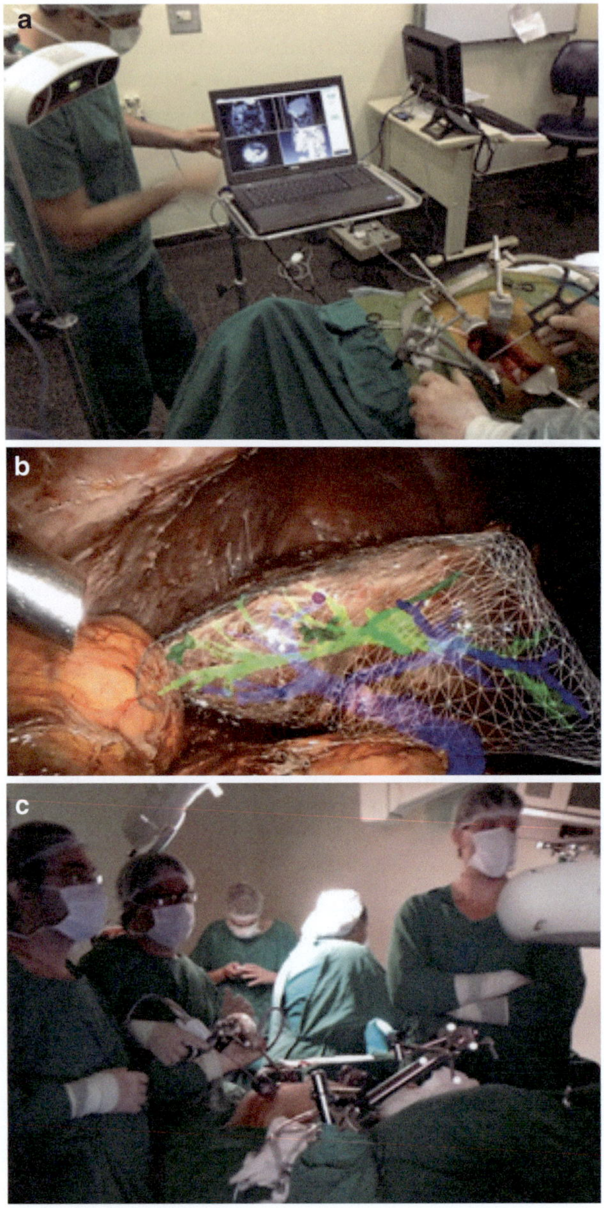

Fig. 30.2 Liver registration and instrument tracking. (**a**) Open rigid optical registration. (**b**) Laparoscopic elastic registration. (**c**) Laparoscopic optical registration

There are many products available around the world (Fig. 30.3), a few commercially, and many only for restricted clinical and/or research use in institutes and universities. Starting the list there is EXPLORER, a navigation system from Pathfinder Therapeutics Inc (PTI, Nashville, TN) that uses Liver Scout, a computer-assisted operation planning tool. The system allows real-time tracking during surgery by mapping various instruments, such as an energy instrument of ablation needle.

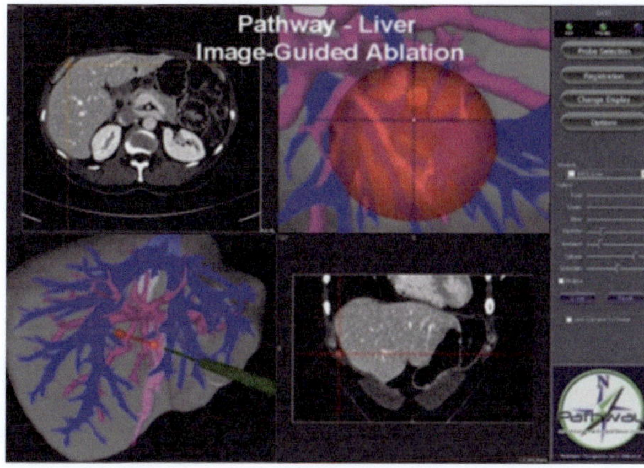

Fig. 30.3 Pathfinder: liver image-guided liver ablation

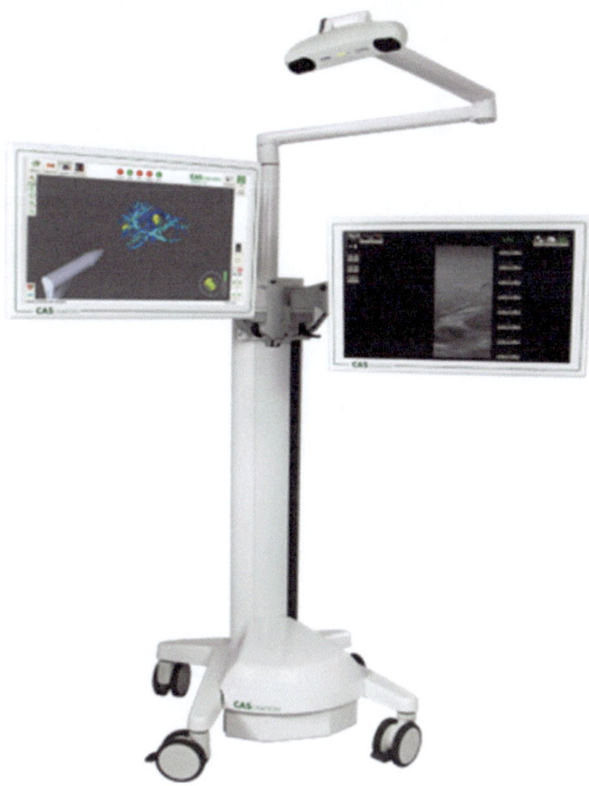

Fig. 30.4 Cascination navigation system

There is also the CAS-ONE Vario System for liver surgery, from CAScination AG (Bern, Switzerland), that uses MeVis Distant Services virtual liver planning system (Fig. 30.4). This platform integrates Ubersound for 3D real-time ultrasound for co-registration. We use the Eximius (Artis Tecnologia, Brasília) (Fig. 30.5) a portable

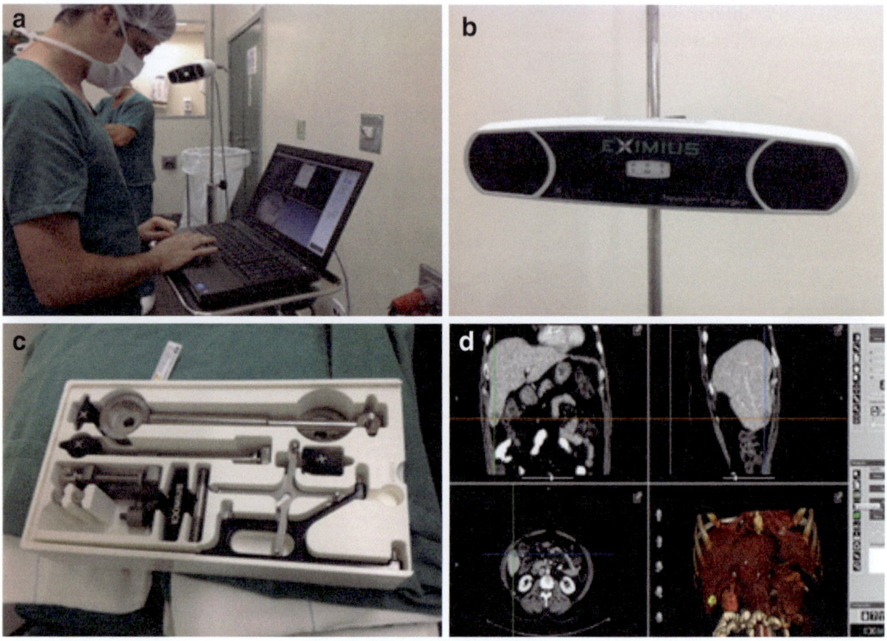

Fig. 30.5 ARTIS navigation system. (**a**) Computer and software. (**b**) Infrared camera. (**c**) Navigation instruments. (**d**) 2D and 3D display of images on the screen

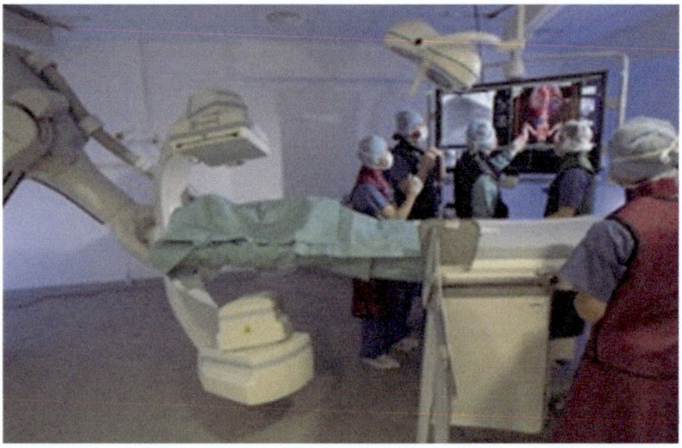

Fig. 30.6 IRCAD: real-time navigation system

platform that allows surgical navigation in different specialities [12]. Other software systems are available, such as OVA (Hitachi Medical Corporation, Japan), Virtual Place (AZE, Japan), mint Liver (Heidelberg, Germany), and VR_Render (IRCAD, France), among others [13]. IRCAD VR-RENDER DICOM viewer is a multiplatform viewer suite that integrates direct volume rendering techniques and surface rendering techniques. It permits to select specific organs or structures inside them to be fused with real patient's images (Fig. 30.6).

Applications and Potential Benefits

There are many theoretical benefits with the use of image-guided techniques in liver surgery:

- Preoperative planning (simulation of transection planes and estimation of liver volumes). Warmann et al. managed to avoid liver transplantation in 12 of 14 patients who theoretically were candidates for this approach by using computer-assisted surgery planning to determine surgical strategies in children with three or four livers sectors affected by hepatoblastoma [14].
- Adequate identification of tumor and vessels with intraoperative navigation based on preoperatively acquired 3D volumes, with or without merging real-time imaging [12, 14–21].
- Guidance, route selection, greater ablative accuracy, and thermal lesion estimation for ablation [22–27].
- Location of missing metastases [12, 28, 29].
- Teaching residents and acceleration of learning curves for all surgeons in laparoscopic and robotic liver resection [12, 30] (Fig. 30.7).
- Increasing safety (less transfusions, adequate liver volumes, more R0 resections, less liver damage) [31].
- Economy (less transfusions, shorter length of stay, less disposable instruments used, less ablation recurrences).

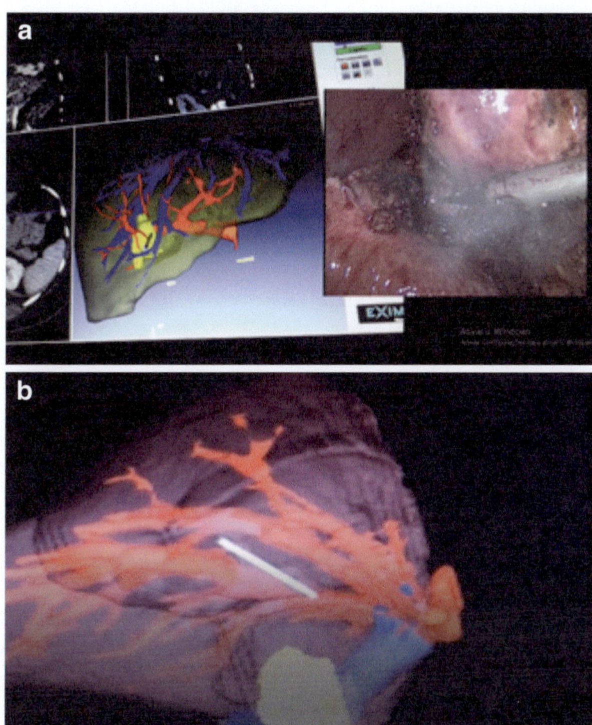

Fig. 30.7 Navigated liver resection (**a**) segment IV, (**b**) segment I

Early Clinical Data

Recent clinical experience is summarized in Table 30.1.

Table 30.1 Summary of recent published clinical experience

Author	Purpose	Platform	Patients and results	Reference
Cash et al. (2007)	Navigation and resection guidance	Optotrack 3020 (Northern Digital, Waterloo, Ontario, Canada) + Realscan 200C (3D Digital Corp, Sandy Hook, CT)	8 pts., 1 to 6 mm registration errors	[32]
Leksell (1983); Beller et al. (2009)	Navigation and ultrasound integration for central liver resections	Intraoperative 3D ultrasound with optoelectronic tracking device (Charite Hospital, Berlin)	54 pts., successful navigation in 96.3%, mean 9 mm resection margin and median error of 8 mm	[33, 34]
Oldhafer et al. (2009)	Navigation and location of missing metastases	MEVIS and image-guided stereotactically navigated ultrasound dissector	Histopathologic workup showed vital tumor cells I the specimen	[28]
Peterhans et al. (2011)	Navigation and resection guidance	Early CAScination system	9 pts., median error per intervention 6.3 mm	[35]
Kingham et al. (2012)	Intraoperative projection of CT images using tracked ultrasound	EXPLORER™ liver guidance system with tracked intraoperative ultrasound	21 pts., tracked US alone provided additional information in 12% of cases	[36]
Kingham et al. (2013)	Laparoscopic liver resection	EXPLORER MIL system	32 pts., laparoscopic registration and errors equivalent to open IGS, overcome	[37]
Hammil et al. (2014)	Laparoscopic navigation and tracked ablation	EXPLORER system	27 pts., tracked needle positioning equal to ultrasound oriented needle positioning	[38]
Correia et al. (2014)	Open and laparoscopic navigation and ablation	EXIMIUS (ARTIS)	10 pts., acceleration of laparoscopic liver resection learning curve, location of missing metastases	[12]
Banz et al. (2016)	Navigation and resection + ablation	CAS-One	65 pts., safety and accuracy improvement	[26]
Aoki et al. (2016)	Route selection for IGLR – MIS	P3DVES and SYNAPSE VINCENT®	38 pts., feasibility and safety confirmed	[24]

Table 30.1 (continued)

Author	Purpose	Platform	Patients and results	Reference
Huber et al. (2016)	Navigation and location of missing metastases	CAS-One	The first laparoscopic computer-assisted 3D-navigated resection of a VLM	[29]
Phutane et al. (2018)	Laparoscopic navigated left hepatectomy	Novel ARGS, Clermont-Ferrand, France	1 case report; safety	[39]

Obstacles

1. Semiautomatic registration methods are time consuming.
2. Lack of studies aiming clinical endpoints and cost-effectiveness.
3. Intraoperative registration methods interfere slightly delay the usual workflow.
4. Deformations of the liver during surgery due to breathing (3 cm error), mobilization, compression, and torsion compromise navigation.
5. Need for tailor-made ergonomic surgical instrument tracking devices.
6. Dependence of technician out of the operating field.
7. Absence of ease integration between technologies for navigation with laparoscopic and robotic systems.
8. Limitation of computational power.

Integration of New Technology

As an attempt to overcome the aforementioned obstacles, several groups have been working to develop smarter segmentation methods; faster, automatic and elastic registration tools; user-friendly image fusion devices; and integrating multiple image sources into the AR vision field.

Some strategies have been initiated to integrate ablation with navigated resection. Hildebrand et al., from the Department of Surgery, University of Schleswig-Holstein, Luebeck, Germany, have developed a prototype of an online navigation system *for laparoscopic RFA* (LapAssistent) that allows electromagnetic ultrasound and needle tracking. A porcine liver was used to produce a perfused tumor-mimic-model. They had a targeting error range between 5 and 7 mm [40].

Wen et al., from the Department of Mechanical Engineering, National University of Singapore, have developed a *hand gesture guided robot* device as an interface with AR. It is a human-robot cooperative mechanism that seems to have improved the accuracy of needle insertion for transcutaneous ablation therapy [41].

Robotic liver resection is performed in many centers but still faces the problem of dealing with tumors inside a solid organ; therefore, navigation seems to be the natural next step to be taken. Peterhans et al., from the ARTORG Center for Biomedical Engineering Research, University of Bern, Switzerland, have developed *augmented environments for robotic liver surgery.* It has been applied for targeting hepatic lesions in two cirrhotic patients, during image-guided robotic liver surgery (DaVinci Surgical System). It was needed to attach optical tracking references to one of the robotic instruments and to the robotic camera. Virtual model of the tracked instrument was superimposed to the endoscopic video image and the resections were performed. The authors suggest that this robotic image guidance might improve surgeon's orientation [35].

Kenngott et al., from the Department of Surgery, University of Heidelberg, Germany, have employed an *intraoperative robotic C-arm cone-beam computed tomography (CBCT) in association with AR* (Syngo iPilot[R] AR system) for laparoscopic liver resection in one patient successfully [42].

Liver deformation during surgery hinders proper tumor location during NS. Shahin et al. (Institute for Robotics and Cognitive Systems, University of Lübeck, Germany) have used *3D ultrasound images to detect and update tumor position* in the navigation system [43]. Sauer et al. (Charité-Universitätsmedizin Berlin, Germany) have developed a *headmounted display for the visualization of anatomical structures during liver resections.* It was used for anatomical reassurance and surgeons reported satisfactory comfort wearing the device [44].

Conclusion

Marescaux and Diana from IHU (image-guided surgery institute) and IRCAD, Strasbourg, France, have published a thought-provoking editorial [10]. In 2001 Jacques Marescaux performed a remote surgical procedure using a robot and in collaboration with NASA and France Telecom. The surgeon was in New York, and the patient was in Strasbourg, and development in data transmission made the lag time for delay reasonable. Since then, this group has been developing technologies to improve MIS and empower the robot's autonomy. They have introduced the concept of the augmented hand for present robotic-assisted surgery, and they presented the concept of the augmented eye, for developing technologies that are aimed for enhancing surgical precision with minimal impact on workflow and comfortable for users. They aim to *see by transparency* ("X-ray" ability); to *see the microscopic,* through confocal laser endomicroscopy to permit "virtual" biopsies; and *to see the invisible,* associating fluorescence image-guided surgery [10].

These challenges are to be met in a multidisciplinary manner by collaborative technology and teaching centers around the world. Today, it is clear that whenever a formal liver resection is not an option, navigated surgery should be considered for aiming a safe, R0, minimally invasive, parenchymal-sparing, tailored procedure. Despite promising results, prospective, randomized controlled trials such as PRONAVIC I will be welcomed to gauge the real impact of navigated liver treatments [45].

The improvement of current navigation platforms, the integration of AR with laparoscopic and robotic liver surgery and the continuous dialogue with upcoming technological medical developments will take us to a time where the present definition of reality might no longer be applicable and where cybernetic surgery will have become a safe option.

Endnote I would like to deeply thank the researchers that have developed with me the 3D LIVER tool for volumetric liver reconstruction which raised my interest for IGLS (Dario Oliveira and Raul Feitosa from the Pontifícia Universidade Católica do Rio e Janeiro); those who helped me understand how navigation works and the challenges we face, such as James D. Stefansic (Pathfinder Radiotherapeutics Inc), Mathias Peterhans (CASCINATION), and Michele Diana (Institute for Hybrid Image-Guided Minimally Invasive Surgery IHU Strasbourg) for sharing with me huge volume of information and finally Bruno Cassaro (EXIMIUS, ARTIS TECNOLOGIA) for initiating IGLS and long-lasting collaboration in NLS in Brazil. Special thanks to Prof Jacques Marescaux for being a formidable example for those who wish to dedicate part of their lives to contribute somehow in tailoring a better future for mankind.

I would also like to thank the special efforts of two coworkers and institutional management leaders whose understanding and dedicated efforts made navigated liver surgery possible in the National Cancer Institute of Brazil, namely, José Paulo de Jesus and Reinaldo Rondinelli.

References

1. Couinaud C. Liver lobes and segments: notes on the anatomical architecture and surgery of the liver. Presse Med. 1954;62(33):709–12.
2. Couinaud C. Le foie: etudes anatomiques et chirurgicales. Paris: Masson; 1957.
3. Enchev Y. Neuronavigation: geneology, reality, and prospects. Neurosurg Focus. 2009;27(3):E11.
4. Mezger U, Jendrewski C, Bartels M. Navigation in surgery. Langenbeck's Arch Surg. 2013;398(4):5–14.
5. Zernov DN. L'encéphalometrie. Rev Gen Clin Ther. 1890;19:302.
6. Roberts DW, Strohbehn JW, Hatch JF, et al. A frameless stereotaxic integration of computerized tomographic imaging and the operating microscope. J Neurosurg. 1986;65(4):545–9.
7. Watanabe E, Watanabe T, Manaka S, et al. Three-dimensional digitizer (neuronavigator): new equipment for computed tomography-guided stereotaxic surgery. Surg Neurol. 1987;27(6):543–7.
8. Bucholz RD. System for indicating the position of a surgical probe within a head on an image of the head. 1995.
9. Bucholz R, McDurmont L. The history, current status, and future of the stealthstation treatment guidance system. In: Lozano AM, Gildenberg PL, Tasker RR, editors. Textbook of stereotactic and functional neurosurgery. Berlin: Springer; 2009.
10. Marescaux J, Diana M, Soler L. Augmented reality and minimally invasive surgery. J Gastroenterol Hepatol Res. 2013;2(5):555–60.
11. Tang SL, Kwoh CK, Teo MY, Sing NW, Ling KV. Augmented reality systems for medical applications. IEEE Eng Med Biol Mag. 1998;17(3):49–58.
12. Correia MM, et al. The introduction of navigation in liver surgery in Brazil. Rev Col Bras Cir. 2014;41(6):451–4.
13. Cloyd JM, et al. Image-guided liver surgery. In: Barrese JC, Henderson JM. The neurosurgical origins of image-guided surgery. Curr Probl Surg. 2015;52:491–7.
14. Warmann, et al. Computer-assisted surgery planning in children with complex liver tumors identifies variability of the classical Couinaud Classification. J Pediatr Surg. 2016;51(11):1801–6.
15. Ryu M, Cho A. [Usefulness of image-navigated surgery in liver surgery]. Nihon Geka Gakkai Zasshi. 2008;109(2):71–6.
16. Zhao J, Zhou XJ, Zhu CZ, et al. 3D simulation assisted resection of giant hepatic mesenchymal hamartoma in children. Comput Assist Surg. 2017;22(1):54–9.

17. Yamanaka J, Okada T, Saito S, et al. Minimally invasive laparoscopic liver resection: 3D MDCT simulation for preoperative planning. J Hepatobiliary Pancreat Surg. 2009;16(6):808–15.
18. Herfarth C, Lamadé W, Fischer L, et al. The effect of virtual reality and training on liver operation planning. Swiss Surg. 2002;8(2):67–73.
19. Högemann D, Stamm G, Shin H, et al. [Individual planning of liver surgery interventions with a virtual model of the liver and its associated structures]. Radiologe. 2000;40(3):267–73.
20. Radtke A, Sotiropoulos GC, Molmenti EP, et al. Computer-assisted surgery planning for complex liver resections: when is it helpful? A single-center experience over an 8-year period. Ann Surg. 2010;252(5):876–83.
21. Fang CH, Li XF, Li Z, et al. Application of a medical image processing system in liver transplantation. Hepatobiliary Pancreat Dis Int. 2010;9(4):370–5.
22. Tinguely P, Fusaglia M, Freedman J, et al. Laparoscopic image-based navigation for microwave ablation of liver tumors-a multi-center study. Surg Endosc. 2017;31(10):4315–24.
23. Baegert C, Villard C, Schreck P, Soler L, Gangi A. Trajectory optimization for the planning of percutaneous radiofrequency ablation of hepatic tumors. Comput Aided Surg. 2007;12(2):82–90.
24. Aoki T, Murakami M, Fujimori A, et al. Routes for virtually guided endoscopic liver resection of subdiaphragmatic liver tumors. Langenbeck's Arch Surg. 2016;401(2):263–73.
25. Freedman J, Nilsson H, Jonas E. New horizons in ablation therapy for hepatocellular carcinoma. Hepat Oncol. 2015;2(4):349–58.
26. Banz VM, Müller PC, Tinguely P, et al. Intraoperative image-guided navigation system: development and applicability in 65 patients undergoing liver surgery. Langenbeck's Arch Surg. 2016;401(4):495–02.
27. Voirin D, Payan Y, Amavizca M, Létoublon C, Troccaz J. Computer-aided hepatic tumour ablation: requirements and preliminary results. C R Biol. 2002;325(4):309–19.
28. Oldhafer KJ, Stavrou GA, Prause G, et al. How to operate a liver tumor you cannot see. Langenbeck's Arch Surg. 2009;394(3):489–94.
29. Huber T, Baumgart J, Peterhans M, et al. Computer-assisted 3D-navigated laparoscopic resection of a vanished colorectal liver metastasis after chemotherapy. Z Gastroenterol. 2016;54(1):40–3.
30. Yeo CT, MacDonald A, Ungi T, et al. Utility of 3D reconstruction of 2D liver computed tomography/magnetic resonance images as a surgical planning tool for residents in liver resection surgery. J Surg Educ. 2017;S1931–7204(17):30384–7.
31. Li H, Shi X, Liang Y, et al. [Application values of computer-assisted preoperative planning of hilar cholangiocarcinoma]. Zhonghua Yi Xue Za Zhi. 2015;95(6):412–15.
32. Cash DM, Miga MI, Glasgow SC, et al. Concepts and preliminary data toward the realization of image-guided liver surgery. J Gastrointest Surg. 2007;11(7):844–59.
33. Leksell L. Stereotactic radiosurgery. J Neurol Neurosurg Psychiatry. 1983;46(9):797–803.
34. Beller S, Eulenstein S, Lange T, et al. Upgrade of an optical navigation system with a permanent electromagnetic position control: a first step towards "navigated control" for liver surgery. J Hepatobiliary Pancreat Surg. 2009;16(2):165–70.
35. Peterhans M, vom Berg A, Dagon B, et al. A navigation system for open liver surgery: design, workflow and first clinical applications. Int J Med Robot. 2011;7(1):7–16.
36. Kingham TP, Scherer MA, Neese BW, et al. Image-guided liver surgery: intraoperative projection of computed tomography images utilizing tracked ultrasound. HPB (Oxford). 2012;14(9):594–603.
37. Kingham TP, Jayaraman S, Clements LW, et al. Evolution of image-guided liver surgery: transition from open to laparoscopic procedures. J Gastrointest Surg. 2013;17(7):1274–82.
38. Hammil CW, Clements LW, Stefansic JD, et al. Evaluation of a minimally invasive image-guided surgery system for hepatic ablation procedures. Surg Innov. 2014;21(4):419–26.
39. Phutane P, Buc E, Poirot K, et al. Preliminary trial of augmented reality performed on a laparoscopic left hepatectomy. Surg Endosc. 2018;32(1):514–5.
40. Hildebrand P, Kleemann M, Schlichting S, et al. Prototype of an online navigation system for laparoscopic radiofrequency ablation. Hepatogastroenterology. 2009;56(96):1710–3.

41. Wen R, Tay WL, Nguyen BP, et al. Hand gesture guided robot-assisted surgery based on a direct augmented reality interface. Comput Methods Prog Biomed. 2014;116(2):68–80.
42. Kenngott HG, Wagner M, Gondan M, et al. Real-time image guidance in laparoscopic liver surgery: first clinical experience with a guidance system based on intraoperative CT imaging. Surg Endosc. 2014;28(3):933–40.
43. Shahin O, Beširević A, Kleemann M, Schlaefer A. Ultrasound-based tumor movement compensation during navigated laparoscopic liver interventions. Surg Endosc. 2014;28(5):1734–41.
44. Sauer IM, Queisner M, Tang P, et al. Mixed reality in visceral surgery: development of a suitable workflow and evaluation of intraoperative use-cases. Ann Surg. 2017;266(5):706–12.
45. Kleemann M, Deichmann S, Esnaashari H, Besirevic A, Shahin O, Bruch HP, Laubert T. Laparoscopic navigated liver resection: technical aspects and clinical practice in benign liver tumors. Case Rep Surg. 2012;2012:265918. https://doi.org/10.1155/2012/265918. Epub 2012 Oct 22.

Staged Hepatectomies for Colorectal Cancer Liver Metastases: When and How

31

Georgios Antonios Margonis and Matthew J. Weiss

Introduction

Hepatic resection remains the only potentially curative treatment option for patients presenting with colorectal liver metastasis (CRLM). Previous resectability criteria precluded surgery in patients with four or more metastases, bilateral disease, extra-hepatic disease, and those with an anticipated R1 resection. As a result, many patients were deemed unresectable and were not offered a chance for cure. The understanding that removing high tumor burden (e.g., multinodular, large, and bilateral disease and limited extrahepatic disease) can lead to acceptable oncological outcomes—even at the cost of an R1 resection, lead to the expansion of indications under the condition that a sufficient future live remnant (FLR) should be achieved to preserve the vital liver functions. In fact, in 2006, a consensus group summarized this paradigm shift in the definition of resectability as a "focus on what will remain after resection rather than on what is to be removed" [1]. Despite the use of portal vein embolization (PVE) and the combination of resection and ablation, some patients with multiple, bilateral CRLM remain ineligible for curative resection due to the lack of a sufficient FLR. Such patients may benefit from a two-stage hepatectomy. TSH consists of an initial procedure to remove part of the metastatic disease, which is followed by a period of time (and possibly PVE) to allow for sufficient hypertrophy of the FLR, before a second procedure is performed to remove all remaining disease, namely a two-stage hepatectomy (TSH).

G. A. Margonis
Department of Surgery, Johns Hopkins University School of Medicine, Baltimore, MD, USA
e-mail: gmargon1@jhu.edu

M. J. Weiss (✉)
Department of Surgery, Johns Hopkins University School of Medicine, Baltimore, MD, USA

Pancreas Cancer Multidisciplinary Clinic, Liver Cancer Multidisciplinary Clinic, Johns Hopkins University, Baltimore, MD, USA
e-mail: mweiss5@jhmi.edu; mweiss8@northwell.edu

M. M. Correia et al. (eds.), *Colorectal Cancer Liver Metastases*,
https://doi.org/10.1007/978-3-030-25486-5_31

First Description of TSH

Although briefly mentioned as early as in 1996, TSH was formally described by Adam et al. in 2000, when they published their initial experience with 16 patients at the Paul Brousse hospital [2]. At the time, it was suggested that a two-stage hepatectomy may be indicated in patients with multinodular bilobar tumors that were (1) stabilized or downstaged by neoadjuvant chemotherapy; (2) preferably without concurrent extrahepatic disease; and (3) were irresectable by a single hepatectomy with or without concurrent radiofrequency ablation (RFA). Almost all patients had received pre-hepatectomy chemotherapy, and for the first stage, the hemiliver with the highest tumor burden was selected to be cleared to minimize tumor growth between the two hepatectomies. Portal vein embolism (PVE) was offered in six patients. To prevent tumor growth, especially in the setting of an increase in growth factor secretion to support liver regeneration, all patients were started on post-stage 1 chemotherapy 3 weeks after liver resection to avoid suppressing liver regeneration. Patients were selected for the second stage only if adequate liver regeneration had occurred and metastatic disease was stable. The median interval between the two stages was 4 months and three patients failed to complete TSH due to disease progression. Two of the 13 patients who completed TSH died after the second stage from liver failure. The 3-year survival rate was 35%. Ultimately, since its first description in 2000, TSH has been widely adopted by many centers worldwide and has undergone several modifications.

The Steps of the Procedure: How

First and second surgical stage of TSH In the first report of TSH Adam et al. supported that clearance of the hemiliver with the higher tumor burden should be performed first, so as to remove as much tumor burden as possible and in turn decrease the chances of tumor growth in the interval between the two stages [2]. In contrast, the Belghiti group suggested that resection of the left hemiliver with concurrent ligation of the right portal vein should always be performed first, as reoperating after a right hepatectomy may lead to increased morbidity. Specifically, a preceding right hepatectomy may cause adhesions of the cut liver surface to the diaphragm and right colon, which can render dissection at the second stage more difficult. In 2004, another group from France proposed that metastases in the FLR (the hemiliver with less tumor burden) should be resected first by performing wedge resections of three or fewer liver metastases with local ablation if more than three metastases were found [3]. After a subsequent PVE, a major hepatic resection of the hemiliver with the highest tumor burden should follow. This modification allows for regeneration in an already cleared hemiliver, which decreases the chances of tumor progression. Interestingly, the Paul Brousse group revisited their initial approach and proposed first clearing the future liver remnant from all metastatic disease (before subjecting it to the hypertrophic stimulus of contralateral PVE), and then embolizing the contralateral portal vein (Fig. 31.1). A similar approach for two-staged hepatectomies has been adopted by our center, MD Anderson and Memorial Sloan Kettering (MSKCC) [4].

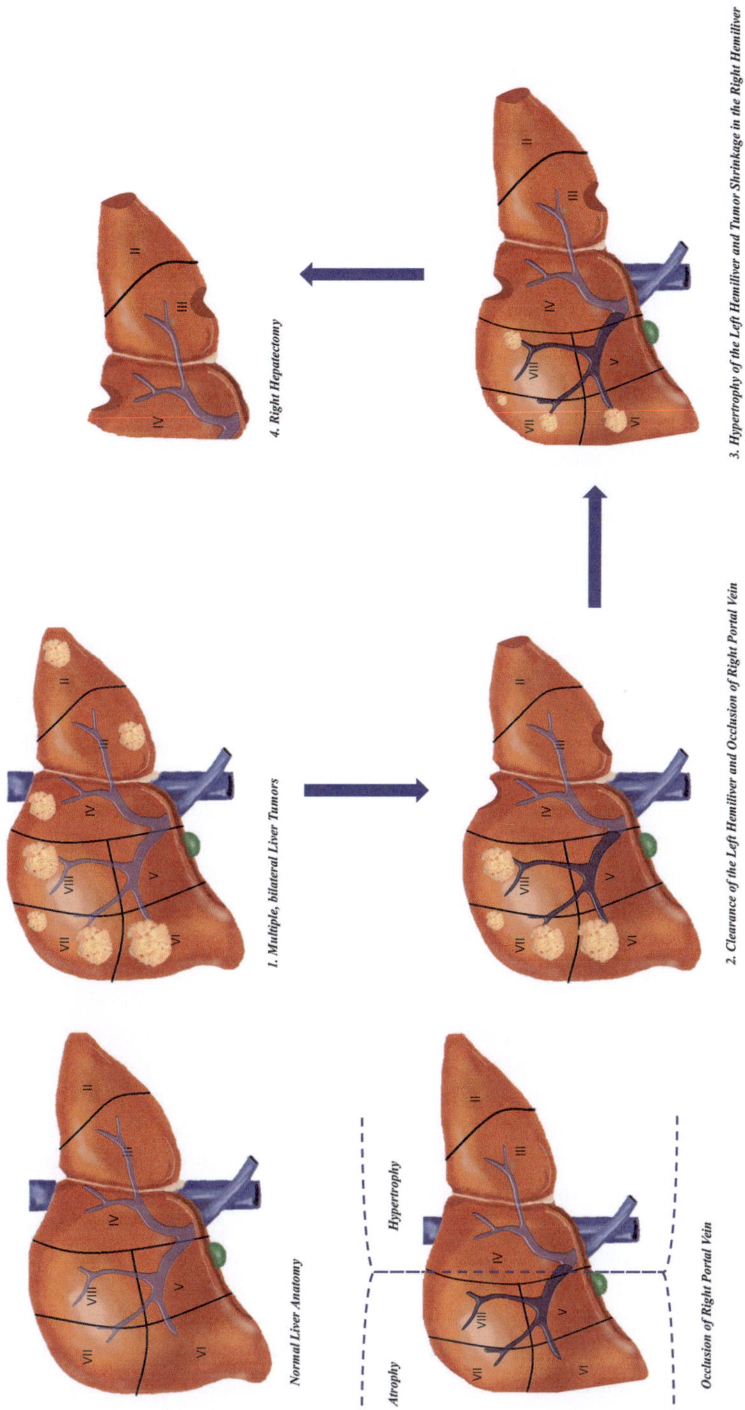

Fig. 31.1 The two stage Hepatectomy

Rate, timing, and PVE versus portal vein ligation (PVL) Although PVL requires general anesthesia and laparotomy, it can be performed during the first stage of TSH, obviating the need for an additional procedure. The issue with PVL is that it may increase the risk of adhesions due to more manipulation of surrounding structures [5]. On the other hand, PVE can be performed percutaneously with local anesthesia. According to a consensus statement, PVE should be considered in patients with normal liver parenchyma and an FLR less than 20%, in patients with a liver pretreated with chemotherapy with an FLR of less than 30% and in those with cirrhotic liver and an FLR of less than 40% [6]. Despite these recommendations, the rates of PVE vary considerably across centers. For example, in a dual institution series of Johns Hopkins and Curry Cabral Hospital, the rate of PVE was 77.8%, while in a recent series from the Paul Brousse group it was 92.8%. In comparison, in the MD Anderson series it was only 62% [7–9].

The timing of PVE varies as well. Some centers perform PVE during the interval between the first- and second-stage resections after disease has been entirely removed from the FLR, which ensures that only non-tumorous FLR is subjected to the cytokine milieu that accompanies regeneration induced by PVE. This is the case with our group, as we favor performing PVE during the interval between the two stages and while patients are on chemotherapy. In comparison, the Paul Brousse group most commonly performed PVE during the first stage of TSH (81.9%) [7, 8].

A recent meta-analysis compared outcomes after a PVE or a PVL procedure [5]. Although both procedures induced a similar rate of liver hypertrophy, significant differences were seen in the proportion of patients who could not undergo a hepatic resection due to an inadequate hypertrophy response (4.3% after PVE and 0% after PVL, $P = 0.002$). A possible explanation is that recanalization of the embolized portal branches or portosystemic shunting (e.g., in patients with portal hypertension) may occur in PVE and in turn cause insufficient embolization of the portal vein [10]. The most recent development in this field has been the new concept of a fast-track TSH pathway which combines the first-stage resection with PVE in a hybrid IR/OR suite [11].

Interval chemotherapy The indications for interval chemotherapy are not clear. This may explain why a recent meta-analysis showed a range of 0–100% for the use of interval chemotherapy with a median of 37% [12]. For example, the MD Anderson group does not routinely administer interval chemotherapy, but only selectively in those with either progressive disease or insufficient growth of FLR following the first stage of TSH [13]. In contrast, our group at Johns Hopkins Hospital and the Paul Brousse group (74.1% in a recent series) support routine administration of interval chemotherapy [7]. Although it is hard to argue against interval chemotherapy in patients with progressive disease following the first stage of TSH, administering chemotherapy in those with stable disease to prevent progression is debatable. Muratore et al. were the first to examine the impact of interval chemotherapy on disease progression and dropout rates between the first and second stages of TSH [14]. Of note, interval chemotherapy did not significantly affect rates of disease progression and dropout. However, the study was relatively small ($n = 47$) and did not allow for stratification by the use of PVE (see next section) or risk factors for progressive disease, which may have allowed the authors to identify a subset of patients who would benefit from interval chemotherapy. Regarding the dosing of interval chemotherapy, although some centers suggest at least three cycles of interval chemotherapy, others argue that administering more cycles than what is needed to control progression may cause an unnecessary delay in performing the second stage of TSH [7]. Lastly, the optimal regimen for interval chemotherapy has not been investigated; the Paul Brousse institutional policy is to administer the same regimen as the one used for preoperative chemotherapy [7].

The interplay of PVE and interval chemotherapy Intuitively, interval chemotherapy could theoretically hinder post-PVE liver hypertrophy but PVE-induced liver hypertrophy may stimulate residual tumor growth and preclude the second stage of the procedure. Regarding the former, although older studies confirmed this theoretical risk, more recent, larger studies support the use of interval chemotherapy (and bevacizumab) between PVE and resection, particularly for patients with colorectal liver metastases [15, 16]. Regarding the latter, this may be particularly important in patients who undergo major resection (e.g., right hepatectomy) first, which subjects the metastatic disease on the left hemiliver to the regenerative cascade. Although not performed in an explicitly TSH cohort, a study by MSKCC in 64 CRLM patients who underwent post-PVE chemotherapy demonstrated a significantly lower rate of disease progression (18.9 vs 34.2%, $P = 0.03$) [17]. Importantly, chemotherapy did not prevent liver hypertrophy following PVE. Similarly, others have found that PVE was associated with increased tumor growth rate and new tumors in the FLR following CRLM resection [18]. Lastly, for the first time, a recent study examined the role of post-PVE chemotherapy and somatic mutations on FLR volume and tumor growth in a mixed cohort of primary and secondary liver malignancies [19]. Chemotherapy was protective against tumor growth without hindering FLR growth. Somatic mutations (e.g., KRAS and TP53) were an independent predictor of tumor growth but did not hinder FLR growth. However, studies that explicitly focus on the impact of somatic mutations on tumor growth and FLR growth in patients with CRLM who undergo TSH are lacking.

Time interval between the two stages Standardized future liver remnant (sFLR) volume and degree of hypertrophy have been used for a long time to assess regeneration and decide the timing of the second stage of TSH [20]. More recently, kinetic growth rate has been proposed as a better marker [21]. Nonetheless, it seems that sufficient liver function can be gained after the first stage of TSH earlier (at 2–3 weeks) than previously estimated by methods assessing the size of FLR. Specifically, a study showed that 23 ± 4.9 days after PVE, the increase in FLR function exceeded the increase in FRL volume, and thus a waiting time of 2–3 weeks may be sufficient between PVE and the second stage of TSH [22]. Others have demonstrated that postoperative liver failure can be predicted more accurately by ^{99m}Tc-mebrofenin hepatobiliary scintigraphy (HBS), a technique that assesses the function of the FLR instead of using volume with CT volumetry [23]. In fact, in another study, HBS could predict what the hypertrophic response would be after PVE, before PVE was even performed [24]. Shortening the time interval between the two stages of the procedure could theoretically decrease the risk of disease progression. On the other hand, we believe that an expedited second stage may only "mask" disease progression until it manifests after the completion of the procedure. In fact, a similar criticism can be made regarding Associating Liver Partition & Portal Vein Ligation (ALPPS), as it does not allow for a time interval to "test" whether the tumor will progress.

Proceeding to the second stage of TSH The decision to proceed with the second operation depends on three criteria: (1) An R0 or even R1 resection can be achieved; (2) The disease left behind after the completion of the first stage is stable; and (3) The volume of FLR is sufficient to preserve liver function. The second-stage hepatectomy should be postponed for patients who present with disease progression after the first-stage hepatectomy. For these patients, systemic chemotherapy should be resumed, and the second stage of the procedure should be postponed until metastatic disease is again under control.

Tips for TSH Although the choice of laparotomy incision is somewhat subjective, in the case of left-sided lesions (the most common scenario in the first stage of TSH as mentioned above) and if technically possible based on body habitus, we prefer a midline incision due to its relatively lower morbidity and postoperative pain. The first stage of TSH starts with real-time evaluation using Intraoperative ultrasound (IOUS) for precise assessment of tumor extent in the left hemiliver. Although, division of the left triangular ligaments is routinely performed in left hepatectomies as it can help to free the liver from the hemidiaphragm this is not the case when "clearing" the left liver from metastases. Rather, we avoid dividing the left triangular ligament to prevent the formation of fibrous adhesions, which would in turn make the second stage of the procedure more difficult. Similarly, we avoid dividing vascular structures in the left liver. Overall, as a rule, the amount of dissection performed on the liver that will be dissected during the second stage should be kept at a minimum. To this end, our center favors the use of minimally invasive surgery (laparoscopic or robotic) for the first stage of TSH to minimize tissue dissection and the subsequent adhesion formation that would make the second procedure (usually a right hepatectomy) more technically challenging. An example of a laparoscopic first-stage procedure followed by an open right hepatectomy is illustrated in Fig. 31.2. The first stage of TSH is completed by clearing the left hemiliver from metastases by performing wedge resections or anatomical segmentectomies with or without concurrent RFA. Parenchymal transection for the first or the second stage of the procedure can be accomplished by numerous methods and devices. Since there is no data indicating that one technique is superior to another, surgeon's experience, training, and personal preference guide this choice. A simple clamp crushing technique is the most conventional approach and is still utilized in many high-volume centers. In our center, we most commonly employ this technique to expose and ligate the larger vessels with clips or ties, while we coagulate

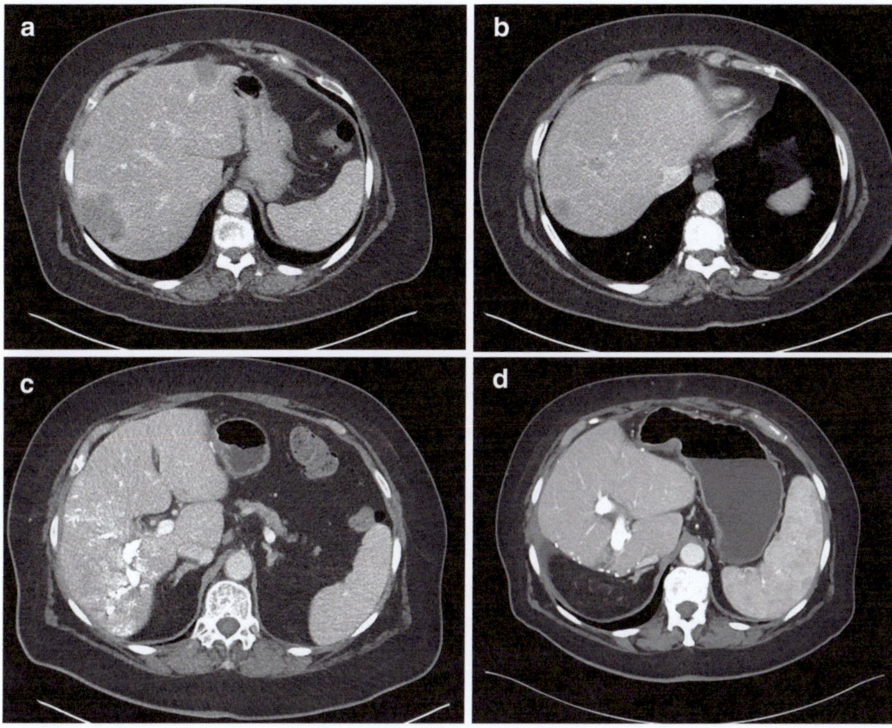

Fig. 31.2 Abdominal Computed tomographic (CT) images of a patient treated at Johns Hopkins Hospital, by neoadjuvant chemotherapy and two-stage hepatectomy. (**a**) Before chemotherapy. (**b**) Just before hepatectomy. (**c**) After the first stage (laparoscopic partial hepatectomy on the left hemi-liver). (**d**) After the second stage (open right hepatectomy 3 months after the first stage). The patient has been disease-free 12 months after the two-stage procedure

smaller structures with radiofrequency ablation using the Aquamantys system (Salient Surgical Technologies, Dover NH). The right portal vein is then embolized to stop flow to the remaining diseased liver. At the conclusion of this procedure, the patient is left with a cleared left hemiliver and a "de-portalized" right hemiliver.

Indications for TSH, When

Why we need to predict TSH failure TSH may be the only curative intent approach for the subset of patients with particularly high tumor burden irresectable by single resection [25]. However, in reality, only about two-thirds of patients ultimately complete the procedure [26]. Predicting who will fail to complete TSH may not only spare them from an invasive procedure, but also allow them to receive systematic chemotherapy earlier. One may argue in favor of attempting TSH regardless, since patients can be switched to chemotherapy anytime if they fail to complete TSH. However, the issue is that patients who complete the first stage of

TSH but fail to proceed to the second stage may actually fare worse than those with similar baseline disease who are treated with chemotherapy only and no surgery. According to a recent meta-analysis in 459 patients, the median survival of the 23% of the cohort who failed to complete TSH was only 16 months, which may be even lower than the survival of patients who undergo palliative chemotherapy [12]. This disturbing fact was also apparent in a more recent study not included in the meta-analysis that demonstrated a median overall survival of 8 months for patients who did not complete the two stages while those treated with chemotherapy alone had a median survival of 21 months ($P = 0.06$) [27]. Similarly, in a study by the Paul Brousse group (which was also not included in the meta-analysis), patients who failed to reach the second stage had an even worse outcome than those receiving chemotherapy alone [7]. Although, similar to the previous study, the chemotherapy-only group was not statistically matched with the TSH failure group, this result is especially concerning given that patients who receive chemotherapy alone often harbor more advanced disease that precluded them from being considered for TSH in the first place. A possible explanation for the dismal prognosis of patients who fail to complete TSH may relate to delays in delivering chemotherapy secondary to post-stage 1 complications, which in turn may negatively impact long-term outcomes. Of note, the authors ruled out post-stage 1 complications as the reason behind the observed worse survival, and thus the cause of these alarming results remains elusive [7].

Predictors of TSH failure TSH was invented as a procedure that should only be offered to patients when a single-stage hepatectomy (with or without concurrent RFA and PVE) cannot completely eradicate liver disease. Adam et al. proposed a classification of multinodular CRLM based on the number, size and location of CRLM, which in turn defined the initial selection criteria for TSH [28]. Unfortunately, on the sole basis of these selection criteria, around one-third of the patients who complete the first stage fail to progress to the second stage. The most common reasons that patients fail to proceed to the second stage include tumor progression, insufficient volume of FLR, poor general condition, and postoperative morbidity/mortality. Therefore, we need to refine the selection criteria by identifying predictors of the causes of TSH dropout. Several scores that predict failure to complete the procedure have been developed and may optimize patient selection. We will report only the ones that were derived by multivariable logistic regression and therefore accounted for confounders. The first score was developed by Narita et al. and demonstrated that "failure to complete TSH was driven by two independent prognostic scenarios: three or more CRLM in the FLR of patients who were over 70 years predicted tumor progression after first-stage hepatectomy, and three or more CRLM in the FLR combined with carcinomatosis at the time of first-stage hepatectomy predicted the development of additional FLR metastases after PVE/PVL" [29]. In a subsequent study, Faitot and colleagues developed a predictive score of TSH failure that included the following variables: male sex, segment 1 metastasis, need for >3 resection(s)/radiofrequency ablation(s), vascular invasion in the primary, need for change in type of chemotherapy, and microscopic biliary invasion by the metastasis

[27]. Although they did not use multivariable logistic regression, it is the first and only study that used histologic information derived from the resected liver tissue from the first stage of TSH. In contrast, a few years later, an Italian multicenter analysis found that tumor progression during pre-hepatectomy chemotherapy was the only independent risk factor that predicted failure to complete TSH [30]. Passot and colleagues identified receipt of more than six cycles of preoperative chemotherapy as the only factor independently associated with failure to complete TSH [13]. Lastly, the most recent study from the Paul Brousse group identified carcinoembryonic antigen >30ng/mL [relative risk (RR) 2.73], tumor size >40 mm (RR 2.89), chemotherapy cycles >12 (RR 3.46), and tumor progression during first-line chemotherapy (RR 6.56) as the only independent predictors of failure [7]. The authors calculated the risks of failure given the number of risk factors: For patients without any factors, the probability of failure was 10.5%, with a 5-year OS rate of 41.9%. The addition of each subsequent factor increased the risk to 43.5, 72.7, 88.5, and 95.5%, and decreased the 5-year OS to 38.8, 29.2, 0, and 0%, respectively, for 1, 2, 3, and 4 factors.

Obviously, predictors identified in each of these scores are not consistent. The differences between predictive scores may reflect heterogeneity in patient selection across different centers. This is problematic if we intend to use them in cohorts different than the ones used to derive them. Indeed, to date none of them has been externally validated. Given the lack of external validation, we do not use any clinical score at our center but instead decide patient eligibility on a case by case basis. We recommend against denying a curative intent TSH on the sole basis of predictive scores as these cases are complex and ideally should be managed in a multi-disciplinary setting.

Predictors of the specific cause of TSH failure All previous studies examined TSH failure as a "yes or no" variable—namely, dropouts vs successful completions of TSH. However, the one-third who will fail can be further divided into those with disease progression (80%) and those who have inadequate remnant liver hypertrophy. It is not unreasonable to consider that patients who experienced each of these two causes of failure should have been treated differently in the first place. For example, failures caused by an insufficiently regenerated FLR may have been prevented by selecting ALPPS instead of TSH, as it is known to induce much faster liver hypertrophy [31]. This likely stems from the liver partition that, in contrast to TSH, prevents any collateral portal blood flow between the two sides of the liver [32]. As such, the FLR receives 100% of the portal in-flow, which stimulates rapid hypertrophy that can be observed as soon as within 1 week. Interestingly, even a "rescue" approach for ALPPS in failed TSH has been suggested by a sub-analysis from the first randomized controlled trial (LIGRO trial) comparing traditional TSH with ALPPS [33]. Specifically, from the 13 eligible patients (27%) in the TSH group who could not proceed to the second stage because of inadequate FLR hypertrophy (i.e., they did not reach a sFLR of 30%), 12 (92%) were treated successfully via crossover to ALPPS. Despite earlier concerns regarding postoperative mortality of

ALPPS, data from a recent study that compared TSH to ALPPS suggest that the strong regenerative effect does not come at the price of increased major morbidity and mortality rates [34]. As such, predictors of TSH failure from insufficiently regenerated FLR could be used to select ALPPS over TSH. However, no study to date has focused on predictors for this scenario.

Although we believe that such predictors could be of value, we await further proof that mortality rates of TSH vs ALPPS are comparable, before recommending ALPPS over TSH in this scenario. For example, although mortality rates of ALPPS and TSH were comparable in the LIGRO trial, the unusually high mortality in the TSH arm (10.7%), which is inconsistent with outcomes from our center and others needs to be verified before any recommendations can be made.

On the other hand, TSH failure due to tumor progression may reflect aggressive tumor biology and thus both TSH and ALPPS may be futile in this scenario. Interestingly, although an ALPPS risk score has been already constructed, it focused only on the short-term outcomes and not on disease progression following ALPPS [35]. An advantage of TSH in this scenario is that the time interval of some weeks between the two stages of TSH can be used to gauge the aggressiveness of the tumor. Patients who progress or develop new disease following the first stage of TSH may be those whose disease harbors aggressive tumor biology and would thus not benefit from any surgery at all because of an underlying aggressive tumor biology. As such, failure to complete TSH may optimize patient selection for surgery in general. In contrast, ALPPS does not allow for enough time to test for tumor aggressiveness, as the interval is only a few days. In turn, this may explain the poor oncological outcomes reported for ALPPS and the significantly inferior overall survival compared to TSH [34, 36]. However, this is a complex problem given that proceeding to TSH instead of offering chemotherapy may impair prognosis even if patients are immediately switched to chemotherapy after failing TSH.

Short-Term Outcomes

The most recent meta-analysis published in 2012 included 10 studies in CRLM patients [12]. In total, 346 patients out of the 459 (75.4%) patients who entered the first stage completed TSH. Regarding the first stage of TSH, postoperative morbidity was 17% (ranged between 0 and 26%) and postoperative mortality was 0%. Postoperative morbidity and mortality rates for the second stage was 40% (20–59%) and 3% (0–7%), respectively. All 11 postoperative deaths were due to liver insufficiency. Unfortunately, the timing of mortality rates (30-, 60-, or 90-days mortality) and the grading of complication according to the Dindo-Clavien system were not reported. These results indicate acceptable morbidity and mortality for TSH.

In a subsequent study, Regimbeau et al. reported in a more detailed fashion on the short-term outcomes following TSH [37]. In this LiverMetSurvey analysis of 869 patients, 625 patients completed TSH (TSH 2/2 group) and 244 aborted the procedure after the first stage (TSH 1/2 group). The 30-, 60-, and 90-day mortality rates were 5.4, 9.2, and 11.3%, respectively in the overall TSH population, 3.8, 7.2, and 9.3% in the TSH (2/2) group, and 9.4, 14.3, and 16.4% in the TSH (1/2) group, respectively. Postoperative morbidity for the first and second stages was 29.1 and 25.1%, respectively. Unfortunately, the cause of perioperative mortality and the grading of complications were not reported. The reported mortality rates are worrisome and may be the result of including 359 centers located in 60 countries with different levels of case volume/experience.

MD Anderson reported a 90-day mortality rate of only 4% [8]. In total, 126 patients entered the first stage of TSH and 92 completed the second stages. In total, 44 out of the 126 patients (35%) developed a postoperative complication, with 18 (14%) of them having a major complication according to the Dindo-Clavien classification. Unfortunately, morbidity and mortality rates separately for each of the two stages were not reported. This TSH cohort was then compared to a group of patients with bilobar CRLM who underwent one-stage major hepatectomy with contralateral resection or ablation. Importantly, patients who underwent TSH were less likely to develop a postoperative major complication (14 vs 26%, $P = 0.03$) or postoperative hepatic insufficiency (6 vs 20%, $P = 0.001$) compared with those who underwent one-stage hepatectomy. These outcomes were confirmed by a study from the University of Zurich that compared postoperative complications following TSH vs one-stage hepatectomies [38]. The risk was similar in both procedures despite the higher baseline risk of the former. Of note, both studies did not match the TSH and one-stage hepatectomy groups prior to comparing their outcomes. In contrast, a case-matched analysis demonstrated that major complications according to Dindo-Clavien were more common in patients who underwent TSH vs one-stage hepatectomy (28 vs 13%, $P = 0.017$). Importantly, mortality rates were almost identical in the matched analysis [39]. Thus, although it seems that mortality rates are comparable, it is unclear whether major morbidity is more common in TSH.

Although no study has compared TSH outcomes in high vs low volume centers, more evidence supporting the importance of accumulated experience emerges when trending short-term outcomes in the same institution over time. In the original description of TSH by Adam et al. in 2000 ($n = 16$), postoperative death rate within 60 days was 0% for the first-stage procedure but as high as 15% for the second stage [2]. Postoperative complication rates were 31 and 45% for the first and the second stages, respectively. In the 2008 report from the same group ($n = 59$), postoperative mortality within 60 days was 0 and 7% after the first and second stage, respectively [40]. Morbidity rates were 20 vs 59% for the first and second stages of TSH. In 2015, they presented their updated experience on 125 patients undergoing TSH [7]. A 90-day mortality was only 0.8 and 2.5% after the first and the second stages of TSH, respectively. Postoperative major complication rates were 14.4 and 33.3% for the first and the second stages, respectively. Although formal comparisons of low- vs high-volume centers are lacking, we favor centralization of TSH particularly to improve perioperative mortality. Studies to confirm the suspected volume-outcomes effect are needed.

Long-term outcomes A recent meta-analysis analyzed the long-term outcomes reported in studies published until 2012 [12]. Median OS in patients who failed to complete both stages of TSH was only 16 months (range: 10–29 months). In contrast, median OS in patients who completed both stages was 37 months (range: 24–44 months). Regarding subsequent studies not included in the meta-analysis, the LiverMetSurvey multi-institutional study reported similar survival rates [37]. Mean OS in patients who failed to complete both stages of TSH was 25 ± 2 months. In contrast, median OS in patients who completed both stages was 40 ± 2 months ($P = 0.007$).

A few studies have compared OS in patients who underwent TSH vs patients who underwent a single-stage major hepatectomy with contralateral resection or ablation for bilobar disease. In the MD Anderson series, patients who completed TSH had a better 5-year OS rate compared with patients who underwent one-stage hepatectomy without (50 vs 20%, $P = 0.023$) or with concurrent RFA (50 vs 24%, $P < 0.0001$) [8]. Another study employed case-matched analysis and compared TSH with one-stage hepatectomy combined with RFA [39]. Their results were slightly different than the previous study. Median OS was very similar among patients undergoing one-stage hepatectomy and those undergoing TSH (37.2 and 34.5 months, $P = 0.6$). Lastly, in a collaborative series from our center and Curry Cabral Hospital, patients who completed TSH had a similar 3-year overall survival compared with patients who were treated with a planned single-stage hepatectomy (58 vs 53%, $P = 0.34$) [9]. Thus, we can conclude that TSH has comparable outcomes to one-stage hepatectomies with or without concurrent RFA for bilobar CRLM. Despite the comparable long-term outcomes, we recommend that a single-stage hepatectomy (with or without concurrent RFA and PVE) should be offered to patients when it can completely eradicate liver disease.

As with the trend in short-term outcomes, the improvement in survival rates over time may be explained by increased experience with the procedure. For example, in the most recent series from MD Anderson, median OS in those who failed to complete the two stages was 24 months while patients who completed both stages had a median OS of 61 months ($P = 0.006$). Of note, this is the highest OS rate reported for TSH by this group [8]. Similarly, long-term outcomes improved in the Paul Brousse series over time. In the original description of TSH the 3-year survival rate was 35% and median survival was 31 months [2]. In 2008, the same group reported that overall 3- and 5-year survivals for patients that completed both hepatectomies were 60 and 42%, respectively [40]. The median survival for completed TSH was 39 vs only 11.4 months for those who failed to complete TSH. Lastly, in 2017, they reported 3- and 5-year survival rates that were significantly better for patients who completed TSH compared to those in patients who failed to complete TSH (69.0 and 44.2% vs 14.0 and 0%, $P < 0.0001$) [7]. Finally, a few studies have demonstrated the safety and efficacy of repeat surgical resection to treat recurrence in patients who have previously undergone TSH [41, 42]. Despite the efficacy of those repeat resections, aggressive tumor biology (i.e., KRAS mutated tumors) was independently associated with poor outcomes in those patients [41]. This is consistent with our group's experience regarding the impact of KRAS and BRAF mutations on long-term outcomes in patients undergoing hepatectomy for CRLM [43, 44].

Conclusion

TSH is a curative intent procedure for multinodular, bilateral disease unresectable by single hepatectomy. Procedural morbidity and mortality have improved over time and are now acceptable. Similarly, overall survival for patients who complete TSH has improved and has been shown to be comparable to that reported for one-stage hepatectomies. Nonetheless, overall survival of patients who fail to complete TSH (around 25%) may be even lower than OS in patients with similar baseline disease treated with chemotherapy alone. As such, there is a need to further refine selection criteria by identifying predictors of TSH failure, which is primarily caused by insufficient liver hypertrophy and disease progression. For the former, recent evidence suggests that ALPPS may be used as rescue therapy in patients who fail to complete TSH due to insufficient liver hypertrophy. For the latter, the use of surrogates of aggressive tumor biology that may predict disease progression after the first stage of TSH should be investigated. Collectively, pushing the limits of technical resectability by using TSH has a role in managing CRLM patients, but only after rigorous patient selection.

References

1. Charnsangavej C, Clary B, Fong Y, Grothey A, Pawlik TM, Choti MA. Selection of patients for resection of hepatic colorectal metastases: expert consensus statement. Ann Surg Oncol. 2006;13:1261–8. https://doi.org/10.1245/s10434-006-9023-y.
2. Adam R, Laurent A, Azoulay D, Castaing D, Bismuth H. Two-stage hepatectomy: a planned strategy to treat irresectable liver tumors. Ann Surg. 2000;232:777–85.
3. Jaeck D, Oussoultzoglou E, Rosso E, Greget M, Weber JC, Bachellier P. A two-stage hepatectomy procedure combined with portal vein embolization to achieve curative resection for initially unresectable multiple and bilobar colorectal liver metastases. Ann Surg. 2004;240:1037–49; discussion 1049-1051.
4. Cardona K, Donataccio D, Kingham TP, Allen PJ, DeMatteo RP, Fong Y, et al. Treatment of extensive metastatic colorectal cancer to the liver with systemic and hepatic arterial infusion chemotherapy and two-stage hepatic resection: the role of salvage therapy for recurrent disease. Ann Surg Oncol. 2014;21:815–21. https://doi.org/10.1245/s10434-013-3351-5.
5. Isfordink CJ, Samim M, Braat M, Almalki AM, Hagendoorn J, Borel Rinkes IHM, et al. Portal vein ligation versus portal vein embolization for induction of hypertrophy of the future liver remnant: a systematic review and meta-analysis. Surg Oncol. 2017;26:257–67. https://doi.org/10.1016/j.suronc.2017.05.001.
6. Adams RB, Aloia TA, Loyer E, Pawlik TM, Taouli B, Vauthey JN, et al. Selection for hepatic resection of colorectal liver metastases: expert consensus statement. HPB (Oxford). 2013;15:91–103. https://doi.org/10.1111/j.1477-2574.2012.00557.x.
7. Imai K, Benitez CC, Allard MA, Vibert E, Cunha AS, Cherqui D, et al. Failure to achieve a 2-stage hepatectomy for colorectal liver metastases: how to prevent it? Ann Surg. 2015;262:772–8. https://doi.org/10.1097/SLA.0000000000001449; discussion 778-779.

8. Mizuno T, Cloyd JM, Omichi K, Chun YS, Conrad C, Tzeng CD, et al. Two-stage hepatectomy vs one-stage major hepatectomy with contralateral resection or ablation for advanced bilobar colorectal liver metastases. J Am Coll Surg. 2018;226:825–34. https://doi.org/10.1016/j.jamcollsurg.2018.01.054.
9. Tsai S, Marques HP, de Jong MC, Mira P, Ribeiro V, Choti MA, et al. Two-stage strategy for patients with extensive bilateral colorectal liver metastases. HPB (Oxford). 2010;12:262–9. https://doi.org/10.1111/j.1477-2574.2010.00161.x.
10. Farges O, Belghiti J, Kianmanesh R, Regimbeau JM, Santoro R, Vilgrain V, et al. Portal vein embolization before right hepatectomy: prospective clinical trial. Ann Surg. 2003;237:208–17. https://doi.org/10.1097/01.SLA.0000048447.16651.7B.
11. Odisio BC, Simoneau E, Holmes AA, Conrad CH, Vauthey JN. Fast-track two-stage hepatectomy using a hybrid interventional radiology/operating suite as alternative option to associated liver partition and portal vein ligation for staged hepatectomy procedure. J Am Coll Surg. 2018;227:e5–e10. https://doi.org/10.1016/j.jamcollsurg.2018.04.027.
12. Lam VW, Laurence JM, Johnston E, Hollands MJ, Pleass HC, Richardson AJ. A systematic review of two-stage hepatectomy in patients with initially unresectable colorectal liver metastases. HPB (Oxford). 2013;15:483–91. https://doi.org/10.1111/j.1477-2574.2012.00607.x.
13. Passot G, Chun YS, Kopetz SE, Zorzi D, Brudvik KW, Kim BJ, et al. Predictors of safety and efficacy of 2-stage hepatectomy for bilateral colorectal liver metastases. J Am Coll Surg. 2016;223:99–108. https://doi.org/10.1016/j.jamcollsurg.2015.12.057.
14. Muratore A, Zimmitti G, Ribero D, Mellano A, Vigano L, Capussotti L. Chemotherapy between the first and second stages of a two-stage hepatectomy for colorectal liver metastases: should we routinely recommend it? Ann Surg Oncol. 2012;19:1310–5. https://doi.org/10.1245/s10434-011-2069-5.
15. Covey AM, Brown KT, Jarnagin WR, Brody LA, Schwartz L, Tuorto S, et al. Combined portal vein embolization and neoadjuvant chemotherapy as a treatment strategy for resectable hepatic colorectal metastases. Ann Surg. 2008;247:451–5. https://doi.org/10.1097/SLA.0b013e31815ed693.
16. Zorzi D, Chun YS, Madoff DC, Abdalla EK, Vauthey JN. Chemotherapy with bevacizumab does not affect liver regeneration after portal vein embolization in the treatment of colorectal liver metastases. Ann Surg Oncol. 2008;15:2765–72. https://doi.org/10.1245/s10434-008-0035-7.
17. Fischer C, Melstrom LG, Arnaoutakis D, Jarnagin W, Brown K, D'Angelica M, et al. Chemotherapy after portal vein embolization to protect against tumor growth during liver hypertrophy before hepatectomy. JAMA Surg. 2013;148:1103–8. https://doi.org/10.1001/jamasurg.2013.2126.
18. Hoekstra LT, van Lienden KP, Doets A, Busch OR, Gouma DJ, van Gulik TM. Tumor progression after preoperative portal vein embolization. Ann Surg. 2012;256:812–7. https://doi.org/10.1097/SLA.0b013e3182733f09; discussion 817-818.
19. Deipolyi AR, Zhang YS, Khademhosseini A, Naidu S, Borad M, Sahin B, et al. Portal vein embolization: impact of chemotherapy and genetic mutations. J Clin Med. 2017;6 https://doi.org/10.3390/jcm6030026.
20. Kishi Y, Abdalla EK, Chun YS, Zorzi D, Madoff DC, Wallace MJ, et al. Three hundred and one consecutive extended right hepatectomies: evaluation of outcome based on systematic liver volumetry. Ann Surg. 2009;250:540–8. https://doi.org/10.1097/SLA.0b013e3181b674df.
21. Shindoh J, Truty MJ, Aloia TA, Curley SA, Zimmitti G, Huang SY, et al. Kinetic growth rate after portal vein embolization predicts posthepatectomy outcomes: toward zero liver-related mortality in patients with colorectal liver metastases and small future liver remnant. J Am Coll Surg. 2013;216:201–9. https://doi.org/10.1016/j.jamcollsurg.2012.10.018.
22. de Graaf W, van Lienden KP, van den Esschert JW, Bennink RJ, van Gulik TM. Increase in future remnant liver function after preoperative portal vein embolization. Br J Surg. 2011;98:825–34. https://doi.org/10.1002/bjs.7456.
23. Cieslak KP, Bennink RJ, de Graaf W, van Lienden KP, Besselink MG, Busch OR, et al. Measurement of liver function using hepatobiliary scintigraphy improves risk assessment

in patients undergoing major liver resection. HPB (Oxford). 2016;18:773–80. https://doi.org/10.1016/j.hpb.2016.06.006.
24. Cieslak KP, Huisman F, Bais T, Bennink RJ, van Lienden KP, Verheij J, et al. Future remnant liver function as predictive factor for the hypertrophy response after portal vein embolization. Surgery. 2017;162:37–47. https://doi.org/10.1016/j.surg.2016.12.031.
25. Qadan M, D'Angelica MI. Complex surgical strategies to improve resectability in borderline-Resectable disease. Curr Colorectal Cancer Rep. 2015;11:369–77. https://doi.org/10.1007/s11888-015-0290-5.
26. Yang C, Rahbari NN, Mees ST, Schaab F, Koch M, Weitz J, et al. Staged resection of bilobar colorectal liver metastases: surgical strategies. Langenbeck's Arch Surg. 2015;400:633–40. https://doi.org/10.1007/s00423-015-1310-2.
27. Faitot F, Soubrane O, Wendum D, Sandrini J, Afchain P, Balladur P, et al. Feasibility and survival of 2-stage hepatectomy for colorectal metastases: definition of a simple and early clinicopathologic predicting score. Surgery. 2015;157:444–53. https://doi.org/10.1016/j.surg.2014.09.033.
28. Adam R, Lucidi V, Bismuth H. Hepatic colorectal metastases: methods of improving resectability. Surg Clin North Am. 2004;84:659–71. https://doi.org/10.1016/j.suc.2003.12.005.
29. Narita M, Oussoultzoglou E, Jaeck D, Fuchschuber P, Rosso E, Pessaux P, et al. Two-stage hepatectomy for multiple bilobar colorectal liver metastases. Br J Surg. 2011;98:1463–75. https://doi.org/10.1002/bjs.7580.
30. Giuliante F, Ardito F, Ferrero A, Aldrighetti L, Ercolani G, Grande G, et al. Tumor progression during preoperative chemotherapy predicts failure to complete 2-stage hepatectomy for colorectal liver metastases: results of an Italian multicenter analysis of 130 patients. J Am Coll Surg. 2014;219:285–94. https://doi.org/10.1016/j.jamcollsurg.2014.01.063.
31. Eshmuminov D, Raptis DA, Linecker M, Wirsching A, Lesurtel M, Clavien PA. Meta-analysis of associating liver partition with portal vein ligation and portal vein occlusion for two-stage hepatectomy. Br J Surg. 2016;103:1768–82. https://doi.org/10.1002/bjs.10290.
32. Alvarez FA, Ardiles V, Sanchez Claria R, Pekolj J, de Santibanes E. Associating liver partition and portal vein ligation for staged hepatectomy (ALPPS): tips and tricks. J Gastrointest Surg. 2013;17:814–21. https://doi.org/10.1007/s11605-012-2092-2.
33. Sandstrom P, Rosok BI, Sparrelid E, Larsen PN, Larsson AL, Lindell G, et al. ALPPS improves resectability compared with conventional two-stage hepatectomy in patients with advanced colorectal liver metastasis: results from a Scandinavian Multicenter Randomized Controlled Trial (LIGRO Trial). Ann Surg. 2018;267:833–40. https://doi.org/10.1097/SLA.0000000000002511.
34. Adam R, Imai K, Castro Benitez C, Allard MA, Vibert E, Sa Cunha A, et al. Outcome after associating liver partition and portal vein ligation for staged hepatectomy and conventional two-stage hepatectomy for colorectal liver metastases. Br J Surg. 2016;103:1521–9. https://doi.org/10.1002/bjs.10256.
35. Linecker M, Stavrou GA, Oldhafer KJ, Jenner RM, Seifert B, Lurje G, et al. The ALPPS risk score: avoiding futile use of ALPPS. Ann Surg. 2016;264:763–71. https://doi.org/10.1097/SLA.0000000000001914.
36. Olthof PB, Huiskens J, Wicherts DA, Huespe PE, Ardiles V, Robles-Campos R, et al. Survival after associating liver partition and portal vein ligation for staged hepatectomy (ALPPS) for advanced colorectal liver metastases: a case-matched comparison with palliative systemic therapy. Surgery. 2017;161:909–19. https://doi.org/10.1016/j.surg.2016.10.032.
37. Regimbeau JM, Cosse C, Kaiser G, Hubert C, Laurent C, Lapointe R, et al. Feasibility, safety and efficacy of two-stage hepatectomy for bilobar liver metastases of colorectal cancer: a LiverMetSurvey analysis. HPB (Oxford). 2017;19:396–405. https://doi.org/10.1016/j.hpb.2017.01.008.
38. Schadde E, Slankamenac K, Breitenstein S, Lesurtel M, De Oliveira M, Beck-Schimmer B, et al. Are two-stage hepatectomies associated with more complications than one-stage procedures? HPB (Oxford). 2013;15:411–7. https://doi.org/10.1111/hpb.12001.

39. Faitot F, Faron M, Adam R, Elias D, Cimino M, Cherqui D, et al. Two-stage hepatectomy versus 1-stage resection combined with radiofrequency for bilobar colorectal metastases: a case-matched analysis of surgical and oncological outcomes. Ann Surg. 2014;260:822–7. https://doi.org/10.1097/SLA.0000000000000976; discussion 827-828.
40. Wicherts DA, Miller R, de Haas RJ, Bitsakou G, Vibert E, Veilhan LA, et al. Long-term results of two-stage hepatectomy for irresectable colorectal cancer liver metastases. Ann Surg. 2008;248:994–1005. https://doi.org/10.1097/SLA.0b013e3181907fd9.
41. Lillemoe HA, Kawaguchi Y, Passot G, Karagkounis G, Simoneau E, You YN, et al. Surgical resection for recurrence after two-stage hepatectomy for colorectal liver metastases is feasible, is safe, and improves survival. J Gastrointest Surg. 2018; https://doi.org/10.1007/s11605-018-3890-y.
42. Imai K, Benitez CC, Allard MA, Vibert E, Cunha AS, Cherqui D, et al. Impact of surgical treatment for recurrence after 2-stage hepatectomy for colorectal liver metastases, on patient outcome. Ann Surg. 2017; https://doi.org/10.1097/SLA.0000000000002472.
43. Margonis GA, Buettner S, Andreatos N, Kim Y, Wagner D, Sasaki K, et al. Association of BRAF mutations with survival and recurrence in surgically treated patients with metastatic colorectal liver Cancer. JAMA Surg. 2018;153:e180996. https://doi.org/10.1001/jamasurg.2018.0996.
44. Margonis GA, Buettner S, Andreatos N, Wagner D, Sasaki K, Barbon C, et al. Prognostic factors change over time after hepatectomy for colorectal liver metastases: a multi-institutional, international analysis of 1099 patients. Ann Surg. 2018; https://doi.org/10.1097/SLA.0000000000002664.

Parenchymal-Sparing Surgery: What Is Behind It?

32

Adriana C. Gamboa and Shishir K. Maithel

Introduction

Treatment strategy for colorectal liver metastases (CRLM) has evolved during the last two decades. Although the number of patients eligible for resection of CLRM remains approximately only 25% despite advances in multidisciplinary approaches, the combination of chemotherapy and surgical resection of liver metastases has resulted in a 5-year survival of approximately 50% [1]. When evaluating CLRM for resectability, both oncologic and technical aspects should be considered including the ability to achieve negative margins, size of future liver remnant (FLR), and necessity for functional vascular inflow and vascular and biliary outflow. In order to maximize the safety of liver surgery by optimizing the FLR and expand the patient population eligible for surgery, several strategies have been developed including portal vein embolization (PVE), two-stage hepatectomy, and associating liver partition and portal vein ligation for staged hepatectomy (ALPPS). The ongoing need to preserve normal liver parenchyma and the expansion of resectability criteria for CRLM have led to the development of parenchymal-sparing liver surgery (PSLS) or parenchymal-sparing hepatectomy (PSH).

The primary goal of PSH is to preserve as much normal liver parenchyma as possible while providing equivalent oncologic benefits when compared to major hepatectomy (MH). This technique includes a variety of resection strategies which necessitate a profound knowledge of liver anatomy and expertise in intraoperative ultrasound (IOUS). PSH includes both segment-oriented and non-segment-oriented variants (also referred to as wedge resections), either as isolated procedures or in combination. PSH has been associated with uncompromised cancer-related outcomes, fewer postoperative complications, and higher feasibility of future resections.

A. C. Gamboa · S. K. Maithel (✉)
Emory University, Atlanta, GA, USA
e-mail: acgambo@emory.edu; smaithe@emory.edu

M. M. Correia et al. (eds.), *Colorectal Cancer Liver Metastases*,
https://doi.org/10.1007/978-3-030-25486-5_32

This chapter reviews the rationale and indications for a parenchymal-sparing approach, and the functional and oncologic benefits and techniques particularly applicable to this approach.

Rationale for Parenchymal-Preserving Techniques for Cancer

Tumor resection avoiding the unnecessary sacrifice of functional parenchyma has been associated with decreased surgical stress, fewer postoperative complications, uncompromised oncologic outcomes, and higher feasibility of future resections.

One of the major benefits of parenchymal-sparing hepatectomies is the ability to maximize functional parenchyma. The literature has shown that up to 80% of the liver can be safely resected in the setting of normal residual liver tissue, while 60% of the liver can be resected with underlying liver disease including cirrhosis or steatohepatitis. Post-hepatectomy liver failure (PLF) is the main cause of death after major hepatectomy, and it is strictly related to the volume and quality of the FLR [2]. It is therefore critically important to accurately determine and optimize the future liver remnant.

Historically, liver volumetry was determined using the patient's height and weight which was an easy method to predict standardized liver volumes but did not necessarily capture volumes at the extremes of the size range. Cross-sectional imaging with computed tomography (CT) or magnetic resonance imaging (MRI) provides a more accurate volume calculation, and this method has been shown to agree with the actual liver volume and mass within 3–5% [3]. Using this technique, volume is calculated by marking cross-sectional images with the planned resection lines which then allows calculation of the surface area. Volume is further derived by multiplying the surface area by the slice thickness. More recently, several software programs have been developed which allow the user to segment the liver, intrahepatic vessels, and tumors to virtually define resection lines and ablation paths in order to calculate the existing functional liver volume and predict post-resection liver volume [4]. Newer developments can also provide three-dimensional (3D) reconstructions of liver structures including branches of the portal vein and hepatic artery, thus enabling the evaluation of the patient's unique intrahepatic anatomy and determining the blood supply to the remnant [5].

Despite these refinements in methods to measure the FLR, the relationship between volume and function can vary and is largely dependent on the histology and quality of the non-tumor-bearing liver parenchyma. It is well known that many patients considered for hepatic resection for malignancy have underlying liver disease secondary to preoperative chemotherapy or intrinsic liver dysfunction. Additionally, hepatic steatosis is the most common chronic liver disease in the Western world as it is largely associated with obesity, diabetes, and metabolic syndrome. A study encompassing 1803 liver resections at Memorial Sloan Kettering Cancer Center (MSKCC) noted that non-tumor-bearing liver histology demonstrated steatosis in 20% of samples, cholestasis and/or inflammation in 15%, and cirrhosis or fibrosis in another 10% [6]. As systemic chemotherapy plays an essential role in the multimodal treatment of patients with CRLM, these findings are not unexpected. Hepatic steatosis is commonly seen with the use of 5-fluorouracil (5-FU), nonalcoholic steatohepatitis is associated with irinotecan, and hepatic sinusoidal obstruction syndrome can be observed with oxaliplatin administration [7]. In a 2006 study in which the median duration of chemotherapy was 16 weeks, patients with chemotherapy-induced steatohepatitis had an increased 90-day mortality after hepatic surgery compared with patients without steatohepatitis (14.7% vs. 1.6%; $P = 0.001$) [8]. Based on the available data, current chemotherapy regimens for patients with resectable CRLM should be limited to a defined period of only 2–3 months per NCCN guidelines to avoid chemotherapy-associated liver injury and increased risk of perioperative morbidity and mortality. Furthermore, hepatic steatosis may have implications on liver regeneration, and it has been shown to be an independent predictor of perioperative complications [9]. However, steatosis alone should not preclude aggressive hepatic resection for neoplasms when indicated, and the anticipated volume of functional liver remaining after resection should largely determine resectability in the setting of underlying liver disease.

Given the importance of background liver function, the optimal assessment of fitness for liver resection would ideally incorporate some measure of FLR volume and function. Additional functional tests to assess the liver remnant should therefore be considered prior to proceeding with a major hepatectomy in the setting of significant background liver disease. Indocyanine green (ICG) clearance is the quantitative measure of hepatic function most used worldwide. ICG is a water-soluble dye that binds to albumin and distributes rapidly and uniformly in the blood after intravenous injection. ICG is exclusively cleared by the liver and then excreted unchanged into bile. ICG clearance tests reflect blood flow-dependent clearance, hepatocyte uptake, and biliary excretion [10]. An ICG retention rate at 15 minutes (ICG R15) of less than 10% is considered to be indicative of normal liver parenchymal function [11]. Some authors have advocated use of adjunct techniques to liver resection, namely, portal vein embolization, in patients with normal liver if the functional liver remnant is less than 40% of the total liver volume or if the remnant is less than 50% in patients with a compromised liver function (10% < ICG R15 < 20%) [12].

With this background, it becomes clear that parenchymal-sparing techniques decrease the risk of liver failure postoperatively. Fisher and colleagues (2013) reported a large, retrospective, multi-institutional study of almost 600 patients undergoing formal right hepatectomy versus a parenchymal-preserving right posterior sectionectomy for benign and malignant disease. In this study, tissue preservation with right posterior sectionectomy was associated with a significantly lower rate of liver failure (1% vs. 8.5%), as defined by hyperbilirubinemia or formation of significant ascites in the postoperative period [13].

Perioperative Outcomes

Nonanatomic limited liver resection minimizes surgical stress and operative risk and should be a basic surgical procedure for colorectal liver metastases.

From a perioperative perspective, several groups have reported better outcomes with the increased use of a parenchymal-sparing technique for CRLM. In 2008, the MSKCC group evaluated a series of 440 patients who underwent resection for bilateral CRLM from 1992 to 2003, dividing the study in four time periods with the purpose of determining trends over time [14]. A significant drop in 90-day mortality (from 6.3% to 1.2%, $P = 0.02$), operative blood loss (from 950 to 490 ml, $P < 0.001$), and length of hospital stay (from 12 to 9 days, $P < 0.001$) was observed occurring simultaneously with the increased application of parenchymal-sparing techniques. Similarly, Torzilli et al. compared systematic extended right posterior sectionectomy (SERPS) with right hepatectomy in patients matched for age and tumor size and number. They found that SERPS resulted in significantly less blood loss, fewer transfusions, reduced portal pedicle clamping with similar operative length, hospital stay, and safety profile [15]. These findings were supported by Ferrero et al. who demonstrated that bisegmentectomy instead of right hepatectomy improves postoperative outcomes, offering similar survival results and increasing the opportunity for re-resection in patients with CRLM of ≤10 cm located in the right liver lobe [16]. In 2013, a comparison study between right posterior sectorectomy (RPS) and formal right hepatectomy (RH) found that there were no significant differences in mean estimated blood loss (697 ml vs. 713 ml, $P = 0.900$), rate of transfusions (19.2% vs. 17.1%, $P = 0.720$), margin-positive resection (9.2% vs. 11.6%, $P = 0.70$), complications (41.8% vs. 42.0%, $P = 1.000$), bile leak (3.0% vs. 4.0%, $P = 1.000$), or length of stay (7.5 days vs. 8.3 days, $P = 0.360$). Additionally, the group did note that postoperative hepatic insufficiency occurred less frequently after RPS (1.0% vs. 8.5%; $P = 0.005$) [13]. The relatively equivalent rate of complications reported in this study may be attributed to the high physiologic impact associated with a posterior sectionectomy in comparison to other series which only reported single segmentectomies or smaller wedge resections.

Oncologic Benefit

Data strongly suggests that parenchyma-sparing liver resection does not compromise oncologic outcomes and may allow improved long-term survival compared to non-parenchymal-sparing approaches.

In addition to demonstrating functional benefits, parenchymal-sparing techniques have also been shown to have equivalent oncologic outcomes to major hepatectomies. The histology of CRLM provides the ideal platform for utilizing PSH techniques. CLRM have been shown to rarely have microscopic deposits in the surrounding parenchyma, even within 10 mm from the metastatic tumor site. Additionally, fibrous pseudocapsule formation is often observed [17]. These two features support nonanatomic hepatic resection with narrow margins as a safe and oncologically sound procedure for CRLM. This same rationale does not necessarily apply to other primary liver tumors, such as hepatocellular carcinoma, and data support the use of an anatomic resection given this tumor's tendency to invade portal vein branches.

Overall Survival and Local Recurrence Rates

In a retrospective study by Mise et al. at MD Anderson Cancer Center (MDACC) of 300 patients with solitary CRLM, PSH did not impact negatively on overall survival (OS), recurrence-free survival, and liver-only recurrence-free survival, compared with non-PSH ($P = 0.53$, $P = 0.97$, and $P = 0.69$, respectively). Liver-only recurrence was observed in 22 patients (14%) in the PSH and 25 (17%) in the non-PSH group ($P = 0.44$). Notably, this group also reported that the use of AR was an independent factor associated with the inability to undergo repeat hepatectomy for recurrent CRLM (HR = 8.18, $P < 0.01$), which may explain the improved survival reported among the PSH group in that particular study [18]. In a separate study that evaluated patients with advanced CRLM (greater than or equal to four tumors), Matsumura et al. reported that 5-year disease-free survival (DFS) was no different among patients who underwent PSH (7.6%) versus AR (6.8%) ($P = 0.597$) [19]. A recent 2016 study by Matsuki et al. compared PSH and major hepatectomy in 63 patients and found that recurrence-free and liver recurrence-free survivals did not differ between the two groups (22.6% vs. 32.4% $P = 0.146$ and 38.4% vs. 45% $P = 0.358$, respectively, Fig. 32.1) [20]. Similarly, Zorsi et al. identified 253 patients who underwent either a wedge or anatomic hepatic resection for CRLM and found that the overall recurrence rates were comparable between the two groups (37.5% vs. 40.3%, $P = 0.4$) with similar patterns of recurrence [21].

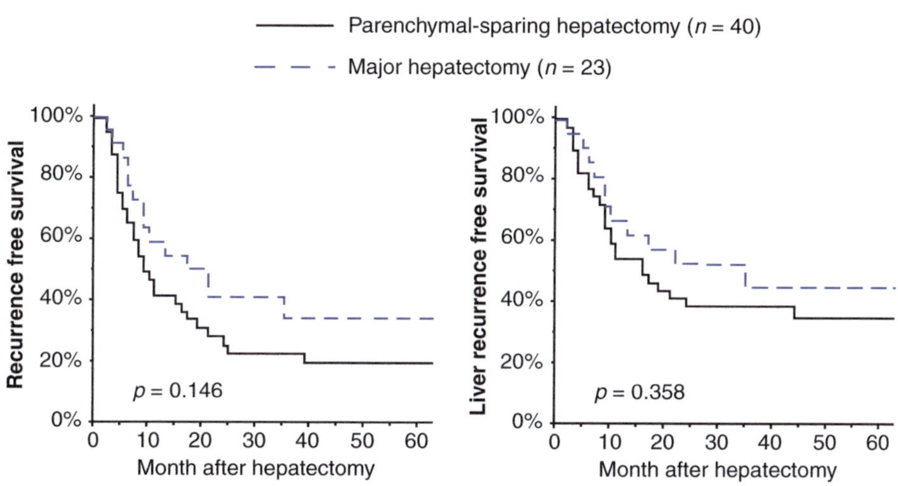

Patients at risk

PSH	40	18	10	9	8	5
MH	23	14	11	7	6	4

Patients at risk

PSH	40	23	15	14	12	7
MH	23	15	12	7	7	4

Fig. 32.1 Recurrence-free survival and liver recurrence-free survival curves comparing 40 patients who underwent parenchymal-sparing hepatectomy with 23 patients who underwent major hepatectomy [20]

In regard to long-term survival, multiple studies have shown no difference in OS between PSH and AR. In 2001, Kokudo and colleagues conducted a retrospective study of 174 patients with CRLM and demonstrated that OS did not differ between anatomic and nonanatomic resection [22]. A number of additional studies have failed to demonstrate a difference in OS among patients undergoing PSH versus AR for CRLM [23–25]. As the data demonstrate no inherent oncologic benefit to an anatomic resection, this further supports the continued use of parenchymal-sparing hepatectomy when clinically appropriate.

Margin Positivity Rates

As parenchymal-preserving techniques were initially gaining attention, there was concern that wedge resection resulted in a higher rate of margin positivity compared with hemi-hepatectomy and trisectionectomy [26]. One of the most important breakthroughs with regard to tumor margins for CRLM was accomplished by Pawlik et al. in 2005, who demonstrated that the width of a negative surgical margin did not affect survival, recurrence risk, or site of recurrence. In this study, which included 557 patients undergoing liver resection for CRLM, negative margins, regardless of margin distance, had similar overall recurrence rates (1–4 mm, 38.7%; 5–9 mm, 41.2%; ≥10 mm, 39.2%, $P = 0.32$) and 5-year overall survival (OS) rates (1–4 mm, 62.3%; 5–9 mm, 71.1%; ≥10 mm, 63.0%, $P = 0.63$, Fig. 32.2) [27]. Advocates of PSH note that a 1 mm margin has been demonstrated to be a sufficient oncological margin among patients with CRLM [28]. In this study, patients with

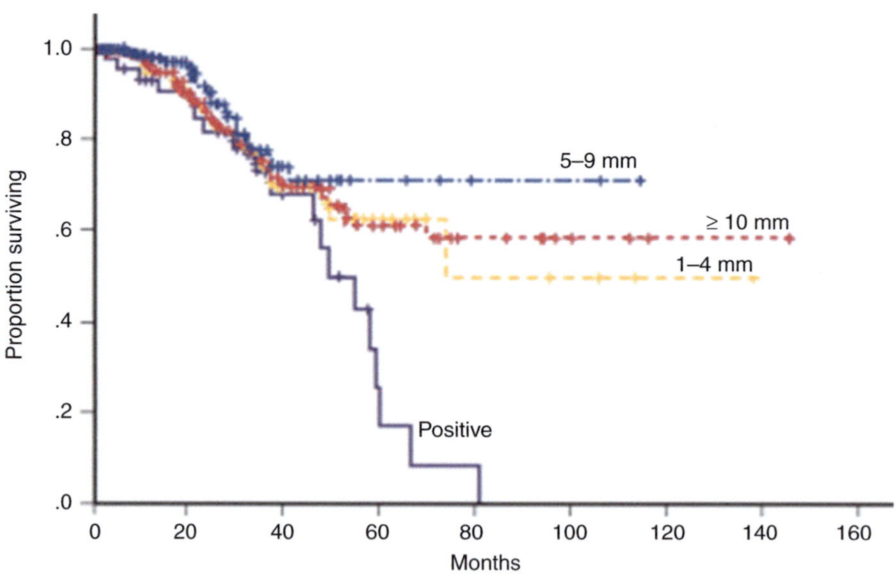

Fig. 32.2 Survival after hepatic resection of colorectal liver metastases, stratified by margin status. Median survival was 49.6 months in patients with positive margins and no significant difference in survival was seen in patients with a negative surgical margin, regardless of the width of the margin (all $P > 0.5$) [27]

margin clearance of 1–4.9 mm had an equivalent OS compared with patients who had a ≥ 5 mm margin [28]. Additionally, in a systematic review by Moris et al. of 2500 patients comprised of data from 12 studies, there was no difference in the incidence of R0 resection among patients undergoing PSH (66.7–100%) versus AR (71.6–98.6%) ($P = 0.58$) [29].

It is also important to note that as more liver parenchyma is resected, there is a potential greater risk for accelerated growth of micrometastases in response to growth factors and cytokines that stimulate liver regeneration. This principle was demonstrated by Tanaka et al. who showed that the prognosis of patients having six or more metastases was worse after major hepatectomy than after multiple smaller resections [30]. Therefore, it seems that tumor biology, as opposed to the extent of margin, is a more robust predictor of intrahepatic recurrence and survival in patients with CRLM.

Repeated Liver Resections

One of the major advantages of parenchymal-sparing hepatectomies is that it enables repeated resections if new metastatic lesions develop. After hepatectomy for metastases from colorectal cancer, approximately 50–70% of patients develop recurrent hepatic metastases. Literature has shown that repeat hepatectomies are feasible and safe and pose similar survival results to those achieved with initial hepatectomies. Although repeat liver resection is technically more challenging due to anatomic alterations involving the vascular and biliary ductal plans, the rates in perioperative morbidity and mortality are unchanged. In 2012, Lopez et al. demonstrated an average perioperative morbidity approaching 20%, an average mortality rate of about 1.5%, median OS ranging from 16 to 56 months, with reported 5-year survival ranging from 16% to 55% after repeat hepatectomy. These results are similar to those observed after an initial hepatectomy [31]. Another series restricted to patients undergoing repeat hepatectomy for CRLM ($n = 246$) demonstrated that significant proportions of well-selected patients may go on to require third (18.7%) and fourth (3.7%) hepatectomies [32].

As previously discussed, tumor biology seems to be the key predictor of intrahepatic recurrence, and new lesions are more likely to occur at different sites than the initial metastasis. Therefore, an initial R0 parenchymal-sparing resection may allow future salvage hepatectomy for liver-only recurrences and may potentially expand the number of CRLM patients eligible for repeat hepatic resection. In the 2016 study by Mise and colleagues, anatomic resection was an independent factor of noncandidacy for repeat hepatectomy, and the survival was significantly better in the parenchymal-sparing hepatectomy group [18]. In a subset analysis of patients with unilobar disease, Kokudo et al. showed an ipsilateral recurrence rate of only 19.6% after wedge resection and concluded that nonanatomic major resection would not have prevented intra- or extrahepatic recurrence. Additionally, 90% of the ipsilateral recurrences were resectable with a second operation, with a 5-year survival rate of 58.3% [22].

A combination of first nonanatomic limited resection followed by second hepatectomy for ipsilateral recurrence appears to be a reasonable choice of surgery for a few unilobar metastases that can be removed without applying major hepatectomy

[22]. With continued improvements in medical therapy and changes in surgical techniques over time, the rate of re-resection of hepatic metastases can be expected to increase.

Parenchymal-Sparing Techniques Expand the Patient Population Eligible for Surgery

One of the key oncologic benefits of PSH is that it can increase the number of patients eligible for surgery by preserving the FLR even for poorly located CLRM. It is notable that in a 2016 study out of Japan, resection volume of PSH was reduced by half compared with that of MH, and 40% of patients undergoing PSH could not have undergone direct MH without PVE due to a small FLR [20]. Although strategies to increase FLR have emerged over the past two decades, previous reports revealed that 15–33% of patients did not benefit from a multistep approach (i.e., PVE or two-stage hepatectomy) due to disease progression or insufficient liver hypertrophy [20]. In addition, PSH reduces the potential oncologic risk that extensive resection of liver parenchyma will stimulate not only liver regeneration but also occult tumor growth.

As previously referenced, in 2008, the MSKCC group evaluated a series of 440 patients operated on for bilateral CRLM from 1992 to 2003, dividing the study in four time periods with the purpose of determining trends over time [14]. They found a significant trend away from large resections in favor of multiple smaller resections despite that patient and tumor variables did not change over time. In concurrence with the increased application of PSH, a significant drop in 90-day mortality (from 6.3% to 1.2%, $P = 0.02$), operative blood loss (from 950 to 490 ml, $P < 0.001$), and length of hospital stay (from 12 to 9 days, $P < 0.001$) was observed [Gold]. Notably, 443 operations were performed for bilateral CRLM over the eleven-year period which accounted for 38% of the total 1150 hepatic resections for CRLM [14]. If parenchymal-preserving techniques were not applied to this population, many would very likely have been ineligible for surgery.

Operative Techniques

In this section, we highlight surgical techniques particularly applicable to parenchymal-sparing approaches. The vascular anatomy of the liver should be thoroughly assessed with imaging methods before PSH. Hepatic venous variants, as well as the pattern of venous drainage into the inferior vena cava (IVC), need to be specifically investigated. The right hepatic vein (RHV) drains hepatic segments V–VIII; the middle hepatic vein (MHV) drains segments IV, V, and VIII; and the left hepatic vein (LHV) drains segments II and III. However, segment VI may have an independent drainage directly into the IVC. An important anatomical variation is the presence of communicating veins, which connect adjacent hepatic veins, and have been demonstrated using IOUS in up to 80% of patients with colorectal liver metastases at the hepatocaval confluence. As described by Torzilli et al., a hepatic vein should be resected only after intraoperatively testing the proper function of these variants [15]. The feeding portal branch of the segment to be spared must preserve hepatopetal blood flow (rather than hepatofugal) on Doppler US when the hepatic vein is occluded by using a clamp or manual compression. PSH includes both segment-oriented and non-segment-oriented variants, either as isolated procedures or in combination.

Use of Intraoperative Ultrasound

Since its first documented use in the late 1970s, IOUS has repeatedly been shown to provide additional detail regarding tumor margins and vascular involvement leading to changes in operative management in spite of advances in preoperative imaging. In early studies, IOUS was found to change the operative strategy in as high as 31–49% of patients undergoing hepatic resection, either by allowing more precise resection or by indicating inoperability because of unsuspected masses or venous invasion [33]. PSH for deep CRLM requires mastery of IOUS and liver anatomy so as to navigate the three-dimensional transection without exposing the tumor and sacrificing major vessels. IOUS evaluation begins with the identification of the main portal pedicle within the hepatoduodenal ligament. The portal pedicles are invested with Glisson's capsule which produces an echogenic covering that helps differentiate them from hepatic vein branches. The pedicle is followed cephalad to the portal bifurcation to the main right and left pedicles. The right branch further bifurcates into an anterior and posterior branch. The right anterior branch gives off separate pedicles to segment V (caudal) and to segment VIII (cephalad). The right posterior branch supplies pedicles to segment VI (caudal) and to segment VII (cephalad). The main left pedicle is usually much longer and courses to the base of the umbilical fissure before branching into various segmental pedicles to segments II, III, IVA, and IVB. At the base of the umbilical fissure, the main left pedicle courses anteriorly toward the round ligament and gives off pedicle branches to segments IVA and IVB laterally toward the right and to segments II and III medially to the left. Variations in portal vein anatomy are seen in approximately 10–20% of patients. If the bare areas around the junction of the hepatic veins and IVC have been well mobilized, the hepatic veins can easily be visualized using intraoperative ultrasonography [34]. Matsuki et al. have shown that despite this added complexity, deep tumors can be removed safely without multistep approaches [20]. With increasing tumor number, bilobar disease, and tumors that are located deep within hepatic parenchyma, IOUS becomes even more important to avoid anatomic resection and achieve an adequate resection while preserving the maximal amount of normal parenchyma.

Anatomic (Segmentectomy) Versus Nonanatomic (Wedge) Resections

Anatomic resection (AR) is defined as complete removal of a hepatic segment (segmentectomy). Traditionally, AR has been reserved for patients with multiple or large tumors within contiguous anatomic segments or when the tumor is invading a

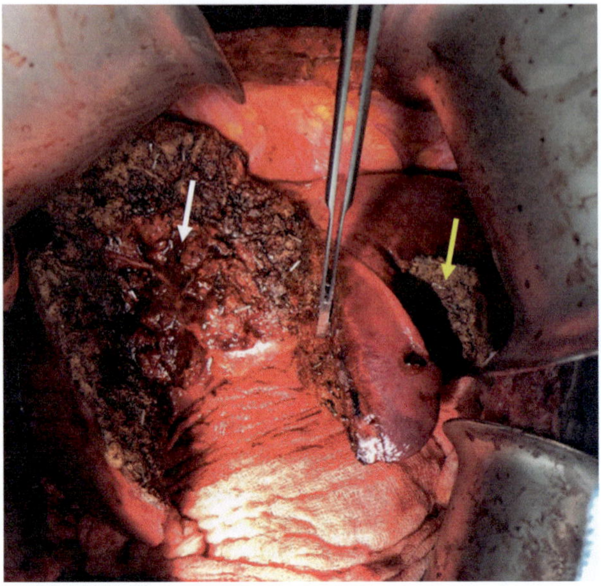

Fig. 32.3 Intraoperative photograph illustrates anatomic central hepatectomy (segments IV, V, and VIII, white arrow) and partial segment III resection (yellow arrow). Blood loss was 200 ml and no transfusion was required

major portal pedicle or hepatic vein [29]. More common segmental resections include resection of segment I, resection of segment IV, and segmentectomy to remove segments IV, V, and VI. Central hepatectomy, comprising resection of segments IV, V, and VIII, is being increasingly performed (Fig. 32.3). Resection of segments VI and VII is referred to as a right posterior sectionectomy, and resection of segments V and VIII is a right anterior sectionectomy.

Nonanatomic resection is defined as tumor resection with a negative tumor margin regardless of segment or section anatomy (Fig. 32.4). Non-segment-oriented resections (also referred to as wedge resections) are usually applied for lesions smaller than 5 cm and located near the liver surface. Since anatomical boundaries are not respected, the use of IOUS to guide this type of resection is paramount to clearly identify all the bile ducts and vascular branches. Additionally, the liver tends to fracture at the interface between tumor and normal parenchyma which may lead to inadequate deep margins. This can be avoided by using IOUS to transect along anatomic planes defined by inflow and outflow structures.

Mini-Mesohepatectomy

In order to avoid major resection, mini-mesohepatectomy (MMH) was initially described by Torzilli et al. in 2008 for tumors involving the middle hepatic vein within 4 cm of the caval confluence [35]. It is defined as the partial removal of segment VIII and/or segment IVa including the involved tract of the middle hepatic

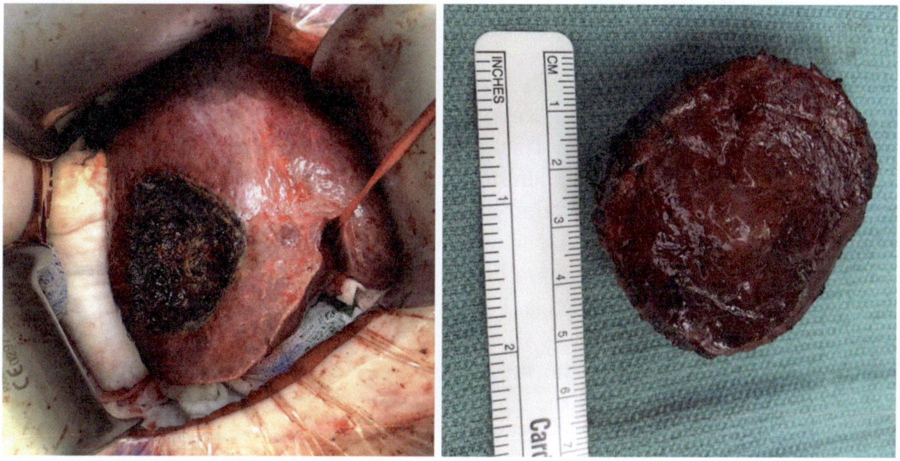

Fig. 32.4 Intraoperative photograph illustrating nonanatomic segment VI resection in a fibrotic liver

Fig. 32.5 Illustration demonstrating a mini-mesohepatectomy with resection of segment VIII and a portion of segment I [36]

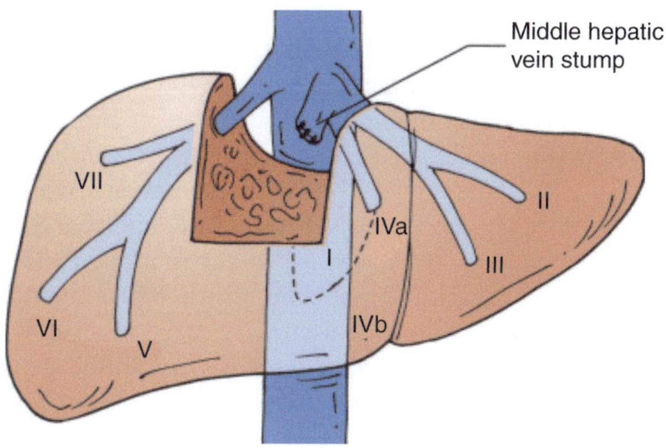

vein (MHV) at the hepatocaval confluence while at the same time preserving the remaining parenchyma of the right anterior section and left median section (Fig. 32.5). To carry out this technique, the anterior surface of the hepatocaval confluence is exposed, and a space between the right and middle hepatic veins is dissected to accommodate a surgeon's fingertip. When the MHV is manually compressed, disappearance or inversion of blood flow through the MHV can be confirmed by IOUS. In the series by Torzilli et al., there were no deaths within 90 days of the operation and no major morbidity; overall morbidity was 18%. There were no instances of significant liver insufficiency, although only six out of the 17 patients in the series had a normal liver. This type of resection is made more feasible with the presence of an accessory RHV draining segment VI [35].

Right Posterior Sectionectomy

A right hepatectomy (RH) is traditionally performed for large right-sided or multiple tumors and those in close proximity to the right hepatic vein (RHV) and/or invading of the either or both first- and second-order portal vein branches. In 2008, Torzilli et al. again described an alternate surgical approach consisting of a systematic extended right posterior sectionectomy (SERPS, Fig. 32.6) with the assistance of contrast-enhanced ultrasound to define tumor-vessel relationships. The main advantage of SERPS is the preservation of most of the liver parenchyma of the right anterior section, despite ligation and division of the RHV. The authors define three main surgical strategies. In cases where first- and second-order portal branches are spared from tumor involvement, the posterior sectionectomy was extended to the right anterior section to allow the complete removal of the tumor with an adequate margin. The dissection line is to the left of the right hepatic vein, which is resected with the specimen, and the right anterior portal branch (P5–8) is not necessarily exposed on the liver cut surface. If the right posterior portal branch (to segments VI and VII, P6–7) is invaded by tumor and the right anterior portal branch (P5–8) is close or in contact with the tumor, the resection is extended to the right anterior section, preserving most of the parenchyma of segment VII, the right hepatic vein, and the left portion of segment V. In this case, P5–8 is not divided but is exposed on the cut surface. Finally, when the tumor involves both the right hepatic vein and P6–7, a sectionectomy combining both strategies is carried out with resection of the right hepatic vein and exposure of P5–8 at the cut surface of the liver. In this study, 21 (10%) patients among 207 consecutive patients who underwent hepatic resection for primary or secondary liver tumors qualified for SERPS based on these criteria. Of those patients, there was no 90-day mortality, and three patients (14%) experienced major morbidity, including pleural effusion requiring thoracentesis and transient mild liver failure with ascites. With a mean follow-up of 24 months, there were no recurrences at the surgical margin, despite four patients with encapsulated HCC exhibiting vascular contact (with P5–8 or from tumor thrombus in P6–7) and

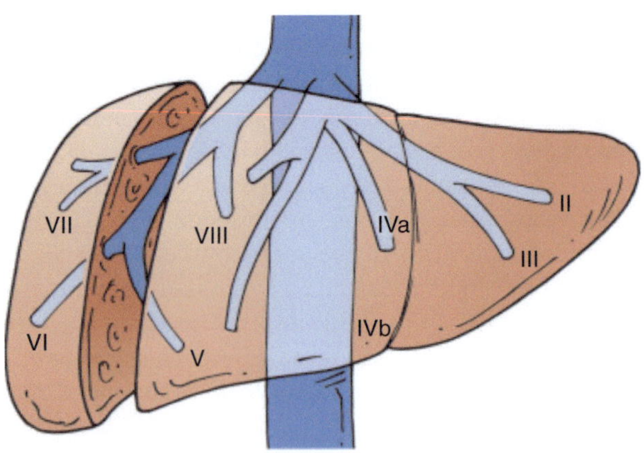

Fig. 32.6 Illustration demonstrating a right posterior sectionectomy [36]

resulting in tumor present at the pathologic margin. Overall median disease-free survival was 10 months, and many patients with remote intrahepatic recurrences have undergone additional resection [15].

Laparoscopic Resection

The first laparoscopic liver resection (LLR) was reported by Gagner et al. [37]. Since then, potential perioperative advantages and favorable oncologic outcomes associated with laparoscopic hepatic surgery have been suggested in the literature. Traditionally, a laparoscopic approach has been reserved for primarily small and subcapsular, peripheral liver lesions located in segments II, III, IVb, and V, thus permitting hepatic parenchymal sparing and allowing the dissection plane to remain distant from the major vessels. However, a minimally invasive technique is increasingly being used to treat central liver lesions or those located in posterior and superior segments. A consensus statement generated in 2008 stated that indications for the use of LLR included solitary lesions less than 5 cm in diameter located in the anterior segment at a distance from the line of transection, the hepatic hilum, and the vena cava [38]. Additionally, the intra-abdominal pressure during pneumoperitoneum has proven to decrease bleeding during liver surgery [39, 40]. Finally, another potential advantage of laparoscopic liver resection for patients with CRLM is that it simplifies subsequent operations.

Despite these advantages, there are clear limitations to the use of laparoscopy for hepatic resections. Manual palpation is not possible, except in the case of hand-assisted LLR. Additionally, the inability to control major bleeding rapidly remains a major challenge. In the largest, multicenter study of 210 major LLR, there were no intraoperative deaths reported, and of the 26 conversions to laparotomy, six cases (23.1%) were related to persistent moderate bleeding during parenchymal division, while three conversions were required for bleeding from a portal vein branch injury, a hepatic vein injury, and a vena cava injury [41]. Additionally, as central venous pressure (CVP) is preferably low during hepatic resections to minimize bleeding, there is a theoretical risk of gas embolism due to the pressure gradient that may exist between insufflation pressure and CVP. Despite these limitations, LLR remains a viable technique to perform PSH.

Conclusion

Parenchymal-sparing hepatectomies reduce perioperative complication, provide adequate oncologic outcomes, and increase the population eligible for initial and additional surgery. This may translate into lower readmission rates, better quality of life, and reduced costs. As surgeons become more comfortable with repeated hepatic resections for recurrences, the population eligible for PSH will continue to grow alongside the development of improved preoperative preparation and intraoperative techniques. The increased availability of data supporting PSH will make prospective studies and clinical trials feasible to test the hypothesis that PSH should be the gold standard of care for CRLM, rather than a technique tailored to a select patient population.

References

1. Berri R, Abdalla E. Curable metastatic colorectal cancer: recommended paradigms. Curr Oncol Rep. 2009;11(3):200–8.
2. Rahbari N, Garden O, Padbury R, Brooke-Smith M, Crawford M, Adam R, Koch M, Makuuchi M, Dematteo R, Christophi C, Banting S, Usatoff V, Nagino M, Maddern G, Hugh T, Vauthey J, Greig P, Rees M, Yokoyama Y, Fan S, Nimura Y, Figueras J, Capussotti L, Büchler M, Weitz J. Posthepatectomy liver failure: a definition and grading by the International Study Group of Liver Surgery (ISGLS). Surgery. 2011;149(5):713–24.
3. Heymsfield SB. Accurate measurement of liver, kidney, and spleen volume and mass by computerized axial tomography. Ann Intern Med. 1979;90(2):185–7.
4. Simpson A, Geller D, Hemming A, Jarnagin W, Clements L, D'Angelica M, Dumpuri P, Gönen M, Zendejas I, Miga M, Stefansic J. Liver planning software accurately predicts postoperative liver volume and measures early regeneration. J Am Coll Surg. 2014;219(2):199–207.
5. Mise Y, Hasegawa K, Satou S, Aoki T, Beck Y, Sugawara Y, Makuuchi M, Kokudo N. Venous reconstruction based on virtual liver resection to avoid congestion in the liver remnant. Br J Surg. 2011;98(12):1742–51.
6. Jarnagin W, Gonen M, Fong Y, DeMatteo R, Ben-Porat L, Little S, Corvera C, Weber S, Blumgart L. Improvement in perioperative outcome after hepatic resection. Ann Surg. 2002;236(4):397–407.
7. Blumgart L, Belghiti J. Surgery of the liver, biliary tract, and pancreas. 6th ed. Philadelphia: Saunders Elsevier; 2017. p. 1065–72.
8. Vauthey J, Pawlik T, Ribero D, Wu T, Zorzi D, Hoff P, Xiong H, Eng C, Lauwers G, Mino-Kenudson M, Risio M, Muratore A, Capussotti L, Curley S, Abdalla E. Chemotherapy regimen predicts steatohepatitis and an increase in 90-day mortality after surgery for hepatic colorectal metastases. J Clin Oncol. 2006;24(13):2065–72.
9. Kooby D. Impact of steatosis on perioperative outcome following hepatic resection. J Gastrointest Surg. 2003;7(8):1034–44.
10. Blumgart L, Belghiti J. Surgery of the liver, biliary tract, and pancreas. 6th ed. Philadelphia: Saunders Elsevier; 2017. p. 60–5.
11. Kubota K. Measurement of liver volume and hepatic functional reserve as a guide to decision-making in resectional surgery for hepatic tumors. Hepatology. 1997;26(5):1176–81.
12. Blumgart L, Belghiti J. Surgery of the liver, biliary tract, and pancreas. 6th ed. Philadelphia: Saunders Elsevier; 2017. p. 1653–63.
13. Fisher S, Kneuertz P, Dodson R, Patel S, Maithel S, Sarmiento J, Russell M, Cardona K, Choti M, Staley C, Pawlik T, Kooby D. A comparison of right posterior sectorectomy with formal right hepatectomy: a dual-institution study. HPB. 2013;15(10):753–62.
14. Gold J, Are C, Kornprat P, Jarnagin W, Gönen M, Fong Y, DeMatteo R, Blumgart L, D'Angelica M. Increased use of parenchymal-sparing surgery for bilateral liver metastases from colorectal cancer is associated with improved mortality without change in oncologic outcome. Ann Surg. 2008;247(1):109–17.
15. Torzilli G, Donadon M, Marconi M, Botea F, Palmisano A, Del Fabbro D, Procopio F, Montorsi M. Systematic extended right posterior sectionectomy. Ann Surg. 2008;247(4):603–11.
16. Ferrero A, Vigan L, Lo Tesoriere R, Russolillo N, Sgotto E, Capussotti L. Bisegmentectomies as alternative to right hepatectomy in the treatment of colorectal liver metastases. Hepatogastroenterology. 2009;56:1429–35.

17. Yamamoto J, Sugihara K, Kosuge T, Takayama T, Shimada K, Yamasaki S, Sakamoto M, Hirohashi S. Pathologic support for limited hepatectomy in the treatment of liver metastases from colorectal cancer. Ann Surg. 1995;221(1):74–8.
18. Mise Y, Aloia T, Brudvik K, Schwarz L, Vauthey J, Conrad C. Parenchymal-sparing hepatectomy in colorectal liver metastasis improves salvageability and survival. Ann Surg. 2016;263(1):146–52.
19. Matsumura M, Mise Y, Saiura A, Inoue Y, Ishizawa T, Ichida H, Matsuki R, Tanaka M, Takeda Y, Takahashi Y. Parenchymal-sparing hepatectomy does not increase intrahepatic recurrence in patients with advanced colorectal liver metastases. Ann Surg Oncol. 2016;23:3718–26.
20. Matsuki R, Mise Y, Saiura A, Inoue Y, Ishizawa T, Takahashi Y. Parenchymal-sparing hepatectomy for deep-placed colorectal liver metastases. Surgery. 2016;160:1256–63.
21. Zorzi D, Mullen JT, Abdalla EK. Comparison between hepatic wedge resection and anatomic resection for colorectal liver metastases. J Gastrointest Surg. 2006;10(1):86–94.
22. Kokudo N, Tada K, Seki M, Ohta H, Azekura K, Ueno M, Matsubara T, Takahashi T, Nakajima T, Muto T. Anatomical major resection versus nonanatomical limited resection for liver metastases from colorectal carcinoma. Am J Surg. 2001;181:153–9.
23. Lalmahomed ZS, Ayez N, Van Der Pool AEM, Verheij J, Ijzermans JNM, Verhoef C. Anatomical versus nonanatomical resection of colorectal liver metastases: is there a difference in surgical and oncological outcome? World J Surg. 2010;35:656–61.
24. Finch RJ, Malik HZ, Hamady ZZ. Effect of type of resection on outcome of hepatic resection for colorectal metastases. Br J Surg. 2007;94(10):1242–8.
25. Stewart G, Osúilleabháin C, Madhavan K, Wigmore S, Parks R, Garden O. The extent of resection influences outcome following hepatectomy for colorectal liver metastases. Eur J Surg Oncol. 2004;30:370–6.
26. Dematteo R. Anatomic segmental hepatic resection is superior to wedge resection as an oncologic operation for colorectal liver metastases. J Gastrointest Surg. 2000;4:178–84.
27. Pawlik TM, Scoggins CR, Zorzi D, et al. Effect of surgical margin status on survival and site of recurrence after hepatic resection for colorectal metastases. Ann Surg. 2005;241:715–24.
28. Hamady ZZR, Lodge JPA, Welsh FK, Toogood GJ, White A, John T, Rees M. One-millimeter cancer-free margin is curative for colorectal liver metastases. Ann Surg. 2014;259:543–8.
29. Moris D, Ronnekleiv-Kelly S, Rahnemai-Azar AA, Felekouras E, Dillhoff M, Schmidt C, Pawlik TM. Parenchymal-sparing versus anatomic liver resection for colorectal liver metastases: a systematic review. J Gastrointest Surg. 2017;21:1076–85.
30. Tanaka K, Shimada H, Matsumoto C, Matsuo K, Takeda K, Nagano Y, Togo S. Impact of the degree of liver resection on survival for patients with multiple liver metastases from colorectal cancer. World J Surg. 2008;32:2057–69.
31. Lopez P, Marzano E, Piardi T, Pessaux P. Repeat hepatectomy for liver metastases from colorectal primary cancer: a review of the literature. J Visc Surg. 2012;149:e97.
32. Jong MCD, Pulitano C, Ferrero A, Strub J, Choti MA, Schulick RD, Mentha G, Capussotti L, Pawlik TM. 807 repeat curative intent liver surgery is safe and effective for recurrent colorectal liver metastases: results from an international multi-institutional analysis. J Gastrointest Surg. 2009;13:2141–51.
33. Rifkin MD, Rosato FE, Branch HM, Foster J, Yang S-L, Barbot DJ, Marks GJ. An important adjunctive tool for decision making in the operating room. Ann Surg. 1987;205:466–72.
34. Paniccia A, Schullick RD. Diagnostic operation of the liver and techniques of hepatic resection. In: Yeo CJ, editor. Shackelford's surgery of the alimentary tract. Philadelphia: Elsevier, Inc. p. 1456–71.
35. Torzilli G, Palmisano A, Procopio F, Cimino M, Botea F, Donadon M, Fabbro DD, Montorsi M. A new systematic small for size resection for liver tumors invading the middle hepatic vein at its caval confluence. Ann Surg. 2010;251:33–9.
36. Blumgart L, Belghiti J. Surgery of the liver, biliary tract, and pancreas. 6th ed. Philadelphia: Saunders Elsevier; 2017. p. 1631–43.

37. Gagner M, Rheault M, Dubuc J. Laparoscopic partial hepatectomy for liver tumor. Surg Endosc. 1992;6:99.
38. Buell JF, Cherqui D, Geller DA. The international position on laparoscopic liver surgery: the Louisville statement. Ann Surg. 2009;250:825–30.
39. Jaskille A, Schechner A, Park K, Williams M, Wang D, Sava J. Abdominal insufflation decreases blood loss and mortality after porcine liver injury. J Trauma. 2005;59:1305–8.
40. Tranchart H, Giuro GD, Lainas P, Pourcher G, Devaquet N, Perlemuter G, Franco D, Dagher I. Laparoscopic liver resection with selective prior vascular control. Am J Surg. 2013;205:8–14.
41. Dagher I, O'rourke N, Geller DA, et al. Laparoscopic major hepatectomy. Ann Surg. 2009;250:856–60.

Resection of the Primary in Unresectable Colorectal Cancer Liver Metastases – Is It Worth?

33

Marcus Valadão, Rinaldo Gonçalves, Rodrigo Araújo, and Roberto de Almeida Gil

Approximately 20% of patients with colorectal cancer present with metastatic disease, which can be challenging to manage [1]. Despite considerable advances in the treatment of metastatic colorectal cancer, in most cases the disease is not curable. Therefore, the treatment goal for most patients is to extend survival and improve the quality of life [2]. Patients with colorectal cancer (CRC) with stage IV disease may manifest various symptoms of their primary tumor and/or metastases, and a palliative resection of the primary tumor before the initiation of systemic treatment is frequently performed [3].

Patients presenting symptoms such as obstruction, perforation, or hemorrhage are clear candidates for surgical resection. On the other hand, the decision to remove the asymptomatic primary colorectal tumor in patients with unresectable metastasis in order to prevent possible complications or to improve survival is more controversial and matter of debate [4].

With recent advances in systemic chemotherapy, the risks and benefits of immediate or deferred surgical strategy have changed. Over the last 10 years, the OS (overall survival) rate has improved from 9 to 24 months (and in some series up to 36 months), which is possibly the result of patient exposition to all available cytotoxic drugs during the course of their disease [5–7]. In contrast to the response rates of 5-FU and leucovorin of approximately 15%, combinations with modern chemotherapy like infusional fluorouracil/leucovorin with oxaliplatin or irinotecan have yielded response rates of 50% and disease control rates of 85% in prospective clinical trials [8, 9]. Furthermore, the addition of the antiangiogenic agent bevacizumab

M. Valadão (✉) · R. Gonçalves · R. Araújo
Department of Abdomino-Pelvic Surgery, Instituto Nacional de Câncer (INCA), Rio de Janeiro, Brazil
e-mail: mvaladao@inca.gov.br; rinaldo.silva@inca.gov.br; raraujo@inca.gov.br

R. de Almeida Gil
Department of Medical Oncology, Instituto Nacional de Câncer (INCA), Rio de Janeiro, Brazil

M. M. Correia et al. (eds.), *Colorectal Cancer Liver Metastases*,
https://doi.org/10.1007/978-3-030-25486-5_33

and/or cetuximab to the above combinations has provided clinically significant improvement in response rates. Several studies have shown that in the era of effective chemotherapy, there is a relative infrequency of complications from unresected primary tumors (less than 15% of the patients required surgical and/or other primary related interventions) [10–14].

Advocates of the deferred surgical approach argue that surgery at diagnosis can delay or even preclude systemic chemotherapy and that most patients will never develop symptoms.

Scheer and colleagues in a review article found that operative mortality was 2.7% (0–4.6%) and postoperative complications were present in 18.8–47.0% of cases, related to obstruction in 13%, hemorrhage in 1.5–2.9%, and sepsis in 2.3–10.6% of patients with unresectable hepatic metastasis submitted to resection of an asymptomatic primary colorectal cancer [10]. In this same paper, the authors reported more favorable results when palliative chemotherapy was delivered without resection of primary tumor, and complications were sparse (obstruction 13.9% and bleeding in 3.0%).

On the other hand, there are several published papers in the literature showing survival benefit for asymptomatic patients that underwent primary tumor resection comparing to patients that were only treated with systemic therapy in the scenario of unresectable CRLM (Table 33.1). Although the NCCN guideline does not recommend resection of the primary tumor in the asymptomatic unresectable CRLM patient, all these aforementioned papers have generated a great debate on the real role of primary tumor resection in unresectable CRLM.

No data from prospective randomized trials are available to compare chemotherapy or resection of the primary tumor in the unresectable CRLM patients with low or absent symptoms of their primary tumor. Venderbosch and colleagues [37] performed a review of the literature regarding this subject (Table 33.1) and identified more than 20 retrospective non-randomized studies performed in a single center. The median OS was improved in resected patients in the majority of the studies. An important limitation of these studies is that few data on the use of systemic therapy were presented, which makes it difficult to assess the contribution of resection on outcome. Venderbosch and colleagues [37] also performed a retrospective analysis of two phase III studies (sequential versus combination chemotherapy with capecitabine, irinotecan, and oxaliplatin in advanced colorectal cancer [CAIRO] and CAIRO2) investigating the prognostic and predictive value of resection of the primary tumor in patients with synchronous CRLM treated with systemic therapy. The analysis compared 547 subjects who underwent a primary tumor resection and 310 subjects who received upfront chemotherapy [38, 39]. As a prognostic factor, primary tumor resection was associated with significantly longer median OS (CAIRO, 16.7 vs 11.4 months; CAIRO2, 20.7 vs 13.4 months). A similar association was found for progression-free survival. The subjects in the two trials received capecitabine, oxaliplatin, and irinotecan regimens as well as biologic therapy. A major limitation of their study is that the decision to resect the primary tumor was made prior to study entry and that they provide no information about the reasons for nonresection, such as nonresectability of the primary tumor, poor performance

Table 33.1 Publications comparing resection vs no resection of palliative resection of primary colorectal tumor

Author	Study period	Resection/no resection	N of patients	OS (months)	*p* value	Reference
Makela	1974–1983	Resection	66	15	–	[15]
		No resection	30	7		
Liu	1986–1991	Resection	57	11	–	[16]
		No resection	6	3		
Konyalian	1991–2002	Resection	62	13	$p < 0.0001$	[17]
		No resection	47	5		
Beham	1993–2003	Resection	46	18	$p < 0.001$	[18]
		No resection	21	8		
Costi	1994–2003	Resection	83	9	$p < 0.001$	[19]
		No resection	47	4		
Law	1996–1999	Resection	150	7	<0.001	[20]
		No resection	30	3		
Mik	1996–2000	Resection	52	21	NS	[21]
		No resection	82	14		
Stelzner	1995–2001	Resection	128	11.4	<0.0001	[22]
		No resection	58	4.6		
Yun	1994–2004	Resection	283	15.3	<0.001	[23]
		No resection	95	5.3		
Frago	2000–2008	Resection	12	23.7	0.008	[24]
		No resection	43	4.4		
Aslam	1998–2007	Resection	366	14.5	<0.005	[25]
		No resection	281	5.83		
Ruo	1996–1999	Resection	127	16	<0.001	[26]
		No resection	103	9		
Kaufman	1998–2003	Resection	115	22	<0.0001	[27]
		No resection	69	3		
Scoggins	1985–1997	Resection	66	14.5	0.59	[12]
		No resection	23	16.6		
Tebbutt	1990–1999	Resection	280	14	0.08	[11]
		No resection	82	8.2		
Michel	1996–1999	Resection	31	21	0.718	[28]
		No resection	23	14		
Benoist	1997–2002	Resection	32	23	–	[29]
		No resection	27	22		
Galizia	1995–2005	Resection	42	15	0.03	[30]
		No resection	23	12.3		
Bajwa	1999–2005	Resection	32	14	0.005	[31]
		No resection	35	6		
Chan	2000–2002	Resection	286	14	<0.001	[32]
		No resection	125	6		
Evans	1999–2006	Resection	45	11	<0.0001	[33]
		No resection	57	2		
Seo	2001–2008	Resection	144	22	0.076	[34]
		No resection	83	14		
Koopman	2003–2004	Resection	297	18	$p < 0.0001$	[35]
		No resection	169	12		
Tol	2005–2006	Resection	329	21	0.0001	[36]
		No resection	149	13		

From Verhoef et al. [4]

status, symptomatic metastases requiring priority for systemic treatment, or absence of symptoms of the primary tumor. For that reasons patients who were and who were not operated on may represent different patient populations. However, when these variables were included in a multivariate analysis, resection of the primary tumor remained a significant prognostic factor in the CAIRO2 study and in the subgroup of patients with one metastatic site in the CAIRO study.

Ahmed and colleagues [40] analyzed patients with stage IV colorectal cancer diagnosed from 2006 to 2010 in Canada. They compared 199 subjects who received chemotherapy and underwent upfront resection to 127 other subjects who also received chemotherapy and did not undergo upfront resection. Ninety-one percent of the patients received FOLFIRI or FOLFOX, and 67% received a biologic agent. The median OS was 27 months in the resection group and 14 months in the nonresection group. However, the longer OS could be a result of selection bias: 54% of the subjects in the nonresection group had stage IVb disease compared with 40% in the resection group, and performance status in the nonresection group was poorer (48%) than in the resection group (25%).

A pooled post hoc analysis [41] of four randomized trials (FFCD-9601, FFCD-2000-05, ML-16987, ACCORD-13) including 816 subjects [42–45] found that primary tumor resection was independently associated with longer OS (median, 19.2 vs 13.3 months) in multivariate analysis (Kaplan-Meier curve). The association of OS with resection of the primary tumor did not differ significantly between the trials or between the types of chemotherapy received. No tumor-specific mutation markers (RAS or BRAF) were available when these studies were conducted, which, in addition to other unmeasured factors, may explain the lower survival in the nonresection group. Despite the adjustments for known potential confounders, it is possible that resections were more likely to be performed in patients with better prognosis.

A meta-analysis of 21 studies including 44,226 subjects [46] found that patients with metastasis who underwent resection of the primary tumor had a lower risk of death than patients who received chemotherapy alone, with a difference in mean OS of 6.4 months (95% CI 5.0–7.9; $p < 0.001$). There might have had some bias in these findings as subjects who underwent resection were more likely to have colon rather than rectal cancer and were less likely to have ≥2 liver metastasis.

Two nationwide population-based studies evaluated the prognostic relevance of primary tumor resection in incurable stage IV colorectal cancer [47, 48]. Tarantino and colleagues [47] analyzed 37,793 stage IV colorectal cancer patients identified in the SEER (Surveillance, Epidemiology, and End Results) database between 1998 and 2009. Of those, 23,004 (60.9%) underwent palliative primary tumor resection. In Cox regression analysis after propensity score matching, primary cancer resection was associated with a significantly improved overall survival and cancer-specific survival. The benefit of palliative primary cancer resection persisted during the time period 1998–2009. The main drawbacks of this analysis are the lack of information on chemotherapeutic drugs or antibodies used, comorbidities, performance status, and site and number of the metastasis. Also it is not deducible from the SEER database whether the primary tumor was truly asymptomatic. On the other hand, the population-based nature of the registry mirrors the real-world outcomes for patients with metastatic colorectal cancer and is associated with a high degree of generalizability. Lam-Boer and colleague [48] analyzed patients with incurable stage IV colorectal cancer identified in the Netherlands Cancer Registry from 2008 to 2011. From a total group of 10,371 patients with stage IV colorectal cancer, 2746 patients (26%) underwent an elective palliative resection of the primary tumor, whether or not followed by systemic therapy, and 3345 patients (32%) were initially treated with palliative systemic therapy. After propensity score matching, median overall survival in these groups were 17.2 months and 11.5 months, respectively. In Cox regression analysis, primary tumor resection was significantly associated with improved survival.

Some studies have been trying to identify predictive markers of better outcome in order to select which patients are good candidates to palliative resection of the primary tumor. He and colleagues [49] evaluated retrospectively 387 patients (254 patients underwent palliative primary tumor resection and 133 did not) with unresectable colorectal liver metastases, showing that only patients with normal lactate dehydrogenase (LDH) levels and with carcinoembryonic antigen (CEA) levels <70 ng/ml benefited from palliative primary tumor resection (median OS, 22.2 months for the resection group and 16.2 months for the nonresection group; $p < 0.001$). Kodaz and colleagues [50] evaluated the survival effect of primary tumor resection in unresectable metastatic colorectal cancer according to KRAS mutation status. Seventy-eight patients were included in the study and the KRAS status was known in all patients. Thirty-four patients had undergone primary tumor resection before the first chemotherapy. The survival was better in the unresectable metastatic colon patients with resected primary tumor, but it was statistically nonsignificant ($p = 0.07$). The median OS was 28 months in KRAS mutant patients who underwent primary tumor resection comparing to 14 months in KRAS mutant patients who did not undergo primary tumor resection ($p = 0.002$); however, the median OS was similar ($p = 0.91$) in the KRAS wild-type patients with and without primary tumor resection.

Dorajoo and colleagues [51] developed a scoring model for predicting survival in order to select patients who are more likely to benefit from the primary tumor resection in incurable stage IV colorectal cancer. The score model was used to classify patients into poor (≥7 points), moderate (≥4 to <7 points), or good (<4 points) survivor groups, using the following predictor variables: age ≥65 years (1 point), poorly or undifferentiated tumor (3 points), moderately differentiated tumors (1 point), metastases to liver (2 points), metastases to lung (1 point), metastases to bone (2 points), carcinomatosis (2 points), albumin <35 g/dl (1 point), and carcinoembryonic antigen levels ≥250 ng/ml (2 points). The study cohort consisted of 482 patients with unresectable stage IV colorectal cancer who had undergone elective primary tumor resection between 1999 and 2007. The scoring model separated patients into three prognostic groups with distinct median survival lengths of 4.8, 12.4, and 18.6 months ($p < 0.0001$). Temporal split-sample validation implied good local generalizability to future patient populations ($p < 0.0001$). The authors [51] concluded that the model-based survival prognostication could support clinical decisions on elective primary tumor resection eligibility.

In our institution we are evolving to an individualized approach, and resection of the asymptomatic primary colorectal tumor in patients presenting unresectable metastatic disease is reserved for patients with good performance status, no other serious clinical illnesses, expected survival of at least 1 year, and tumors deemed favorable to surgical resection (no need of permanent stoma or adjacent organ involvement).

Summary

The dogma that an asymptomatic primary tumor should never be resected in patients with unresectable colorectal liver metastases must be questioned. Besides all the bias related to retrospective analysis, the majority of these studies (including retrospective single center cohort studies, meta-analysis, population-based studies, retrospective analysis of prospective randomized trials) favor resection of the primary in unresectable CRLM due to improved survival. Identifying incurable colorectal stage IV patients with better prognosis to undergo primary tumor resection might be the key to benefit selected patients among all palliative treatment patients. Prospective randomized clinical trials such as CAIRO4, CAIRO5, and the French Research Group of Rectal Cancer Surgery (GRECCAR) 8 trial are currently being conducted in Europe to explicitly address this question.

References

1. Jemal A, Murray T, Ward E, et al. Cancer statistics, 2005. CA Cancer J Clin. 2005;55(1):10–30.
2. Feo L, Polcino M, Nash G. Resection of the primary tumor in stage IV colorectal cancer: when is it necessary? Surg Clin North Am. 2017;97:657–69.
3. Cook AD, Single R, McCahill LE. Surgical resection of primary tumors in patients who present with stage IV colorectal cancer: an analysis of Surveillance, Epidemiology, and End Results data, 1988 to 2000. Ann Surg Oncol. 2005;12:637–45.
4. Verhoef C, Wilt J, Burger J, et al. Surgery of the primary in stage IV colorectal cancer with unresectable metastases. Eur J Cancer. 2011 Sep;47(Suppl 3):S61–6.
5. Grothey A, Sargent D, Goldberg RM, Schmoll HJ. Survival of patients with advanced colorectal cancer improves with the availability of fluorouracil–leucovorin, irinotecan, and oxaliplatin in the course of treatment. J Clin Oncol. 2004;22:1209–14.
6. Hurwitz H, Fehrenbacher L, Novotny W, et al. Bevacizumab plus irinotecan, fluorouracil, and leucovorin for metastatic colorectal cancer. N Engl J Med. 2004;350:2335–42.
7. Bokemeyer C, Bondarenko I, Makhson A, et al. Fluorouracil, leucovorin, and oxaliplatin with and without cetuximab in the first line treatment of metastatic colorectal cancer. J Clin Oncol. 2009;27:663–71.
8. Tournigand C, Andre T, Achille E, et al. FOLFIRI followed by FOLFOX6 or the reverse sequence in advanced colorectal cancer: a randomized GERCOR study. J Clin Oncol. 2004;22(2):229–37.
9. Goldberg RM, Sargent DJ, Morton RF, et al. A randomized controlled trial of fluorouracil plus leucovorin, irinotecan, and oxaliplatin combinations in patients with previously untreated metastatic colorectal cancer. J Clin Oncol. 2004;22(1):23–30.
10. Scheer MG, Sloots CE, van der Wilt GJ, Ruers TJ. Management of patients with asymptomatic colorectal cancer and synchronous irresectable metastases. Ann Oncol. 2008;19(11):1829–35.

https://doi.org/10.1093/annonc/mdn398. Epub 2008 Jul 28; Poultsides GA, Servais EL, Saltz LB, et al. Outcome of primary tumor in patients with synchronous stage IV colorectal cancer receiving combination chemotherapy without surgery as initial treatment. J Clin Oncol. 2009;27(20):3379–84.
11. Tebbutt NC, Norman AR, Cunningham D, et al. Intestinal complications after chemotherapy for patients with unresected primary colorectal cancer and synchronous metastases. Gut. 2003;52(4):568–73.
12. Scoggins CR, Meszoely IM, Blanke CD, et al. Nonoperative management of primary colorectal cancer in patients with stage IV disease. Ann Surg Oncol. 1999;6(7):651–7.
13. Mahteme H, Pahlman L, Glimelius B, Graf W. Prognosis after surgery in patients with incurable rectal cancer: a population based study. Br J Surg. 1996;83(8):1116–20.
14. Crane CH, Janjan NA, Abbruzzese JL, et al. Effective pelvic symptom control using initial chemoradiation without colostomy in metastatic rectal cancer. Int J Radiat Oncol Biol Phys. 2001;49(1):107–16.
15. Makela J, Haukipuro K, Laitinen S, Kairaluoma MI. Palliative operations for colorectal cancer. Dis Colon Rectum. 1990;33(10):846–50.
16. Liu SK, Church JM, Lavery IC, Fazio VW. Operation in patients with incurable colon cancer – is it worthwhile? Dis Colon Rectum. 1997;40(1):11–4.
17. Konyalian VR, Rosing DK, Haukoos JS, et al. The role of primary tumour resection in patients with stage IV colorectal cancer. Color Dis. 2007;9(5):430–7.
18. Beham A, Rentsch M, Pullmann K, et al. Survival benefit in patients after palliative resection vs non-resection colon cancer surgery. World J Gastroenterol. 2006;12(41):6634–8.
19. Costi R, Mazzeo A, Di Mauro D, et al. Palliative resection of colorectal cancer: does it prolong survival? Ann Surg Oncol. 2007;14(9):2567–76.
20. Law WL, Chan WF, Lee YM, Chu KW. Non-curative surgery for colorectal cancer: critical appraisal of outcomes. Int J Color Dis. 2004;19(3):197–202.
21. Mik M, Dziki L, Galbfach P, et al. Resection of the primary tumour or other palliative procedures in incurable stage IV colorectal cancer patients? Color Dis. 2010;12(7 Online):e61–7.
22. Stelzner S, Hellmich G, Koch R, Ludwig K. Factors predicting survival in stage IV colorectal carcinoma patients after palliative treatment: a multivariate analysis. J Surg Oncol. 2005;89(4):211–7.
23. Yun HR, Lee WY, Lee WS, et al. The prognostic factors of stage IV colorectal cancer and assessment of proper treatment according to the patient's status. Int J Color Dis. 2007;22(11):1301–10.
24. Frago R, Kreisler E, Biondo S, et al. Outcomes in the management of obstructive unresectable stage IV colorectal cancer. Eur J Surg Oncol. 2010;36(12):1187–94.
25. Aslam MI, Kelkar A, Sharpe D, Jameson JS. Ten years experience of managing the primary tumours in patients with stage IV colorectal cancers. Int J Surg. 2010;8(4):305–13.
26. Ruo L, Gougoutas C, Paty PB, et al. Elective bowel resection for incurable stage IV colorectal cancer: prognostic variables for asymptomatic patients. J Am Coll Surg. 2003;196(5):722–8.
27. Kaufman MS, Radhakrishnan N, Roy R, et al. Influence of palliative surgical resection on overall survival in patients with advanced colorectal cancer: a retrospective single institutional study. Color Dis. 2008;10(5):498–502.
28. Michel P, Roque I, Di Fiore F, et al. Colorectal cancer with nonresectable synchronous metastases: should the primary tumor be resected? Gastroenterol Clin Biol. 2004;28(5):434–7.
29. Benoist S, Pautrat K, Mitry E, et al. Treatment strategy for patients with colorectal cancer and synchronous irresectable liver metastases. Br J Surg. 2005;92(9):1155–60.
30. Galizia G, Lieto E, Orditura M, et al. First-line chemotherapy vs bowel tumor resection plus chemotherapy for patients with unresectable synchronous colorectal hepatic metastases. Arch Surg. 2008;143(4):352–8; discussion: 358.
31. Bajwa A, Blunt N, Vyas S, et al. Primary tumour resection and survival in the palliative management of metastatic colorectal cancer. Eur J Surg Oncol. 2009;35(2):164–7.

32. Chan TW, Brown C, Ho CC, Gill S. Primary tumor resection in patients presenting with metastatic colorectal cancer: analysis of a provincial population-based cohort. Am J Clin Oncol. 2010;33(1):52–5.
33. Evans MD, Escofet X, Karandikar SS, Stamatakis JD. Outcomes of resection and non-resection strategies in management of patients with advanced colorectal cancer. World J Surg Oncol. 2009;7:28.
34. Seo GJ, Park JW, Yoo SB, et al. Intestinal complications after palliative treatment for asymptomatic patients with unresectable stage IV colorectal cancer. J Surg Oncol. 2010;102(1):94–9.
35. Koopman M, Antonini NF, Douma J, et al. Sequential versus combination chemotherapy with capecitabine, irinotecan, and oxaliplatin in advanced colorectal cancer (CAIRO): a phase III randomised controlled trial. Lancet. 2007;370(9582):135–42.
36. Tol J, Koopman M, Cats A, et al. Chemotherapy, bevacizumab, and cetuximab in metastatic colorectal cancer. N Engl J Med. 2009;360(6):563–72.
37. Venderbosch S, de Wilt JH, Teerenstra S, et al. Prognostic value of resection of primary tumor in patients with stage IV colorectal cancer: retrospective analysis of two randomized studies and a review of the literature. Ann Surg Oncol. 2011 Nov;18(12):3252–60.
38. Koopman M, Antonini NF, Douma J, et al. Sequential versus combination therapy with capecitabine, irinotecan, and oxaliplatin in advanced colorectal cancer (CAIRO): a phase III randomized controlled trial. Lancet. 2007;370:135–42.
39. Tol J, Koopman M, Rodenburg CJ, et al. A randomized phase III study on capecitabine, oxaliplatin and bevacizumab with or without cetuximab in first-line advanced colorectal cancer: the CAIRO2 study of the Dutch Colorectal Cancer Group (DCCG). An interim analysis of toxicity. Ann Oncol. 2008;19:734–8.
40. Ahmed S, Leis A, Chandra-Kanthan S, et al. Surgical management of the primary tumor in stage IV colorectal cancer: a confirmatory retrospective cohort study. J Cancer. 2016;7:837–45.
41. Faron M, Pignon JP, Malka D, et al. Is primary tumor resection associated with survival improvement in patients with colorectal cancer and unresectable synchronous metastases? A pooled analysis of individual data from four randomized trials. Eur J Cancer. 2015;51:166–76.
42. Ducreux M, Bouche O, Pignon JP, et al. Randomized trial comparing three different schedules of infusional 5FU and raltitrexed alone as first-line therapy in metastatic colorectal cancer. Final results of the Federation Francophone de Cancerologie Digestive (FFCD) 9601 trial. Oncology. 2006;70:222–30.
43. Ducreux M, Malka D, Mendiboure J, et al. Sequential versus combination chemotherapy for the treatment of advanced colorectal cancer (FFCD 2000-05): an open-label, randomized, phase 3 trial. Lancet Oncol. 2011;12:1032–44.
44. Ducreux M, Adenis A, Mendiboure J, et al. Efficacy and safety of bevacizumab (BEV)-based combination regimens in patients with metastatic colorectal cancer (mCRC): randomized phase II study of BEV1FOLFIRI versus BEV1XELIRI (FNCLCC ACCORD-13/0503). Abstr Annu Meet Am Soc Clin Oncol. 2009;27:4086.
45. Ducreux M, Bennouna J, Hebbar M, et al. Capecitabine plus oxaliplatin (XELOX) versus 5-fluorouracil/leucovorin plus oxaliplatin (FOLFOX-6) as first-line treatment for metastatic colorectal cancer. Int J Cancer. 2011;128:682–90.
46. Clancy C, Burke JP, Barry M, et al. A meta-analysis to determine the effect of primary tumor resection for stage IV colorectal cancer with unresectable metastases on patient survival. Ann Surg Oncol. 2014;21:3900–8.
47. Tarantino I, Warschkow R, Worni M, et al. Prognostic relevance of palliative primary tumor removal in 37,793 metastatic colorectal cancer patients. A population-based, propensity score-adjusted trend analysis. Ann Surg. 2015;262:112–20.
48. Lam-Boer J, Van der Geest L, Verhoef C, et al. Palliative resection of the primary tumor is associated with improved overall survival in incurable stage IV colorectal cancer: a nationwide population-based propensity-score adjusted study in the Netherlands. Int J Cancer. 2016;139:2082–94.

49. He WZ, Rong YM, Jiang C, et al. Palliative primary tumor resection provides survival benefits for the patients with metastatic colorectal cancer and low circulating levels of dehydrogenase and carcinoembryonic antigen. Chin J Cancer. 2016;35(1):58–65.
50. Kodaz H, Erdogan B, Hacibekiroglu I, et al. Primary tumor resection offers higher survival advantage in KRAS mutant metastatic colorectal cancer patients. Hepatogastroenterology. 2015;62(140):876–9.
51. Dorajoo SR, Tan WJ, Koo SX, et al. A scoring model for predicting survival following primary tumour resection in stage IV colorectal patients with unresectable metastasis. Int J Color Dis. 2016;31(2):235–45.

Liver Pedicle Lymphadenectomy: How and When?

34

Jaime A. P. Krüger and Paulo Herman

Introduction—What History Tells

Resection of colorectal liver metastases (CLM) has been considered the optimal treatment for CLM, offering the possibility of long-term survival and, in some instances, cure. According to various risk factors, the association of high- quality staging, effective chemotherapy, and modern surgical strategies has led to 5-year survival rates of 36–58% in published series [1, 15, 33].

Extra-hepatic disease has been historically known to negatively impact prognosis in the setting of CLM. Although prognostic implications of extra-hepatic disease vary widely depending on the location (i.e., lung metastatic patients live longer than patients with peritoneal metastases), the poor outcomes of patients with CLM and extra-hepatic disease led many authors contraindicate liver resection in the presence of additional tumor deposits outside the liver [4, 8, 11, 16].

Among extra-hepatic disease, hepatic hilar metastases (which generally includes nodes along the hepatoduodenal ligament, superior retropancreatic chain, hepatic artery, and celiac axis) seemed to represent advanced disease, implying in dismal survival and thus liver resection was not justified in that circumstance. In a large dataset of patients published in the late 1980s, The Registry of Hepatic Metastasis [16], a multicenter study with 859 patients, identified 24 patients that underwent hepatectomy with positive hilar lymph nodes (LNs). Despite having gross disease cleared, all those patients recurred on follow-up, 17 of them with early recurrences and there was no 5-year survivor. Almost 10 years later Beckurts studied 126 consecutive patients undergoing hepatectomy for CLM [4]. They performed routine lymphadenectomy of the hepatoduodenal ligament in all patients, and identified 35 (28%) patients bearing positive lymph nodes. Patients with R0 hepatic resection and

J. A. P. Krüger (✉) · P. Herman
Liver Surgery Unit, Hospital das Clínicas (HC) and Instituto do Câncer do Estado de São Paulo (ICESP), University of São Paulo Medical School, São Paulo, SP, Brazil
e-mail: jaime.kruger@hc.fm.usp.br

M. M. Correia et al. (eds.), *Colorectal Cancer Liver Metastases*,
https://doi.org/10.1007/978-3-030-25486-5_34

no metastatic lymph nodes had 3- and 5-year survival rates of 48% and 22%, respectively, whereas lymph node positive patients had 3% and 0% survival at 3- and 5-year follow-up.

The discouraging clinical data was supported by the pathophysiological understanding that metastatic disease to hepatic hilar lymph nodes was a sign of aggressive disease. In 1985, August et al. analyzed a series of patients with CLM considered for liver resection [3]. They studied 81 patients referred to the National Institutes of Health (NIH) from years 1976 to 1983. Of those, after what was considered optimal staging, 51 patients were considered resectable and went to laparotomy. Thirteen patients had unresectable disease identified intraoperatively, 5 of them bearing secondary lymph nodes. This paper brought an interesting concept of hepatic hilar involvement as tertiary disease [14], since those patients didn't have any other evidence of lymphatic spread. In other words, lymph nodes spread to liver hilum indicated metastatic disease that originated from metastatic hepatic nodes (CLM), so lymphatic disease represented remetastases. This was an indication of aggressive disease that was not amenable to control through hepatic resection.

The landscape of managing hepatic hilar metastases began to change in the transition of the late 1990s to early 2000s. Nakamura et al. overlooked a 20-year period managing CLM [25]. The authors performed routine pedicle lymphadenectomy during their early experience (1978–1989) and afterward (1990–1998) lymph nodes were dissected only when clinically suspicious. Overall 43 patients had lymphadenectomy (41 at first operation and 2 at repeat hepatectomy). Interestingly, lymph node metastases were not found as having prognostic implication, and the 7 patients bearing positive nodes had a 42% 5-year survival. This study should be carefully interpreted, since it evaluated a limited number of patients, most of them having micrometastic disease, clinically unsuspected and found during routine hilar lymphadenectomy. Moreover, the results presented strongly disagree with previous published data, but despite methodological criticism, it suggested that long-term survival could be achieved in hilar lymph node positive patients.

Hepatic hilar lymph node remetastases were in the spot light. Seeking better understanding of their prognostic impact, Rodgers and McCall conducted a systematic review published in 2000 in the British Journal of Surgery, gathering data from 15 studies [34]. They concluded that long-term survival was rare at that time, only 5 patients out of 145 node positive individuals were still alive after 5 years. Moreover, there was only one disease-free individual. Long-term survival was possible, although rare, in the setting of metastatic hepatic lymph nodes. Probably the most important feature in the paper was written on the last paragraph: the call for effective adjuvant systemic treatment, unavailable at that moment. In the early 2000s the initial papers on the use of modern chemotherapy were published and the results of treatment employing irinotecan and oxaliplatin improved substantially the survival in colorectal metastatic patients [7, 35]. Hepatic surgery also proved to be safer and progressively associated with low morbidity and mortality [18]. The association of aggressive but safe strategies to resect CLM and effective chemotherapy began to change the landscape of managing CLM and hepatic lymph node metastases.

Micrometastatic Versus Macrometastatic Disease

In the management of hepatic hilar metastases there seems to be different implications in treating patients with micrometastatic disease, in which hilar nodes are found incidentally during routine en bloc lymphadenectomy, and managing patients with grossly infiltrated (clinically evident) lymph nodes.

Many of the abovementioned studies were made public at a time in which preoperative staging was less effective than modern techniques employed today. Macroscopic hepatic nodal involvement was found in around 10% of cases during laparotomy for a planned liver resection [3, 11]. More than indicative of a less effective preoperative staging, the presence of macroscopic disease suggests that there was a bigger tumor burden than expected, explaining the dismal, if none, benefit of lymphadenectomy in remetastatic CLM.

On the other hand, authors have planned routine hilar lymphadenectomy, with the intent to study the incidence and clinical relevance of hepatic hilar nodes remetastases. The incidence of microscopic lymph nodal disease varies from 7% to 24% [4, 5, 36]. A well-designed prospective multicenter French study from Elias in which 114 consecutive patients underwent planned routine hepatoduodenal ligament lymphadenectomy [9]. Eight patients with operative finding of macroscopic nodes were excluded and additional 6 patients with insufficient lymph node yield were also excluded from analysis, leaving 100 patients in the study group. There were 14 patients (14%) with confirmed metastases to lymph nodes, with positive nodes found in primary chains near the *porta hepatis*, in secondary chains along the hepatic artery and retropancreatic nodes and also in tertiary chains on the celiac axis. *Probably the most relevant information in this study was the fact that nodal involvement was not continuous along primary, secondary, and tertiary chains. In other words, a skip metastases pattern was found, with metastatic lymph nodes found in secondary or tertiary drainage levels without any node positivity in primary and/or secondary chains.* The authors also investigated the risk factors related to lymph node involvement. Hepatic hilar node positive patients had a higher level of carcinoembrionic antigen (CEA), higher number of liver metastases, higher percentage of parenchymal involvement, and undergone more frequently to major resections.

In another prospective study, Jaeck et al. evaluated 160 consecutive patients undergoing routine hilar lymphadenectomy [17]. Seventeen patients (10.6%) had positive hepatic lymph nodes and lymph node metastases had prognostic impact, being 3-year survival 62% for node negative patients and 19% for node positive patients. Beyond analyzing the effect of node positivity, the study also sought the effect of lymph node location on survival. Lymphatic spread to primary chains (i.e., along hepatoduodenal ligament and retro pancreatic chain) had a better outcome (3-year survival: 38%) than distal lymphatic metastasis (0% 3-year survival in patients with positive nodes on proximal hepatic artery and celiac axis). Risk factors for hepatic lymph node metastases were: more than three liver metastases, metastases located on segments 4 and 5, and poorly differentiated histology.

Laurent et al. also published their experience on consecutive patients undergoing systematic routine hilar lymphadenectomy [20]. There were 156 patients with 23 (15%) bearing microscopically positive lymph nodes. Patients with positive nodes had a higher rate of recurrence (21/23, 91%) compared to node negative patients (79/133, 59%), but the sites of recurrence were similar between the two groups. In multivariate analysis, positive lymph nodes were independent predictors of survival. In disagreement to the abovementioned papers, Laurent et al. found no risk factor associated with microscopic nodal involvement in the hepatic hilum.

In a different approach, a group of patients from the Memorial Sloan Kettering Cancer Center (MSKCC) underwent selective hepatic hilar lymph node sampling during hepatic resection for CLM [5]. Differently from above cited studies, the patients did not undergo a complete hilar lymphadenectomy. The study focused on increasing the yield of positive nodes through the use of special staining methods. Immunohistochemistry (IHC) increased the detection of metastatic lymph nodes, raising the yield from 14% to 24% when compared to regular hematoxylin–eosin (HE) staining. Another paper from Viana et al. made a similar investigation on patients undergoing a thorough hilar lymphadenectomy. Hematoxylin–eosin found micrometastatic nodes in 7% of patients, a number that raised to 18% when specific IHC staining was employed [36].

Diagnosis of Hilar Lymph Nodes Metastasis

The preoperative diagnosis of metastatic lymph nodes is often difficult. Most institutions apply computed tomography (CT) and magnetic resonance imaging (MRI) as a routine tool for oncological follow-up and in the preoperative planning for resection of colorectal liver metastases [10]. Positron emission computed tomography (PET-CT), despite having limited application on liver-only metastatic patients [24], can be useful in the staging of patients with CLM and extra-hepatic disease.

Grobmyer et al. analyzed the performance of preoperative staging on the diagnosis of metastatic lymph nodes on 100 patients with primary or metastatic liver tumors, 75 of them with CLM, undergoing lymph node sampling during liver resection [12]. Nodes were obtained from three areas: portocaval, pancreatoduodenal, and common hepatic artery. After histological detection of metastatic disease, the preoperative imaging studies were blindly reviewed. Intraoperative assessment of hepatic lymph nodes had 90% sensitivity, 87% specificity, 39% positive predictive value, and 99% negative predictive value. CT showed 40% sensitivity, 92% specificity, 30% positive predictive value, and 95% negative predictive value. PET scan numbers were 57% sensitivity, 100% specificity, 100% positive predictive value, and 88% negative predictive value. All patients in the series undergone CT scans and intraoperative assessment, 66 underwent a preoperative PET scan.

Few years later a French study from Beaujon Hospital evaluated 76 patients with CLM submitted to liver resection and systematic hilar lymphadenectomy [31]. Similarly they compared the results of preoperative CT and intraoperative findings with histology. Sensitivity, specificity, positive predictive value, and negative predictive value were 33%, 93%, 56%, and 85% for computed tomography and 67%, 79%, 43%, and 91% for intraoperative assessment. Lymph node size was not statistically significant when metastatic and non-metastatic nodes were compared (11.7 vs 7.8 mm, $p = 0.08$) but round-shaped nodes were significantly associated with secondary disease (40% vs 6.5%, $p = 0.004$).

Adam et al. evaluated the indication for lymph node resection when there was evidence of metastatic disease [2]. The paper was not designed to address the issue of preoperative staging, but revealed interesting information on the topic. Forty-seven cases had histological confirmation of lymphatic metastases, of whom 19 patients were diagnosed before surgery (40%) and 28 patients were diagnosed intra-operatively. All patients underwent CT scans and in selected cases PET-CT was indicated. From the lymph node positive group of patients there were 6 undergoing PET-CT, which suspected secondary disease in four cases confirmed on pathology.

Hodgson et al. also analyzed their experience in similar fashion to Adam et al., applying CT as a routine procedure, MRI for most patients undergoing hepatectomy and PET-CT in selected cases [13]. They performed lymphadenectomy in 76 patients and found 38 patients with histologically proved positive lymph nodes. CT identified 7 out of 38 patients, MRI identified 13 out of 36 patients, and PET-CT 4 out of 4 patients. Importantly PET-CT was negative in other 7 patients with suspicious enlarged nodes that were resected, but were negative on final pathology.

Recently, Okuno et al. reviewed a large dataset of patients bearing colorectal liver metastases and undergoing hepatic hilum lymphadenectomy [27]. Once again the accuracy of diagnostic methods was compared to final pathology. In their 1485 CLM patients' experience, 174 patients undergone lymphadenectomy for suspected disease and in 54 (31%) lymph node metastases were histologically proven to be positive. Preoperative imaging showed suspected lymph nodes in 98 patients, of those 39 (40%) were proved positive. In 1387 patients preoperative imaging was negative, but 76 patients had suspicious lymph nodes found during operative assessment and 15 of those (20%) were confirmed on final pathology.

The above-cited literature suggests that relying only in one preoperative imaging method might be misleading on the diagnosis of metastatic hepatic lymph nodes. *To adequately confirm the presence of secondary lymphatic disease the surgeon must know the risk factors for metastatic hilar nodes and associate preoperative imaging studies, including PET-CT in the search for equivocal extra-hepatic disease, with operative assessment.* In experienced centers lymphadenectomy is carried out with minimal complication rate and when suspected, lymph node dissection should be carried out as it offers opportunity for prolonged disease control (see further information on this chapter) (Fig. 34.1).

Current Indication for Hilar Lymphadenectomy

With modern staging, effective chemotherapy, and optimal results of liver resection (low morbidity, low mortality, and parenchymal preservation), the results of managing CLM in patients with extra-hepatic disease began to change. Selected patients

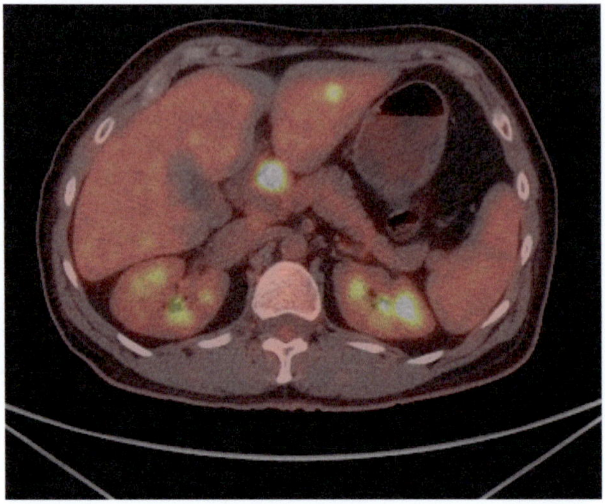

Fig. 34.1 PET-CT in a patient with colorectal liver metastases and a positive lymph node along the common hepatic artery

can benefit from surgery, being the goals of treatment an effective systemic control associated with complete clearance of all tumor sites. Such association has led to improved survival, up to 26% in 5 years [6, 29], in a stage which multicentric disease would be expected to have no long-term survivors.

Better management of extra-hepatic disease also had impact on hilar lymph nodes treatment. Oussoultzoglou et al. published an interesting paper on hilar lymphadenectomy in patients with risk factors for unsuspected microscopic lymph node metastases [28]. According to a previous publication from the same group, patients with multiple hepatic nodules (three or more metastases), nodules located on segments 4 and 5 and patients with elevated CEA (over 20 μg/dl) were at risk for microscopic lymph nodes metastases. They performed lymphadenectomy in 45 patients selected with the abovementioned criteria, at the same time of liver resection. Those patients had adjuvant chemotherapy in 36 cases (25 oxaliplatin based, 6 irinotecan based, and 4 other regimens). Overall survival for 3- and 5-year follow-up was 29.7% and 17.3%, respectively. Median survival was 20.9 months. Those numbers indicate that lymphatic hepatic disease might worsen survival if compared to liver-only metastatic patients, but long-term survival could be achieved and the survival rates were better than those cited on this chapter's Introduction.

Another approach to lymph node metastases was undertaken by Bennett et al. form MSKCC [5]. In their paper a risk score for seeking positive lymph nodes in hepatic malignancies was employed, so this was not a paper seeking management of occult disease, but looking after nodes that were clinically macroscopically or microscopically suspicious. In their series they did not perform complete lymphadenectomy, rather applying lymph node sampling. In the sample nodes their final objective and main purpose of their study was to analyze how could IHC identify more positive nodes than regular HE staining. In 65 patients HE positive nodes were found in 8 (14%) patients and IHC positive nodes were identified in 14 (24%) patients. Despite mixing clinically suspicious with actual microscopic lymph nodal disease, this paper offers some interesting analysis. The patients bearing IHC positive nodes had smaller tumor burden, confirming they had real microscopic disease, and their survival curves were similar to those of lymph node negative patients and better than HE positive lymph node patients. This is an important information suggesting that those patients with microscopic disease and very small amount of tumor cells will have similar outcome of patients without positive lymph nodes or with microscopic lymph nodes that were not discovered during surgery. *This raises the argument for effective management of micrometastatic disease through effective chemotherapy in association with adequate resection of all measurable disease.*

In such understanding the paper published from Paul Brousse was the first to describe the management of clinically evident lymph node disease discovered on oncological follow-up or preoperative assessment for hepatic surgery for colorectal metastases [2]. At that time they sought their database of 763 patients operated for CLM, being 53 of them (7%) treated with additional lymphadenectomy, in 47 cases there was histological confirmation of lymphatic metastases. There were 19 patients diagnosed presurgery (40%) and 28 patients diagnosed intraoperatively. All patients received chemotherapy prior to liver surgery, most patients having oxaliplatin-based treatment. Overall survival at 3 and 5 years was 38% and 18% for the LN positive group versus 68% and 53% for the lymph node negative patients. Survival varied not only with the presence of lymph nodes but was related to their location. At 5 years 25% of patients with pedicle lymph nodes were alive, but no one survived when nodes were located at celiac axis and para-aortic region. On multivariate analysis celiac location of lymph node metastases were confirmed as independent prognostic factors. For hepatic lymph node metastases, multimodal treatment and location of secondary lymph nodes are key matters on the management of those patients.

A broader study was performed by Pulitano and co-workers, performing a multi-institutional analysis on the concept of surgery for hepatic lymph node metastases in modern multimodal management [30]. They analyzed 1629 patients treated for CLM, 171 with extra-hepatic, being 61 with positive hilar LNs. Sixty-nine percent of patients received preoperative chemotherapy and the majority, 65%, also received adjuvant treatment. Most patients, 52%, had combined therapy with irinotecan- or oxaliplatin-based regimens. Patients with preoperative or intraoperative suspected lymph nodes underwent complete nodal clearance in the following areas: hepatoduodenal ligament and retropancreatic (area 1, 28 patients), common hepatic artery and celiac axis (area 2, 17 patients), and para-aortic (area 3, 16 patients). Overall survival for LN positive patients was 32 months, being 3 and 5 years survival 35% and 18%, respectively. Location of lymph nodes strongly affected the survival, with median survival being 37 and 32 months in patients with affected lymph nodes in areas 1 and 2, opposed to 17 months survival in patients with metastatic area 3 nodes. Of note, confirming the relevance of lymph node location, 5-year survival was 30% for patients in area 1 while para-aortic nodes remained independent risk factor for survival on multivariate analysis.

Modern series are still paying attention to the results of aggressive management of hilar lymphatic spread. Over a 20-year period Hodgson et al. analyzed 2082 patients with CLM, of those 76 patients had lymphadenectomy (4%), half of them (38 patients) had confirmed metastases on pathology [13]. Patients underwent staging with MRI, CT, and recent cases had also PET-CT included in the preoperative work-up. Overall survival reached reasonable numbers of 44% and 31% in 3 and 5 years, respectively, for patients with metastatic lymph nodes. Those good results suggest that modern management with newer chemotherapy agents, adequate staging, and complete resection of all measurable secondary disease results in prolonged survival.

Another recent study compared 1311 patients undergoing hepatectomy with 174 patients undergoing hepatectomy and lymphadenectomy [27]. Of those 31% (54 patients) had LN metastases confirmed histologically. The majority of those patients underwent preoperative chemotherapy, being 76% oxaliplatin based and 70% also had targeted therapy with bevacizumab. Among patients receiving lymphadenectomy at the time of liver resection, several features were associated with lymph node positivity: number of metastases (multiple metastasis: 73% vs 52.7%), larger hepatic tumor diameter (lesion over 30 mm: 52.9% vs 33.9%), and greater likelihood of preoperative chemotherapy (88.5% vs 81.8%). Those clinical features are associated with a bigger tumor load on the liver and also had implications on the operative characteristics, since lymphadenectomy patients had more staged hepatectomies associated with portal vein embolization, more major resections, prolonged operative times, and longer hospital stay. Independent risk factors for lymph node metastasis were LN positive primary tumor and intrahepatic recurrence requiring rehepatectomy. For patients undergoing lymphadenectomy, median relapse free survival was 5.3 months for those with positive nodes versus 13.8 months for those without metastatic lymph nodes. Overall survival was 20.5 months versus 71.3 months. Of the 54 patients with histologically proven LN metastases, 34 had disease restricted to the hepatoduodenal ligament, 8 had disease along hepatic artery and celiac axis, and 12 had para-aortic lymph nodes. Disease free and overall survival was 4.5 and 15.5 months for the first group; 6.1 and 23 months for the second and 5.1 and 58.2 months for the later, without statistical difference (p = 0.233) among groups, in disagreement with previous publications, location of lymph nodes did not seem relevant. This probably reflects the systemic management of patients included in the study, most of them treated with aggressive chemotherapic regimens. Beyond location, the study also analyzed the number of lymph nodes bearing disease. Forty-two patients had one or two positive nodes, with median survival of 25.4 months; 12 patients had three or more nodes and their survival was significantly worse, 16.3 months (p = 0.039).

Hepatic Lymphatic Anatomy [21–23, 26]

The liver produces a large amount of lymphatic fluid, around 1–3 liters daily, which represents about 25–50% of all lymphatic fluid produced in the body. This fluid comes from the perisinusoidal spaces of Disse, located between hepatocytes and sinusoids, a space where small lymphatic capillaries collect interstitial fluid rich in substances exchanged from sinusoidal blood and hepatocytes. The small capillaries converge to thicker lymph vessels and communicate to broader lymphatic systems in the liver: the deep lymphatic system and the superficial lymphatic system.

Both systems form a complex network and are further divided according to their anatomy. Superficial lymphatic system runs in the subserosa connective tissue of the liver surface. The superficial system of the convex (diaphragmatic) surface of the liver will drain through falciform, triangular and coronary ligaments to thoracic lymph nodes and the superficial system of the liver inferior (visceral) surface converges toward the hepatic hilum.

The deep lymphatic system is composed of two subdivisions, the venous hepatic and periportal lymphatic systems. The venous hepatic lymphatic system drains lymph along the vena cava to the general lymphatic system of the posterior mediastinum and the periportal network runs in Glisson's sheath along with portal vein, hepatic artery, and bile duct. The periportal lymphatic flow runs in the same direction as bile, converging to the hepatic hilum. *Of extreme importance is the fact that 80% of all hepatic lymph drains* via *the periportal system, so surgeons must pay special attention to hepatic pedicle lymph nodes when operating on liver malignancies.* Hilar LNs will then connect to celiac nodes, juxtacardic nodes, and gastrocardiac nodes in one route and to retropancreatic and superior mesenteric nodes in another route. Celiac and superior mesenteric nodes will connect to the cisterna chyli.

Lymphatic anatomy of the hilum is highly relevant, since it represents the topography where lymphatic spread will be apparent, and technically it is the place where surgeons will have access to resect metastatic lymph nodes during hepatectomy (Fig. 34.2). Along the hepatic hilum the superficial inferior lymphatic network converges with deep portal lymphatic system to drain most (>80%) of the lymph produced inside the liver. The hilar drainage occurs via three separate dominant lymph nodal routes. There is a right route along the bile duct, present in almost all patients; there is a left route along hepatic artery, noticeable in 50% of patients and a third route, present in few patients (5%) between those two previously mentioned.

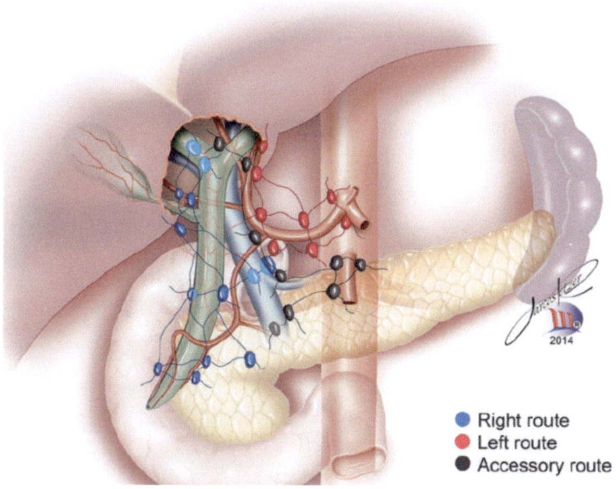

Fig. 34.2 Hilar hepatic lymphatic anatomy. From lymphatic drainage of the liver and its implications in the management of colorectal cancer liver metastases. (Lupinacci et al., Updates in Surgery [21]. With permission of Springer Nature # 4396240447350)

Technique [23]

The hepatic pedicle contains structures of the portal triad (hepatic artery, portal vein, and bile duct) surrounded by connective, fatty, and lymphatic tissue (Fig. 34.3). The lymphadenectomy can be performed applying the same patient positioning and incision utilized for a conventional liver resection. The intention is to clear all connective, fatty, and lymphatic tissue preserving the integrity of the portal triad. It is important to remove all lymphatic tissue surrounding the bile duct without complete skeletonization of hepatic and choledocal ducts, in order to preserve biliary vasculature and to avoid postoperative strictures.

After laparotomy, section and division of round and falciform ligaments associated to gentle verticalization of the visceral (inferior) surface of the liver along with gentle traction of the round ligament allow for pedicle exposure. The pars falcisa is opened, giving access to the hepatic artery and nodes along it. Assistant's traction caudal toward patient's feet will help to complete exposure.

Procedure starts with cholecystectomy and is planned to be performed in a counterclockwise fashion. Lymphadenectomy begins with section of pyloric vessels and clearance of suprapyloric nodes up to left gastric vein and common hepatic artery which are the medial limits of the lymphadenectomy. The hepatic artery is cleared up to the emergence of left gastric and/or splenic arteries. To ease nodal clearance from proper hepatic artery and its branches, they should be encircled with surgical tapes and gentle traction must be applied in a manner not to occlude vessels. To better expose vessels in the portal triad a small Cushing retractor is very useful for gentle retraction. Small arterial branches should be carefully managed to avoid bleeding or hematomas and subsequent arterial thrombosis.

Dissection continues along the inferior border of the liver close to porta hepatis toward the right side of the pedicle. Dissection on the right side begins with the cystic lymph node and progresses downward to retroduodenal and suprapancreatic nodes. After accomplished retroportal nodes are harvested and the en bloc specimen should be free enough to be rotated behind the pedicle and end the dissection.

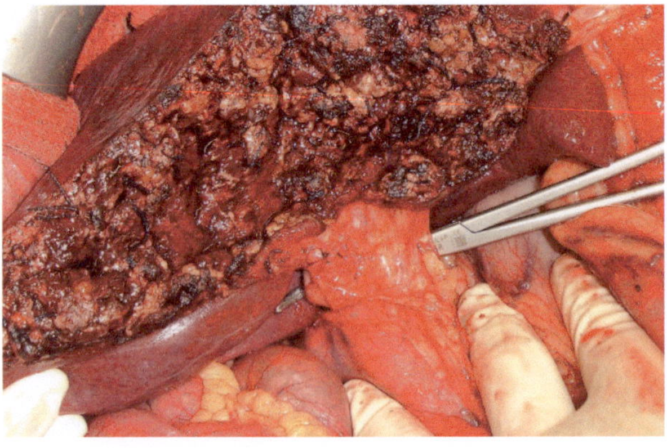

Fig. 34.3 Normal view of the hepatic hilum after a left hepatectomy

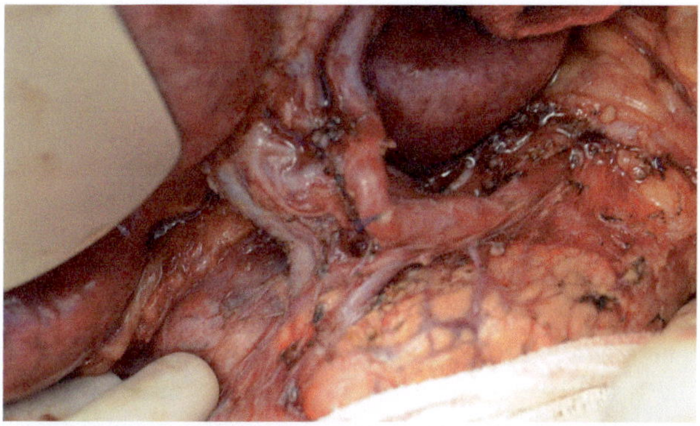

Fig. 34.4 The same patient on Fig. 34.1. After proper chemotherapy hepatic resection and lymphadenectomy were carried out. Final aspect of hilar lymph node clearance is shown

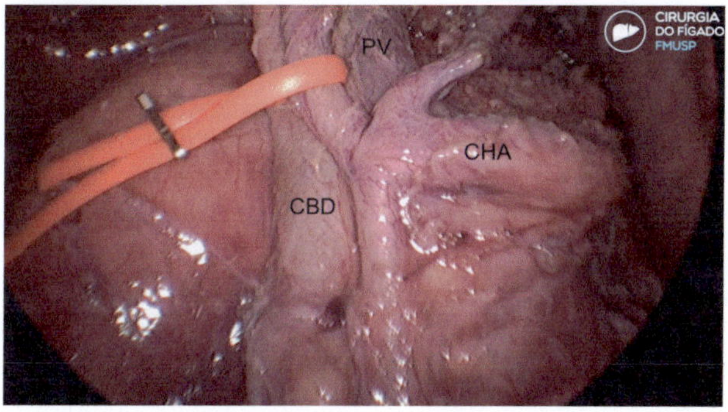

Fig. 34.5 Final aspect of laparoscopic hilar lymphadenectomy in patient with a segment VI CLM and a positive hilar lymph node. CHA common hepatic artery, CBD common bile duct, PV portal vein

Special attention should be paid to a right replaced hepatic artery during retroportal dissection (Figs. 34.4 and 34.5).

Lymph Node Retrieval and Complications of Lymphadenectomy

The number of harvested nodes is a frequent concern in surgery for malignant disease. The number of nodes obtained during hepatic pedicle dissection varies according to the technique employed. In lymph node sampling the mean number of nodes varies from 2.4 to 3.2 [12, 19]. When complete lymphadenectomy is performed the mean number of lymph nodes rises to 3.2–8.6 [9, 20, 31, 32, 36].

There is some debate among authors that suggest that systematic hilar lymphadenectomy would aid to control microscopic metastatic disease versus the fact that lymphadenectomy would not be beneficial in many cases (more than 80% of patients will have negative nodes) and the extension of surgery would imply in higher morbidity. *Most papers derive from experienced centers and general complications of liver resection were not increased when patients had lymphadenectomy. Some papers indicate an increased operative time and presence of lymphatic leakage as the main problems associated with lymphadenectomy, without any major clinical impact on patient's outcomes* [4, 20, 31, 32, 36]. It seems justified to perform nodal dissection to achieve complete resection of CLM patients, but special attention should be on biliary vascularization since biliary stenosis had been described after hepatic hilar lymphadenectomy, especially in cases of extensive devascularization (e.g., lymphadenectomy for hilar cholangiocarcinoma).

Conclusion

The management of hepatic lymphatic metastases has changed substantially along the last 20 years. The early experience indicated hilar lymph node metastases as indicators of poor prognosis, precluding hepatic resection, and further lymphadenectomy. As hepatic surgery became safer, staging offered better operative planning and systemic treatment resulted in better disease control, the numbers on survival improved and selected patients can benefit from resection of secondary and tertiary disease.

Those patients should be carefully sought for extra-hepatic disease, with staging utilizing computed tomography, liver magnetic resonance imaging, and whole body PET-CT to obtain a full picture of local and distant spread of disease. After considering a patient resectable, it is essential to test for biological behavior and response to systemic treatment, employing effective drugs, so that operation is offered under controlled disease for good responders. As a complex procedure, liver surgery must be performed along with hilar lymphadenectomy in excellence centers by surgeons aware of modern hepatic surgical techniques and the complex hepatic lymphatic anatomy.

References

1. Abdalla EK, Vauthey J-N, Ellis LM, et al. Recurrence and outcomes following hepatic resection, radiofrequency ablation, and combined resection/ablation for colorectal liver metastases. Ann Surg. 2004;239:818–25; discussion 825–7.
2. Adam R, de Haas RJ, Wicherts DA, et al. Is hepatic resection justified after chemotherapy in patients with colorectal liver metastases and lymph node involvement? J Clin Oncol. 2008;26:3672–80. https://doi.org/10.1200/JCO.2007.15.7297.
3. August DA, Sugarbaker PH, Schneider PD. Lymphatic dissemination of hepatic metastases. Implications for the follow-up and treatment of patients with colorectal cancer. Cancer. 1985;55:1490–4.
4. Beckurts KT, Hölscher AH, Thorban S, et al. Significance of lymph node involvement at the hepatic hilum in the resection of colorectal liver metastases. Br J Surg. 1997;84:1081–4.
5. Bennett JJ, Schmidt CR, Klimstra DS, et al. Perihepatic lymph node micrometastases impact outcome after partial hepatectomy for colorectal metastases. Ann Surg Oncol. 2008;15:1130–6. https://doi.org/10.1245/s10434-007-9802-0.
6. Carpizo DR, D'Angelica M. Liver resection for metastatic colorectal cancer in the presence of extra-hepatic disease. Lancet Oncol. 2009;10:801–9. https://doi.org/10.1016/S1470-2045(09)70081-6.
7. de Gramont A, Figer A, Seymour M, et al. Leucovorin and fluorouracil with or without oxaliplatin as first-line treatment in advanced colorectal cancer. J Clin Oncol. 2000;18:2938–47. doi: papers://4253D9C4-4004-42F3-8ABE-9698C59DDEF8/Paper/p1472.

8. Ekberg H, Tranberg KG, Andersson R, et al. Determinants of survival in liver resection for colorectal secondaries. Br J Surg. 1986;73:727–31.
9. Elias D, Saric J, Jaeck D, et al. Prospective study of microscopic lymph node involvement of the hepatic pedicle during curative hepatectomy for colorectal metastases. Br J Surg. 1996;83:942–5.
10. Fowler KJ, Linehan DC, Menias CO. Colorectal liver metastases: state of the art imaging. Ann Surg Oncol. 2012;20:1185–93. https://doi.org/10.1245/s10434-012-2730-7.
11. Gibbs JF, Weber TK, Rodriguez-Bigas MA, et al. Intraoperative determinants of unresectability for patients with colorectal hepatic metastases. Cancer. 1998;82:1244–9.
12. Grobmyer SR, Wang L, Gonen M, et al. Perihepatic lymph node assessment in patients undergoing partial hepatectomy for malignancy. Ann Surg. 2006;244:260–4. https://doi.org/10.1097/01.sla.0000217606.59625.9d.
13. Hodgson R, Sethi H, Ling AH, Lodge P. Combined hepatectomy and hepatic pedicle lymphadenectomy in colorectal liver metastases is justified. HPB (Oxford). 2017;19:525–9. https://doi.org/10.1016/j.hpb.2017.01.025.
14. Hoover HC, Ketcham AS. Metastasis of metastases. Am J Surg. 1975;130:405–11.
15. House MG, Ito H, Gönen M, et al. Survival after hepatic resection for metastatic colorectal cancer: trends in outcomes for 1,600 patients during two decades at a single institution. J Am Coll Surg. 2010;210:744–52, 752–5. https://doi.org/10.1016/j.jamcollsurg.2009.12.040.
16. Hughes KS, Rosenstein RB, Songhorabodi S, et al. Resection of the liver for colorectal carcinoma metastases. A multi-institutional study of long-term survivors. Dis Colon Rectum. 1988;31:1–4.
17. Jaeck D, Nakano H, Bachellier P, et al. Significance of hepatic pedicle lymph node involvement in patients with colorectal liver metastases: a prospective study. Ann Surg Oncol. 2002;9:430–8.
18. Jarnagin WR, Gonen M, Fong Y, et al. Improvement in perioperative outcome after hepatic resection: analysis of 1,803 consecutive cases over the past decade. Ann Surg. 2002;236:397–406; discussion 406–7. https://doi.org/10.1097/01.SLA.0000029003.66466.B3.
19. Kokudo N, Sato T, Seki M, et al. Hepatic lymph node involvement in resected cases of liver metastases from colorectal cancer. Dis Colon Rectum. 1999;42:1285–90; discussion 1290–1.
20. Laurent C, Sa Cunha A, Rullier E, et al. Impact of microscopic hepatic lymph node involvement on survival after resection of colorectal liver metastasis. J Am Coll Surg. 2004;198:884–91. https://doi.org/10.1016/j.jamcollsurg.2004.01.017.
21. Lupinacci RM, Paye F, Coelho FF, et al. Lymphatic drainage of the liver and its implications in the management of colorectal cancer liver metastases. Updat Surg. 2014;66:239–45. https://doi.org/10.1007/s13304-014-0265-0.
22. Morine Y, Shimada M. The value of systematic lymph node dissection for intrahepatic cholangiocarcinoma from the viewpoint of liver lymphatics. J Gastroenterol. 2015;50:913–27. https://doi.org/10.1007/s00535-015-1071-2.
23. Moszkowicz D, Cauchy F, Dokmak S, Belghiti J. Routine pedicular lymphadenectomy for colorectal liver metastases. J Am Coll Surg. 2012;214:e39–45. https://doi.org/10.1016/j.jamcollsurg.2012.02.015.
24. Moulton C-A, Gu C-S, Law CH, et al. Effect of PET before liver resection on surgical management for colorectal adenocarcinoma metastases: a randomized clinical trial. JAMA. 2014;311:1863–9. https://doi.org/10.1001/jama.2014.3740.
25. Nakamura S, Suzuki S, Konno H. Resection of hepatic metastases of colorectal carcinoma: 20 years' experience. J Hepato-Biliary-Pancreat Surg. 1999;6:16–22.
26. Ohtani O, Ohtani Y. Lymph circulation in the liver. Anat Rec Adv Integr Anat Evol Biol. 2008;291:643–52. https://doi.org/10.1002/ar.20681.
27. Okuno M, Goumard C, Mizuno T, et al. Prognostic impact of perihepatic lymph node metastases in patients with resectable colorectal liver metastases. Br J Surg. 2018;105:1200–9. https://doi.org/10.1002/bjs.10822.

28. Oussoultzoglou E, Romain B, Panaro F, et al. Long-term survival after liver resection for colorectal liver metastases in patients with hepatic pedicle lymph nodes involvement in the era of new chemotherapy regimens. Ann Surg. 2009;249:879–86. https://doi.org/10.1097/SLA.0b013e3181a334d9.
29. Pulitanò C, Bodingbauer M, Aldrighetti L, et al. Liver resection for colorectal metastases in presence of extra-hepatic disease: results from an international multi-institutional analysis. Ann Surg Oncol. 2011;18:1380–8. https://doi.org/10.1245/s10434-010-1459-4.
30. Pulitanò C, Bodingbauer M, Aldrighetti L, et al. Colorectal liver metastasis in the setting of lymph node metastasis: defining the benefit of surgical resection. Ann Surg Oncol. 2012;19:435–42. https://doi.org/10.1245/s10434-011-1902-1.
31. Rau C, Blanc B, Ronot M, et al. Neither preoperative computed tomography nor intraoperative examination can predict metastatic lymph node in the hepatic pedicle in patients with colorectal liver metastasis. Ann Surg Oncol. 2012;19:163–8. https://doi.org/10.1245/s10434-011-1994-7.
32. Ravaioli M, Ercolani G, Grazi GL, et al. Safety and prognostic role of regional lymphadenectomy for primary and metastatic liver tumors. Updat Surg. 2010;62:27–34. https://doi.org/10.1007/s13304-010-0008-9.
33. Rees M, Tekkis PP, Welsh FKS, et al. Evaluation of long-term survival after hepatic resection for metastatic colorectal Cancer. Ann Surg. 2008;247:125–35. https://doi.org/10.1097/SLA.0b013e31815aa2c2.
34. Rodgers MS, McCall JL. Surgery for colorectal liver metastases with hepatic lymph node involvement: a systematic review. Br J Surg. 2000;87:1142–55. https://doi.org/10.1046/j.1365-2168.2000.01580.x.
35. Rougier P, Van Cutsem E, Bajetta E, et al. Randomised trial of irinotecan versus fluorouracil by continuous infusion after fluorouracil failure in patients with metastatic colorectal cancer. Lancet. 1998;352:1407–12. https://doi.org/10.1016/S0140-6736(98)03085-2.
36. Viana EF, Herman P, Siqueira SC, et al. Lymphadenectomy in colorectal cancer liver metastases resection: incidence of hilar limph nodes micrometastasis. J Surg Oncol. 2009;100:534–7. https://doi.org/10.1002/jso.21357.

ALPPS for Colorectal Cancer Liver Metastases—Short and Long-Term Results

35

Kerollos Nashat Wanis, Bao Tram Nghiem, and Roberto Hernandez-Alejandro

The definition of resectability in liver surgery for colorectal liver metastases (CRLM) has undergone considerable evolution in the last few years. While previously characterized by conditions based on the number and size of metastases, resectability is now mainly determined by the ability to preserve a well-perfused and adequately functioning future liver remnant (FLR), with adequate biliary drainage [1, 2]. Advances in imaging, surgical technology, knowledge of hepatic anatomy, portal vein occlusion techniques, adjuvant therapies, and the understanding of liver regeneration have facilitated more aggressive treatment of CRLM. To address the specific limitation of a small predicted FLR, several strategies have been applied, including two-staged resection and portal vein occlusion.

Two-staged hepatectomy (TSH) for primarily unresectable colorectal liver metastases (CRLM) was first introduced in the 1990s and developed over the subsequent two decades. In 2000, Adam and colleagues published results from a series of patients who underwent TSH [3]. Prior to this, portal vein embolization (PVE) had been described, initially by Makuuchi in Japan, as a strategy for generating liver regeneration [4]. It was soon realized by Jaeck and colleagues that these techniques could be used in a complementary fashion, with PVE performed to accelerate hypertrophy of the FLR prior to the second stage of TSH [5].

While conventional TSH with PVE has facilitated successful curative resection in many patients with advanced CRLM, it has been limited because of its prolonged interstage waiting period (typically, 6–8 weeks) and the technical difficulty of successfully embolizing the right portal vein and segment IV portal vein branch. During

K. N. Wanis
Western University, London, ON, Canada
e-mail: Knwanis@g.harvard.edu

B. T. Nghiem · R. Hernandez-Alejandro (✉)
University of Rochester, Rochester, NY, USA
e-mail: cassie_nghiem@urmc.rochester.edu; roberto_hernandez@urmc.rochester.edu

M. M. Correia et al. (eds.), *Colorectal Cancer Liver Metastases*,
https://doi.org/10.1007/978-3-030-25486-5_35

the interstage period, following PVE, which typically takes 4–8 weeks, hypertrophy of the FLR occurs. Unfortunately, in approximately 30% of cases, the second stage of conventional TSH cannot be completed because of inadequate growth of the FLR or, more commonly, tumor progression during the interstage period, precluding curative resection [6, 7]. It has been suggested, but not proven, that short-interval disease progression allows for selection of only those patients with favorable tumor biology. Consequently, much attention has been devoted to improving the feasibility of TSH.

Within the past decade, associating liver partition and portal vein ligation for staged hepatectomy (ALPPS) has emerged as a modification of TSH with PVE, with the purpose of reducing the time interval between stages by accelerating and intensifying FLR hypertrophy. It addresses the main limitation of conventional TSH with PVE by ensuring that almost all patients can achieve the necessary hypertrophy and complete the second stage. Before it was formally elucidated in 2011 [8–10], ALPPS had been first performed unintentionally in 2007 during what was initially planned as an extended right hepatectomy for a perihilar cholangiocarcinoma [11]. Numerous centers have subsequently adopted the ALPPS technique in order to improve the feasibility of two-staged resection, and many modifications of the original technique have been proposed [12–15].

Operative Technique

The authors' description of classical ALPPS (Fig. 35.1) outlines the general approach. In stage I, exploratory laparotomy is performed with intraoperative assessment of resectability using intraoperative liver ultrasonography. If the metastases are resectable, cholecystectomy is performed followed by complete mobilization of the right lobe and caudate lobe, including ligation and division of small venous branches of the posterior segments and caudate lobe which drain directly into the inferior vena cava. At this point, the FLR (typically, the left lateral section) is cleared of metastases if necessary, and the right portal vein is ligated by approaching from behind the common hepatic duct, avoiding dissection of the hepatoduodenal ligament and preserving the right hepatic artery branches. In instances of portal vein trifurcation, the right posterior portal vein will usually be encountered before the right anterior and can be ligated. The right anterior portal vein can then often be encircled with careful dissection in the hilar plate, but occasionally it cannot be ligated safely using the hilar plate approach. In these cases, the parenchymal division should be started and the right anterior portal vein can be ligated as it is encountered during the liver transection. During ligation of the right portal vein, it is essential to avoid encircling and injuring the left portal vein.

The parenchymal division is begun just to the right of the falciform ligament, between segment IV and the left lateral section, targeting the right hilar plate and transecting all of the liver parenchyma until the retrohepatic inferior vena cava is visualized. Once the transection has been completed, the right and middle hepatic veins are preserved and encircled with vessel loops to aid dissection during the

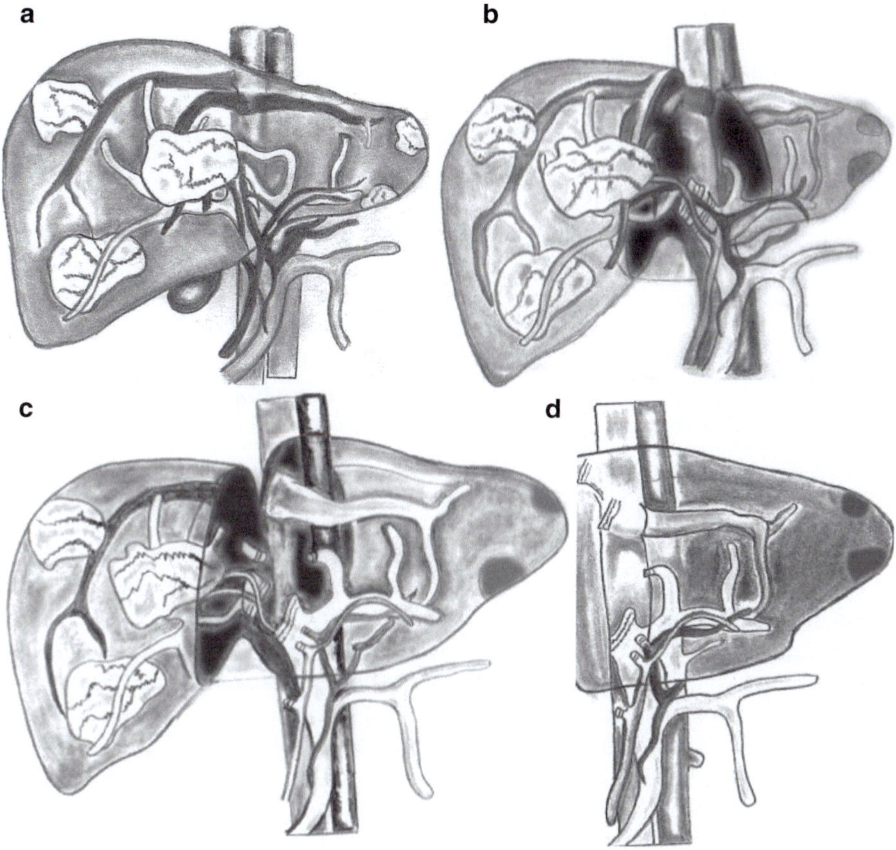

Fig. 35.1 (**a**) Extensive, challenging colorectal liver metastases, with a large central tumor and a small future liver remnant (FLR). Resection of the metastasis in the FLR (left lateral section) is required, with subsequent right trisectionectomy. ALPPS facilitates the necessary rapid hypertrophy of the FLR. (**b**) During ALPPS stage I, the metastasis in the left lateral section has been resected with a nonanatomic wedge resection, and an in situ parenchymal division has been performed starting anteriorly between segment IV and the left lateral section, targeting the right hilar plate. The right portal vein has been ligated along with the segment IV portal vein branch. Cholecystectomy is performed during the first stage. (**c**) Hypertrophy of the future liver remnant occurs during the interstage period. (**d**) Right trisectionectomy has been completed during stage II of ALPPS. The middle hepatic vein, right hepatic vein, right bile duct, and right hepatic artery have been ligated

second stage while avoiding congestion of the deportalized liver. Special attention should be paid to junction of middle and left hepatic vein, and intraoperative ultrasound is indispensable for defining the hepatic vein anatomy. Knowing that the left hepatic vein will be the only vein draining the FLR after completion of ALPPS, it may sometimes be prudent to leave a bridge of parenchyma in this junction to prevent injury. During the second stage, after confirming liver hypertrophy, division of the right hilar plate is performed followed by division of the right and middle hepatic veins. The extended right hepatectomy is then completed. Finally, the left lateral section is fixed to the anterior abdominal wall to prevent torsion and kinking of the vascular inflow or outflow of the liver. At this point, the patient has had complete resection of the metastatic disease.

Publication of the initial ALPPS technique generated considerable interest within the international hepatobiliary community. Many centers adopted the strategy in order to replicate the remarkable FLR hypertrophy and improve the feasibility of two-staged resection. The initial excitement was followed by controversy due to reports of unacceptable morbidity and mortality in many of the first published case series. Nonetheless, several centers continued to apply ALPPS, despite the initially concerning results, because of the possibility of completing the second stage of TSH in more patients. Over time, results improved in conjunction with modifications in diagnostic modalities, surgical technique, refinement of patient selection criteria, risk assessment during interstage management, and the introduction of technical variants.

Technique Variants

Several technical variations of the original ALPPS technique have been described, with the intention of minimizing short-term morbidity and mortality, while preserving the rapid and extensive hypertrophy achieved with portal vein ligation and complete parenchymal transection [14]. One of the challenges in in the classical ALPPS technique is avoidance of segment IV ischemia, and the resultant cascade of ischemia, necrosis, biliary leak, severe sepsis, and death. Segment IV receives its arterial supply from the left, middle, and right hepatic arteries, and is at high risk of ischemia following parenchymal transection [16]. Minimizing dissection of the hepatoduodenal ligament during stage I in order to preserve the middle hepatic artery or its branches, and prevent dearterialization of segment IV, especially IVb, is advocated [17]. Furthermore, three of the general ALPPS variants—the partial ALPPS, mini-ALPPS, and ALPPS with preservation of portal pedicles—can be considered in order to reduce the risk of segment IV necrosis, the technical difficulty of stage I, and, potentially, the morbidity of the overall operation; however, regarding techniques that focus on preservation of portal pedicles, it is worth noting that one of the main causes of inadequate hypertrophy following PVE is incomplete occlusion of the segment IV branches [18].

Partial ALPPS involves partial transection, usually at least 50% of the liver parenchyma, along the transection plane [19, 20]. Its advocates posit that the remarkable hypertrophy observed between ALPPS stages is mainly due to the production of circulating proliferative factors as a result of hepatic injury, and that partial transection generates an adequate growth stimulus without the major trauma of complete division [21, 22]. The caveat is that the transection must be completed later, making the second stage more difficult compared to classical ALPPS. Mini-ALPPS was subsequently proposed, and further reduces the dissection required during the first stage by combining partial transection with intraoperative portal vein embolization in order to minimize trauma to the hilar plate [23]. The rationale of this approach is to perform a more limited operation in the first stage, with the major operation reserved for the second stage—the inverse of classical ALPPS. Another approach, focusing on preserving the portal pedicles supplying segment IV, has been proposed [24]. In this technique, the portal pedicles are identified during parenchymal transection and their division is avoided with the intention of preventing segment IV necrosis. This is in contrast to TSH with PVE, in which specific occlusion of the segment IV portal vein branch is advocated in order to improve left lateral section hypertrophy and is tolerated without segment IV ischemia due to the absence of parenchymal division [18]. Lastly, in both classical ALPPS and its modifications, preservation of the middle hepatic vein in order to prevent postoperative venous congestion is advocated.

Other ALPPS modifications have further innovated beyond traditional liver parenchymal transection. A tourniquet modification, termed associating liver tourniquet and portal ligation for staged hepatectomy (ALTPS), involves positioning of a tourniquet around the liver at the level of the typical transection plane. Occlusion of collateral vessels is then confirmed with intraoperative ultrasound, and the entire parenchymal transection is reserved for the second stage [25]. Other alternatives, including microwave and radiofrequency ablation along the transection plane, have also been proposed and applied [14]. Of all the ALPPS variations proposed, only outcomes following the classical approach and partial ALPPS have been reported in the literature by multiple independent centers, and it is difficult to recommend any one approach over another. Nonetheless, several experts have advised that the extent of resection during the first stage should be minimized, with more centers tending to perform partial ALPPS in recent years [26, 27]. Despite this, the classical technique is still most widely used, and both of the common approaches (i.e., classical ALPPS and partial ALPPS) can be performed with acceptable morbidity and mortality in experienced centers following careful patient selection. The authors believe that while techniques focused on minimizing stage I reduce the surgical trauma of the first stage, the physiological insult (i.e., hepatic function) is not exacerbated with complete ALPPS since the deportalized liver remains inside the patient, providing some function, until the second stage in both cases.

Laparoscopic ALPPS

Laparoscopic and hand-assisted laparoscopic liver resection is considered feasible, safe, and similarly efficacious compared to open surgery for the treatment of CRLM [28–30]. Much less has been reported regarding the safety of laparoscopic ALPPS; however, laparoscopy has been used in one or both stages at some centers [31, 32]. Advantages to the laparoscopic approach include reducing the extent of adhesions following stage I, potentially reducing morbidity and minimizing the trauma of stage I, and improving visualization of the transection plane. Little evidence is available to confirm the safety and efficacy of laparoscopic ALPPS, and its application should be limited to centers with extensive experience in complex liver surgery and advanced hepatobiliary laparoscopy.

Simultaneous ALPPS and Colorectal Surgery

In patients with synchronously discovered colorectal cancer and liver metastases, multiple theoretical advantages of a simultaneous resection of the colorectal primary tumor and the CRLM exist. Simultaneous resection might reduce total treatment time, minimize the potential for disease progression, reduce overall anesthetic time, reduce length of hospital stay, and minimize the total time of chemotherapy. This approach to synchronous metastases has been usually reserved for patients without extensive hepatic tumors, and with good functional status, limiting the inferences possible from studies comparing simultaneous and staged resection [33, 34].

When ALPPS is combined with colorectal surgery, morbidity and mortality appear to be higher than after ALPPS alone, and this approach cannot be recommended [35]. It should only be considered at high-volume ALPPS centers, in select cases. Typically, a reverse approach (liver resection first) will be more appropriate in patients with synchronous metastasis, leaving the colorectal primary tumor to be addressed at a later date after the patient has recovered from ALPPS. In some cases, the primary tumor may even have complete clinical and pathological response to chemotherapy.

FLR Growth in ALPPS

Since ALPPS was discovered by accident and innovated in human patients, prior to development in experimental models, there has been great interest in replicating the accelerated FLR growth in the laboratory setting. Various animal models have now been explored in order to elucidate the mechanisms underlying the rapid FLR hypertrophy seen during the ALPPS interstage period. Several hypotheses have been proposed and tested without a consensus. The remarkable growth is likely due to a combination of factors, including an increase in circulating proliferative factors due to hepatic injury, prevention of collateral formation across the parenchymal divide, increase in contralateral portal vein flow and pressure, and venous congestion in the devitalized liver [21, 36–38]. In addition, the mechanisms previously understood in the context of partial hepatectomy and portal vein occlusion, which involve major hemodynamic shifts in both the arterial and portal venous systems, are also important mediators of cellular hyperplasia following ALPPS [39–41].

In one of the earliest models of ALPPS, Schelgel and colleagues injected plasma obtained from mice that had undergone complete parenchymal transection during ALPPS into mice that had undergone portal vein occlusion alone [21]. In the latter mice, injection of the ALPPS mouse plasma induced a comparable degree of hepatic hyperplasia as in the ALPPS mice themselves. Moreover, in mice that underwent portal vein occlusion and extrahepatic injury, such as ablation of the kidney, spleen, or lung, the FLR grew to a similar size as those who underwent hepatic transection. These findings have pointed to systemic release of proliferative markers as one of the major stimuli of regeneration following ALPPS stage I.

The rapid and robust liver regeneration seen in ALPPS has led to concerns about the possibility of accelerated tumor growth in the devitalized lobe. Moreover, there is disagreement within the hepatobiliary community regarding the advantages and disadvantages of the shortened interstage interval. While ostensibly desirable, some surgeons have argued that condensing the growth interval prevents the "test of time" and hinders clinical assessment of tumor biology. This hypothesis posits that patients who experience short interval disease progression in conventional two-staged hepatectomy, and do not proceed to the second stage, would have otherwise experienced early cancer recurrence, and therefore would not benefit from liver resection. The alternative viewpoint holds that completing the resection before major tumor progression can occur affords more patients the opportunity for potentially curative surgery.

Since we cannot identify which patients would have developed short-interval disease progression had they undergone conventional TSH with PVE rather than ALPPS, the "test of time" hypothesis remains unproven. Nonetheless, investigation of the histopathological features of tumors in the deportalized liver lobe has yielded insights into the oncological sequelae of liver partition. Currently, there is no evidence that tumor progression, as measured by immunohistochemical and histopathological markers of cellular proliferation, occurs differentially in ALPPS compared to conventional liver resection, or compared to liver resection following PVE, which may itself be associated with tumor growth [42–45].

Patient Selection

The trend in patient selection for ALPPS has followed an atypical pattern. During the initial learning curve for a new procedure, conservative selection criteria should be expected until the safety of the technique is proven. A different trend occurred following introduction of ALPPS, with many surgeons applying ALPPS in patients with fibrosis, in older patients, in patients who did not receive neoadjuvant chemotherapy, in those with high-risk non-CRLM tumors including primary hepatobiliary cancers, and in patients who did not require major FLR hypertrophy [12, 13, 27]. All of these factors contributed to the high morbidity and mortality initially reported by several centers. Over time, more caution has been applied leading to more stringent selection criteria for patients who might benefit from ALPPS with minimal risk [26].

Patient selection in ALPPS follows the same principles as for TSH with PVE. As for major hepatectomy in general, resectability in TSH requires preservation of two contiguous hepatic segments, preservation of adequate vascular inflow, outflow, and biliary drainage, and preserving >30% FLR after completion of both stages [1]. Other important oncological considerations in patients with CRLM include the feasibility of complete tumor resection with pathologically cancer-free margins, and the absence of extrahepatic disease, except for resectable lung metastases in selected patients. The intensified and accelerated hypertrophy generated by the ALPPS approach has subverted some of these considerations and, in some cases, a single healthy liver segment may be sufficient. These heterogenous resections have been classified as monosegment ALPPS, and the variations are named after the segment constituting the FLR [46].

Specific criteria for ALPPS include oncological factors, patient characteristics, and technical considerations. Besides the absence of nonresectable extrahepatic metastases, patients should have radiographical and biochemical (serum carcinoembryonic antigen, CEA, level) evidence of response to systemic chemotherapy after 4–6 cycles in order to justify two major operations, excellent functional status, and absence of major medical comorbidities. The technical considerations in ALPPS are the same as for TSH with PVE. Patients typically have bilateral, extensive CRLM with an FLR initially less than 30%, requiring significant hypertrophy in order to achieve curative resection. Response to chemotherapy is an important marker prior to liver resection for CRLM, and especially for patients who are undergoing ALPPS since the truncated interstage period limits assessment of tumor biology. Patients who experience progression while receiving chemotherapy are at high risk of recurrence, and ALPPS cannot be recommended [47]. Moreover, neoadjuvant treatment should generally be limited to 4–6 cycles of chemotherapy to limit the possibility of parenchymal injury and decrease the postoperative complication rate. If more cycles of systemic chemotherapy are planned, they can be completed following the second stage.

In addition to the previously mentioned selection factors, evidence and expert opinion suggest that older patients, over the age of 67 years, have significantly worse outcomes [12, 27]. Supporting this, a trend towards selection of younger patients, and those with CRLM, as opposed to primary hepatobiliary tumors, has been correlated with a dramatic yearly reduction in morbidity and mortality rates at centers with considerable ALPPS experience. In some cases, ALPPS can be justified in older patients with excellent performance status and no major comorbidities. At the senior author's center, a handful of patients above the age of 70 years, selected with excellent functional status, have undergone ALPPS with minimal morbidity and no mortality. Better refinement in patient selection may be possible with tools such as KRAS mutation status, which has been shown to predict recurrence-free and overall survival in patients with CRLM. This may be particularly useful for patients with extensive metastases for whom two-staged resection is being contemplated [48].

Interstage Management

The interstage period is a sensitive interval in the treatment of patients undergoing ALPPS. Data from several ALPPS centers have indicated that patients who suffer major complications following the first stage are at significantly increased risk of death if they proceed to the second stage [12, 13, 35, 49]. In one multicenter study, 36% of patients who had a major complication in stage I died following stage II [49]. As expected, based on these reports, major trends at experienced centers towards reducing interstage complications over time have been associated with vastly improved overall outcomes [27]. Other important interstage markers besides major complications have also been shown to predict stage II outcomes. Patients with a model for end-stage liver disease (MELD) score of at least 10, or liver failure by the International Study Group for Liver Surgery criteria, during the interstage interval have an elevated risk of mortality. Furthermore, major elevations in bilirubin and creatinine levels before the second stage might be predictors of mortality, even if liver failure criteria are not met. However, most patients experience minor, transient increases in bilirubin and/or creatinine, so these laboratory values should be interpreted within the broader clinical context [12]. Whether it is in a high-risk patient's best interest to proceed to the second stage rather than abandon completion of ALPPS is a matter of ongoing controversy; however, delaying or abandoning stage II should be contemplated for those who suffer major complications and/or have definitive evidence of liver failure.

Accelerated hypertrophy in ALPPS, due to the mechanisms hypothesized and discussed earlier in this chapter, allows for truncation of the several-week hypertrophy time usually seen in conventional TSH with PVE. The rapid and extensive FLR growth is similar to the growth rate observed in living liver donors and can often facilitate completion of the two-staged resection in as little as several days, and typically within 2 weeks [50]. While this is a major advantage of ALPPS as a modification on the conventional TSH technique, it remains unclear whether the FLR volume regeneration during the interstage period correlates with an appropriate increase in remnant liver function. How FLR volume and function can be most accurately measured prior to the second stage is an area of active investigation.

Computed tomography (CT) volumetry or magnetic resonance imaging should be used to measure the absolute volume of the FLR and calculate the standardized FLR, which is the proportion defined as the FLR volume divided by the estimated total liver volume (TLV) [51]. The TLV can be estimated using CT volumetry, but often formula-based estimates using body surface area or body weight are used as they are more accurate when multiple liver lesions, potentially with ill-defined borders, are present [52–54]. CT imaging should be obtained both before the first stage and before the planned second stage, in order to estimate the FLR growth and should be combined with an assessment of the FLR function. Typically, a near-doubling in the FLR volume can be observed within 1 week of stage I completion [12, 50, 55].

Quantitative assessment of FLR function using hepatobiliary scintigraphy is emerging as an important component of preoperative decision making in major liver resection, and has potential as a tool to complement clinical decision making in the ALPPS interstage period [56, 57]. While there is consensus on a target FLR volume of 30%, there is insufficient evidence on which to base a recommended FLR function threshold beyond which the second stage can be safely completed [58, 59]. Uptake in the use of hepatobiliary scintigraphy (HBS) at several high-volume ALPPS centers has uncovered a concerning lack of correlation between FLR volume growth and function gain [55]. Moreover, volume gains far outpace increases in FLR function as measured by scintigraphy. This is particularly concerning since the majority of patients who suffer perioperative mortality following ALPPS have evidence of liver failure by one of the accepted liver failure definitions [12]. HBS using 99-Technetium-labeled (99mTc)-Mebrofenin has been used to predict postoperative liver failure when planning liver resection, and is being explored as a useful adjunct to volume measurement in ALPPS [57, 60, 61].

Expanded use of existing tools for measuring FLR function and development of other techniques will be necessary to better improve the safety profile of major liver resection, including conventional TSH and ALPPS. Indocyanine green (ICG) retention rate at 15 minutes is one such technique. It has been used preoperatively to identify patients, with and without chronic liver disease, who can safely undergo liver resection [62, 63]. More recently, an intraoperative protocol has been described which provides real-time information for decision making [64]. The procedure involves measurement of ICG plasma disappearance rate after clamping of the arterial and portal inflow to the segments that will be resected. The FLR function measurements during clamping correlate well with measurements following actual resection, which implies that trial clamping and ICG measurement can be used to predict posthepatectomy liver failure prior to committing to resection. This has yet to be applied in the two-staged hepatectomy setting, but might facilitate identification of patients for whom stage II should be delayed or abandoned. Ultimately, there remains a paucity of data regarding quantitative assessment of FLR function in ALPPS, but several institutions are actively engaged in investigating this topic and more data is anticipated.

Short-Term Outcomes

During the early period of ALPPS adoption, several single-institution studies were published reporting high morbidity and mortality [65–68]. Larger, multicenter and registry-based studies also raised concerns about perioperative outcomes, with 90-day mortality reported at 9–17% [13, 27, 69]. Because of these concerns, the role of ALPPS in the treatment of patients with initially unresectable CRLM has continued to be controversial. During this time period, other institutions described their experiences with ALPPS, with some cohorts experiencing minimal severe morbidity and zero perioperative mortality while achieving near-100% feasibility of second-stage completion and high R0 resection rates [17, 22, 70–72]. Much of the subsequent literature has been focused on identifying patient selection criteria and operative techniques that can facilitate safe resection, with low morbidity and mortality, while taking advantage of the improved feasibility of ALPPS compared to classical TSH (Table 35.1).

Data from the International ALPPS Registry has helped to guide recommendations by shedding light on important risk factors for mortality following ALPPS. The main preoperative predictors of perioperative death are age greater than 67 years and resection for primary hepatobiliary tumors [12, 13, 73]. We and others have argued that many of the poor outcomes initially reported were due to application of ALPPS in patients with non-CRLM tumors and in too many older patients with suboptimal functional or comorbid status (elevated eastern cooperative oncology group (ECOG) or american society of anesthesiologists (ASA) status). Most institutions have now adjusted their approach to patient selection for ALPPS, and recent evidence

Table 35.1 Short-term outcomes from multicenter studies and major ALPPS registry reports

Author	Year of publication[a]	Morbidity[b]	Mortality[d]
Wanis et al.	2017	12/58 (21%)	0 (0%)
Sandström et al.	2017	19/44 (43%)[c]	4/48 (8.3%)
Linecker et al.	2017	14/68 (21%)	7/68 (10%)
Linecker et al.	2016	–	47/528 (8.9%)
Kambakamba et al.	2016	9/43 (21%)	5/43 (12%)
Serenari et al.	2016	27/50 (54%)[c]	20/50 (20%)
Björnsson et al.	2016	3/22 (14%)	1/22 (4.5%)
Røsok et al.	2016	4/36 (11%)	1/36 (2.8%)
Schadde et al.	2015	–	28/320 (8.8%)
Truant et al.	2015	25/62 (40%)[c]	8/62 (13%)
Ratti et al.	2015	5/12 (42%)[c]	1/12 (8.3%)
Schadde et al.	2014	56/202 (28%)	19/202 (9.4%)
Schadde et al.	2014	–	7/48 (15%)
Torres et al.	2013	23/39 (59%)	5/39 (13%)
Schnitzbauer et al.	2012	9/25 (36%)	3/25 (12%)

[a]Year of first availability online if still in press
[b]Clavien–Dindo ≥3b unless otherwise indicated with [c]
[c]Clavien–Dindo ≥3a
[d]90-day or in-hospital perioperative mortality—the higher of the two is displayed if both were reported

demonstrates a trend towards younger patients, fewer patients with biliary tumors, and greater consideration of comorbid and functional assessments. This trend is correlated with dramatic improvements in perioperative outcomes, with 90-day mortality dropping from 17% in the first year of reported cases to 3.8% in 2015 [27]. As such, if ALPPS is contemplated for non-CRLM indications or in older patients, it should be considered on a case-by-case basis with multidisciplinary input in order to ensure that high-risk patients are not undergoing ALPPS for little potential benefit.

ALPPS Compared to Conventional TSH

Directly comparing conventional TSH with ALPPS is difficult because some surgeons, and even institutions, perform one but not the other, and at centers where both procedures are performed, selection criteria usually vary. This makes adjustment for provider and patient differences challenging and likely confounds comparisons of observational data. Moreover, ALPPS is a new technique still in relative infancy and variations in outcomes over time due to the learning curve may lead to conflicting results depending on which data, and from what time period, is used for comparison to TSH. Two recent meta-analyses have compared the approaches and have concluded that ALPPS has significantly better FLR kinetic growth rate and second-stage completion rate, but at the cost of higher morbidity and mortality [74, 75]. In light of these preliminary comparisons, both ALPPS and conventional TSH seem to be useful strategies, with unique advantages and disadvantages, for increasing the feasibility of resection in patients with bilobar, extensive CRLM when it is oncologically justified.

Until currently, there was no experimental evidence comparing ALPPS with conventional TSH; however, a recent multicenter randomized controlled trial, recruiting 92 patients, found no difference in major complications or 90-day mortality comparing the two approaches [76]. Furthermore, 92% of patients in the ALPPS arm achieved the standardized FLR volume target of 30% prior to the second stage, while only 57% of those in the conventional TSH arm achieved the target. Most of those who failed to reach the volume target underwent salvage ALPPS, a strategy in which parenchymal transection is used to stimulate FLR growth in patients for whom PVE was inadequate [77]. More data is anticipated from ongoing randomized trials, with long-term outcome comparisons forthcoming.

Long-Term Outcomes

Although much has been said about perioperative outcomes, less is known about long-term survival following ALPPS. Data from single-institution cohorts suggest that oncological outcomes are similar to those following TSH with PVE. Studies of conventional TSH report median survivals of 24–44 months, with disease-free survivals of 6–27% at 3 years following surgery [6]. Likewise, in two studies reporting intermediate-term survival, patients who underwent ALPPS for CRLM had 59% 2-year and 50% 3-year overall survival with 13% 3-year disease-free survival from the date of surgery [78, 79]. Reassuringly, patients who complete ALPPS have similar quality of life at follow-up compared to the general population, consistent with the experience of other patients who undergo less extensive liver resection [79–82].

Further Innovation

In some patients, neither ALPPS nor conventional TSH would achieve complete resection of all liver metastases. For these cases, the only option has traditionally been palliative chemotherapy; however, in recent years, Norweigan investigators have leveraged their fortunate organ donor situation to explore the potential for total hepatectomy and liver transplantation in selected patients. Despite high rates of early recurrence (median disease-free survival (DFS) of 10 months), an overall survival of 56–60% was observed at 5 years posttransplant [83, 84]. Nonetheless, liver transplantation for CRLM is not popular due to the shortage of grafts in most countries.

Recent developments, integrating concepts learned from ALPPS, may challenge existing practices. An innovative approach termed resection and partial liver segment II/III transplantation with delayed total hepatectomy (RAPID) was described in 2015. It extrapolates on the concept of split liver transplantation, in which an extended right graft is allocated to an adult recipient while the complementary segments II and III are transplanted in a pediatric recipient. When a pediatric recipient is not available, the segment II/III graft may be allocated to an adult with nonresectable CRLM. In the first operation, segments I–III are resected, the segment II/III graft is implanted, and the right portal vein is ligated. Right extended hepatectomy is later performed after the graft achieves adequate volume and function [85]. Nadalin and colleagues have extended this same concept to living donor liver donation, using a segment II/III graft from a live donor [86]. While these kinds of innovations require further scientific and ethical scrutiny, they are examples of potential surgical solutions for patients with extensive metastatic colorectal cancer, and illustrate how the principles learned from ALPPS might even be applied to solve nononcological problems.

Conclusion

ALPPS is an innovative modification on the conventional TSH with portal vein occlusion technique that increases resectability. Despite initial controversy, recent data suggests considerable improvements in morbidity and mortality with assiduous patient selection, risk factor assessment in the interstage period, and alterations in operative technique. While many approaches exist (e.g., partial ALPPS, mini ALPPS, complete ALPPS), outcomes can be optimized regardless of the technique chosen if interstage complications are minimized. ALPPS expands the feasibility of two-staged resection to almost all patients who are candidates for the procedure, and at experienced centers it can be performed with low perioperative morbidity and minimal mortality, resulting in good patient survival with preserved quality of life, as recent evidence has shown.

References

1. Charnsangavej C, Clary B, Fong Y, Grothey A, Pawlik TM, Choti MA. Selection of patients for resection of hepatic colorectal metastases: expert consensus statement. Ann Surg Oncol. 2006;13:1261–8.
2. Rocha FG, Helton WS. Resectability of colorectal liver metastases: an evolving definition. HPB. 2012;14:283–4.
3. Adam R, Laurent A, Azoulay D, Castaing D, Bismuth H. Two-stage hepatectomy: a planned strategy to treat irresectable liver tumors. Ann Surg. 2000;232:777–85.
4. Makuuchi M, Thai BL, Takayasu K, Takayama T, Kosuge T, Gunvén P, Yamazaki S, Hasegawa H, Ozaki H. Preoperative portal embolization to increase safety of major hepatectomy for hilar bile duct carcinoma: a preliminary report. Surgery. 1990;107:521–7.
5. Jaeck D, Oussoultzoglou E, Rosso E, Greget M, Weber J-C, Bachellier P. A two-stage hepatectomy procedure combined with portal vein embolization to achieve curative resection for initially unresectable multiple and bilobar colorectal liver metastases. Ann Surg. 2004;240:1037–51.
6. Lam VWT, Laurence JM, Johnston E, Hollands MJ, Pleass HCC, Richardson AJ. A systematic review of two-stage hepatectomy in patients with initially unresectable colorectal liver metastases. HPB. 2013;15:483–91.
7. Chua TC, Liauw W, Chu F, Morris DL. Summary outcomes of two-stage resection for advanced colorectal liver metastases: two-stage resection of CLM. J Surg Oncol. 2013;107:211–6.
8. Baumgart J, Lang S, Lang H. A new method for induction of liver hypertrophy prior to right trisectionectomy: a report of three cases. HPB (Oxford). 2011;13(suppl 2):1–145.

9. de Santibañes E, Alvarez FA, Ardiles V. How to avoid postoperative liver failure: a novel method. World J Surg. 2011;36:125–8.
10. Schnitzbauer AA, Lang SA, Goessmann H, et al. Right portal vein ligation combined with in situ splitting induces rapid left lateral liver lobe hypertrophy enabling 2-staged extended right hepatic resection in small-for-size settings. Ann Surg. 2012;255:405–14.
11. de Santibañes E, Clavien P-A. Playing Play-Doh to prevent postoperative liver failure: the "ALPPS" approach. Ann Surg. 2012;255:415–7.
12. Schadde E, Raptis DA, Schnitzbauer AA, et al. Prediction of mortality after ALPPS stage-1: an analysis of 320 patients from the International ALPPS Registry. Ann Surg. 2015;262:780–6.
13. Schadde E, Ardiles V, Robles-Campos R, et al. Early survival and safety of Associating Liver Partition and Portal Vein Ligation for Staged Hepatectomy (ALPPS): first report of the International ALPPS Registry. Ann Surg. 2014;260:829–38.
14. Peng S-Y, Wang X-A, Huang C-Y, Zhang Y-Y, Li J-T, Hong D-F, Cai X-J. Evolution of associating liver partition and portal vein ligation for staged hepatectomy: simpler, safer and equally effective methods. World J Gastroenterol. 2017;23:4140.
15. Edmondson MJ, Sodergren MH, Pucher PH, Darzi A, Li J, Petrowsky H, Campos RR, Serrablo A, Jiao LR. Variations and adaptations of associated liver partition and portal vein ligation for staged hepatectomy (ALPPS): many routes to the summit. Surgery. 2016;159:1058–72.
16. Alghamdi T, Viebahn C, Justinger C, Lorf T. Arterial blood supply of liver segment IV and its possible surgical consequences. Am J Transplant. 2017;17:1064–70.
17. Hernandez-Alejandro R, Bertens KA, Pineda-Solis K, Croome KP. Can we improve the morbidity and mortality associated with the associating liver partition with portal vein ligation for staged hepatectomy (ALPPS) procedure in the management of colorectal liver metastases? Surgery. 2015;157:194–201.
18. Mise Y, Aloia TA, Conrad C, Huang SY, Wallace MJ, Vauthey J-N. Volume regeneration of segments 2 and 3 after right portal vein embolization in patients undergoing two-stage hepatectomy. J Gastrointest Surg. 2015;19:133–41.
19. Petrowsky H, Györi G, de Oliveira M, Lesurtel M, Clavien P-A. Is partial-ALPPS safer than ALPPS? A single-center experience. Ann Surg. 2015;261:e90–2.
20. Linecker M, Kambakamba P, Reiner CS, et al. How much liver needs to be transected in ALPPS? A translational study investigating the concept of less invasiveness. Surgery. 2017;161:453–64.
21. Schlegel A, Lesurtel M, Melloul E, Limani P, Tschuor C, Graf R, Humar B, Clavien PA. Associating Liver Partition and Portal Vein Ligation for Staged Hepatectomy (ALPPS): from human to mice highlighting accelerated and novel mechanisms of liver regeneration. Ann Surg. 2014;260:839–47.
22. Alvarez FA, Ardiles V, de Santibañes M, Pekolj J, de Santibañes E. Associating liver partition and portal vein ligation for staged hepatectomy offers high oncological feasibility with adequate patient safety: a prospective study at a single center. Ann Surg. 2015;261:723–32.
23. de Santibañes E, Alvarez FA, Ardiles V, Pekolj J, de Santibañes M. Inverting the ALPPS paradigm by minimizing first stage impact: the Mini-ALPPS technique. Langenbeck's Arch Surg. 2016;401:557–63.
24. Tanaka K, Kikuchi Y, Kawaguchi D, Murakami T, Hiroshima Y, Matsuo K. Modified ALPPS procedures avoiding division of portal pedicles. Ann Surg. 2017;265:e14–20.
25. Robles R, Parrilla P, López-Conesa A, Brusadin R, de la Peña J, Fuster M, García-López JA, Hernández E. Tourniquet modification of the associating liver partition and portal ligation for staged hepatectomy procedure. Br J Surg. 2014;101:1129–34.
26. Oldhafer KJ, Stavrou GA, van Gulik TM. ALPPS—where do we stand, where do we go?: eight recommendations from the first international expert meeting. Ann Surg. 2016;263:839–41.
27. Linecker M, Björnsson B, Stavrou GA, et al. Risk adjustment in ALPPS is associated with a dramatic decrease in early mortality and morbidity. Ann Surg. 2017;266:779–86.
28. Schiffman SC, Kim KH, Tsung A, Marsh JW, Geller DA. Laparoscopic versus open liver resection for metastatic colorectal cancer: a metaanalysis of 610 patients. Surgery. 2015;157:211–22.

29. Nachmany I, Pencovich N, Zohar N, Ben-Yehuda A, Binyamin C, Goykhman Y, Lubezky N, Nakache R, Klausner JM. Laparoscopic versus open liver resection for metastatic colorectal cancer. Eur J Surg Oncol. 2015;41:1615–20.
30. Parks KR, Kuo Y, Davis JM, O'Brien B, Hagopian EJ. Laparoscopic versus open liver resection: a meta-analysis of long-term outcome. HPB. 2014;16:109–18.
31. Machado MAC, Makdissi FF, Surjan RC. Totally laparoscopic ALPPS is feasible and may be worthwhile. Ann Surg. 2012;256:e13; author reply e16–19.
32. Machado MAC, Makdissi FF, Surjan RC, Basseres T, Schadde E. Transition from open to laparoscopic ALPPS for patients with very small FLR: the initial experience. HPB. 2017;19:59–66.
33. Yin Z, Liu C, Chen Y, Bai Y, Shang C, Yin R, Yin D, Wang J. Timing of hepatectomy in resectable synchronous colorectal liver metastases (SCRLM): simultaneous or delayed? Hepatology. 2013;57:2346–57.
34. Kelly ME, Spolverato G, Lê GN, Mavros MN, Doyle F, Pawlik TM, Winter DC. Synchronous colorectal liver metastasis: a network meta-analysis review comparing classical, combined, and liver-first surgical strategies: synchronous colorectal liver metastasis. J Surg Oncol. 2015;111:341–51.
35. Wanis KN, Buac S, Linecker M, Ardiles V, Tun-Abraham ME, Robles-Campos R, Malago M, de Santibañes E, Clavien P-A, Hernandez-Alejandro R. Patient survival after simultaneous ALPPS and colorectal resection. World J Surg. 2016;41:1119–25.
36. Andersen KJ, Knudsen AR, Jepsen BN, Meier M, Gunnarsson APA, Jensen UB, Nyengaard JR, Hamilton-Dutoit S, Mortensen FV. A new technique for accelerated liver regeneration: an experimental study in rats. Surgery. 2017;162:233–47.
37. Deal R, Frederiks C, Williams L, Olthof PB, Dirscherl K, Keutgen X, Chan E, Deziel D, Hertl M, Schadde E. Rapid liver hypertrophy after portal vein occlusion correlates with the degree of collateralization between lobes—a study in pigs. J Gastrointest Surg. 2018;22:203–13.
38. Kawaguchi D, Hiroshima Y, Kikuchi Y, Matsuo K, Tanaka K. Associating liver partition and portal vein occlusion, including venous congestion, induction in rats. Anticancer Res. 2017;37:2919–25.
39. Michalopoulos GK. Liver regeneration. J Cell Physiol. 2007;213:286–300.
40. Kito Y, Nagino M, Nimura Y. Doppler sonography of hepatic arterial blood flow velocity after percutaneous transhepatic portal vein embolization. Am J Roentgenol. 2001;176:909–12.
41. Eipel C. Regulation of hepatic blood flow: the hepatic arterial buffer response revisited. World J Gastroenterol. 2010;16:6046.
42. Tanaka K, Endo I. Associating Liver Partition and Portal Vein Ligation for Staged Hepatectomy (ALPPS): short-term outcome and functional changes in the future liver remnant. Ann Surg. 2014;262:e88–9.
43. de Graaf W, van den Esschert JW, van Lienden KP, van Gulik TM. Induction of tumor growth after preoperative portal vein embolization: is it a real problem? Ann Surg Oncol. 2009;16:423–30.
44. Joechle K, Moser C, Ruemmele P, Schmidt KM, Werner JM, Geissler EK, Schlitt HJ, Lang SA. ALPPS (associating liver partition and portal vein ligation for staged hepatectomy) does not affect proliferation, apoptosis, or angiogenesis as compared to standard liver resection for colorectal liver metastases. World J Surg Oncol. 2017;15:57. https://doi.org/10.1186/s12957-017-1121-8.
45. Kambakamba P, Linecker M, Schneider M, et al. Impact of associating liver partition and portal vein ligation for staged hepatectomy (ALPPS) on growth of colorectal liver metastases. Surgery. 2017;15:57.
46. Schadde E, Malagó M, Hernandez-Alejandro R, Li J, Abdalla E, Ardiles V, Lurje G, Vyas S, Machado MA, de Santibañes E. Monosegment ALPPS hepatectomy: extending resectability by rapid hypertrophy. Surgery. 2015;157:676–89.
47. Adam R, Pascal G, Castaing D, Azoulay D, Delvart V, Paule B, Levi F, Bismuth H. Tumor progression while on chemotherapy: a contraindication to liver resection for multiple colorectal metastases? Ann Surg. 2004;240:1052–64.

48. Brudvik KW, Kopetz SE, Li L, Conrad C, Aloia TA, Vauthey J-N. Meta-analysis of *KRAS* mutations and survival after resection of colorectal liver metastases: *KRAS* status and survival after resection of colorectal liver metastases. Br J Surg. 2015;102:1175–83.
49. Truant S, Scatton O, Dokmak S, et al. Associating liver partition and portal vein ligation for staged hepatectomy (ALPPS): impact of the inter-stages course on morbi-mortality and implications for management. Eur J Surg Oncol. 2015;41:674–82.
50. Croome KP, Hernandez-Alejandro R, Parker M, Heimbach J, Rosen C, Nagorney DM. Is the liver kinetic growth rate in ALPPS unprecedented when compared with PVE and living donor liver transplant? A multicentre analysis. HPB. 2015;17:477–84.
51. Heymsfield SB, Fulenwider T, Nordlinger B, Barlow R, Sones P, Kutner M. Accurate measurement of liver, kidney, and spleen volume and mass by computerized axial tomography. Ann Intern Med. 1979;90:185–7.
52. Pomposelli JJ, Tongyoo A, Wald C, Pomfret EA. Variability of standard liver volume estimation versus software-assisted total liver volume measurement. Liver Transpl. 2012;18:1083–92.
53. Vauthey J-N, Abdalla EK, Doherty DA, et al. Body surface area and body weight predict total liver volume in Western adults. Liver Transpl. 2002;8:233–40.
54. Johnson TN, Tucker GT, Tanner MS, Rostami-Hodjegan A. Changes in liver volume from birth to adulthood: a meta-analysis. Liver Transpl. 2005;11:1481–93.
55. Olthof PB, Tomassini F, Huespe PE, et al. Hepatobiliary scintigraphy to evaluate liver function in associating liver partition and portal vein ligation for staged hepatectomy: liver volume overestimates liver function. Surgery. 2017;162:775–83.
56. Chapelle T, Op De Beeck B, Huyghe I, Francque S, Driessen A, Roeyen G, Ysebaert D, De Greef K. Future remnant liver function estimated by combining liver volumetry on magnetic resonance imaging with total liver function on 99mTc-mebrofenin hepatobiliary scintigraphy: can this tool predict post-hepatectomy liver failure? HPB. 2016;18:494–503.
57. de Graaf W, van Lienden KP, Dinant S, Roelofs JJTH, Busch ORC, Gouma DJ, Bennink RJ, van Gulik TM. Assessment of future remnant liver function using hepatobiliary scintigraphy in patients undergoing major liver resection. J Gastrointest Surg. 2010;14:369–78.
58. Kishi Y, Abdalla EK, Chun YS, Zorzi D, Madoff DC, Wallace MJ, Curley SA, Vauthey J-N. Three hundred and one consecutive extended right hepatectomies: evaluation of outcome based on systematic liver volumetry. Trans Meet Am Surg Assoc. 2009;127:171–9.
59. Shindoh J, Vauthey J-N, Zimmitti G, Curley SA, Huang SY, Mahvash A, Gupta S, Wallace MJ, Aloia TA. Analysis of the efficacy of portal vein embolization for patients with extensive liver malignancy and very low future liver remnant volume, including a comparison with the associating liver partition with portal vein ligation for staged hepatectomy approach. J Am Coll Surg. 2013;217:126–33.
60. Bennink RJ, Dinant S, Erdogan D, Heijnen BH, Straatsburg IH, van Vliet AK, van Gulik TM. Preoperative assessment of postoperative remnant liver function using hepatobiliary scintigraphy. J Nucl Med. 2004;45:965–71.
61. Serenari M, Collaud C, Alvarez FA, de Santibañes M, Giunta D, Pekolj J, Ardiles V, de Santibañes E. Interstage assessment of remnant liver function in ALPPS using hepatobiliary scintigraphy: prediction of posthepatectomy liver failure and introduction of the HIBA index. Ann Surg. 2018;267:1141. https://doi.org/10.1097/SLA.0000000000002150.
62. de Liguori CN, O'Reilly DA, Dajani K, Ghaneh P, Poston GJ, Wu AV. Perioperative use of the LiMON method of indocyanine green elimination measurement for the prediction and early detection of post-hepatectomy liver failure. Eur J Surg Oncol. 2009;35:957–62.
63. Cheung TT, Chan SC, Chok KSH, Chan ACY, Yu WC, Poon RTP, Lo CM, Fan ST. Rapid measurement of indocyanine green retention by pulse spectrophotometry: a validation study in 70 patients with Child-Pugh A cirrhosis before hepatectomy for hepatocellular carcinoma. Hepatobiliary Pancreat Dis Int. 2012;11:267–71.
64. Thomas MN, Weninger E, Angele M, et al. Intraoperative simulation of remnant liver function during anatomic liver resection with indocyanine green clearance (LiMON) measurements. HPB. 2015;17:471–6.

65. Ratti F, Cipriani F, Gagliano A, Catena M, Paganelli M, Aldrighetti L. Defining indications to ALPPS procedure: technical aspects and open issues. Updat Surg. 2013;66:41–9.
66. Torres OJM, Fernandes Ede SM, CVC O, Lima CX, Waechter FL, JMA M-J, Linhares MM, Pinto RD, Herman P, MAC M. Associating liver partition and portal vein ligation for staged hepatectomy (ALPPS): the Brazilian experience. Arq Bras Cir Dig. 2013;26:40–3.
67. Li J, Girotti P, Königsrainer I, Ladurner R, Königsrainer A, Nadalin S. ALPPS in right trisectionectomy: a safe procedure to avoid postoperative liver failure? J Gastrointest Surg. 2013;17:956–61.
68. Nadalin S, Capobianco I, Li J, Girotti P, Königsrainer I, Königsrainer A. Indications and limits for associating liver partition and portal vein ligation for staged hepatectomy (ALPPS). Lessons Learned from 15 cases at a single centre. Z Gastroenterol. 2014;52:35–42.
69. Schadde E, Ardiles V, Slankamenac K, et al. ALPPS offers a better chance of complete resection in patients with primarily unresectable liver tumors compared with conventional-staged hepatectomies: results of a multicenter analysis. World J Surg. 2014;38:1510–9.
70. Sala S, Ardiles V, Ulla M, Alvarez F, Pekolj J, de Santibañes E. Our initial experience with ALPPS technique: encouraging results. Updat Surg. 2012;64:167–72.
71. Oldhafer KJ, Donati M, Jenner RM, Stang A, Stavrou GA. ALPPS for patients with colorectal liver metastases: effective liver hypertrophy, but early tumor recurrence. World J Surg. 2013;38:1504–9.
72. Røsok BI, Björnsson B, Sparrelid E, Hasselgren K, Pomianowska E, Gasslander T, Bjørnbeth BA, Isaksson B, Sandström P. Scandinavian multicenter study on the safety and feasibility of the associating liver partition and portal vein ligation for staged hepatectomy procedure. Surgery. 2016;159:1279–86.
73. Linecker M, Stavrou GA, Oldhafer KJ, et al. The ALPPS risk score: avoiding futile use of ALPPS. Ann Surg. 2016;264:763–71.
74. Eshmuminov D, Raptis DA, Linecker M, Wirsching A, Lesurtel M, Clavien P-A. Meta-analysis of associating liver partition with portal vein ligation and portal vein occlusion for two-stage hepatectomy: ALPPS *versus* portal vein occlusion for staged hepatectomy. Br J Surg. 2016;103:1768–82.
75. Moris D, Ronnekleiv-Kelly S, Kostakis ID, Tsilimigras DI, Beal EW, Papalampros A, Dimitroulis D, Felekouras E, Pawlik TM. Operative results and oncologic outcomes of Associating Liver Partition and Portal Vein Ligation for Staged Hepatectomy (ALPPS) versus two-stage hepatectomy (TSH) in patients with unresectable colorectal liver metastases: a systematic review and meta-analysis. World J Surg. 2018;42:806–15.
76. Sandström P, Røsok BI, Sparrelid E, et al. ALPPS improves resectability compared with conventional two-stage hepatectomy in patients with advanced colorectal liver metastasis: results from a Scandinavian Multicenter Randomized Controlled Trial (LIGRO Trial). Ann Surg. 2018;267:833. https://doi.org/10.1097/SLA.0000000000002511.
77. Tschuor C, Croome KP, Sergeant G, et al. Salvage parenchymal liver transection for patients with insufficient volume increase after portal vein occlusion – an extension of the ALPPS approach. Eur J Surg Oncol. 2013;39:1230–5.
78. Björnsson B, Sparrelid E, Røsok B, Pomianowska E, Hasselgren K, Gasslander T, Bjørnbeth BA, Isaksson B, Sandström P. Associating liver partition and portal vein ligation for staged hepatectomy in patients with colorectal liver metastases – intermediate oncological results. Eur J Surg Oncol. 2016;42:531–7.
79. Wanis KN, Ardiles V, Alvarez FA, Tun-Abraham ME, Linehan D, de Santibañes E, Hernandez-Alejandro R. Intermediate-term survival and quality of life outcomes in patients with advanced colorectal liver metastases undergoing associating liver partition and portal vein ligation for staged hepatectomy. Surgery. 2018;163:691–7.
80. Rees JR, Blazeby JM, Brookes ST, John T, Welsh FK, Rees M. Patient-reported outcomes in long-term survivors of metastatic colorectal cancer needing liver resection. Br J Surg. 2014;101:1468–74.
81. Langenhoff BS, Krabbe PFM, Peerenboom L, Wobbes T, Ruers TJM. Quality of life after surgical treatment of colorectal liver metastases. Br J Surg. 2006;93:1007–14.

82. Rees JR, Blazeby JM, Fayers P, Friend EA, Welsh FKS, John TG, Rees M. Patient-reported outcomes after hepatic resection of colorectal cancer metastases. J Clin Oncol. 2012;30:1364–70.
83. Hagness M, Foss A, Line P-D, et al. Liver transplantation for nonresectable liver metastases from colorectal cancer. Ann Surg. 2013;257:800–6.
84. Dueland S, Guren TK, Hagness M, Glimelius B, Line P-D, Pfeiffer P, Foss A, Tveit KM. Chemotherapy or liver transplantation for nonresectable liver metastases from colorectal cancer? Ann Surg. 2015;261:956–60.
85. Line P-D, Hagness M, Berstad AE, Foss A, Dueland S. A novel concept for partial liver transplantation in nonresectable colorectal liver metastases: the RAPID concept. Ann Surg. 2015;262:e5–9.
86. Nadalin S, Templin S, Koenigsrainer I, Capobianco I, Kopp H-G, Zender L, Sipos B, Kanz L, Wagner S, Konigsrainer A. Living Donor APOLT-ALPPS: paradigm shift in the management of irresectable colorectal liver metastases. Presented at the 12th Biennial E-AHPBA Congress 2017, Mainz, Germany, May 23–May 26, 2017.

Ablative Techniques for CRLM: Alone or in Association

36

Mariana I. Chavez, Christopher Coon, and T. Clark Gamblin

Introduction

Approximately half of the patients diagnosed with colon cancer will suffer from colorectal liver metastasis (CRLM) during their management. Currently, the standard treatment for hepatic metastasis is surgical resection with a potential curative intent. When surgery is not feasible, patients may undergo systemic treatment to downstage lesions and allow them to become eligible surgical candidates. Despite improved systemic therapies, surgical techniques, and perioperative care, most of the patients still remain ineligible for surgical resection and hence the reason for alternative techniques for local control of the disease.

Ablative techniques for the treatment of CRLM offer a less invasive treatment route than hepatic resection and can be used alone or in association with resection and/or chemotherapy.

In general, ablative techniques for CRLM can be divided into thermal and non-thermal techniques. Thermal techniques rely on differing mechanisms of delivering energy to the tumor site in order to increase or decrease local temperatures to cytotoxic levels. Thermal techniques examined in this chapter include laser-induced thermotherapy (LITT), high-intensity focused ultrasound ablation (HIFU), radiofrequency ablation (RFA), microwave ablation (MWA), and cryoablation. In techniques using thermal energy to increase tissue temperature, energy loss may occur due to local blood flow. This heat-sink effect is more pronounced in tumors located near major blood vessels [1]. Cryoablation, on the other hand, uses the opposite effect—quickly lowering temperatures to cytotoxic levels.

Nonthermal techniques that will be reviewed include chemoablation, which refers to ethanol or acetic acid ablation; irreversible electroporation (IRE) which uses electrical current to irreversibly damage the cell membrane causing cellular

M. I. Chavez · C. Coon · T. C. Gamblin (✉)
Division of Surgical Oncology, Medical College of Wisconsin, Milwaukee, WI, USA
e-mail: ccoon@mcw.edu; tcgamblin@mcw.edu

M. M. Correia et al. (eds.), *Colorectal Cancer Liver Metastases*,
https://doi.org/10.1007/978-3-030-25486-5_36

Table 36.1 Classification of liver ablative techniques by method of action

Liver ablation techniques
Thermal techniques
Coagulatives
Laser-induced thermotherapy (LITT)
High-intensity focused ultrasound ablation (HIFU)
Radiofrequency ablation (RFA)
Microwave ablation (MWA)
Cryoablation
Nonthermal techniques
Chemical ablation
Ethanol injection
Acetic acid
Irreversible electrophoresis (IRE)
Stereotactic body radiation therapy (SBRT)

apoptosis; and stereotactic body radiation therapy. See Table 36.1 for classification of ablative techniques by method of action.

This chapter will focus on describing current available ablative techniques in the treatment of CRLM and will discuss the evidence of outcomes when used alone or in association with other techniques.

Types of Ablative Techniques

Thermal Techniques

Laser-Induced Thermotherapy (LITT)

- LITT requires laser fibers to be inserted into target tissue.
- Ablation size is limited to 1–1.5 cm unless multiple-applicator arrays are used.
- Usually well tolerated with low risk of major complications.

LITT, also known as laser ablation, requires laser fibers to be inserted into the target tissue. LITT systems usually consist of a generator connected to a neodymium:yttrium aluminum garnet diode laser (wavelength of 1064 nm) [2]. The light energy from the fiberoptic applicator tip is absorbed by the target tissue and converted into heat when the photons are absorbed by naturally occurring chromophores [2, 3]. This heat is used to increase tissue temperatures to cytotoxic levels. Charred and desiccated tissue limits penetration of the photons, limiting ablation size in LITT to 1–1.5 cm. Slow heating and multiple-applicator arrays can be used to address this limitation and increase ablation zone size limitations [2].

The benefits of LITT closely resemble those of other thermal ablative techniques. It can be combined with resection to minimize the extent of resection required [4]. One early study from 2003 examined the use of transarterial chemoembolization (TACE) to downsize unresectable hepatic tumors prior to MRI-guided LITT. It was found that TACE combined with LITT produced significantly better median survival than TACE alone (26.2 and 12.8 months, respectively) [5].

According to Knavel et al., one major benefit of LITT over other ablative techniques is that most LITT systems are MRI compatible, allowing for intraprocedural temperature monitoring, though the authors do acknowledge the increased cost and limited availability of these options [3].

The major complication rate of LITT is acceptably low, with reported rates of 0.1–3.5% [4].

Originally, the intention of LITT was limited to palliative control of CRLM, but survival data have shown that it is comparable to resection in survival rates with decreased morbidity and mortality in selected cases [4]. As with other ablative techniques, Vogl et al. found that the number and size of tumors were significant prognostic indicators of overall and progression free survival (PFS) in patients treated with LITT. Median survival in 594 patients with CRLM was 25 months and median PFS was 13 months [6]. A recent review reported median survival ranging from 14.8–54 months, though combined median survival from all studies examined was 33.7 months [4].

A prospective study of 44 patients published in 2006 by Pacella et al. analyzed percutaneous LITT for treatment of unresectable CRLM. The authors found an overall survival of 30.0 ± 12.7 months in patients with complete ablation and no major complications during the study. Incomplete tumor ablation was associated with a significantly lower overall survival (20.2 ± 10.2 months). Tumor diameter <3 cm was a strong predictor of complete ablation [7]. However, more robust data are lacking. According to a review of available and future ablative techniques by Facciorusso et al. from 2016, the limited availability of LITT data limits its use until it can be further studied [8].

High-Intensity Focused Ultrasound Ablation (HIFU)

- HIFU is a noninvasive technique.
- Better to use on superficial tumors rather than deep ones.

HIFU is a completely noninvasive technique. HIFU uses a transducer to generate ultrasound waves like those used in diagnostic ultrasound imaging, but with increased intensity (720 mW/cm^2 diagnostic vs. 100–10,000 W/cm^2 HIFU) [9]. The ablative effect of HIFU is a result of heat generation from the conversion of acoustic energy into thermal energy, but some cavitation collapse sends shock waves into surrounding tissue as well [3, 10]. HIFU devices focus the ultrasound waves on a focal point. This focus and the rapid increase in temperature helps preserve tissue that is between the focal point and the transducer from thermal damage. Temperatures at the focal point reach 60 °C rapidly and coagulative necrosis occurs within a few seconds [10]. HIFU is limited by ultrasound penetrance and thermal energy that may build up along the path of travel—thus, superficial tumors are better candidates for HIFU ablation than deeper areas of disease [3].

The obvious benefit of HIFU compared to other ablative techniques is its noninvasive status. Additionally, there are both ultrasound- and MRI-guided systems available for intraoperative assessment of treatment [9]. Investigations into the use of HIFU for CRLM were lacking in the current literature, but recent studies of HIFU treatment of hepatocellular carcinoma can give some indication of its potential. A study conducted by Zhang et al. in 2009 demonstrated that hepatocellular carcinoma tumors adjacent to major blood vessels could be safely and completely ablated by HIFU with no major blood vessel injury observed on follow-up in 39 patients (median follow-up 23.8 ± 17.2 months) [11].

A study of 50 patients by Wu et al. found that HIFU could be safely combined with TACE and provided survival benefits (combined therapy median survival: 11.3 months, TACE only: 4 months) in the treatment of advanced-stage hepatocellular carcinoma [12].

Studies into the risks of HIFU have shown that the ultrasound waves can reflect or scatter, causing thermal damage to nearby structures. Skin burns, peripheral nerve damage, bowel injury, and pleural effusion have all been documented [13–16]. Further study of this technique to assess its safety and efficacy is needed.

A phase I-IIa clinical trial conducted in France examining HIFU safety and efficacy for CRLM showed promising results, with 30 ablations in 15 patients causing no damage to neighboring tissue and conducted with a precision of 1–2 mm [17].

Radiofrequency Ablation (RFA)

- RFA requires placement of electrodes which can be done with the guidance of US, CT, or MRI and using laparoscopy, open, or percutaneous approach.
- Usually well tolerated with low complication rates.
- Benefits have been demonstrated when using this technique combined with others and/or surgical resection.
- Higher local tumor recurrence when tumor >3 cm.
- *Use of RFA should be avoided when the target zone is immediately adjacent to vital structures such as the bile duct, major vessels, diaphragm, or bowel due to increased risk of damage.*
- Postablation syndrome present in 1/3 of patients.

RFA is an ablative technique that uses thermal energy derived from the application of electrical current to the targeted tissue. RFA can be performed using open, laparoscopic, or percutaneous approaches. The goal of RFA is complete ablation of the tumor and a surrounding margin [18].

RFA uses alternating current in the range of 450–500 kHz to cause agitation of the ions within the target tissue [19]. Once the resulting frictional heat causes temperatures to reach 60–100 °C, coagulative necrosis occurs due to the irreversible damage to both mitochondrial and cytosolic enzymes within the cells [20]. If temperatures reach 100 °C or above, evaporation causes instantaneous cell death, but the resulting tissue charring by the heated gasses hinders the continued effectiveness of RFA due to insulating properties of the carbonized tissue [21]. The aim is to achieve temperatures of 50°–100 °C for 4–6 minutes in the entire target volume. Because of the risk of charring and evaporation, slow heating of the target tissue is preferable. Due to the nature of heat conduction in the tissue, this allows a larger target volume to reach desired temperatures [22]. The resulting increase in circuit impedance, thus limiting current flow, is an important limitation on increasing RFA ablative zone size [23].

RFA electrodes (usually 14–21 gauge) are placed directly in the target tissue with the help of imaging such as ultrasound (US), computed tomography (CT), or magnetic resonance imaging (MRI) [24]. A reference electrode in the form of grounding pads is also placed on the patient's skin to disperse heat and prevent cutaneous burns at the pad site [22]. It should be noted that newer systems utilizing a bipolar probe do not require a grounding pad. Because of the low heat conductance of tissue, a single needle electrode has a small effective zone of necrosis. Solutions to this problem include multipronged electrodes, expandable electrodes, interstitial saline cooling, internal cooling of the electrode, and pulsing of the electrical current [25].

RFA shows low complication rates when used to treat cancers of the liver. Koda et al. conducted a multicenter study of the use of RFA to treat hepatocellular carcinoma, which examined 16,346 treated nodules in 13,283 patients, and found a complication rate of 3.5% and a complication-related death rate of just 0.04% [26]. Similar studies of RFA use for liver tumors have reported rates of major complications ranging from 1.9% to 5.7%, with those delineating between CRLM and other hepatic tumors showing similar complication rates for the two diseases [27–31].

RFA can be administered in combination with several other treatment techniques such as traditional resection and chemotherapy. Van Amerongen et al. found that RFA combined with resection to treat CRLM exhibited no increase in morbidity or mortality compared to resection alone and allowed treatment of patients that would have been otherwise considered inoperable [32]. A 2012 study of patients with unresectable CRLM found a significantly increased median PFS time in those treated with RFA plus systemic treatment (16.8 months) compared to those treated with systemic treatment alone (9.9 months) [33]. The investigators continued to publish a 2017 study of the same patients showing increased 3-, 5-, and 8-year overall survival (OS) in those undergoing the combined treatments compared to systemic treatment alone [34]. Chemotherapy can also be used prior to RFA to downstage initially untreatable tumors to a treatable size [35].

Patients with recurrent CRLM may be good candidates for RFA to avoid the technical difficulties of performing reoperative surgery. A study by Valls et al. demonstrated that RFA provides survival benefits in patients with recurrent CRLM of 3 cm or less. Patients with tumors larger than 3 cm experienced a recurrence rate of over 50%, and may be better served with other therapies [36].

However, the risks associated with RFA must be taken into considerations. Local tumor recurrence rates between 18% and 84% have been reported, with other reports varying extensively and are heavily dependent on lesion size [36–40]. A recent study performed by Tanis et al. demonstrated that the local recurrence rate in RFA was comparable to that of resection when tumor size was limited to 3 cm [41].

Postablation syndrome occurs in approximately one-third of patients and is an important consideration for postoperative management [42, 43]. Postablation syndrome manifests as flu-like symptoms, with patients exhibiting malaise, fever, chills, and/or nausea. It is believed that this may be a result of increased cytokine release and immune system activation in response to necrotic tissue [44–46]. Dodd et al. found that lesion size and volume ablated were significant predictors of postablation syndrome [43].

An additional risk consideration for RFA is tumor location. Adjacency to important structures such as the gallbladder or bile ducts, blood vessels, the diaphragm, and the bowel complicate the procedure, making significant bleeding, pleural effusion, bile peritonitis, thrombosis of vessels, and perforation of nonhepatic structures among others a concern [47–51]. Lu et al. found that vessels >3 mm contiguous with the target tumor were a dominant predictor of incomplete tumor destruction or local recurrence. Incomplete destruction or local recurrence occurred at a rate of 7% in the nonperivascular group compared to 48% in the perivascular group [48].

One risk of RFA that seems to have been addressed with newer systems is the risk of superficial burns at the grounding pad site. In order to produce the current used by the electrode, an equal amount of current, and therefore heat, is deposited at the grounding pad site. A review by Rhim et al. notes that second- and third-degree grounding pad site burns are relatively rare when sufficiently large grounding pad area is used [52]. Severe burns can be avoided with careful grounding pad placement [53].

When considered holistically, the benefits and potential of RFA can outweigh the risks. RFA is a safe, well-tolerated procedure that provides alternatives to resection or chemotherapy alone and can be an option for patients whose disease is otherwise inoperable. The recurrence rate, in particular, should be considered however, and candidacy should be evaluated on a case-by-case basis.

The widely accepted ideal size of ≤3 cm is supported by a multitude of studies that show RFA provides comparable survival outcomes to resection alone in tumors of this size [36, 38, 54–57]. A propensity score analysis performed by Lee et al. in 2015 states that survival curves for RFA are comparable to those of resection in tumors ≤2 cm, but asserts that resection provides better outcomes in larger tumors [58]. Two studies conducted by Gillams et al. and Oshowo et al. examined the use of RFA to treat solitary CRLM of up to 5 cm (mean tumor size: 3.9 cm) and 10 cm (mean tumor size: 3 cm), respectively, showed comparable survival outcomes to resection [59, 60]. In addition to tumor size, number of tumors and uncontrolled extrahepatic disease were significant indicators of poorer survivability after RFA [61].

RFA is often conducted as an adjunct to resection and/or systemic chemotherapy. A review conducted by Boame et al. demonstrated that RFA, when used as an adjunct to resection to treat CRLM, does not decrease overall survival [62]. In addition to the studies conducted by Ruers et al. mentioned above, a 2012 study presented data supporting the conclusion that adding RFA to systemic chemotherapy improves overall survival compared to systemic chemotherapy alone [33, 34, 63]. See Table 36.2 for summarizing data of RFA versus liver resection (LR) for CRLM.

Table 36.2 Survival data of RFA versus liver resection (LR) for CRLM

Author	Type of study	Treatment	No. of patients	Morbidity (%)	Mortality (%)	Local recurrence (%)	Median follow-up (months)	Five-year overall survival (%)
Hur et al. [55]	Retrospective	LR	42	14	0	9.5	42	50
		RFA	25	0	0	28		25.5
Otto et al. [64]	Retrospective	LR	82	36.5	0	4	NR	51
		RFA	28	25	0	32		48
Reuter et al. [65]	Retrospective	LR	126	29	NR	2	20	23
		RFA	66	10		17		21
Kim KH et al. [54]	Retrospective	LR	278	21.2	0	NR	NR	51
		RFA	177	6	0			51
Lee et al. [66]	Retrospective	LR	25	4	3.5	8	NR	44
		RFA	28	3.5	0	42.9		17.9
Ko et al. [67]	Retrospective	LR	12	NR	NR	NR	NR	66.7
		RFA	17					37.8

Microwave Ablation (MWA)

- MWA requires placement of electrodes which can be done with the guidance of US, CT, or MRI and using laparoscopy, open or percutaneous approach.
- Faster ablation and less heat-sink effect.
- Usually well tolerated with low complication rates.
- Benefits have been demonstrated when using this technique combined with others and/or surgical resection.

MWA is quite similar in concept and application to RFA, with an electromagnetic wave-producing probe providing energy to heat the target tissue to cytotoxic levels, but does provide some benefits over its predecessor counterpart. A growing body of literature assessing safety, efficacy, and comparisons to RFA has presented several possible advantages to the newer system [3, 68]. The advantages of MWA over RFA and other ablative techniques discussed in this section imply a role for MWA in treatment strategies for CRLM.

The key differences between MWA and RFA systems are the frequency of waves produced and the use of microwaves versus electrical current, respectively. MWA systems generate waves with significantly higher frequencies than RFA, with most systems using either 915 MHz or 2.45 GHz and 45–80 W [69, 70]. Unlike RFA, MWA systems do not need a grounding pad [71]. Microwaves passing through tissue induce oscillation in water molecules acting as dipoles as they attempt to align opposite electromagnetic charges [72]. The oscillation transforms electrical energy into thermal energy through friction, heating surrounding tissue [18]. Most systems on the market today utilize 14- to 17-gauge antennae with a water or CO_2 active antennae cooling system to reduce unwanted heating around the probe length and prevent skin burns at the site of insertion [3, 71, 73].

Compared to RFA, which relies heavily on thermal conduction for heat dissipation further than a few millimeters from the probe, MWA creates an elliptical field that can reach up to 2 cm from the probe tip, allowing for a larger ablation zones and more uniform coagulative necrosis [72].

Many of the same risks associated with RFA should be considered when employing MWA. Incidental healthy tissue ablation can be avoided with careful application. Skin burns at the site of antennae insertion, though largely avoided by the internal cooling element of today's MWA instruments, can also occur [71]. As a type of thermal ablation, MWA is susceptible to the same heat-sink effect as other thermal modalities [74].

As with RFA, a risk of MWA is local tumor recurrence. Groeschl et al. conducted a multi-institutional analysis of MWA for hepatic malignancies and found a local recurrence rate of 5.2% for CRLM in 393 ablated tumors [75].

MWA is comparable to resection for the treatment of multiple metastases. An early study by Shibata et al. demonstrated that MWA is equally effective as resection for treatment of multiple hepatic metastases while causing a lower amount of intraoperative blood loss (median overall survival of 27 and 25 months, respectively) [76].

Surgical approach for application of MWA in hepatic malignancies—open, laparoscopic, or percutaneous—was examined by Groeschl et al. who found no difference in morbidity or survival between the three in 473 procedures but did find higher rates of local recurrence from percutaneous operations (14.1% vs. 6.0% overall). These recurrence rates were given for all hepatic malignancies, not CRLM specifically. The same study showed median overall survival of patients treated with MWA for CRLM was 32.1 months [75].

MWA as it compares to RFA is of particular interest as the techniques have significant crossover in patient candidacy. A meta-analysis performed by Huo et al. in 2015 examined 16 studies comparing the outcomes of MWA and RFA for hepatic lesions. The investigators found that patients who underwent MWA exhibited a significant increase in 6-year overall survival compared to RFA (odds ratio (OR): 1.64, 95% confidence interval (CI): 1.15–2.35); however, this was based on only 3 of the 16 studies. The same meta-analysis found MWA and RFA comparable in a number of measures including: 1–5-year overall survival, disease-free survival, local recurrence rate, and adverse events [70]. See Table 36.3 for a summary of some important studies into the safety and efficacy of MWA.

Cryoablation

- Cryoablation allows visualization of affected tissue being ablated under US or CT guidance, which helps in monitoring margins.
- Risk of complications is high compared to other hepatic ablation techniques.
- No benefits are seen when associated with other ablative techniques or surgical resection.

Table 36.3 Summary of some important studies into the safety and efficacy of MWA

Author	No. of patients	Type of study	CRLM specific (Y/N)	Morbidity (%)	Mortality (%)	Local recurrence (%)	Median follow-up (months)
Liu et al. [77]	35	Randomized	N	1.1	0	8.6	32.2
Correa-Gallego et al. [78]	67	Matched cohort	Y	27	0	6	18
Martin et al. [79]	20	Prospective	N	4	0	11.3	5
Iannitti et al. [80]	33	Prospective	Y	19	0	2.7	19
Zhou et al. [81]	35	Prospective	N	NR	NR	11.3	5

Cryoablation can be performed percutaneously with image guidance or laparoscopically. Cryoablative devices lower cell temperatures to cytotoxic levels through the formation of ice crystals. The ones used today employ the Joule-Thompson process to cool argon gas as it passes through a probe that is inserted into the target tissue [82]. During the freezing cycle, an "ice ball" that encompasses the tumor along with a 1 cm margin is formed, with multiple probes being used simultaneously for larger lesions [83, 84]. Like thermal ablation types, cryoablation is susceptible to a thermal sink effect; however in cryoablation, the risk stems from blood vessels bringing new, warm blood to the target tissue, hindering the effectiveness of the cooling.

The mechanism of cell death is multifaceted. The initial freezing event creates intracellular ice crystals, which disrupt the cell membrane [85]. These intracellular ice crystals also deplete the cells of water, causing multiple harmful effects. Additionally, the formation of ice in blood vessels can lead to ischemic injury [86].

The main advantage of cryoablation over other thermal ablative techniques is the clear visualization of the ice ball on ultrasound imaging or CT scan [82]. This allows for easy intraoperative monitoring of ablation margins.

While cryoablation is one of the oldest forms of ablation, the risk of complications is high compared to other techniques. Complications stemming from parenchyma shearing due to cracks forming in the ice ball include hemorrhage, biliary injury, and abscess formation [87]. Multiple studies have placed cryoablation-related complication rates between 20% and 30% for the treatment of CRLM [83, 88–90]. Additionally, a rare but serious risk of cryoablation is cryoshock syndrome [91]. Cryoshock is a cytokine-mediated systemic shock that, although rare overall, has been documented in multiple studies [84, 92, 93].

Comparisons between RFA and cryoablation have shown that recurrence rates tend to be higher in patients who underwent cryoablation versus those who underwent RFA for treatment of hepatic malignancies [83, 94]. See Table 36.4 for some of the important studies of cryoablation for hepatic tumors.

Table 36.4 Summary of some important studies into the safety and efficacy of cryoablation

Author	No. of patients	Type of study	CRLM specific (Y/N)	Morbidity (%)	Mortality (%)	Local recurrence (%)	Median follow-up (months)
Rivoire et al. [90]	24	Retrospective	Y	21	0	18	48
Yan et al. [88]	172	Prospective	Y	28	0	NR	23
Paganini et al. [89]	64 (49 open; 15 laparoscopic)	Retrospective	Y	26.2 (open); 6.7 (lap.)	4.1 (open); 0 (lap.)	0	39.3 (open); 87.1 (lap.)
Adam et al. [83]	31	Prospective	N	29	3.2	53	21.2
Bageacu et al. [84]	53	Retrospective	Y	66	3.8	22.6	24.8
Xu et al. [92]	326	Retrospective	Y	5.8	2.1	15.3	32
Pearson et al. [94]	54	Prospective	N	40.7	1.8	22.2	15
Kerkar et al. [93]	56	Retrospective	Y	11	11	NR	54

Nonthermal Techniques

Chemical Ablation

- Ethanol-ablation is simple and well tolerated.
- Presents high risk of local recurrence, requires multiple sessions, and ablation zone is variable.
- Limited value on CRLM due to its dense and infiltrative nature.

These techniques are useful to destroy tissues chemically with the use of either acetic acid or more commonly sterile ethanol. Percutaneous ethanol injection, also known as ethanol ablation, is a well-established and highly used ablation technique. Ethanol ablation involves the injection of ethanol directly into the target tissue. It requires no special equipment besides the injection needle and is usually conducted under the guidance of ultrasound [20, 85]. Small (20–22 gauge) needles are used to inject 95–100% ethanol [95]. The mechanism of cell death in ethanol ablation is dehydration of the cytoplasm, protein denaturation, and microvascular thrombosis [85, 96, 97].

The main benefit of ethanol ablation compared to the other modalities is its simplicity. Ethanol ablation is usually performed without general or local anesthetic and is well tolerated in the vast majority of patients. High local tumor progression rates and, although rare, hepatic necrosis are two main risk factors when considering ethanol ablation [98–100]. One relatively common side effect of ethanol ablation is nausea, and patients are instructed to fast prior to treatment [20].

Ethanol ablation safety has been well established for decades, but variable ablation zone size, the necessity of multiple sessions, and high local tumor progression rate compared to more modern techniques has led to it only being used in cases where tumor characteristics preclude the use of other modalities [85].

Irreversible Electrophoresis (IRE)

- IRE works with high-voltage pulses of electrical current to cause nanopore defects in the lipid bilayer of cell membranes.
- Requires general anesthesia combined with paralytic agents.
- It creates very sharp ablation margins and preservation of nearby vital structures.
- High major morbidity rate, safety, and efficacy still under study.

IRE is a newer form of surgical ablation. It was approved by the FDA for soft tissue ablation in 2006 [101]. The principle of IRE is to cause cell death through the application of electrical energy. IRE does not cause cell death through the same mechanism of any previously discussed techniques. Rather, IRE devices used today employ multiple electrodes inserted into the target tissue to apply short, high-voltage pulses of electrical current to cause nanopore defects in the lipid bilayer of cell membranes [85, 101]. The devices used typically deliver 90 pulses of 2–3 kV/cm for periods of a few milliseconds [85, 87]. Several studies have shown that the nanopores created led to cell death through both destabilization of the cell membrane and an increase in permeability [102–104].

Interestingly, the pores created by the electrical current application are extremely short-lived and often reversible if a certain threshold of electrical current is not met. Melikov et al. demonstrated that nanopores remained open for an average of just 3 +/− 0.8 ms at 250 mV [105]. The higher voltage used by IRE devices causes irreversible and persistent pores [85, 105].

IRE progress can be measured intraoperatively with ultrasound, but imaging changes to the ablation area can take several minutes to appear [106]. The technique also requires general anesthesia combined with paralytic agents to inhibit muscle activation by the electrical current [107].

There are several potential advantages IRE may hold. Because IRE utilizes effects of electrical current to directly damage cell membranes, it is not subject to the same heat-sink effect of the thermal modalities [87]. IRE has also been shown to create very sharp ablation margins and preservation of nearby vital structures, such as bile ducts and blood vessels, while showing successful ablation [108–111].

Hosein et al. conducted a retrospective analysis of IRE in CRLM in which 25 out of 29 patients had an absolute or relative contraindication to thermal ablation based on tumor size and location and found the procedure both safe and effective at destroying the tumor while preserving vital structures [112].

Complications of IRE were examined in a large systematic review conducted by Scheffer et al. in 2014. This review looked at the use of IRE in multiple organs, but found only minor complications reported for liver tumors treated with IRE [101]. However, some major complications associated with IRE have been reported. One study from 2016 of 65 malignant liver tumors in 34 patients reported major complications in 6 patients: 1 patient had diffuse intraperitoneal bleeding, 1 experienced partial thrombosis of the portal vein, and liver abscesses appeared in 4 patients [113].

Due to its recent surge in public interest, the literature on outcomes of IRE has mostly focused on assessing efficacy and safety. The review article published by Scheffer et al. mentioned previously concluded that IRE is safe and effective in otherwise untreatable liver tumors, but emphasizes that further study is needed to more thoroughly assess the possible role of IRE as a treatment option [101]. A more recent single-center study from 2017 reported that IRE was a safe treatment modality for liver tumors and achieved high local tumor control out to 6 months postoperatively [114].

Stereotactic Body Radiation Therapy (SBRT)

- SBRT implies delivery of high dosing, few fractions of radiation to a focal area of the liver.
- Well tolerated with minimal toxicity.
- Further studies needed to compare efficacy.

SBRT is also a relatively new form of surgical ablation. It allows delivery of higher doses in fewer fractions of radiation to discrete individual liver metastases, while sparing the normal hepatic tissue and surrounding organs [115]. The main challenge of SBRT to deliver radiation to the liver is managing respiratory movements. Various breathing control strategies such as respiratory gating and motion management techniques have been implemented to overcome this limitation, including the CyberKnife system (Accuracy Inc), which performs real-time tumor tracking. This allows for a high level of precision while treating the patient in free breathing and maintaining patient comfort [116].

Benefits from this technique include good local control of the disease with relatively low risks for major complications or toxicity. A recent retrospective study by Mahadevan et al. showed 427 patients with 568 liver metastases treated, with reasonable overall survival (median 22 months) and local control (median 52 months) on patients where most of the tumors were of colorectal origin [115]. Higher SBRT doses and smaller tumor volumes were associated with improved local control and overall survival. Because of the focal area of radiation delivered, toxicity from this technique has been reported as minimal in the literature, but includes anorexia, fatigue, and some nausea, especially when left lobe of the liver is treated [117]. Due to the lack of randomized trials and comparative studies, further studies will be needed to compare the efficacies of SBRT with those of surgical resection or radiofrequency ablation.

Combining Surgical Resection with Ablative Techniques

As previously stated, the current standard of care involves surgical removal of CRLM as the only potential cure. However, whenever patients were not surgical candidates for curative resection due to major comorbidities, inadequate functional hepatic reserve, multifocal disease or a combination of these, most of the mentioned locoregional therapies are utilized as palliative treatment. Combining hepatectomy with ablative techniques allows the removal of the largest tumors while simultaneously ablating smaller residual tumors [118].

Recent studies have associated combined treatments including surgery and ablation, mostly using comparisons with RFA, but the information regarding outcomes may lack external validity since these are mostly limited to single-center studies. A meta-analysis published in 2015 on RFA versus liver resection on survival outcomes for CRLM concluded that liver resection was superior to RFA in survival outcomes and ablation should be reserved for patients who are not optimal candidates for resection until new supportive evidence is obtained from large randomized control trials [119].

More recently in 2016, Pawlik et al. conducted a study based on ACS-NSQIP database including patients undergoing liver resection and examined the patterns of these resections in North America, making emphasis on concurrent wedge resections and ablations [118]. The use of concurrent wedge surgical resection was observed in 56% of patients, more commonly among patients undergoing partial lobectomy compared to major hepatectomy. Concurrent ablations were performed in 14.2% of patients, also more often associated with partial resections. Prolonged length of stay, increased requirements of blood transfusions, and postoperative morbidity and mortality were more related to major hepatectomies than to ablative techniques. These results suggest that hepatectomy can be safely performed with concurrent ablation and could allow for more patients to undergo potentially curative therapy.

Conclusions and Recommendations

A large variety of ablative techniques are available to assist in the management of CRLM. Such techniques also expand the treatment options for disease recurrence in patients whose liver remnant is inadequate for surgical resection. General and liver-related comorbidities are common contraindications to hepatic resection and are often independent of the extent of disease or proposed operation. Many technical factors make hepatic malignancies unresectable, including insufficient future liver remnant, involvement of all three hepatic veins, and involvement of portal inflow to both lobes of the liver. Many techniques to deal with technically unresectable tumors have been developed, such as portal vein embolization and two-stage operations. Nonetheless, most liver tumors are still unresectable. Currently, the most common ablative techniques include RFA and MWA. MWA has increased in utilization due to less heat-sink, the potential to address larger lesions, and lower operative time.

References

1. Pillai K, Akhter J, Chua TC, et al. Heat sink effect on tumor ablation characteristics as observed in monopolar radiofrequency, bipolar radiofrequency, and microwave, using ex vivo calf liver model. Medicine (Baltimore). 2015;94(9):e580. https://doi.org/10.1097/MD.0000000000000580.
2. Garrean S, Hering J, Helton WS, Espat NJ. A primer on transarterial, chemical, and thermal ablative therapies for hepatic tumors. Am J Surg. 2007;194(1):79–88. https://doi.org/10.1016/j.amjsurg.2006.11.025.
3. Knavel EM, Brace CL. Tumor ablation: common modalities and general practices. Tech Vasc Interv Radiol. 2013;16(4):192–200. https://doi.org/10.1053/j.tvir.2013.08.002.
4. Vogl TJ, Farshid P, Naguib NNN, et al. Thermal ablation of liver metastases from colorectal cancer: radiofrequency, microwave and laser ablation therapies. Radiol Med (Torino). 2014;119(7):451–61. https://doi.org/10.1007/s11547-014-0415-y.
5. Vogl TJ, Mack MG, Balzer JO, et al. Liver metastases: neoadjuvant downsizing with transarterial chemoembolization before laser-induced thermotherapy. Radiology. 2003;229(2):457–64. https://doi.org/10.1148/radiol.2292021329.
6. Vogl TJ, Dommermuth A, Heinle B, et al. Colorectal cancer liver metastases: long-term survival and progression-free survival after thermal ablation using magnetic resonance–guided laser-induced interstitial thermotherapy in 594 patients. Investig Radiol. 2014;49(1):48–56. https://doi.org/10.1097/RLI.0b013e3182a6094e.
7. Pacella CM, Valle D, Bizzarri G, et al. Percutaneous laser ablation in patients with isolated unresectable liver metastases from colorectal cancer: results of a phase II study. Acta Oncol. 2006;45(1):77–83. https://doi.org/10.1080/02841860500438029.
8. Facciorusso A, Serviddio G, Muscatiello N. Local ablative treatments for hepatocellular carcinoma: an updated review. World J Gastrointest Pharmacol Ther. 2016;7(4):477–89. https://doi.org/10.4292/wjgpt.v7.i4.477.
9. Zhou Y-F. High intensity focused ultrasound in clinical tumor ablation. World J Clin Oncol. 2011;2(1):8–27. https://doi.org/10.5306/wjco.v2.i1.8.
10. Srikanth P, Martinie JB, Iannitti David A. Liver tumor ablation: percutaneous and open approaches. J Surg Oncol. 2009;100(8):619–34. https://doi.org/10.1002/jso.21364.
11. Zhang L, Zhu H, Jin C, et al. High-intensity focused ultrasound (HIFU): effective and safe therapy for hepatocellular carcinoma adjacent to major hepatic veins. Eur Radiol. 2009;19(2):437. https://doi.org/10.1007/s00330-008-1137-0.
12. Wu F, Wang Z-B, Chen W-Z, et al. Advanced hepatocellular carcinoma: treatment with high-intensity focused ultrasound ablation combined with transcatheter arterial embolization. Radiology. 2005;235(2):659–67. https://doi.org/10.1148/radiol.2352030916.
13. Chan ACY, Cheung TT, Fan ST, et al. Survival analysis of high-intensity focused ultrasound therapy versus radiofrequency ablation in the treatment of recurrent hepatocellular carcinoma. Ann Surg. 2013;257(4):686–92. https://doi.org/10.1097/SLA.0b013e3182822c02.

14. Kim Y, Rhim H, Choi MJ, Lim HK, Choi D. High-intensity focused ultrasound therapy: an overview for radiologists. Korean J Radiol. 2008;9(4):291–302. https://doi.org/10.3348/kjr.2008.9.4.291.
15. Li J-J, Xu G-L, Gu M-F, et al. Complications of high intensity focused ultrasound in patients with recurrent and metastatic abdominal tumors. World J Gastroenterol WJG. 2007;13(19):2747–51. https://doi.org/10.3748/wjg.v13.i19.2747.
16. Jung SE, Cho SH, Jang JH, Han J-Y. High-intensity focused ultrasound ablation in hepatic and pancreatic cancer: complications. Abdom Imaging. 2011;36(2):185–95. https://doi.org/10.1007/s00261-010-9628-2.
17. Dupré A, Melodelima D, Pérol D, et al. First clinical experience of intra-operative high intensity focused ultrasound in patients with colorectal liver metastases: a phase I-IIa study. PLoS ONE. 2015;10(2):e0118212. https://doi.org/10.1371/journal.pone.0118212.
18. Petre EN, Sofocleous C. Thermal ablation in the management of colorectal cancer patients with oligometastatic liver disease. Visc Med. 2017;33(1):62–8. https://doi.org/10.1159/000454697.
19. Haemmerich D, Schutt DJ. Radiofrequency ablation at low frequencies for targeted tumor heating: in-vitro and computational modeling results. IEEE Trans Biomed Eng. 2011;58(2):404–10. https://doi.org/10.1109/TBME.2010.2085081.
20. VanSonnenberg E, McMullen W, Solbiati L, editors. Tumor ablation: principles and practice. New York: Springer; 2004.
21. Hong K, Georgiades CS. Radiofrequency ablation: mechanism of action and devices. In: Hong K, Georgiades CS, editors. Percutaneous tumor ablation. 2011th ed. Stuttgart: Georg Thieme Verlag; 2011. https://doi.org/10.1055/b-0034-81499.
22. Hong K, Georgiades CS. Percutaneous tumor ablation: strategies and techniques. New York: Thieme; 2011. http://public.eblib.com/choice/publicfullrecord.aspx?p=1250509. Accessed April 2, 2018.
23. Gazelle GS, Goldberg SN, Solbiati L, Livraghi T. Tumor ablation with radio-frequency energy. Radiology. 2000;217(3):633–46. https://doi.org/10.1148/radiology.217.3.r00dc26633.
24. Nahum Goldberg S, Dupuy DE. Image-guided radiofrequency tumor ablation: challenges and opportunities--part I. J Vasc Interv Radiol JVIR. 2001;12(9):1021–32.
25. Geschwind J-FH, Soulen MC. Interventional oncology: principles and practice of image-guided cancer therapy. Cambridge: Cambridge University Press; 2016.
26. Koda M, Murawaki Y, Hirooka Y, et al. Complications of radiofrequency ablation for hepatocellular carcinoma in a multicenter study: an analysis of 16 346 treated nodules in 13 283 patients. Hepatol Res Off J Jpn Soc Hepatol. 2012;42(11):1058–64. https://doi.org/10.1111/j.1872-034X.2012.01025.x.
27. de Baère T, Risse O, Kuoch V, et al. Adverse events during radiofrequency treatment of 582 hepatic tumors. AJR Am J Roentgenol. 2003;181(3):695–700. https://doi.org/10.2214/ajr.181.3.1810695.
28. Livraghi T, Solbiati L, Meloni MF, Gazelle GS, Halpern EF, Goldberg SN. Treatment of focal liver tumors with percutaneous radio-frequency ablation: complications encountered in a multicenter study. Radiology. 2003;226(2):441–51. https://doi.org/10.1148/radiol.2262012198.
29. Choi D, Lim HK, Rhim H, et al. Percutaneous radiofrequency ablation for early-stage hepatocellular carcinoma as a first-line treatment: long-term results and prognostic factors in a large single-institution series. Eur Radiol. 2007;17(3):684–92. https://doi.org/10.1007/s00330-006-0461-5.
30. Curley SA, Izzo F, Delrio P, et al. Radiofrequency ablation of unresectable primary and metastatic hepatic malignancies. Ann Surg. 1999;230(1):1.
31. Hildebrand P, Kleemann M, Roblick UJ, et al. Radiofrequency-ablation of unresectable primary and secondary liver tumors: results in 88 patients. Langenbeck's Arch Surg. 2006;391(2):118–23. https://doi.org/10.1007/s00423-006-0024-x.
32. van Amerongen MJ, van der Stok EP, Fütterer JJ, et al. Short term and long term results of patients with colorectal liver metastases undergoing surgery with or without radiofrequency

ablation. Eur J Surg Oncol J Eur Soc Surg Oncol Br Assoc Surg Oncol. 2016;42(4):523–30. https://doi.org/10.1016/j.ejso.2016.01.013.
33. Ruers T, Punt C, Van Coevorden F, et al. Radiofrequency ablation combined with systemic treatment versus systemic treatment alone in patients with non-resectable colorectal liver metastases: a randomized EORTC intergroup phase II study (EORTC 40004). Ann Oncol. 2012;23(10):2619–26. https://doi.org/10.1093/annonc/mds053.
34. Ruers T, Van Coevorden F, Punt CJA, et al. Local treatment of unresectable colorectal liver metastases: results of a randomized phase II trial. JNCI J Natl Cancer Inst. 2017;109(9) https://doi.org/10.1093/jnci/djx015.
35. Nielsen K, Scheffer HJ, Volders JH, et al. Radiofrequency ablation to improve survival after conversion chemotherapy for colorectal liver metastases. World J Surg. 2016;40(8):1951–8. https://doi.org/10.1007/s00268-016-3554-6.
36. Valls C, Ramos E, Leiva D, Ruiz S, Martinez L, Rafecas A. Safety and efficacy of ultrasound-guided radiofrequency ablation of recurrent colorectal cancer liver metastases after hepatectomy. Scand J Surg SJS Off Organ Finn Surg Soc Scand Surg Soc. 2015;104(3):169–75. https://doi.org/10.1177/1457496914553147.
37. Sucandy I, Cheek S, Golas BJ, Tsung A, Geller DA, Marsh JW. Longterm survival outcomes of patients undergoing treatment with radiofrequency ablation for hepatocellular carcinoma and metastatic colorectal cancer liver tumors. HPB. 2016;18(9):756–63. https://doi.org/10.1016/j.hpb.2016.06.010.
38. Eltawil KM, Boame N, Mimeault R, et al. Patterns of recurrence following selective intraoperative radiofrequency ablation as an adjunct to hepatic resection for colorectal liver metastases. J Surg Oncol. 2014;110(6):734–8. https://doi.org/10.1002/jso.23689.
39. Liu C-H, Yu C-Y, Chang W-C, Dai M-S, Hsiao C-W, Chou Y-C. Radiofrequency ablation of hepatic metastases: factors influencing local tumor progression. Ann Surg Oncol. 2014;21(9):3090–5. https://doi.org/10.1245/s10434-014-3738-y.
40. Hof J, Wertenbroek MWJL a E, PMJG P, Widder J, Sieders E, de Jong KP. Outcomes after resection and/or radiofrequency ablation for recurrence after treatment of colorectal liver metastases. Br J Surg. 2016;103(8):1055–62. https://doi.org/10.1002/bjs.10162.
41. Tanis E, Nordlinger B, Mauer M, et al. Local recurrence rates after radiofrequency ablation or resection of colorectal liver metastases. Analysis of the European Organisation for Research and Treatment of Cancer #40004 and #40983. Eur J Cancer Oxf Engl 1990. 2014;50(5):912–9. https://doi.org/10.1016/j.ejca.2013.12.008.
42. Wah TM, Arellano RS, Gervais DA, et al. Image-guided percutaneous radiofrequency ablation and incidence of post-radiofrequency ablation syndrome: prospective survey. Radiology. 2005;237(3):1097–102. https://doi.org/10.1148/radiol.2373042008.
43. Dodd GD, Napier D, Schoolfield JD, Hubbard L. Percutaneous radiofrequency ablation of hepatic tumors: postablation syndrome. AJR Am J Roentgenol. 2005;185(1):51–7. https://doi.org/10.2214/ajr.185.1.01850051.
44. Ikei S, Ogawa M, Beppu T, et al. Changes in IL-6, IL-8, C-reactive protein and pancreatic secretory trypsin inhibitor after transcatheter arterial chemo-embolization therapy for hepato-cellular carcinoma. Cytokine. 1992;4(6):581–4. https://doi.org/10.1016/1043-4666(92)90023-K.
45. Yoshito I, Takeshi O, Naoki O, et al. Hepatic damage induced by transcatheter arterial chemoembolization elevates serum concentrations of macrophage-colony stimulating factor. Liver. 2007;19(2):97–103. https://doi.org/10.1111/j.1478-3231.1999.tb00017.x.
46. Yukihiko M, Sumio K, Toshihiko N, et al. Interleukin-6 in transcatheter arterial embolization for patients with hepatocellular carcinoma. Effects of serine protease inhibitor. Cancer. 2006;73(1):53–7. https://doi.org/10.1002/1097-0142(19940101)73:1<53::AID-CNCR2820730111>3.0.CO;2-W.
47. McDermott S, Gervais DA. Radiofrequency ablation of liver tumors. Semin Interv Radiol. 2013;30(1):49–55. https://doi.org/10.1055/s-0033-1333653.
48. Lu DSK, Raman SS, Limanond P, et al. Influence of large peritumoral vessels on outcome of radiofrequency ablation of liver tumors. J Vasc Interv Radiol JVIR. 2003;14(10):1267–74.

49. Howenstein MJ, Sato KT. Complications of radiofrequency ablation of hepatic, pulmonary, and renal neoplasms. Semin Interv Radiol. 2010;27(3):285–95. https://doi.org/10.1055/s-0030-1261787.
50. Kwon H-J, Kim PN, Byun JH, et al. Various complications of percutaneous radiofrequency ablation for hepatic tumors: radiologic findings and technical tips. Acta Radiol. 2014;55(9):1082–92. https://doi.org/10.1177/0284185113513893.
51. Kim KR, Thomas S. Complications of image-guided thermal ablation of liver and kidney neoplasms. Semin Interv Radiol. 2014;31(2):138–48. https://doi.org/10.1055/s-0034-1373789.
52. Rhim H, Dodd GD, Chintapalli KN, et al. Radiofrequency thermal ablation of abdominal tumors: lessons learned from complications. Radiographics. 2004;24(1):41–52. https://doi.org/10.1148/rg.241025144.
53. Goldberg SN, Solbiati L, Halpern EF, Gazelle GS. Variables affecting proper system grounding for radiofrequency ablation in an animal model. J Vasc Interv Radiol. 2000;11(8):1069–75. https://doi.org/10.1016/S1051-0443(07)61341-4.
54. Kim KH, Yoon YS, Yu CS, et al. Comparative analysis of radiofrequency ablation and surgical resection for colorectal liver metastases. J Korean Surg Soc. 2011;81(1):25–34. https://doi.org/10.4174/jkss.2011.81.1.25.
55. Hur H, Ko YT, Min BS, et al. Comparative study of resection and radiofrequency ablation in the treatment of solitary colorectal liver metastases. Am J Surg. 2009;197(6):728–36. https://doi.org/10.1016/j.amjsurg.2008.04.013.
56. Van Tilborg AAJM, Meijerink MR, Sietses C, et al. Long-term results of radiofrequency ablation for unresectable colorectal liver metastases: a potentially curative intervention. Br J Radiol. 2011;84(1002):556–65. https://doi.org/10.1259/bjr/78268814.
57. Veltri A, Guarnieri T, Gazzera C, et al. Long-term outcome of radiofrequency thermal ablation (RFA) of liver metastases from colorectal cancer (CRC): size as the leading prognostic factor for survival. Radiol Med (Torino). 2012;117(7):1139–51. https://doi.org/10.1007/s11547-012-0803-3.
58. Lee H, Heo JS, Cho YB, et al. Hepatectomy vs radiofrequency ablation for colorectal liver metastasis: a propensity score analysis. World J Gastroenterol. 2015;21(11):3300–7. https://doi.org/10.3748/wjg.v21.i11.3300.
59. Oshowo A, Gillams A, Harrison E, Lees WR, Taylor I. Comparison of resection and radiofrequency ablation for treatment of solitary colorectal liver metastases. Br J Surg. 2003;90(10):1240–3. https://doi.org/10.1002/bjs.4264.
60. Gillams AR, Lees WR. Radio-frequency ablation of colorectal liver metastases in 167 patients. Eur Radiol. 2004;14(12):2261–7. https://doi.org/10.1007/s00330-004-2416-z.
61. Hamada A, Yamakado K, Nakatsuka A, et al. Radiofrequency ablation for colorectal liver metastases: prognostic factors in non-surgical candidates. Jpn J Radiol. 2012;30(7):567–74. https://doi.org/10.1007/s11604-012-0089-0.
62. Boame N, Gresham G, Jonker D, Martel G, Balaa F, Asmis T. Use of chemotherapy and radiofrequency ablation to treat colorectal cancer metastases: a retrospective review of the Ottawa Hospital Cancer Centre over 7 years. Curr Oncol. 2014;21(4):e557–63. https://doi.org/10.3747/co.21.1929.
63. Solbiati L, Ahmed M, Cova L, Ierace T, Brioschi M, Goldberg SN. Small liver colorectal metastases treated with percutaneous radiofrequency ablation: local response rate and long-term survival with up to 10-year follow-up. Radiology. 2012;265(3):958–68. https://doi.org/10.1148/radiol.12111851.
64. Otto G, Düber C, Hoppe-Lotichius M, König J, Heise M, Pitton MB. Radiofrequency ablation as first-line treatment in patients with early colorectal liver metastases amenable to surgery. Ann Surg. 2010;251(5):796–803. https://doi.org/10.1097/SLA.0b013e3181bc9fae.
65. Reuter NP, Woodall CE, Scoggins CR, McMasters KM, Martin RCG. Radiofrequency ablation vs. resection for hepatic colorectal metastasis: therapeutically equivalent? J Gastrointest Surg Off J Soc Surg Aliment Tract. 2009;13(3):486–91. https://doi.org/10.1007/s11605-008-0727-0.

66. Lee KH, Kim HO, Yoo CH, et al. Comparison of radiofrequency ablation and resection for hepatic metastasis from colorectal cancer. Korean J Gastroenterol Taehan Sohwagi Hakhoe Chi. 2012;59(3):218–23.
67. Ko S, Jo H, Yun S, Park E, Kim S, Seo H-I. Comparative analysis of radiofrequency ablation and resection for resectable colorectal liver metastases. World J Gastroenterol WJG. 2014;20(2):525–31. https://doi.org/10.3748/wjg.v20.i2.525.
68. Brace CL. Radiofrequency and microwave ablation of the liver, lung, kidney and bone: what are the differences. Curr Probl Diagn Radiol. 2009;38(3):135–43. https://doi.org/10.1067/j.cpradiol.2007.10.001.
69. de Baere T, Deschamps F. New tumor ablation techniques for cancer treatment (microwave, electroporation). Diagn Interv Imaging. 2014;95(7–8):677–82. https://doi.org/10.1016/j.diii.2014.04.001.
70. Huo YR, Eslick GD. Microwave ablation compared to radiofrequency ablation for hepatic lesions: a meta-analysis. J Vasc Interv Radiol. 2015;26(8):1139–1146.e2. https://doi.org/10.1016/j.jvir.2015.04.004.
71. Poulou LS, Botsa E, Thanou I, Ziakas PD, Thanos L. Percutaneous microwave ablation vs radiofrequency ablation in the treatment of hepatocellular carcinoma. World J Hepatol. 2015;7(8):1054–63. https://doi.org/10.4254/wjh.v7.i8.1054.
72. Wolf F, Dupuy DE. Microwave ablation: mechanism of action and devices. In: Hong K, Georgiades CS, editors. Percutaneous tumor ablation. 2011th ed. Stuttgart: Georg Thieme Verlag; 2011. https://doi.org/10.1055/b-0034-81501.
73. Brace CL. Microwave ablation technology: what every use should know. Curr Probl Diagn Radiol. 2009;38(2):61–7. https://doi.org/10.1067/j.cpradiol.2007.08.011.
74. Ringe KI, Lutat C, Rieder C, Schenk A, Wacker F, Raatschen H-J. Experimental evaluation of the heat sink effect in hepatic microwave ablation. PLoS ONE. 2015;10(7):e0134301. https://doi.org/10.1371/journal.pone.0134301.
75. Groeschl RT, Pilgrim CHC, Hanna EM, et al. Microwave ablation for hepatic malignancies: a multiinstitutional analysis. Ann Surg. 2014;259(6):1195–200. https://doi.org/10.1097/SLA.0000000000000234.
76. Shibata T, Niinobu T, Ogata N, Takami M. Microwave coagulation therapy for multiple hepatic metastases from colorectal carcinoma. Cancer. 2000;89(2):276–84.
77. Liu Y, Li S, Wan X, et al. Efficacy and safety of thermal ablation in patients with liver metastases. Eur J Gastroenterol Hepatol. 2013;25(4):442–6. https://doi.org/10.1097/MEG.0b013e32835cb566.
78. Correa-Gallego C, Fong Y, Gonen M, et al. A retrospective comparison of microwave ablation vs. radiofrequency ablation for colorectal cancer hepatic metastases. Ann Surg Oncol. 2014;21(13):4278–83. https://doi.org/10.1245/s10434-014-3817-0.
79. Martin RCG, Scoggins CR, McMasters KM. Microwave hepatic ablation: initial experience of safety and efficacy. J Surg Oncol. 2007;96(6):481–6. https://doi.org/10.1002/jso.20750.
80. Iannitti DA, Martin RCG, Simon CJ, et al. Hepatic tumor ablation with clustered microwave antennae: the US Phase II Trial. HPB. 2007;9(2):120–4. https://doi.org/10.1080/13651820701222677.
81. Zhou P, Liang P, Yu X, Wang Y, Dong B. Percutaneous microwave ablation of liver cancer adjacent to the gastrointestinal tract. J Gastrointest Surg. 2009;13(2):318. https://doi.org/10.1007/s11605-008-0710-9.
82. Sag AA, Selcukbiricik F, Mandel NM. Evidence-based medical oncology and interventional radiology paradigms for liver-dominant colorectal cancer metastases. World J Gastroenterol. 2016;22(11):3127–49. https://doi.org/10.3748/wjg.v22.i11.3127.
83. Adam R, Hagopian EJ, Linhares M, et al. A comparison of percutaneous cryosurgery and percutaneous radiofrequency for unresectable hepatic malignancies. Arch Surg. 2002;137(12):1332–9. https://doi.org/10.1001/archsurg.137.12.1332.
84. Bageacu S, Kaczmarek D, Lacroix M, Dubois J, Forest J, Porcheron J. Cryosurgery for resectable and unresectable hepatic metastases from colorectal cancer. Eur J Surg Oncol EJSO. 2007;33(5):590–6. https://doi.org/10.1016/j.ejso.2007.01.003.

85. Yu H, Burke CT. Comparison of percutaneous ablation technologies in the treatment of malignant liver tumors. Semin Interv Radiol. 2014;31(2):129–37. https://doi.org/10.1055/s-0034-1373788.
86. Baust JG, Gage AA. The molecular basis of cryosurgery. BJU Int. 2005;95(9):1187–91. https://doi.org/10.1111/j.1464-410X.2005.05502.x.
87. Ryan MJ, Willatt J, Majdalany BS, et al. Ablation techniques for primary and metastatic liver tumors. World J Hepatol. 2016;8(3):191–9. https://doi.org/10.4254/wjh.v8.i3.191.
88. Bo YD, Philip C, Morris David L. Hepatic cryotherapy and regional chemotherapy with or without resection for liver metastases from colorectal carcinoma. Cancer. 2003;98(2):320–30. https://doi.org/10.1002/cncr.11498.
89. Paganini AM, Rotundo A, Barchetti L, Lezoche E. Cryosurgical ablation of hepatic colorectal metastases. Surg Oncol. 2007;16:137–40. https://doi.org/10.1016/j.suronc.2007.10.031.
90. Michel R, Franco DC, Pierre M, Sylvie N, Henri S, Pierre K. Combination of neoadjuvant chemotherapy with cryotherapy and surgical resection for the treatment of unresectable liver metastases from colorectal carcinoma. Cancer. 2002;95(11):2283–92. https://doi.org/10.1002/cncr.10973.
91. Seifert JK, Morris DL. World survey on the complications of hepatic and prostate cryotherapy. World J Surg. 1999;23(2):109–14. https://doi.org/10.1007/PL00013173.
92. Xu K-C, Niu L-Z, He W-B, Hu Y-Z, Zuo J-S. Percutaneous cryosurgery for the treatment of hepatic colorectal metastases. World J Gastroenterol WJG. 2008;14(9):1430–6. https://doi.org/10.3748/wjg.14.1430.
93. Kerkar S, Carlin AM, Sohn RL, et al. Long-term follow up and prognostic factors for cryotherapy of malignant liver tumors. Surgery. 2004;136(4):770–9. https://doi.org/10.1016/j.surg.2004.07.001.
94. Pearson AS, Izzo F, Fleming RY, et al. Intraoperative radiofrequency ablation or cryoablation for hepatic malignancies. Am J Surg. 1999;178(6):592–9.
95. Evans J. Ablative and catheter-delivered therapies for colorectal liver metastases (CRLM). Eur J Surg Oncol EJSO. 2007;33:S64–75. https://doi.org/10.1016/j.ejso.2007.09.027.
96. Clark TWI, Soulen MC. Chemical ablation of hepatocellular carcinoma. J Vasc Interv Radiol JVIR. 2002;13(9 Pt 2):S245–52.
97. Shiina S, Tagawa K, Unuma T, et al. Percutaneous ethanol injection therapy for hepatocellular carcinoma. A histopathologic study. Cancer. 1991;68(7):1524–30.
98. Da Ines D, Buc E, Petitcolin V, et al. Massive hepatic necrosis with gastric, splenic, and pancreatic infarctions after ethanol ablation for hepatocellular carcinoma. J Vasc Interv Radiol JVIR. 2010;21(8):1301–5. https://doi.org/10.1016/j.jvir.2010.04.011.
99. Hasegawa S, Yamasaki N, Hiwaki T, et al. Factors that predict intrahepatic recurrence of hepatocellular carcinoma in 81 patients initially treated by percutaneous ethanol injection. Cancer. 1999;86(9):1682–90.
100. Masahiko K, Yoshikazu M, Akeri M, et al. Predictive factors for intrahepatic recurrence after percutaneous ethanol injection therapy for small hepatocellular carcinoma. Cancer. 2000;88(3):529–37. https://doi.org/10.1002/(SICI)1097-0142(20000201)88:3<529::AID-CNCR6>3.0.CO;2-M.
101. Scheffer HJ, Nielsen K, de Jong MC, et al. Irreversible electroporation for nonthermal tumor ablation in the clinical setting: a systematic review of safety and efficacy. J Vasc Interv Radiol JVIR. 2014;25(7):997–1011; quiz 1011. https://doi.org/10.1016/j.jvir.2014.01.028.
102. Davalos RV, Mir ILM, Rubinsky B. Tissue ablation with irreversible electroporation. Ann Biomed Eng. 2005;33(2):223–31.
103. Miller L, Leor J, Rubinsky B. Cancer cells ablation with irreversible electroporation. Technol Cancer Res Treat. 2005;4(6):699–705. https://doi.org/10.1177/153303460500400615.
104. Edd JF, Horowitz L, Davalos RV, Mir LM, Rubinsky B. In vivo results of a new focal tissue ablation technique: irreversible electroporation. IEEE Trans Biomed Eng. 2006;53(7):1409–15. https://doi.org/10.1109/TBME.2006.873745.
105. Melikov KC, Frolov VA, Shcherbakov A, Samsonov AV, Chizmadzhev YA, Chernomordik LV. Voltage-induced nonconductive pre-pores and metastable single pores in

unmodified planar lipid bilayer. Biophys J. 2001;80(4):1829–36. https://doi.org/10.1016/S0006-3495(01)76153-X.
106. Schmidt CR, Shires P, Mootoo M. Real-time ultrasound imaging of irreversible electroporation in a porcine liver model adequately characterizes the zone of cellular necrosis. HPB. 2012;14(2):98–102. https://doi.org/10.1111/j.1477-2574.2011.00409.x.
107. Thomson KR, Cheung W, Ellis SJ, et al. Investigation of the safety of irreversible electroporation in humans. J Vasc Interv Radiol JVIR. 2011;22(5):611–21. https://doi.org/10.1016/j.jvir.2010.12.014.
108. Kos B, Voigt P, Miklavcic D, Moche M. Careful treatment planning enables safe ablation of liver tumors adjacent to major blood vessels by percutaneous irreversible electroporation (IRE). Radiol Oncol. 2015;49(3):234–41. https://doi.org/10.1515/raon-2015-0031.
109. Cannon R, Ellis S, Hayes D, Narayanan G, Martin RCG. Safety and early efficacy of irreversible electroporation for hepatic tumors in proximity to vital structures. J Surg Oncol. 2013;107(5):544–9. https://doi.org/10.1002/jso.23280.
110. Kingham TP, Karkar AM, D'Angelica MI, et al. Ablation of perivascular hepatic malignant tumors with irreversible electroporation. J Am Coll Surg. 2012;215(3):379–87. https://doi.org/10.1016/j.jamcollsurg.2012.04.029.
111. Silk MT, Wimmer T, Lee KS, et al. Percutaneous ablation of peribiliary tumors with irreversible electroporation. J Vasc Interv Radiol JVIR. 2014;25(1):112–8. https://doi.org/10.1016/j.jvir.2013.10.012.
112. Hosein PJ, Echenique A, Loaiza-Bonilla A, et al. Percutaneous irreversible electroporation for the treatment of colorectal cancer liver metastases with a proposal for a new response evaluation system. J Vasc Interv Radiol. 2014;25(8):1233–1239.e2. https://doi.org/10.1016/j.jvir.2014.04.007.
113. Niessen C, Beyer LP, Pregler B, et al. Percutaneous ablation of hepatic tumors using irreversible electroporation: a prospective safety and midterm efficacy study in 34 patients. J Vasc Interv Radiol JVIR. 2016;27(4):480–6. https://doi.org/10.1016/j.jvir.2015.12.025.
114. Frühling P, Nilsson A, Duraj F, Haglund U, Norén A. Single-center nonrandomized clinical trial to assess the safety and efficacy of irreversible electroporation (IRE) ablation of liver tumors in humans: short to mid-term results. Eur J Surg Oncol J Eur Soc Surg Oncol Br Assoc Surg Oncol. 2017;43(4):751–7. https://doi.org/10.1016/j.ejso.2016.12.004.
115. Mahadevan A, Blanck O, Lanciano R, et al. Stereotactic body radiotherapy (SBRT) for liver metastasis – clinical outcomes from the international multi-institutional RSSearch® patient registry. Radiat Oncol Lond Engl. 2018;13:26. https://doi.org/10.1186/s13014-018-0969-2.
116. Berkovic P, Gulyban A, Nguyen PV, et al. Stereotactic robotic body radiotherapy for patients with unresectable hepatic oligorecurrence. Clin Colorectal Cancer. 2017;16(4):349–357.e1. https://doi.org/10.1016/j.clcc.2017.03.006.
117. Joo JH, Park J, Kim JC, et al. Local control outcomes using stereotactic body radiation therapy for liver metastases from colorectal cancer. Int J Radiat Oncol. 2017;99(4):876–83. https://doi.org/10.1016/j.ijrobp.2017.07.030.
118. Gani F, Thompson VM, Bentrem DJ, Hall BL, Pitt HA, Pawlik TM. Patterns of hepatic resections in North America: use of concurrent partial resections and ablations. HPB. 2016;18(10):813–20. https://doi.org/10.1016/j.hpb.2016.06.002.
119. Bai H, Huangz X, Jing L, Zeng Q, Han L. The effect of radiofrequency ablation vs. liver resection on survival outcome of colorectal liver metastases (CRLM): a meta-analysis. Hepato-Gastroenterology. 2015;62(138):373–7.

Chemoembolization for Colorectal Liver Metastases

37

José Hugo Mendes Luz

Introduction

The combination of drug injection and targeted embolic occlusion through a catheter is known as transarterial chemoembolization (TACE) and has been extensively used for the treatment of hypervascular tumors such as hepatocellular carcinoma and neuroendocrine liver metastases [1, 2]. A little over a decade ago, Drug-Eluting Beads TACE (DEB-TACE) were reported and consisted of TACE using microspheres capable of absorbing the chemotherapeutic drug and slowly releasing it once inside the tumor vascular supply [3–5]. Promising results were shown in the treatment of HCC with this new concept of chemoembolization, doxorubicin DEB-TACE [6], and concurrently reports demonstrated its usefulness in colorectal metastases adopting microspheres loaded with irinotecan [7]. This TACE modality, in which drug-eluting beads are loaded with irinotecan, is called DEBIRI, and it allows sustained drug release after the beads are trapped in the tumoral circulation [7]. Over the years there was an increasing body of data over DEBIRI from clinical trials and systematic reviews, enabling the evaluation of the efficacy and safety of this therapeutic modality in the treatment of colorectal liver metastases (CRLM).

Rationale

TACE has been used for decades in the treatment of liver malignancy. Its principle arises from two principle milestones. First of all the liver has a unique circulation in which its blood supply comes from the portal vein and the hepatic artery, preventing

J. H. M. Luz (✉)
Head Interventional Radiology Unit, Radiology Department, INCA – Brazilian National Cancer Institute, Rio de Janeiro, Brazil

M. M. Correia et al. (eds.), *Colorectal Cancer Liver Metastases*,
https://doi.org/10.1007/978-3-030-25486-5_37

major organ necrosis after occlusion of its arterial supply. Second, in contrast to normal healthy liver tissue, which is supplied mostly by the portal vein, liver tumors (primary and metastatic) receive their blood supply almost exclusively from the artery, which can then be exploited for anatomical targeting and treatment. The concept of TACE comprises the infusion of the chemotherapeutic agents followed by an embolic agent into the hepatic arteries supplying the liver tumors while sparing the surrounding normal hepatic parenchyma. The chemotherapy is usually mixed with an oil-based contrast medium (Lipiodol Ultrafiltrate, Laboratoire Guerbert, France), which serves as a drug carrier. This water-in-oil emulsion obtained (drug plus Lipiodol) is selectively delivered to the tumor-feeding artery through a microcatheter, followed by the infusion of the elected embolic material. Lipiodol is the primary component of conventional TACE (cTACE), and due to the high vascularization of most liver tumors and the absence of Kupffer cells inside the tumors, Lipiodol can persist within tumor nodules, thus exposing it to the chemotherapeutic agent.

This type of approach was the first described technique, known as cTACE, and also the first one to demonstrate survival benefit in the treatment of the hepatocellular carcinoma [8, 9]. DEB-TACE has been derived from cTACE, where Lipiodol is substituted for a polymer-based microparticles, which results in enhanced drug delivery when compared to conventional cTACE. DEB-TACE was suggested to improve cTACE efficacy by means of its slow drug-release capability, thus prolonging the duration of tumor exposure to high concentrations of chemotherapy, with reduced systemic bioavailability. The high first-pass effect of chemotherapy, augmented by prolonged exposure time with high drug levels from embolic effects on the tumor vasculature, produces a significant increase of the pharmacological advantage for regional drug delivery [10]. For the treatment of hepatocellular carcinoma (HCC), cTACE has generated solid evidence along the years, established as a recognized treatment option in international guidelines such as the BCLC algorithm [11]. While this holds true for TACE in the treatment of HCC, it is not well acknowledged for TACE in the treatment of colorectal liver metastases. The disappointing performance for TACE in CRLM was mainly due to two factors: the liver lesions were not as vascularized as HCC, and the available drugs were not highly active against this type of malignancy. DEB-TACE with irinotecan (DEBIRI) brought the opportunity to use a drug that is part of the arsenal of the systemic treatment of colorectal cancer. This generated a relative awareness and adoption of DEBIRI in the treatment of CRLM, which, initially, was also based on the known evidence and widespread use of doxorubicin DEB-TACE in the treatment of HCC. Besides the research and clinical interest in DEBIRI, a fundamental paradox exists specifically with irinotecan in this type of treatment. After eluded in the beads, this drug is directly injected and targeted to the tumor vascularity. However, it is known that irinotecan requires activation within the normal liver parenchyma to become an active drug. Based on this knowledge, the question remains as to whether our understanding of tumoral metabolism is incorrect, or whether alternate mechanisms of administration provide a more optimal method of therapeutic payload delivery [12].

Technical Aspects and Recommendations

Patient Selection

Patients suitable for TACE are the ones who are not candidates for curative therapy such as surgical resection, have a tumor burden not greater than 60%, and have liver dominant disease with minimal extrahepatic disease [13–15]. In spite of the aforementioned recommendations, some isolated reports have described DEBIRI as a downstage approach to liver metastases prior to surgical resection and even in upfront surgical candidates [16]. Patients should have an Eastern Cooperative Oncology Group performance status of 0 or 1 and a well-compensated liver function. It has been shown that patients with bilirubin levels above 2 mg/dL and more than 50% tumor liver burden have longer hospital permanence and more adverse events [17]. Patient selection should finally follow multidisciplinary discussion and thoroughly clinical, laboratorial, and imaging assessment.

Procedural Description

Patients are admitted to the hospital prior to the procedure for clinical and laboratory review and pre-procedure medication. Periprocedural care is of vital importance, mainly focused to control pain and nauseas and vomiting. The procedure might be accomplished with venous analgesia or through paravertebral block, at the discretion of the executing radiologist. Arterial access is established through transfemoral or trans-radial vascular sheath positioning. Celiac and superior mesenteric angiograms are acquired for anatomy delineation and tumor distribution. A microcatheter is advanced co-axially to the right or left hepatic artery for the DEB-TACE administration. In patients with bilobar liver disease, each lobe is treated separately, and the untreated lobe is scheduled for treatment within 2 weeks. In this situation 100 mg of irinotecan is administrated with the DEB in each session, and a total of four sessions are accomplished – two sessions in the right lobe and two in the left. For unilobar disease a total of two sessions are scheduled with 2-week interval, and similarly 100 mg of irinotecan is administrated in each session. A whole-liver treatment in a single session through selective right and left lobar injections and total administration of 200 mg irinotecan loaded in the DEB has been described although it should be employed in selected patients since it is associated with higher toxicity [18]. After the procedure all patients are admitted for at least 24 h in-hospital observation for pain and nausea control. Figures 37.1, 37.2, and 37.3.

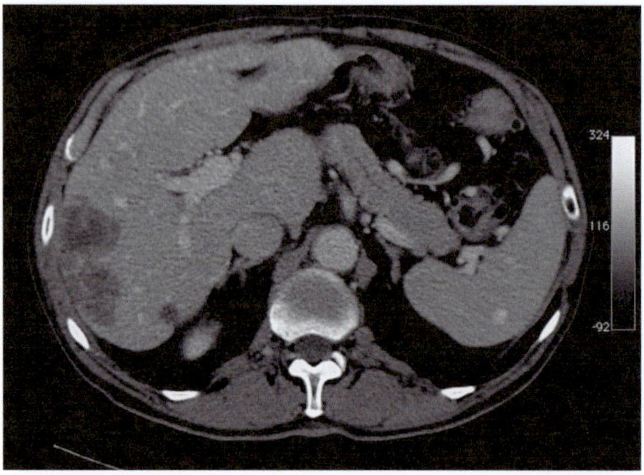

Fig. 37.1 62-year-old male patient with colorectal liver metastases already submitted to two lines of systemic chemotherapy. Computed tomography with intravenous contrast showing a metastatic lesion in the right lobe of the liver

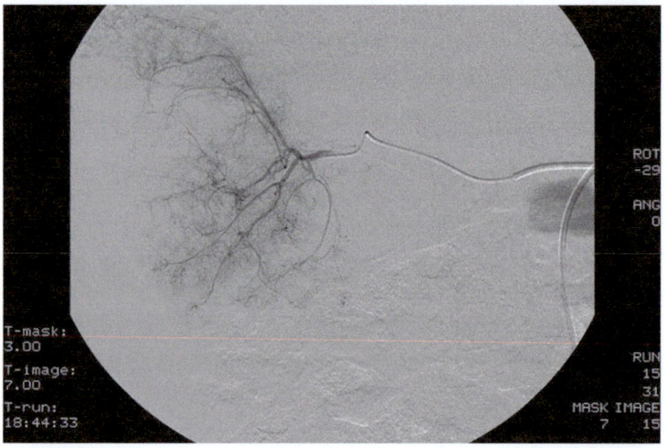

Fig. 37.2 Selective arteriography with a microcatheter right before accomplishing TACE with drug-eluting beads loaded with irinotecan – DEBIRI

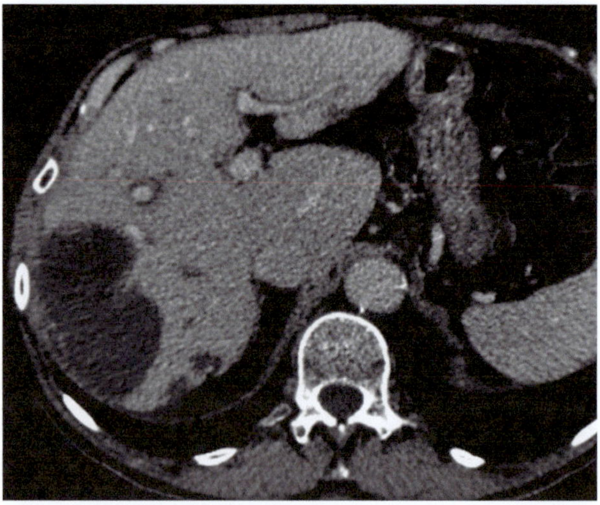

Fig. 37.3 Contrasted computed tomography 9 months after the first DEBIRI session. The metastatic lesion is now markedly hypodense and with minimal contrast enhancement (the patient also demonstrated a persistent and significant reduction in CEA values)

TACE Associated with Percutaneous Ablation

Few reports have addressed the associative treatment of TACE and ablation in the CRLM treatment, as it has been more widely reported in the hepatocellular carcinoma scenario. Previous studies demonstrated that microwave ablation combined with TACE therapy for HCC resulted in a high complete response rate [19, 20]. There are some potential and rational explanations for combining these two treatment modalities. Through the reduction in blood flow to the liver tumor area, TACE can enlarge the thermal coagulation area of ablation by attenuating the cooling effect of the hepatic circulation. Meanwhile it is speculated that thermal ablation can increase pooling and sensitize tumor cells to chemotherapy, thus decreasing the total number of TACE sessions and allowing chemotherapy dose reduction. This can ultimately reduce adverse reactions in the liver and might influence patient prognosis [21]. In a study conducted to evaluate percutaneous microwave ablation combined with synchronous TACE for the treatment of colorectal liver metastases, they administered an average dose of Lipiodol of only 1.5–10 mL, while in most publications related to Lipiodol-TACE, the reported dose can be as high as 20 mL [22]. In this combined treatment study, the objective response rate was 83.4%, which compares favorably with the highest achieved objective response rate for the DEBIRI treatment, reported at 70% [7]. Authors of this study also described no major complications or treatment-related mortality and suggested that MWA combined with synchronous TACE is a safe and well-tolerated procedure for CRLM patients. Figures 37.4, 37.5, 37.6, 37.7, 37.8, and 37.9.

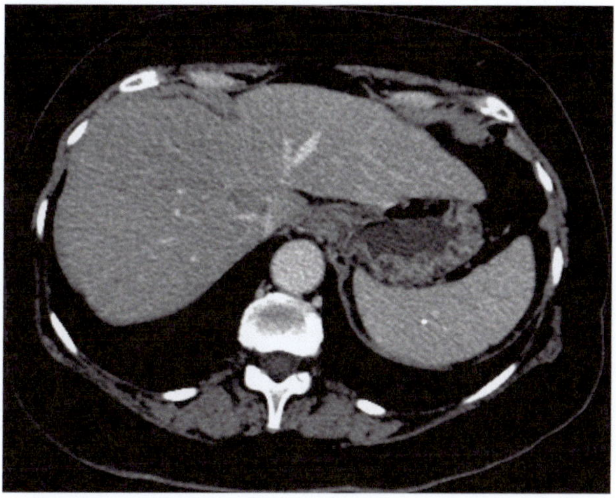

Fig. 37.4 An 83-year-old female patient with colorectal liver metastases, PS of 1, heavely treated with two lines of systemic chemotherapy, presented with a new liver lesion. A multidisciplinary decision was not for surgery, and she was fowered to perform ablation followed by DEB-TACE (the combined treatment was chosen based in the new lesion proximity to the right and middle hepatic veins)

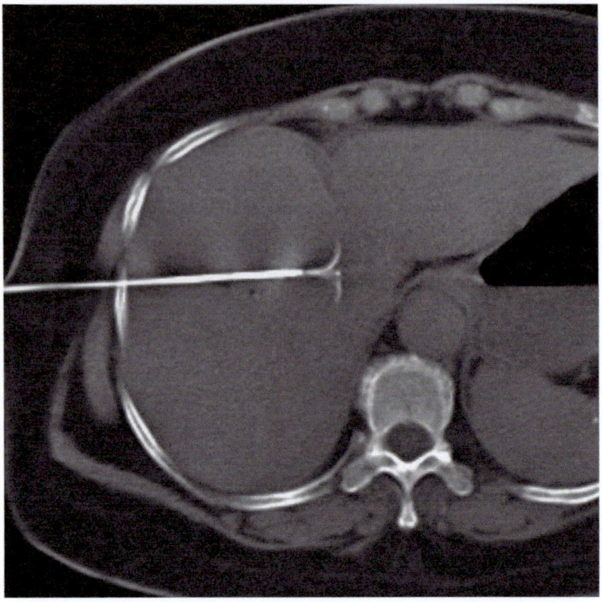

Fig. 37.5 Computed tomography imaging of the ablation procedure shows the radiofrequency ablation needle properly positioned inside the liver lesion

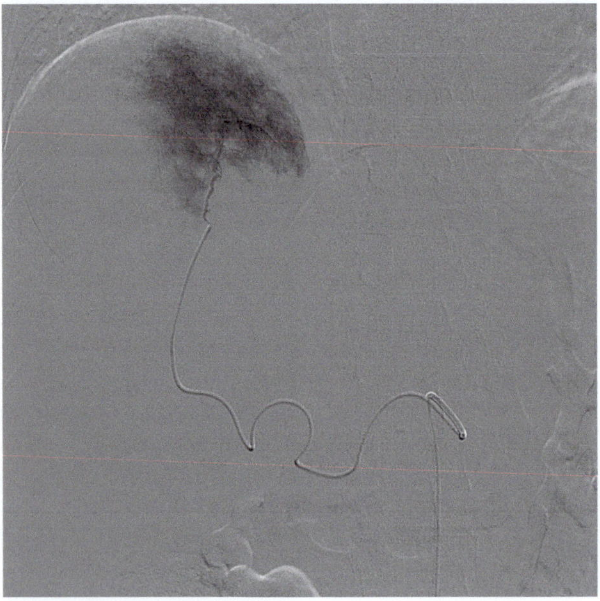

Fig. 37.6 Two days later the patient was submitted to DEBIRI. Selective angiography performed to confirm the adequate location for DEBIRI administration

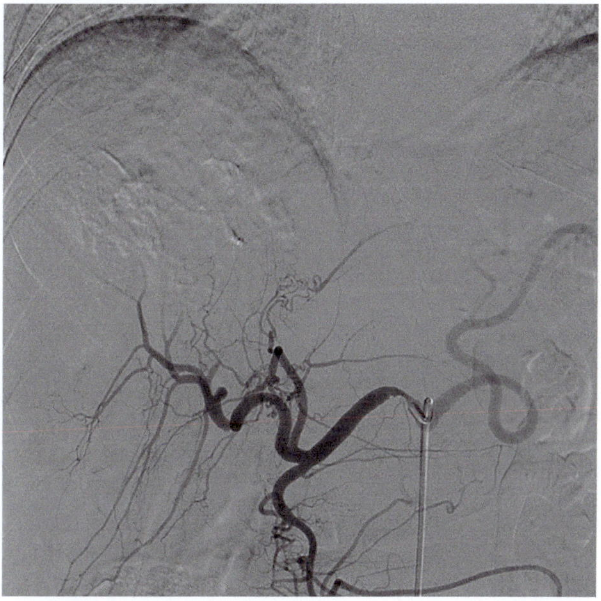

Fig. 37.7 Control angiography after DEBIRI showing devascularization of the area occupied by the liver metastases

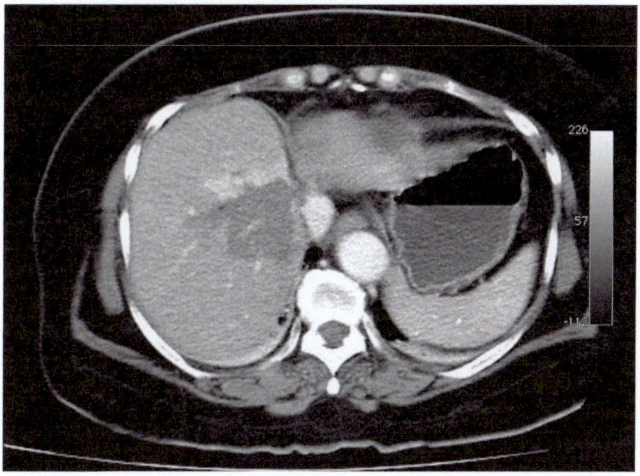

Fig. 37.8 Contrasted computed tomography one day after DEBIRI showing an adequate, large hypodense area corresponding to the result of the two treatments

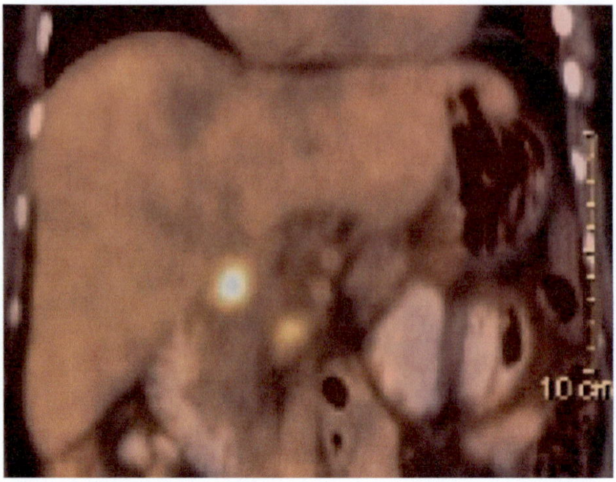

Fig. 37.9 Positron emission tomography scan of the abdomen 2 years after the combined procedures (TACE plus ablation) depicted an avid augmented ganglia in the hepatic hilum. The liver lesion did not show any enhancement by the nuclear medicine radiotracer

Treatment Response and Adverse Events

Tumor response was used as an outcome in most of the publications related to TACE in the CRLM. When scrutinizing this literature, an important aspect is to identify which radiological response criterion was used. Studies adopting the Response Evaluation Criteria in Solid Tumors (RECIST) [23] guideline will base tumor response mainly on lesion size changes, while other radiological imaging criteria such as the modified RECIST (mRECIST) [24] and the EASL criteria [25] will determine tumor response also through tumor enhancement variations. EASL and mRECIST are then considered functional imaging biomarkers, while RECIST is an anatomic imaging biomarker. Several studies have shown good to excellent inter-rater correlation between mRECIST and EASL [26]. Of the studies pooled in a recent systematic review [27], eight utilized mRECIST/EASL criteria for response assessment, which yielded 51.1% (weighted averages), and seven studies utilized RECIST, with that group yielding a response of 56.2% (weighted averages). The study with the highest rate of responders reported 70% of patients showing response after DEBIRI treatment [28]. In contrast, studies with low rates of response, as low as 10%, were also seen [29]. Some studies reported on biological markers such as CEA and whether or not patients showed a decreased level of CEA compared to pretreatment levels. Two studies reported a 100% decrease in CEA level after DEBIRI treatment [7, 30]. Of the four studies that reported on CEA reduction, the percentage ranged from 42% to 100% of patients, though most studies did not report on this laboratory value.

Most studies reporting the use of DEBIRI used the CTCAE criteria to assess toxicity. All grade toxicity for these studies ranged from 6% to 100% with an average of 35.2% [27]. The most commonly reported adverse events were pain and nausea and vomiting, present in all publications. High-grade toxicity can get as high as 32% with most of the reported events related to abdominal pain and liver dysfunction. Very few cases of death were reported across all studies with only two events in which death might have been credited to treatment complications [31, 32]. Few studies reported that the DEBIRI treatments were done on an outpatient basis though most studies did report regular hospitalizations, averaging 2.3 days of hospital stay [30, 33, 34]. A specific study showed factors independently associated with DEBIRI toxicity such as not using intra-arterial lidocaine in the hepatic-feeding vessel immediately before TACE, three treatments or more, complete arterial stasis in the control angiography immediate after TACE, more than 100 mg of DEBIRI in one treatment, bilirubin higher than 2 mg/dl, and more than 50% liver involvement [17].

Survival, Progression-Free Survival, and Time to Progression

In 15 studies included in a recent systematic review, progression-free survival, described in months, was reported in 12 of them. This outcome varied from 4 to 15.3 months with a calculated average of 8.1 months. Two studies reported time to progression of 5 months [33, 35]. Median overall survival in months was reported in 11 of the 15 studies. The results reported for DEBIRI treatment for the shortest and longest median overall survival were 5.4 months [36] and 20.4 months, respectively [37]. When analyzing TACE results for CRLM, it is critical to carefully acknowledge the study population. For instance, of the total patients treated with DEBIRI in the studies included in a recent systematic review, 33% had extrahepatic disease and 43% of patients had prior liver surgery or ablation. Other primordial aspect is the pre-TACE exposure to systemic chemotherapy. In the majority of the studies, the number of prior systemic treatment lines was two, which serves as an indirect measure of the advanced disease stage of patients that are typically referred for DEBIRI treatment. Subgroup analyses were performed without reaching relevance, except for toxicity, in which patients with extrahepatic disease experienced significant more adverse events.

Authors also explored the clinical utility of TACE in combinations with systemic chemotherapy, which can be particularly beneficial in the group of patients with extrahepatic disease. Capecitabine, an oral chemotherapeutic drug, has been addressed concomitant with DEBIRI [32]. Authors compared DEBIRI alone versus DEBIRI plus capecitabine and demonstrated no additional toxicity when adding this drug to this TACE modality. In spite of that, survival benefit with concurrent capecitabine was not statistically significant although there was a trend towards improved survival. A randomized controlled trial (RCT) compared DEBIRI to systemic FOLFIRI (a chemotherapy regimen composed of folinic acid, fluorouracil, and irinotecan) in a pretreated population, mainly patients submitted to one or two systemic chemotherapeutic regimens. This RCT showed a statistically significant difference between DEBIRI and systemic FOLFIRI for three different outcomes. DEBIRI demonstrated better overall survival, longer progression-free survival, and enhanced quality of life. Furthermore, a 4-month significant improvement in time to extrahepatic progression was observed for DEBIRI, a reversal of the expectation for a regional treatment. While limitations have been alluded, due to the study population and the lack of oxaliplatin, bevacizumab, cetuximab, or panitumumab in the FOLFIRI arm, this RCT does suggest a benefit of DEBIRI treatment over standard chemotherapy and serves to establish the expected difference between these two treatment options for planning future large randomized studies [30]. The second RCT consisted of two treatment arms containing DEBIRI with systemic FOLFOX6 versus systemic FOLFOX6. Bevacizumab could be added accordingly to the investigator discretion. Authors concluded that simultaneous mFOLFOX6 and DEBIRI did not cause more chemotherapy delivery delays nor increased chemotherapy toxicity. In addition, simultaneous use of FOLFOX and DEBIRI leads to improved overall response rates, improved hepatic progression-free survival, and more durable overall progression-free survival in patients downsized to resection [28].

Current Evidence and Conclusions

In the last decade most of the relevant literature to support TACE in the treatment of CRLM came from reports using the drug-eluting carrier-based delivery treatment. More specifically, DEBIRI has the majority of the data in this context and is the only TACE treatment with a reported phase III study and two published systematic reviews. The combination of TACE and thermal ablation has potential synergistic benefits although it has been scarcely exploited in the literature. Scheduled TACE administration with concurrent systemic chemotherapy seems promising, and two randomized controlled trials exploiting this association have been published. Although different TACE modalities can show high tumor response rate and adequate progression-free survival rate or overall survival, the optimal intra-arterial approach to CRLM has not been established, and recognized competitive modalities such as radioembolization and intra-arterial chemotherapy treatment must be addressed in a head-to-head comparison to TACE.

References

1. Yao KA, Talamonti MS, Nemcek A, Angelos P, Chrisman H, Skarda J, Benson AB, Rao S, Joehl RJ. Indications and results of liver resection and hepatic chemoembolization for metastatic gastrointestinal neuroendocrine tumors. Surgery. 2001;130(4):677–82; discussion 682–5.
2. Bruix J, Sherman M, Practice Guidelines Committee, A. e. A. f. t. S. o. L. D. Management of hepatocellular carcinoma. Hepatology. 2005;42(5):1208–36.
3. Lewis AL, Taylor RR, Hall B, Gonzalez MV, Willis SL, Stratford PW. Pharmacokinetic and safety study of doxorubicin-eluting beads in a porcine model of hepatic arterial embolization. J Vasc Interv Radiol. 2006;17(8):1335–43.
4. Varela M, Real MI, Burrel M, Forner A, Sala M, Brunet M, Ayuso C, Castells L, Montañá X, Llovet JM, Bruix J. Chemoembolization of hepatocellular carcinoma with drug eluting beads: efficacy and doxorubicin pharmacokinetics. J Hepatol. 2007;46(3):474–81.
5. Poon RT, Tso WK, Pang RW, Ng KK, Woo R, Tai KS, Fan ST. A phase I/II trial of chemoembolization for hepatocellular carcinoma using a novel intra-arterial drug-eluting bead. Clin Gastroenterol Hepatol. 2007;5(9):1100–8.

6. Lammer J, Malagari K, Vogl T, Pilleul F, Denys A, Watkinson A, Pitton M, Sergent G, Pfammatter T, Terraz S, Benhamou Y, Avajon Y, Gruenberger T, Pomoni M, Langenberger H, Schuchmann M, Dumortier J, Mueller C, Chevallier P, Lencioni R, Investigators PV. Prospective randomized study of doxorubicin-eluting-bead embolization in the treatment of hepatocellular carcinoma: results of the PRECISION V study. Cardiovasc Intervent Radiol. 2010;33(1):41–52.
7. Aliberti C, Tilli M, Benea G, Fiorentini G. Trans-arterial chemoembolization (TACE) of liver metastases from colorectal cancer using irinotecan-eluting beads: preliminary results. Anticancer Res. 2006;26(5B):3793–5.
8. Llovet JM, Bruix J. Systematic review of randomized trials for unresectable hepatocellular carcinoma: chemoembolization improves survival. Hepatology. 2003;37(2):429–42.
9. Llovet JM, Real MI, Montaña X, Planas R, Coll S, Aponte J, Ayuso C, Sala M, Muchart J, Solà R, Rodés J, Bruix J, Group, B. L. C. Arterial embolisation or chemoembolisation versus symptomatic treatment in patients with unresectable hepatocellular carcinoma: a randomised controlled trial. Lancet. 2002;359(9319):1734–9.
10. Collins JM. Pharmacologic rationale for regional drug delivery. J Clin Oncol. 1984;2(5):498–504.
11. Forner A, Gilabert M, Bruix J, Raoul JL. Treatment of intermediate-stage hepatocellular carcinoma. Nat Rev Clin Oncol. 2014;11(9):525–35.
12. Liu DM, Thakor AS, Baerlocher M, Alshammari MT, Lim H, Kos S, Kennedy AS, Wasan H. A review of conventional and drug-eluting chemoembolization in the treatment of colorectal liver metastases: principles and proof. Future Oncol. 2015;11(9):1421–8.
13. Richardson AJ, Laurence JM, Lam VW. Transarterial chemoembolization with irinotecan beads in the treatment of colorectal liver metastases: systematic review. J Vasc Interv Radiol. 2013;24(8):1209–17.
14. Bower M, Metzger T, Robbins K, Tomalty D, Válek V, Boudný J, Andrasina T, Tatum C, Martin RC. Surgical downstaging and neo-adjuvant therapy in metastatic colorectal carcinoma with irinotecan drug-eluting beads: a multi-institutional study. HPB (Oxford). 2010;12(1):31–6.
15. Brown RE, Bower MR, Metzger TL, Scoggins CR, McMasters KM, Hahl MJ, Tatum C, Martin RC. Hepatectomy after hepatic arterial therapy with either yttrium-90 or drug-eluting bead chemotherapy: is it safe? HPB (Oxford). 2011;13(2):91–5.
16. Jones RP, Malik HZ, Fenwick SW, Terlizzo M, O'Grady E, Stremitzer S, Gruenberger T, Rees M, Plant G, Figueras J, Albiol M, Adam R, Awad S, Poston GJ. PARAGON II – a single arm multicentre phase II study of neoadjuvant therapy using irinotecan bead in patients with resectable liver metastases from colorectal cancer. Eur J Surg Oncol. 2016;42(12):1866–72.
17. Martin RC, Howard J, Tomalty D, Robbins K, Padr R, Bosnjakovic PM, Tatum C. Toxicity of irinotecan-eluting beads in the treatment of hepatic malignancies: results of a multi-institutional registry. Cardiovasc Intervent Radiol. 2010;33(5):960–6.
18. Lencioni R, Aliberti C, de Baere T, Garcia-Monaco R, Narayanan G, O'Grady E, Rilling WS, Walker D, Martin RC. Transarterial treatment of colorectal cancer liver metastases with irinotecan-loaded drug-eluting beads: technical recommendations. J Vasc Interv Radiol. 2014;25(3):365–9.
19. Li S, Zhang L, Huang ZM, Wu PH. Transcatheter arterial chemoembolization combined with CT-guided percutaneous thermal ablation versus hepatectomy in the treatment of hepatocellular carcinoma. Chin J Cancer. 2015;34(6):254–63.
20. Yang GW, Zhao Q, Qian S, Zhu L, Qu XD, Zhang W, Yan ZP, Cheng JM, Liu QX, Liu R, Wang JH. Percutaneous microwave ablation combined with simultaneous transarterial chemoembolization for the treatment of advanced intrahepatic cholangiocarcinoma. Onco Targets Ther. 2015;8:1245–50.
21. Liu HC, Shan EB, Zhou L, Jin H, Cui PY, Tan Y, Lu YM. Combination of percutaneous radiofrequency ablation with transarterial chemoembolization for hepatocellular carcinoma: observation of clinical effects. Chin J Cancer Res. 2014;26(4):471–7.
22. Wu ZB, Si ZM, Qian S, Liu LX, Qu XD, Zhou B, Zhang W, Wang GZ, Liu R, Wang JH. Percutaneous microwave ablation combined with synchronous transcatheter arterial

chemoembolization for the treatment of colorectal liver metastases: results from a follow-up cohort. Onco Targets Ther. 2016;9:3783–9.
23. Therasse P, Arbuck SG, Eisenhauer EA, Wanders J, Kaplan RS, Rubinstein L, Verweij J, Van Glabbeke M, van Oosterom AT, Christian MC, Gwyther SG. New guidelines to evaluate the response to treatment in solid tumors. European Organization for Research and Treatment of Cancer, National Cancer Institute of the United States, National Cancer Institute of Canada. J Natl Cancer Inst. 2000;92(3):205–16.
24. Lencioni R, Llovet JM. Modified RECIST (mRECIST) assessment for hepatocellular carcinoma. Semin Liver Dis. 2010;30(1):52–60.
25. Bruix J, Sherman M, Llovet JM, Beaugrand M, Lencioni R, Burroughs AK, Christensen E, Pagliaro L, Colombo M, Rodés J, HCC EP o E o. Clinical management of hepatocellular carcinoma. Conclusions of the Barcelona-2000 EASL conference. European Association for the Study of the Liver. J Hepatol. 2001;35(3):421–30.
26. Gillmore R, Stuart S, Kirkwood A, Hameeduddin A, Woodward N, Burroughs AK, Meyer T. EASL and mRECIST responses are independent prognostic factors for survival in hepatocellular cancer patients treated with transarterial embolization. J Hepatol. 2011;55(6):1309–16.
27. Akinwande O, Dendy M, Ludwig JM, Kim HS. Hepatic intra-arterial injection of irinotecan drug eluting beads (DEBIRI) for patients with unresectable colorectal liver metastases: a systematic review. Surg Oncol. 2017;26(3):268–75.
28. Martin RC, Scoggins CR, Schreeder M, Rilling WS, Laing CJ, Tatum CM, Kelly LR, Garcia-Monaco RD, Sharma VR, Crocenzi TS, Strasberg SM. Randomized controlled trial of irinotecan drug-eluting beads with simultaneous FOLFOX and bevacizumab for patients with unresectable colorectal liver-limited metastasis. Cancer. 2015;121(20):3649–58.
29. Iezzi R, Marsico VA, Guerra A, Cerchiaro E, Cassano A, Basso M, Devicienti E, Rodolfino E, Barone C, Bonomo L. Trans-arterial chemoembolization with irinotecan-loaded drug-eluting beads (DEBIRI) and capecitabine in refractory liver prevalent colorectal metastases: a phase II single-center study. Cardiovasc Intervent Radiol. 2015;38(6):1523–31.
30. Fiorentini G, Aliberti C, Tilli M, Mulazzani L, Graziano F, Giordani P, Mambrini A, Montagnani F, Alessandroni P, Catalano V, Coschiera P. Intra-arterial infusion of irinotecan-loaded drug-eluting beads (DEBIRI) versus intravenous therapy (FOLFIRI) for hepatic metastases from colorectal cancer: final results of a phase III study. Anticancer Res. 2012;32(4):1387–95.
31. Martin RC, Joshi J, Robbins K, Tomalty D, Bosnjakovik P, Derner M, Padr R, Rocek M, Scupchenko A, Tatum C. Hepatic intra-arterial injection of drug-eluting bead, irinotecan (DEBIRI) in unresectable colorectal liver metastases refractory to systemic chemotherapy: results of multi-institutional study. Ann Surg Oncol. 2011;18(1):192–8.
32. Akinwande O, Miller A, Hayes D, O'Hara R, Tomalty D, Martin RC. Concomitant capecitabine with hepatic delivery of drug eluting beads in metastatic colorectal cancer. Anticancer Res. 2014;34(12):7239–45.
33. Eichler K, Zangos S, Mack MG, Hammerstingl R, Gruber-Rouh T, Gallus C, Vogl TJ. First human study in treatment of unresectable liver metastases from colorectal cancer with irinotecan-loaded beads (DEBIRI). Int J Oncol. 2012;41(4):1213–20.
34. Narayanan G, Barbery K, Suthar R, Guerrero G, Arora G. Transarterial chemoembolization using DEBIRI for treatment of hepatic metastases from colorectal cancer. Anticancer Res. 2013;33(5):2077–83.
35. Huppert P, Wenzel T, Wietholtz H. Transcatheter arterial chemoembolization (TACE) of colorectal cancer liver metastases by irinotecan-eluting microspheres in a salvage patient population. Cardiovasc Intervent Radiol. 2014;37(1):154–64.
36. Stutz M, Mamo A, Valenti D, Hausvater A, Cabrera T, Metrakos P, Chaudhury P, Steacy G, Garoufalis E, Kavan P. Real-life report on chemoembolization using DEBIRI for liver metastases from colorectal cancer. Gastroenterol Res Pract. 2015;2015:715102.
37. Aliberti C, Fiorentini G, Muzzio PC, Pomerri F, Tilli M, Dallara S, Benea G. Trans-arterial chemoembolization of metastatic colorectal carcinoma to the liver adopting DC Bead®, drug-eluting bead loaded with irinotecan: results of a phase II clinical study. Anticancer Res. 2011;31(12):4581–7.

Role of Y90 Radioembolization in Hepatic Metastatic Colorectal Carcinoma

38

Rehan Ali, Ahmed Gabr, Ronald Mora, Ahsun Riaz, and Robert Lewandowski

Introduction

In the United States, nearly 20% of patients with colorectal cancer (CRC) present with stage IV disease with distant metastases at diagnosis (synchronous) [1]. Forty percent of these metastases are in the liver. An additional 35–60% of patients develop hepatic metastases during the course of their disease [2]. Five-year survival in patients with distant disease at diagnosis is estimated at 13.1%, and the majority of deaths from metastatic colorectal cancer (mCRC) are thought to be secondary to hepatic involvement and progression [3, 4].

Major advances in systemic chemotherapy regimen and biological agents, like the introduction of oxaliplatin, irinotecan, and targeted therapies including vascular endothelial growth factor (VEGF) and epidermal growth factor receptor (EGFR) inhibitors alongside surgery, have substantially improved survival in select patients [5]. The main issue in choosing these options is whether the metastases are curable or incurable. Patients who are not candidates for surgical resection at the time of diagnosis or presentation are considered for systemic therapy with biological agents as neoadjuvant or definitive treatment. Most colorectal cancer metastases eventually

R. Ali · A. Gabr · R. Mora · A. Riaz
Department of Radiology, Section of Interventional Radiology, Northwestern Memorial Hospital, Chicago, IL, USA
e-mail: ahmed.gabr@northwestern.edu; ahsun-riaz@northwestern.edu

R. Lewandowski (✉)
Department of Radiology, Section of Interventional Radiology, Northwestern Memorial Hospital, Chicago, IL, USA

Department of Medicine, Division of Hematology and Oncology, Northwestern University, Chicago, IL, USA

Department of Surgery, Northwestern University, Chicago, IL, USA
e-mail: r-lewandowski@northwestern.edu

M. M. Correia et al. (eds.), *Colorectal Cancer Liver Metastases*,
https://doi.org/10.1007/978-3-030-25486-5_38

become refractory or resistant to chemotherapy and biological agents, decreasing the overall survival (OS) to less than 6 months (<6 mo) [6]. Moreover, many patients do not tolerate treatment and eventually have to discontinue chemotherapy secondary to toxicities and subsequent decreased quality of life.

Role of Locoregional Liver Therapies (LRT)

While surgical resection is considered the most definitive locoregional therapy for patients with mCRC to the liver, the majority of patients are not operative candidates. For those with oligometastatic disease, thermal-based ablative technologies can be considered [7]. However, these therapies are best applied to a small percentage of patients with mCRC to the liver secondary to the limitations of the technology. Ideally, patients have ≤3 tumors, all ≤3 cm in diameter. Further, many patients treated with ablation will ultimately demonstrate residual or progressive disease [8].

The majority of patients with metastatic colorectal cancer (mCRC) in the liver present outside criteria for surgical resection and/or thermal ablation. These patients often have multifocal bilobar tumors. These tumors tend to be best approached via an intra-arterial route. The success behind this paradigm lies in the dual blood supply of the liver through the hepatic arteries and portal venous system. Hepatic parenchyma is dependent on portal blood system, while tumors are mainly perfused from hepatic arteries [9]. Metastatic colorectal tumors are often hypo-vascular relative to surrounding hepatic parenchyma on imaging; the role of macro-embolic therapies such as bland or chemoembolization has not demonstrated reproducibly good results against this disease. There is growing interest in drug-eluting embolic chemoembolization with irinotecan for mCRC to the liver, but there is no consensus as to the value of this therapy at this time. Radioembolization with yttrium-90 (Y90) is employed to treat these mCRC hepatic metastases that are not candidates for surgical resection or thermal ablation. Radioembolization has been most commonly utilized in the salvage setting where patients have progressed on standard lines of therapy. This treatment has proven beneficial with good tumor control rates, low toxicity, and consistent survival from time of first treatment of around 10 months [6, 10–12]. Metastatic colorectal cancer cells are highly radiosensitive and do not exhibit any cross-resistance to radiation despite being chemotherapy-refractory.

Principles of Radioembolization

Radioembolization is a well-tolerated outpatient transcatheter intra-arterial brachytherapy which delivers radioactive particles to hepatic tumor(s) via its feeding arteries. The agent used for hepatic radioembolization is the high-radiation beta-emitter, yttrium-90 (Y90). Y90 has a half-life of 64.1 h and an average energy of 0.94 mega-electron volt (MeV). As the average tissue penetration of Y90 is 2.5 mm with maximum penetration of 1.1 cm, the adjacent normal liver parenchyma is spared and 94% of the dose is delivered within the first 11 days following administration [13].

Y90-labled resin microspheres (SIR-Speheres®, Sirtex Medical Ltd., North Sydney, Australia) and Y90-labeled glass microspheres (TheraSphere®, BTG International, UK) are two different delivery systems with slightly different characteristics. SIR-Spheres® are resin-based microspheres with size of 20–60 micron coated with Y90 leading to lower density and specific activity (radiation dose per microsphere). On the contrary, TheraSphere® is glass-based microspheres in which Y90 is a component of the glass with size of 15–35 micron leading to higher specific activity than SIR-Spheres® (2500 Bq vs. 50 Bq at time of calibration). In 2002, the FDA approved SIR-Spheres® as internal brachytherapy device for the treatment of unresectable metastatic CRC with adjuvant hepatic artery infusion of floxuridine, while TheraSphere® is used under the humanitarian device exemption in the United States. The outcomes from both of these delivery systems for the treatment of mCRC to the liver appear similar and consistent, although no comparative trial has been conducted.

Successful intratumoral administration of Y90 microspheres involves: (1) appropriate patient selection, (2) meticulous pretherapy assessment and mapping of the feeding hepatic arteries and lung shunt fraction (LSF) calculation, (3) dosimetry calculation, and (4) intra-arterial delivery of the microspheres [14]. Inclusion criteria for radioembolization include patient, tumor, and alternative therapy consideration. The patients should have liver-only or liver-dominant metastatic disease not amendable to surgery or thermal ablation, and they should either not be a candidate for or have failed standard-of-care systemic therapy options. The patients should have preserved performance status, often graded according to the Eastern Cooperative Oncology Group (ECOG) system. They should have an ECOG performance status ≤2 (out of bed more than half the day) and a life expectancy of >6 weeks. Patients should also have preserved liver function, manifested by normal serum bilirubin as well as appropriate renal function for angiography. Patients with poor performance status, inadequate hepatic reserve (Child Pugh-C), and widespread multiorgan metastases are poor candidates for this therapy.

A separate planning angiogram is performed to: a) delineate tumor perfusing hepatic arteries to plan for delivery of the microspheres and b) to isolate hepatic perfusion to a few arteries and to identify vessels that may be at risk of nontargeted delivery of the microspheres. The hepatic arterial branches that are at risk of nontarget delivery are occluded (coil embolized) to mitigate risk of complications if clinically indicated. The degree of LSF is estimated through the intra-arterial infusion of technetium-99 m macro-aggregated albumin (MAA) and subsequent distribution and measurement of activity in the lungs and liver through nuclear medicine planar and single-photon emission computed tomography (SPECT) imaging. Presence of an increased LSF is not considered a contraindication for radioembolization with Y90 microspheres as long as the radiation dose per treatment to the lungs does not exceed 30 Gray or the cumulative dose to the lungs is below 50 Gray.

Dose calculation for SIR-Spheres® is based on the tumor volume in the liver and body surface area (BSA) [14]. Approach of lobar treatment versus whole liver treatment with SIR-Spheres microspheres is based on the locations of visible tumor on pretreatment cross-sectional imaging. For visible unilobar disease, SIR-Spheres®

microspheres should be administered to that lobe only sparing the contralateral lobe from unnecessary internal radiation. For whole liver treatment, prescribed activity of SIR-Spheres® microspheres (GBq) can be calculated using (BSA − 0.2) + [(V_T /V_T + V_{NL})] where V_T is the total volume of tumor in the liver and V_{NL} is the volume of the nontumor liver tissue. In patients who receive lobar or segmental/superselective treatment with SIR-Spheres® microspheres, the prescribed activity must be reduced in accordance with the size of the portion of the liver being treated, and specific activity can be calculated using = [BSA − 0.2 + (tV_L/TV_L)] × [TV_L/Total liver volume], where tV_L is the volume of tumor present in the lobe, TV_L is the total volume of the lobe including the tumor in the lobe, and total liver volume is the total volume of the liver including the tumor [15]. The dose calculations for TheraSphere® are based on partition model with an intent to deliver 80–150 Gy (8000 rad to 15,000 rad) of radiation dose to the treated volume of the liver. The desired dose for required radioactivity to deliver to the liver may be calculated using the formula [{Desired Dose (Gy) × Liver Mass (kg)}]/50 [16]. Liver volume and corresponding liver mass may be calculated using cross-sectional imaging such as CT or MRI scans.

Postinfusion imaging of the liver through SPECT or positron-emission tomography (PET) is often performed to assess the hepatic uptake pattern of the microspheres. Clinical toxicities are assessed at 1–2 weeks follow-up and laboratory toxicities are assessed at 1-month and 3-month period following radioembolization. For bilobar disease, Y-90 radioembolization of the contralateral lobe is performed at 4–6 weeks following initial therapy. Tumor response is assessed at 3-month intervals with cross-sectional imaging such as CT or MRI. Additional Y-90 infusions are not routinely performed but can be considered if tumors recur.

Radioembolization Outcomes in Hepatic mCRC

The role of Y90 radioembolization can be assessed as a salvage treatment for chemotherapy-refractory disease or in combination with second-/third-line therapy and/or first-line therapy.

Yttrium-90 Radioembolization for Chemotherapy-Refractory/ Salvage Disease

Radioembolization has been increasingly used for patients with mCRC with liver-only or liver-dominant disease refractory to chemotherapy.

Saxena et al. published the outcome of 302 patients who underwent Y90 radioembolization for unresectable chemorefractory hepatic metastatic CRC and demonstrated OS of 10.5 months from the date of radioembolization with an objective response of 39% [6]. This was consistent with the previously published retrospective multicenter data by Kennedy et al. of 506 and 208 patients, where median OS of 10.1 months and 10.5 months was demonstrated, respectively [14, 17].

A retrospective case control study was conducted by Bester et al. to evaluate the effect of Y90 radioembolization ($n = 224$) versus best supportive care ($n = 51$) in patients with chemorefractory liver metastases [18]. This study compared Y-90 to best supportive care and reported median OS of 11.6 months versus 6.3 months, respectively. The incidence of duodenal/gastric ulceration was 3.2% among patients who received radioembolization.

In 2014, a review of trans-arterial radioembolization for chemorefractory mCRC disease showed that studies on radioembolization include patients with advanced disease who have failed a median of three different chemotherapy regimens and tend to have bilobar disease, and one-third of these studies had patients with extra-hepatic metastatic disease leading to lowering of survival due to selection bias [19]. In spite of this, it was found that the median OS after radioembolization treatment was 12 months, median TTP was 4.9 months, and median time to intra-hepatic disease progression was 9 months [19]. Despite these, radioembolization previously remained a category 3 recommendation in the National Comprehensive Cancer Network (NCCN®) guidelines [20]. Recently, by consensus in the latest NCCN® Clinical Practice Guidelines in Oncology, SIRT (SIR-Spheres® Y-90 resin microspheres) has been upgraded as a category 2A recommended treatment for liver-dominant, chemotherapy-resistant colorectal disease (mCRC) [21]. Moreover, in 2014, the European Society of Medical Oncology (ESMO) incorporated radioembolization as a treatment option for patients with liver-limited metastases that have failed/exhausted available chemotherapeutic options [22].

While the bias of selecting patients healthy enough to undergo radioembolization may influence these results, the median OS for patients with chemorefractory disease treated with radioembolization is generally better than the reported median survival rates for salvage chemotherapies.

To date, the largest series using resin microspheres, the Metastatic colorectal cancer liver metastases Outcomes after RadioEmbolization (MORE) study, included 606 patients and demonstrated an overall survival of 9.6 months [23]. Regarding survival outcome, this study revealed that patients with extra-hepatic disease benefit less from radioembolization: 35% of patients in the MORE study had extra-hepatic disease, and it was concluded that survival for patients without extra-hepatic disease was significantly longer than those with extra-hepatic disease (12.1 vs. 7.4 months respectively; $p < 0.001$).

Most of the above-mentioned studies were based on resin-based Y90 microspheres. A single-center study of 214 patients using glass microsphere radioembolization for unresectable, chemorefractory disease generated results very similar to that for resin microspheres with reported median OS of 10.6 months from the time of radioembolization [11]. Another multicenter study by Hickey et al. reported survival and safety outcome from 531 patients with hepatic mCRC treated with Y90 using glass microspheres. Median OS was 10.6 months and safety profile was similar and consistent with prior published studies using resin microspheres [24].

Yttrium-90 Radioembolization in Combination with Second- or Third-Line Chemotherapy for Hepatic mCRC

Van Hazel et al. reported the results of 25 patients who initially failed initial 5-FU chemotherapy and later received concomitant Y-90 radioembolization with systemic irinotecan [25]. It was a prospective dose-escalation study in which 48% patients had partial response (PR) and 39% patients had stable disease (SD), with median overall survival of 12.2 months. Only 12 patients reported grade 3/4 toxicities.

Another study published by Lim et al. reported on a heterogeneous group of 30 patients who were treated with 5-FU as first-line chemotherapy. In this prospective study, all patients failed initial 5-FU chemotherapy and later were treated with radioembolization ($n = 21$), oxaliplatin, and/or irinotecan [26]. Treatment with SIR-Spheres demonstrated encouraging activity with partial response observed in 38% patients with TTP of 5.3 months. Thirteen percent adverse events were recorded due to nontarget embolization by Yttrium-90 microspheres.

Yttrium-90 Radioembolization as First-Line Therapy for Hepatic mCRC

Gray et al. analyzed 70 patients in a randomized prospective phase III trial in which patients received Y90 radioembolization plus hepatic arterial chemoinfusion (HAC) with floxuridine ($n = 36$) versus HAC with floxuridine ($n = 34$) [27]. This first prospective study led to FDA registration of SIR-Spheres® for the treatment of hepatic metastases from CRC and concluded that there was significantly higher objective response rate in patients who received Y-90 microsphere therapy in addition to HAC compared to those who received HAC alone with 50% or more reduction in elevated carcinoembryonic antigen (CEA) levels following therapy (72.2 vs. 47.1%, $p = 0.004$). Median time to tumor progression (TTP) was longer in the group that received Y-90 (15.9 vs. 9.7 months; $p = 0.001$) with no significant differences in the incidence of grade 3/4 adverse events in either group. This study demonstrated safety, response, and TTP of Y-90 radioembolization without significant survival advantage due to low number of cohort.

Following this study, Van Hazel et al. published a phase 2 study where patients ($n = 21$) were randomized to receive systemic chemotherapy with 5-fluorouracil and leucovorin alone or in combination with a single hepatic artery infusion of Y-90 SIR-Spheres®. It was concluded that the addition of single infusion of Y-90 microspheres resulted in significantly higher objective response rate ($p < 0.001$), longer TTP (18.6 vs. 3.6 months; $p < 0.0005$), and better median survival (29.4 vs. 12.8 months; $p = 0.025$) [28]. There was no difference in quality of life but with limited number of patients. Hendlisz et al. also concluded the similar outcome that radioembolization with Y90 resin microspheres plus fluorouracil (FU) was well tolerated and significantly improved time to liver progression (TTLP) and time to progression (TTP) as compared with FU alone [29].

With the development of oxaliplatin and irinotecan approval for mCRC, radioembolization studies combined with these systemic therapies were performed. A phase 1 study by Sharma et al. assessed the synergistic effect of Y90 radioembolization and the radio-sensitizing chemotherapy oxaliplatin [30] and concluded the maximum tolerated dose of oxaliplatin (60 mg/m^2) during the first three cycles of chemotherapy (FOLFOX) as radiation sensitizer for Y-90 therapy with standard dose oxaliplatin onward [30]. Adverse events attributable to this combination were little with a 90% partial response (PR) rate at 3 months, median TTP of 12.3 months, median PFS of 9.3, and 14.2 months in patients with and without extra-hepatic disease, respectively. On the contrary, median PFS and OS for only FOLFOX regimen used as first-line chemotherapy without Y-90 radioembolization ranges from 7.6 to 9.0 months and 16.2 to 19.5 months, respectively. This study demonstrated the safety of combining Y-90 therapy with standard first-line systemic chemotherapy (FOLFOX); but without a randomization arm, conclusions on the effectiveness of such combination therapy were not generatable. The above-mentioned Van Hazel et al. study was performed to evaluate the maximum tolerable dose of irinotecan with radioembolization in FU-refractory patients with hepatic mCRC, and recommended dose of irinotecan was 100 mg/m^2 on day-1 and day-8 of a 3-week cycle though maximum tolerable dose was not achieved in this particular setting [25].

SIRFLOX

SIRFLOX (randomized comparative study of FOLFOX6m plus SIR-Spheres microspheres versus FOLFOX6m alone as first-line treatment in patients with nonresectable liver metastases from primary colorectal carcinoma) is a recently published randomized, multinational, multicenter phase III trial designed to assess the efficacy and safety of adding Y90 resin microspheres to standard fluorouracil-, leucovorin-, and oxaloplatin (FOLFOX)-based chemotherapy in patients with metastatic CRC [31]. The primary endpoint of the study was progression-free survival (PFS), while secondary endpoints included were progression-free survival in the liver, tumor response rate in the liver, tumor response rate at any site, hepatic resection rate, and toxicity. Patients with liver-dominant, but extra-hepatic disease (40%) were included and nearly 45% of patients in the study had intact primary tumor(s). This study analyzed 530 patients with liver-dominant mCRC and concluded that there was no improvement in progression-free survival (PFS) by adding systemic internal radiation therapy (SIRT) to FOLFOX-based first-line chemotherapy. This may be explained by an uncertain impact of intact primary tumors (approximately 45%) on endpoint of PFS leading to inferior survivals outcome. There was 7.9 months improvement (median 20.5 months vs. median 12.6 months) observed in median PFS in the liver (local disease control) due to radioembolization, resulting in a 31% risk reduction of local hepatic progression.

There is interest in considering this first-line combination approach in patients with right-sided colon cancer. A secondary analysis of the SIRFLOX and FOXFIRE Global trials suggested that patients with right-sided colon cancers had a 4.9 months increase in survival ($p = 0.007$) [32] when radioembolization was added to first-line chemotherapy despite the fact that right-sided colon cancer is notorious for having different mutations, worse survival, and less response to chemotherapy as compared to left-sided colon cancers [33, 34].

SIRFLOX, FOXFIRE, and FOXFIRE Global Studies

Combined, SIRFLOX, FOXFIRE (an open-label randomized phase III trial of 5-fluorouracil, oxaliplatin, and folinic acid +/− interventional radioembolization as first-line treatment for patients with unresectable liver-only or liver-predominant metastatic colorectal cancer), and FOXFIRE Global (assessment of overall survival of FOLFOX6m plus SIR-Spheres microspheres versus FOLFOX6m alone as first-line treatment in patients with nonresectable liver metastases from primary colorectal carcinoma in a randomized clinical study) studies recruited >1100 patients with adequate power to detect a survival advantage. Based on these studies, the potential long-term impact on overall survival from integrating radioembolization into first-line treatment of mCRC was not evident, concluding that the addition of radioembolization to first-line FOLFOX chemotherapy for patients with liver-only and liver-dominant metastatic colorectal cancer did not improve OS compared to that for FOLFOX alone [32].

Summary

Current Trends

Based on these and many other publications, the median OS for patients with hepatic mCRC treated with radioembolization in the salvage setting is in the range of 10–12 months with response rates of 31% PR and 41% SD. The presence of large volume disease (>25% of liver volume), extra-hepatic disease, poor response to radioembolization, and ≥3 lines of prior chemotherapy portend poor prognosis. Hickey et al. showed that preserved performance status, tumor burden <25%, having received ≤2 chemotherapeutic agents, and a lack of extra-hepatic metastases all projected better survival outcomes [35]. Given that the median survival of patients who failed third-line chemotherapy is in the range of 4–6 months, radioembolization may improve survival outcomes.

Recommendations

According to latest NCCN guidelines, Y90 radioembolization is a category 2A recommendation in the treatment of mCRC [21], while per ESMO guidelines, Y90 radioembolization is a treatment option for patients with liver-limited mCRC who failed available chemotherapeutic options [22]. Despite potential bias of selecting healthier patients to undergo radioembolization, median OS is better for these refractory patients treated with radioembolization than with salvage chemotherapies. Use of radioembolization is not recommended in patients with extensive extrahepatic disease or extensive bilobar hepatic involvement. Likewise, mCRC patients with poor performance status (ECOG PS >2) are not candidate for Y-90 therapy.

Limitations of Current Data

Currently available data demonstrates that radioembolization is safe for the treatment of mCRC to the liver. Many studies, including the SIRFLOX data, further suggest safety of concurrent radioembolization and full-dose chemotherapy. When placing the level 1 evidence for radioembolization of mCRC hepatic metastases into perspective, it is important to acknowledge that radioembolization is a procedure that requires a learning curve. Some of the centers involved in the SIRFLOX trial had very limited experience, possibly accounting for the reported GI ulcer rate. Also, overall PFS may be a poor choice of a surrogate endpoint in patients with extra-hepatic sites of metastases (as was the case in SIRFLOX where 40% patients had extra-hepatic disease) as radioembolization does not target extra-hepatic disease. Despite these limitations, FOXFIRE and FOXFIRE Global studies did not demonstrate overall survival benefit of radioembolization plus first-line chemotherapeutics to first-line chemotherapeutics alone. This may in part be due to therapy crossover, the fact that not all patients in the radioembolization arm received this therapy, or that patients who were treated with radioembolization had fewer subsequent therapies [32].

Future Goals/Directions

Concurrent use of radioembolization combined with first- and second-line chemotherapies requires more rigorous data with inclusion of centers experienced in this treatment modality. Patients with right-sided colon cancers (worse outcomes with standard therapies) may be a subgroup that may benefit from radioembolization earlier in their treatment course and should be the focus of future studies. Long-term effects of radioembolization on hepatotoxicity and portal hypertension need to be studied. Future trials need to focus on identifying specific target populations who may benefit most from this therapy. One clincal trial, that has recently completed enrollment, employs radioembolization with glass microspheres in combination with second-line systemic therapy (EPOCH trial). Results are yet to be reported [36].

References

1. Siegel RL, Miller KD, Jemal A. Cancer statistics, 2018. CA Cancer J Clin. 2018;68(1):7–30.
2. Lee WS, Yun SH, Chun HK, Lee WY, Yun HR, Kim J, et al. Pulmonary resection for metastases from colorectal cancer: prognostic factors and survival. Int J Color Dis. 2007;22(6):699–704.

3. Howlader N, NA KM, Garshell J, Miller D, Altekruse S, Kosary C, et al. SEER cancer statistics review, 1975–2011. Bethesda: National Cancer Institute; 2014.
4. Welch JP, Donaldson GA. The clinical correlation of an autopsy study of recurrent colorectal cancer. Ann Surg. 1979;189(4):496–502.
5. Simmonds PC. Palliative chemotherapy for advanced colorectal cancer: systematic review and meta-analysis. Colorectal Cancer Collaborative Group. BMJ. 2000;321(7260):531–5.
6. Saxena A, Meteling B, Kapoor J, Golani S, Morris DL, Bester L. Is yttrium-90 radioembolization a viable treatment option for unresectable, chemorefractory colorectal cancer liver metastases? A large single-center experience of 302 patients. Ann Surg Oncol. 2015;22(3):794–802.
7. Vogl TJ, Farshid P, Naguib NN, Darvishi A, Bazrafshan B, Mbalisike E, et al. Thermal ablation of liver metastases from colorectal cancer: radiofrequency, microwave and laser ablation therapies. Radiol Med. 2014;119(7):451–61.
8. Lee KF, Wong J, Hui JW, Cheung YS, Chong CC, Fong AK, et al. Long-term outcomes of microwave versus radiofrequency ablation for hepatocellular carcinoma by surgical approach: a retrospective comparative study. Asian J Surg. 2017;40(4):301–8.
9. Breedis C, Young G. The blood supply of neoplasms in the liver. Am J Pathol. 1954;30(5):969–77.
10. Sangha BS, Nimeiri H, Hickey R, Salem R, Lewandowski RJ. Radioembolization as a treatment strategy for metastatic colorectal cancer to the liver: what can we learn from the SIRFLOX trial? Curr Treat Options in Oncol. 2016;17(6):26.
11. Lewandowski RJ, Memon K, Mulcahy MF, Hickey R, Marshall K, Williams M, et al. Twelve-year experience of radioembolization for colorectal hepatic metastases in 214 patients: survival by era and chemotherapy. Eur J Nucl Med Mol Imaging. 2014;41(10):1861–9.
12. Raval M, Bande D, Pillai AK, Blaszkowsky LS, Ganguli S, Beg MS, et al. Yttrium-90 radioembolization of hepatic metastases from colorectal cancer. Front Oncol. 2014;4:120.
13. Kalva SP, Thabet A, Wicky S. Recent advances in transarterial therapy of primary and secondary liver malignancies. Radiographics. 2008;28(1):101–17.
14. Kennedy AS, Ball D, Cohen SJ, Cohn M, Coldwell DM, Drooz A, et al. US patients receiving resin 90Y microspheres for unresectable colorectal liver metastases: a multicenter study of 506 patients. American Society of Clinical Oncology; 2012.
15. Yttrium S-S. Resin microspheres [package insert]. North Sydney: SirTex Medical; 2013.
16. Nordion M. TheraSphere yttrium-90 microspheres package insert. Kanata: MDS Nordion; 2004.
17. Kennedy AS, Coldwell D, Nutting C, Murthy R, Wertman DE Jr, Loehr SP, et al. Resin 90Y-microsphere brachytherapy for unresectable colorectal liver metastases: modern USA experience. Int J Radiat Oncol Biol Phys. 2006;65(2):412–25.
18. Bester L, Meteling B, Pocock N, Pavlakis N, Chua TC, Saxena A, et al. Radioembolization versus standard care of hepatic metastases: comparative retrospective cohort study of survival outcomes and adverse events in salvage patients. J Vasc Interv Radiol. 2012;23(1):96–105.
19. Saxena A, Bester L, Shan L, Perera M, Gibbs P, Meteling B, et al. A systematic review on the safety and efficacy of yttrium-90 radioembolization for unresectable, chemorefractory colorectal cancer liver metastases. J Cancer Res Clin Oncol. 2014;140(4):537–47.
20. Network N. NCCN guidelines colon cancer version 1.2017. 2016.
21. Benson AB, Venook AP, Cederquist L, Chan E, Chen Y-J, Cooper HS, et al. Colon cancer, version 1.2017, NCCN clinical practice guidelines in oncology. J Natl Compr Cancer Netw. 2017;15(3):370–98.
22. Van Cutsem E, Cervantes A, Nordlinger B, Arnold D. Metastatic colorectal cancer: ESMO clinical practice guidelines for diagnosis, treatment and follow-up. Ann Oncol. 2014;25(Suppl 3):iii1–9.
23. Kennedy AS, Ball D, Cohen SJ, Cohn M, Coldwell DM, Drooz A, et al. Multicenter evaluation of the safety and efficacy of radioembolization in patients with unresectable colorectal liver metastases selected as candidates for (90)Y resin microspheres. J Gastrointest Oncol. 2015;6(2):134–42.

24. Hickey R, Lewandowski RJ, Prudhomme T, Ehrenwald E, Baigorri B, Critchfield J, et al. 90Y radioembolization of colorectal hepatic metastases using glass microspheres: safety and survival outcomes from a 531-patient multicenter study. J Nucl Med. 2016;57(5):665–71.
25. van Hazel GA, Pavlakis N, Goldstein D, Olver IN, Tapner MJ, Price D, et al. Treatment of fluorouracil-refractory patients with liver metastases from colorectal cancer by using yttrium-90 resin microspheres plus concomitant systemic irinotecan chemotherapy. J Clin Oncol. 2009;27(25):4089–95.
26. Lim L, Gibbs P, Yip D, Shapiro JD, Dowling R, Smith D, et al. A prospective evaluation of treatment with Selective Internal Radiation Therapy (SIR-spheres) in patients with unresectable liver metastases from colorectal cancer previously treated with 5-FU based chemotherapy. BMC Cancer. 2005;5:132.
27. Gray B, Van Hazel G, Hope M, Burton M, Moroz P, Anderson J, et al. Randomised trial of SIR-Spheres plus chemotherapy vs. chemotherapy alone for treating patients with liver metastases from primary large bowel cancer. Ann Oncol. 2001;12(12):1711–20.
28. Van Hazel G, Blackwell A, Anderson J, Price D, Moroz P, Bower G, et al. Randomised phase 2 trial of SIR-Spheres plus fluorouracil/leucovorin chemotherapy versus fluorouracil/leucovorin chemotherapy alone in advanced colorectal cancer. J Surg Oncol. 2004;88(2):78–85.
29. Hendlisz A, Van den Eynde M, Peeters M, Maleux G, Lambert B, Vannoote J, et al. Phase III trial comparing protracted intravenous fluorouracil infusion alone or with yttrium-90 resin microspheres radioembolization for liver-limited metastatic colorectal cancer refractory to standard chemotherapy. J Clin Oncol. 2010;28(23):3687–94.
30. Sharma RA, Van Hazel GA, Morgan B, Berry DP, Blanshard K, Price D, et al. Radioembolization of liver metastases from colorectal cancer using yttrium-90 microspheres with concomitant systemic oxaliplatin, fluorouracil, and leucovorin chemotherapy. J Clin Oncol. 2007;25(9):1099–106.
31. van Hazel GA, Heinemann V, Sharma NK, Findlay MP, Ricke J, Peeters M, et al. SIRFLOX: randomized phase III trial comparing first-line mFOLFOX6 (plus or minus Bevacizumab) versus mFOLFOX6 (plus or minus Bevacizumab) plus selective internal radiation therapy in patients with metastatic colorectal cancer. J Clin Oncol. 2016;34(15):1723–31.
32. Wasan HS, Gibbs P, Sharma NK, Taieb J, Heinemann V, Ricke J, et al. First-line selective internal radiotherapy plus chemotherapy versus chemotherapy alone in patients with liver metastases from colorectal cancer (FOXFIRE, SIRFLOX, and FOXFIRE-Global): a combined analysis of three multicentre, randomised, phase 3 trials. Lancet Oncol. 2017;18(9):1159–71.
33. Lee MS, Menter DG, Kopetz S. Right versus left colon cancer biology: integrating the consensus molecular subtypes. J Natl Compr Cancer Netw. 2017;15(3):411–9.
34. Arnold D, Lueza B, Douillard JY, Peeters M, Lenz HJ, Venook A, et al. Prognostic and predictive value of primary tumour side in patients with RAS wild-type metastatic colorectal cancer treated with chemotherapy and EGFR directed antibodies in six randomized trials. Ann Oncol. 2017;28(8):1713–29.
35. Hickey R, Lewandowski RJ, Prudhomme T, Ehrenwald E, Baigorri B, Critchfield J, et al. Radioembolization of colorectal hepatic metastases using glass microspheres: safety and survival outcomes from a. 2016.
36. Chauhan N, Mulcahy MF, Salem R, Benson III AB, Boucher E, Bukovcan J, Cosgrove D, Laframboise C, Lewandowski RJ, Master F, El-Rayes B. TheraSphere Yttrium-90 Glass Microspheres Combined With Chemotherapy Versus Chemotherapy Alone in Second-Line Treatment of Patients With Metastatic Colorectal Carcinoma of the Liver: Protocol for the EPOCH Phase 3 Randomized Clinical Trial. JMIR Res Protoc. 2019;8(1):e11545.

Liver Transplantation for CRLM—Is It Ever Indicated?

39

Pål-Dag Line, Morten Hagness, and Svein Dueland

Background

Colorectal cancer (CRC) has a high prevalence worldwide, and about half of the patients will develop metastases, most frequently in the liver and lung. Consequently, colorectal liver metastases (CRLM) represents a major source of cancer-associated morbidity and mortality.

By the introduction of the currently available chemotherapeutic regimens, the overall survival (OS) has doubled from 12 to 24 months after the start of first-line therapy. Oncological treatment alone is however not curative, and the best 5-year OS rates are around 10% [1, 2]. Over time, patients undergoing chemotherapy will usually experience treatment failure and have to switch chemotherapy regimen. The overall survival after the start of second line is typically in the range of 10–12 months [3], and after third line about 6–8 months [4]. Despite tremendous progress with regard to chemotherapy for colorectal cancer in general, the only potential curative treatment remains radical surgical removal of all metastatic deposits.

The concept of surgical resectability has evolved dynamically since 1986, when Ekberg and coworkers proposed that liver resection was only indicated when the number of tumors was less than 4 and resection margins over 10 mm could be anticipated [5]. In the modern era of liver surgery for CRLM, a far more aggressive

P.-D. Line (✉)
Department of Transplantation Medicine, Oslo University Hospital, Oslo, Norway

Institute of Clinical Medicine, University of Oslo, Oslo, Norway
e-mail: p.d.line@medisin.uio.no

M. Hagness
Department of Transplantation Medicine, Oslo University Hospital, Oslo, Norway
e-mail: morten.hagness@ous-hf.no

S. Dueland
Department of Oncology, Oslo University Hospital, Oslo, Norway
e-mail: svein.dueland@ous-hf.no

M. M. Correia et al. (eds.), *Colorectal Cancer Liver Metastases*,
https://doi.org/10.1007/978-3-030-25486-5_39

approach has been shown to be beneficial. Essentially, any tumor number can be resected as long as there is a liver remnant of sufficient volume and parenchymal quality. The free margin requirement is considered to be >1 mm. In situations with a large number of metastases or small liver remnant, techniques like two-stage hepatectomy and portal vein embolization has become standard of care to provide patients with a surgical option [6–8]. Thus, to simplify, resectability could currently be defined as the ability to perform an R0 resection with a reliable functioning liver remnant of sufficient size [9].

Outcome after liver resection for CRLM is dependent on an array of clinicopathological factors, as well as patient selection but the reported 5-year OS lies between 16% and 74% [10],

Despite the advances in surgical approach, only about 20–25% of the patients with CRLM are amenable to liver resection [11]. Consequently, there is a large demand for other surgical options in this patient cohort, and one alternative could be the ultimate liver resection—liver transplantation.

Historic Overview

Offering liver transplantation to patients with unresectable metastases from colorectal cancer is not new. Early attempts were performed during the initial development of liver replacement as a clinical treatment [12, 13]. During this pioneering era, the operations were hampered by unsolved technical challenges and limited experience, and prolonged postoperative survival was a rarity due to severe complications and lack of effective immunosuppression. Later on, as transplant technique matured somewhat more, patients with liver metastases were still offered transplantation. Between 1983 and 1994, the University of Vienna transplanted 24 patients for nonresectable CRLM. The overall survival at 1, 3, and 5 years was 76%, 32%, and 12%, respectively [14]. The postoperative mortality after liver transplantation in general was substantially higher in this period and more than 40% of these patients died from causes unrelated to cancer recurrence. Smaller series were done elsewhere in Europe. In the European Liver Transplant Registry (ELTR), a total of 55 patients were identified having undergone liver transplantation for CRLM up to 2007, including the patients published by the Vienna group. One- and 5-year OS in this expanded cohort was 62% and 18%, respectively [15]. Due to the inferior outcomes in general, liver transplantation in patients with CRLM was abandoned and internationally considered a contraindication. Since oncology, imaging modalities, and clinical liver transplantation have undergone tremendous improvements in the last 20 years and a significant proportion of the early experiences with transplantation of CRLM patients were hampered by high morbidity and mortality of noncancer origin, it is not possible to assess the clinical efficacy of liver transplantation in patients with nonresectable CRLM based on these data.

The Concept

Although the historical experience could indicate that liver transplantation for CRLM does not yield satisfactory long-term results, there are a number of casuistic reports in the literature suggesting that sustained survival can be obtained in selected cases. Two patients contained in the data from the ELTR registry survived for 9 and 21 years posttransplant [15], and other reports on treatment success in single or a few patients have been published [16–18]. Therefore, one might hypothesize that long-term survival and possible cure can be obtained in a small cohort of carefully selected patients with colorectal liver metastases. If so, this is quite similar to the situation the liver transplantation community faced with regard to outcomes for patients transplanted for hepatocellular carcinoma (HCC) in the late eighties and early nineties. The results were disappointing, and the role of transplantation for HCC as main indication was eagerly discussed [19, 20]. The urgent problem was to select the proper candidates for the procedure. The pivotal change came about when Mazzaferro and coworkers in Milan demonstrated that when limiting liver transplantation to patients with either single tumor up to 5 cm in diameter or three tumors up to 3 cm in diameter, survival rates comparable to that obtained in patients with benign disease could be achieved [21]. These findings constitute the MILAN criteria for transplantation in HCC. In order to elucidate whether good OS can be achieved in patients with nonresectable CRLM, and to obtain data regarding improved patient selection, systematic studies are needed.

In 2006, the secondary cancer (SECA) I study was launched at Oslo University Hospital. This was an open, prospective pilot study to explore the possibility of long-term OS in patients with nonresectable CRLM.

Inclusion criteria were fairly wide. Patients had to have undergone a radical resection of the primary tumor, have a good performance status, and received at least 6 weeks of chemotherapy prior to transplant. As one might anticipate, the study population was very heterogeneous with respect to pretransplant carcinoembryonic antigen (CEA) levels, the number of lesions, maximal tumor size, stage of the primary tumor, and the objective response to chemotherapy. The results after transplantation of 21 patients were reported in 2013 when the first patient had been observed for 5 years and the median observation time in the cohort was 27 months. The estimated 1-, 3-, and 5-year OS was 98%, 68%, and 60%, respectively, and the patients experienced excellent quality of life (QoL) [22, 23]. After longer observation time and a median follow-up of 65 months, OS at 5 years was 56% [24]. The results obtained are far better than any available alternative treatment for nonresectable colorectal metastases and even compares favorably with outcomes following liver resection, keeping in mind that all these patients were found nonresectable at the institutional multidisciplinary meeting. When interpreting these results, it is quite important to recognize the SECA I trial as a “proof of concept” study. As such, it renders some similarity to the introduction of the MILAN criteria for HCC as mentioned earlier. But unlike the Mazzaferro study that sought to document the effect of optimal patient selection on survival, the SECA I trial contained a heterogeneous patient cohort and despite the encouraging results, further studies would be needed to clarify what is the optimal selection criterion for liver transplantation in CRLM.

Barriers and Limitations

Recurrence

One of the main limitations experienced in liver transplantation of patients with nonresectable CRLM is recurrence of disease. In the SECA I trial, recurrence was almost universal, and the disease-free survival (DFS) was only 35% at 1 year [22]. It is worth noting, however, that the majority of patients relapsed in the lungs (68%) whereas the remainder got recurrence in the liver, lymph nodes, and peripheral sites as well as one patient with recurrence of the primary tumor [25]. There was a marked difference in survival between lung-only metastases and patients with recurrence in the liver and/or other sites. Six of the seven patients who developed metastasis to the transplanted graft died from recurrent disease. Lung metastases proved to be clinically slow growing, and no chemotherapy was in general given. The lung tumors that were resectable were observed until they reached a size of minimum 10–15 mm, whereby they got referred to lung resection. An example of a patient with typically slow-growing resectable lung metastasis is given in Fig. 39.1.

Patients with relapse confined only to the lung had a 5-year survival of 100%, whereas those with lung relapse followed by other sites of relapse later on had a 5-year survival of 72% [25]. On careful retrospective examination of pretransplant CT scans in the patients with lung metastases, it became evident that out of 17 patients, 7 had lung metastases prior to transplant. This indicates that lung relapse in many of the patients is a consequence of a staging error that is related to insufficient sensitivity and specificity in the pretransplant thoracic CT investigations. Thus, it appears important to focus on pattern of recurrence and to distinguish between pulmonary metastases alone versus extrapulmonary sites, since the latter might signal systemic relapse more often, which carries a much worse prognosis.

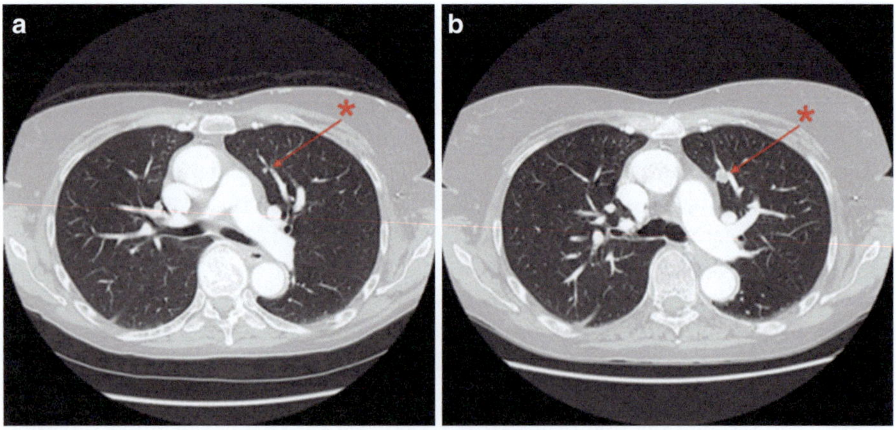

Fig. 39.1 Chest CT scan of a patient transplanted for CRLM in 2007. (**a**) Small metastatic nodule was noted on follow-up CT scan in 2009, 2 years posttransplant (∗ and arrow). (**b**) The lesion was observed with no specific treatment until 2011, 4 years posttransplant (∗ and arrow). The patient then underwent lung resection and is without evidence of disease

Immunosuppression

It is well documented that transplant recipients have an increased risk for cancer development in the posttransplant period. This has been mainly attributed to the chronic immunosuppression but may for liver-transplanted patients partly also be related to the underlying disease [26, 27]. Based on this, a natural empiric assumption would be that patients transplanted for CRLM that relapse might experience accelerated tumor growth and, as a consequence, a reduced survival. In our experience with about 50 transplants for CRLM, we have not been able to demonstrate that this is the case. On the contrary, when comparing growth rate of resected lung metastases in the SECA I population with a population of rectal cancer patients who had lung metastases only and were treated with resection, there was no difference in growth rate between the two groups, even though the transplanted population was on immunosuppression [28]. In a comparative study between the SECA I population and patients enrolled in the NORDIC VII chemotherapy trial, both groups had similar disease and progression-free survival of 8–10 months. The survival after relapse and progression of disease was, however, markedly different with only 9% of the NORDIC VII patients alive at 5 years whereas the corresponding figure in the liver-transplanted patients was 56%. This suggests that the immunosuppression did not adversely affect outcome. The regimen used has been sirolimus, mycophenolate mofetil, and steroids, with steroid tapering whenever possible. Sirolimus was chosen because of its possible antineoplastic properties [29, 30]. There are no data to determine whether the use of sirolimus itself might explain the somewhat unexpected missing negative impact of the immunosuppression on growth of pulmonary metastases and survival after relapse. All transplanted patients have also received aspirin once daily for the whole posttransplant period. Interestingly, there are some pieces of new evidence suggesting a positive effect on survival for patients with colorectal cancer who receive aspirin [31–33]. Whether this has had any significant effect on the patients transplanted for CRLM is currently not possible to ascertain. Based on the experience with the utilized immunosupressive regimen so far, there is no data indicating an accelerated metastatic growth in the transplanted population.

Patient Selection

A prerequisite for successful transplantation of patients with non-resectable CRLM is proper selection of candidates. In essence, what the selection process is aimed at is to identify patients with liver-only disease who have a favorable tumor biology.

Even though substantial progress has been made in modern imaging techniques, there are clear limitations as to whether metastatic deposits in other sites than the liver can be detected reliably. Thus, it is difficult to avoid extrahepatic disease in 100% of the cases. Based on more than 10 years of experience, it appears essential that the pretransplant work-up consists of more than one modality. At Oslo University Hospital, we have combined thoracic and abdominal CT scans in all patients. In addition, F^{18} fluorodeoxyglucose positron emission tomography in combination with computed tomography (FDG PET/CT) has been performed. At the time of transplant, all patients have undergone an exploratory laparotomy. Before proceeding to engraftment, frozen section of lymph nodes in the hepatoduodenal ligament has been taken to ensure that the patients do not have extrahepatic disease. In our total experience, findings from 5 out of 50 laparotomies have been positive. In a recent study it has been demonstrated that the combination of these three modalities is required since relying on only one of them would not have detected all cases of extrahepatic disease [34].

There is no single parameter that can provide a good assessment of tumor aggressiveness or what in popular terms is called unfavorable tumor biology. It is well documented that patients with BRAF mutations and microsatellite instability (MSI-H) have a worse prognosis, but population-based data are not always easily applicable in clinical selection of individual patients [35, 36]. In the SECA trials discussed here, BRAF-mutated patients have not been included, but routine testing for MSI-H has not been performed.

In the SECA I study, four factors that had significant impact on overall survival could be identified. Pretransplant maximum tumor size exceeding 5.5 cm, CEA levels >80 μg/l, time interval from resection of the primary tumor to transplant <2 years, and progressive disease on chemotherapy were all factors associated with inferior survival after transplantation (Fig. 39.2). In order to construct a usable scoring system, each of the factors was assigned the value of 1, and the summary score (OSLO Score) could predict patients who would not reach 5-year survival due to recurrent cancer [22].

Patients with metachronous disease have a very favorable prognosis with 100% 5-year survival [22]. Stable disease over time and good response to treatment are both clinically robust criteria for biologically less aggressive disease.

In a recent publication, Toso and coworkers reported a series of 12 patients who were transplanted on varying clinical indications at different European centers affiliated to the "Compagnons Hépato-Biliaires," which originates from the Poul Brousse Hospital in Paris [37]. Nine had synchronous disease, median CEA level pretransplant was 16.9 μg/l, only one patient had maximal tumor diameter exceeding 5.5 cm, all responded to chemotherapy, and 10 out of 12 patients had undergone at least one liver resection prior to transplant. Liver transplantation was performed median 41 months after resection of the primary (range 12–97). Overall patient survival at 1, 3, and 5 years was 83%, 62%, and 50%, respectively, after a median follow-up of 26 months (0–108 months). Corresponding DFS was 56%, 38%, and 38% at the same time intervals. A total of six patients experienced recurrence. Relapses were located in the lung ($n = 5$), liver ($n = 3$), and peritoneum ($n = 1$). Six patients transplanted for upfront clinical emergency or as a compassionate indication did significantly worse than the reminder patients and experienced recurrence within 18 months in most cases [37]. Since this is a small clinical series outside of any study and without proper uniform selection criteria, the results obtained must be interpreted with caution. The report does, however, seem to support the significance of prolonged time interval from resection of the primary to transplant, maximal tumor diameter, and pretransplant CEA level as well as response to therapy as important selection criteria. Unlike the SECA I study, prolonged DFS was obtained in 38%.

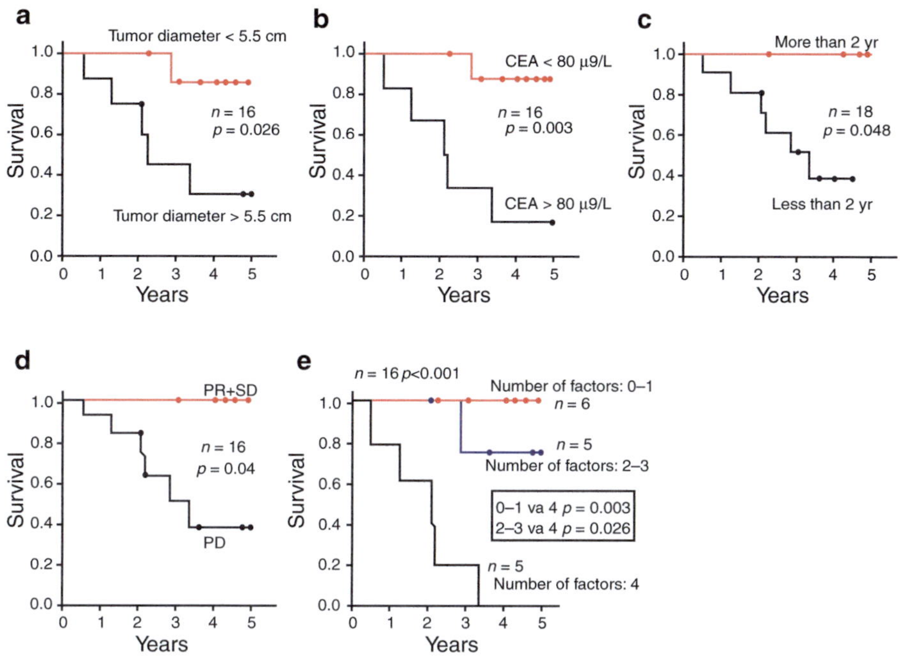

Fig. 39.2 (**a–e**) Preoperative factors affecting survival. (**a**) Kaplan–Meier plots for patients with maximum tumor diameter above and below the median diameter of 5.5 cm. (**b**) Kaplan–Meier plots with CEA levels before transplantation above and below 80 μg/l. (**c**) Kaplan–Meier plots for patients with time from primary surgery to liver transplantation more than 2 years and less than 2 years. (**d**) The number of patients who had progressive disease (PD) on chemotherapy at the time of liver transplantation was plotted against the number of patients with stable disease (SD) or had partial response to chemotherapy (PR). The factors displayed in panels A–D present in each patient was summed up, giving scores from 0 to 4 (OSLO score). (**e**) Kaplan–Meier plots for three groups of patients, those having OSLO score 0–1, OSLO score 2–3, or OSLO score = 4. Log-rank method was used for the calculation of *p* values in all panels

Investigations with FDG PET/CT have been shown to be of value for staging and prognostic assessment in colorectal cancer [38, 39]. In a recent study we have studied the relationship between FDG PET/CT data done during pretransplant work-up and posttransplant survival. Maximum standardized uptake value (SUVmax), average SUV (SUVmean), peak SUV (SUVpeak), tumor-to-background ratio (T/B ratio), metabolic tumor volume (MTV), and total lesion glycolysis (TLG) of the liver metastases were measured and registered. Total MTV and TLG under cutoff values determined by receiver operating characteristic (ROC) analysis were significantly correlated to improved OS at 3 and 5 years and DFS (Fig. 39.3b, c) [40]. Examples of two patients with MTV and TLG values under and over the cutoff values, respectively, are illustrated in Fig. 39.4. These results suggest that the utilization of FDG PET/CT may play a role in the selection of optimal candidates to liver transplantation for nonresectable CRLM.

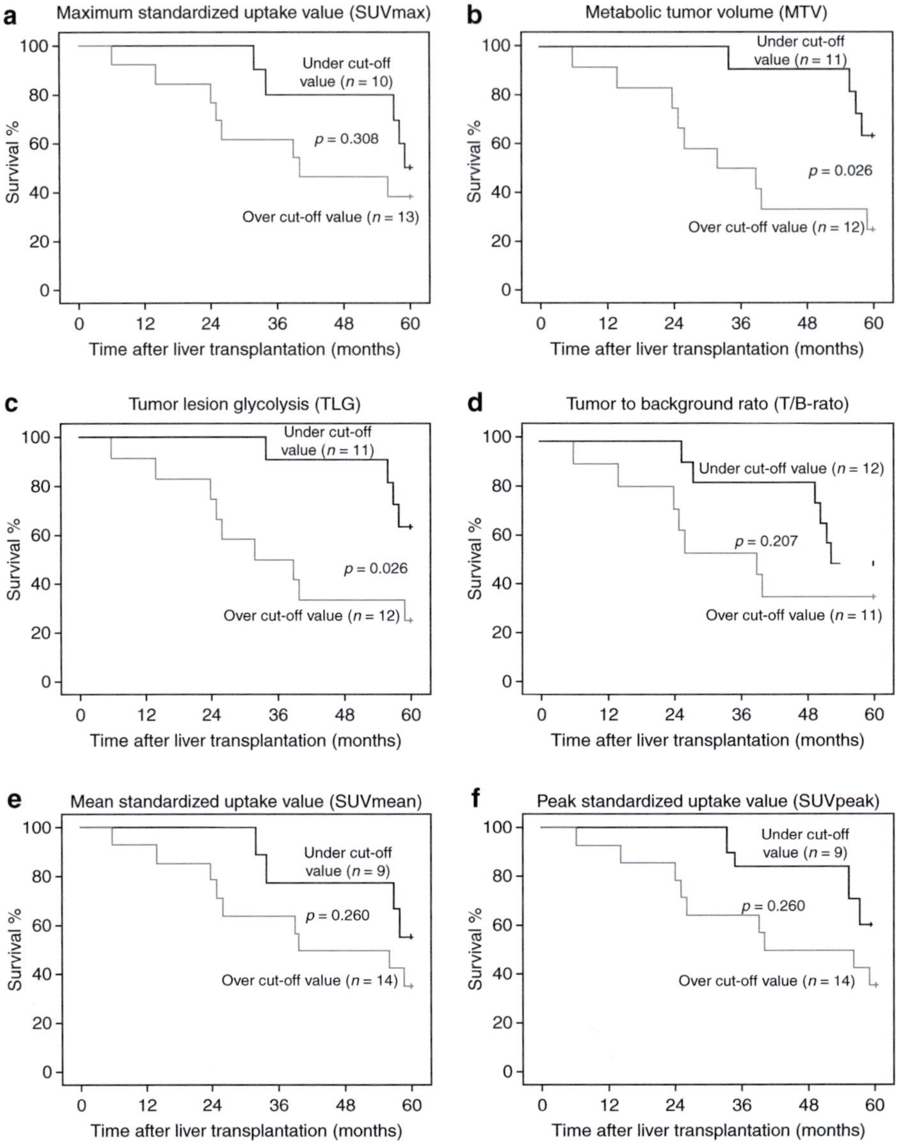

Fig. 39.3 (**a**–**f**) Kaplan–Meier 5-year overall survival (OS) plot. Patients with total metabolic tumor volume (**b**) and total lesion glycolysis (**c**) under cutoff value had significantly longer 5-year OS than patients over cutoff value ($p = 0.027$ and 0.026, log-rank test). Maximum standardized uptake value (**a**), tumor-to-background ratio (**d**), mean standardized uptake value (**e**), and peak standardized uptake value (**f**) were not significantly correlated to OS

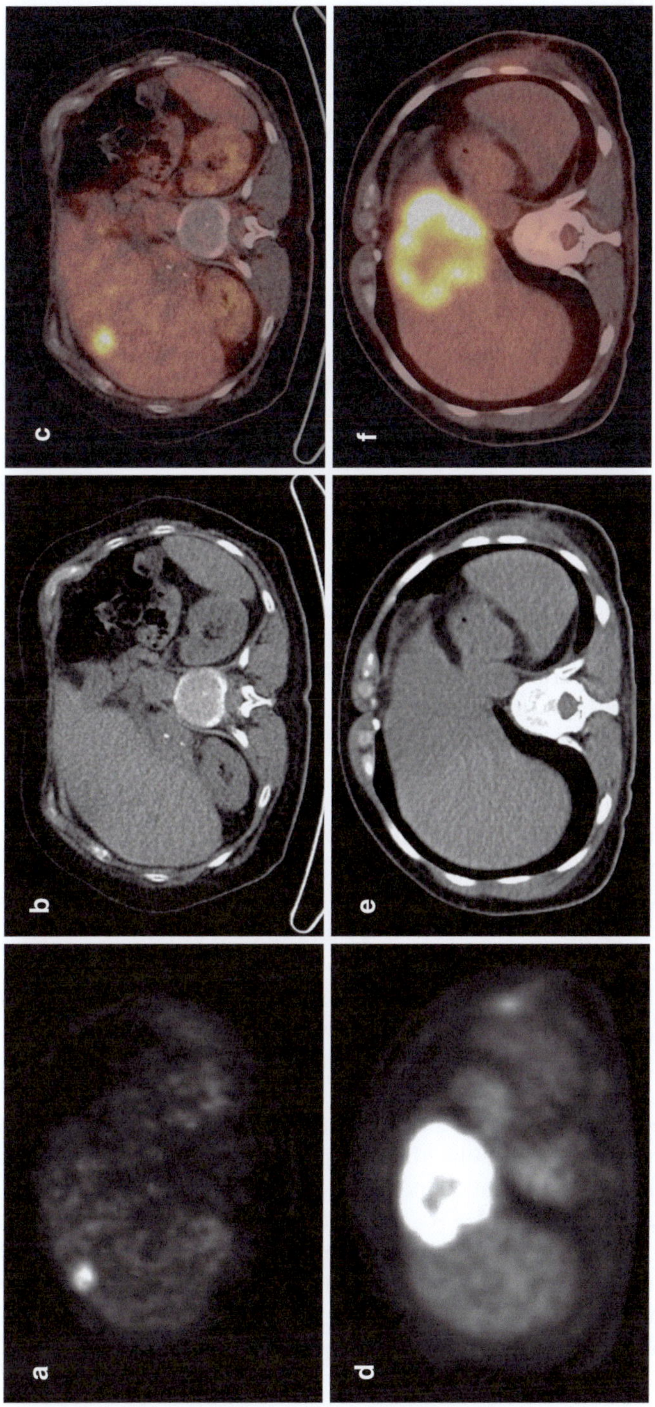

Fig. 39.4 (**a–c**) FDG PET, CT, and fused FDG PET /CT images of a patient with total metabolic tumor volume (MTV) and total lesion glycolysis (TLG) under the cutoff value. The patient is still alive 10 years after liver transplantation. (**d–f**) FDG PET, CT, and fused FDG PET/CT images of a patient with total MTV and TLG over the cutoff value. The patient died from recurrent disease 2 years after transplantation

Updated Status

Since 2012, a follow-up trial to the SECA I study has been ongoing, named the SECA II trial (Clinical Trials.gov: NCT01479608). The aim of this study was to investigate whether improved selection may improve OS and DFS after liver transplantation for CRLM. The main inclusion criteria were liver-only disease by CT / MRI scans and PET/CT scan, no prior extrahepatic metastases, or local relapse of the primary tumor. Primary tumor should have been treated and resected according to standard procedure for curative treatment. Required time from diagnosis to being listed for LT should be at least 1 year. At the time of listing for transplantation, the patients should have at least 10% response to chemotherapy according to RECIST response criteria. Only patients with good performance status (ECOG 0–1) were included and although not listed as formal inclusion criteria, maximal tumor diameter less than 5.5 cm and CEA levels well below 80 μg/l were aimed for when screening potential candidates.

The first 5-year results from the study are pending publication shortly and can therefore not be presented in detail in this chapter. Briefly, preliminary analysis shows that overall survival after 5 years is fully comparable with what is seen after transplantation for benign disease or liver transplantation for HCC within the MILAN criteria. Disease-free survival is also substantially improved compared with all other reports in the literature on liver transplantation for CRLM.

DFS is a common parameter to measure efficacy of treatment after oncological surgery. Since a high proportion of the observed relapses after transplantation are small, slow-growing and often resectable lung metastases, one might speculate whether DFS is a good outcome variable for assessment of treatment efficacy in liver transplantation for nonresectable CRLM. We have compared OS and DFS and survival after recurrence between patients transplanted for HCC and for colorectal liver metastasis at our center. HCC patients were classified as within and outside the MILAN criteria and colorectal metastasis patients were stratified into low risk (OSLO score 0–3) and high risk (OSLO score 4). The 5-year OS rate in patients with colorectal cancer in the low- and high-risk groups was 75% and 0%, respectively. The corresponding figure for HCC patients within MILAN criteria was 76% and for those outside 56% [41]. Patients in the high-risk CRC group had a median OS from time of relapse of 21 months ($p = 0.002$ versus median OS in the low-risk group) (Fig. 39.5c). In the low-risk CRC group, median OS from the time of recurrence was not reached, with 12 of 15 patients alive at 20–58 months after relapse. In contrast, median survival in HCC patients after relapse, independent of MILAN criteria, was significantly shorter than that in the low-risk CRC group (Fig. 39.5c). On this background, it seems justified to propose that OS is the most important outcome measure to assess efficacy of liver transplantation for CRLM, and that disease-free survival first and foremost has a significant impact on 5-year survival in high-risk patients with OSLO score 4.

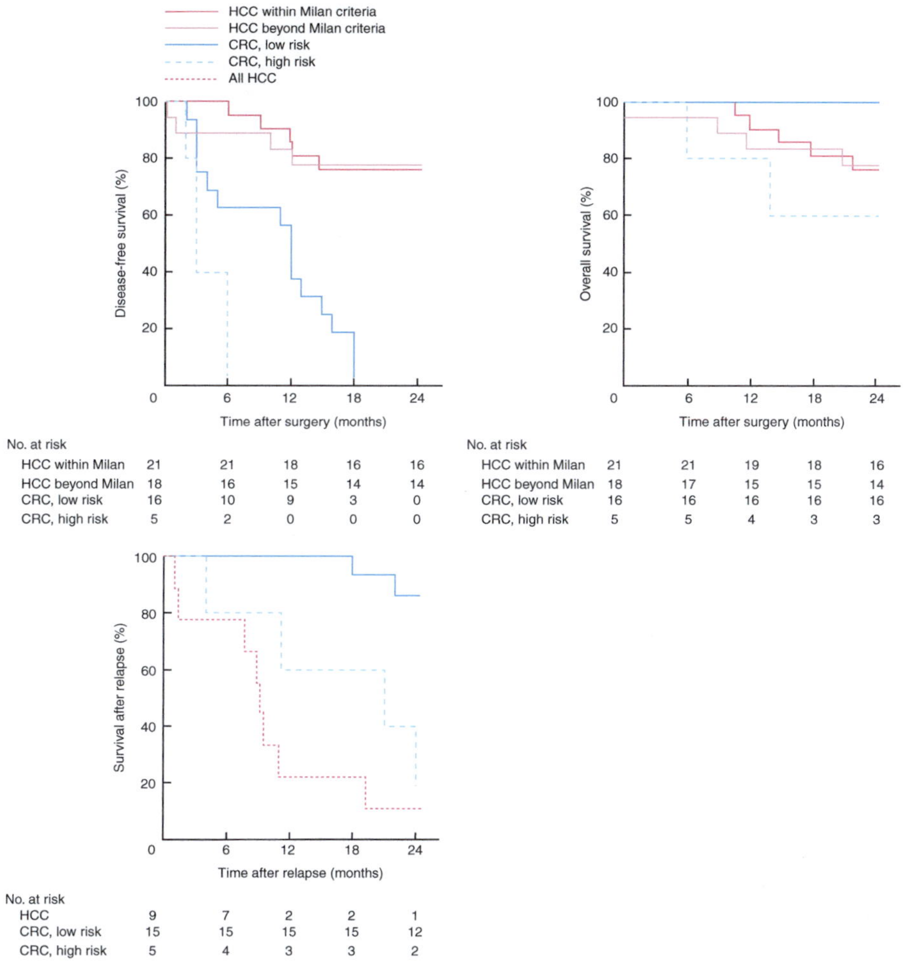

Fig. 39.5 Kaplan–Meier estimated survival in patients with hepatocellular carcinoma (HCC), stratified according to Milan criteria and patients with colorectal liver metastases (CRC) stratified according to OSLO score low/high. (**a**): Disease-free survival, Milan versus CRC low-risk group ($p < 0.001$), CRC low-risk versus high-risk group ($p < 0.02$) (**b**): Overall survival, CRC low-risk group versus Milan ($p = 0.040$), CRC low-risk versus high-risk group ($p = 0.008$). (**c**): Overall survival calculated from time of relapse after liver transplantation, CRC low-risk group versus HCC ($p < 0.001$), CRC low-risk versus high-risk group ($p = 0.002$). (All comparisons by log-rank test)

Future Perspectives

During the last years, the concept of liver transplantation as a possible treatment option for highly selected patients with nonresectable colorectal liver metastases has gained renewed interest and popularity [42]. Following the success of liver transplantation as treatment for a wide range of serious and most often

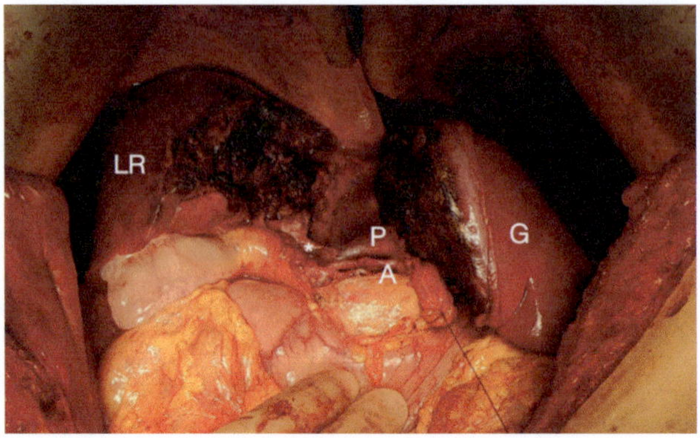

Fig. 39.6 Photograph showing the completion of stage 1 of the RAPID procedure. (*G* S2–3 graft, *LR* liver remnant, *P* graft portal vein, *A* graft hepatic artery, ∗liver remnant portal vein closed with staples

life-threatening liver diseases, there has been a substantial increase in the demand for liver grafts in most countries [43]. A significant obstacle to broader application of colorectal liver metastasis as a transplant indication is therefore the scarcity of liver grafts. Our group has pioneered a novel approach where the goal is to utilize left lateral segment split grafts as a surplus liver for patients with CRLM. This is called the RAPID concept and it is briefly done by combining liver resection and segment 2–3 auxiliary transplantation at the initial first stage with modulation of graft portal inflow under pressure guidance while ligating the portal vein to the liver remnant. An example of a finished first-stage operation is given in Fig. 39.6.

Graft volume is assessed weekly by volumetry, and the delayed second-stage hepatectomy of the liver remnant with metastasis is performed once the graft has reached a volume of 35–40% of standard liver volume [44]. This is part of an ongoing trial at Oslo University Hospital (Clinicaltrials.gov; NCT02215889). The primary aim is to test safety and the number of patients who can reach second-stage hepatectomy within 4 weeks after liver transplantation. Three patients have been operated so far and received grafts weighing 250–330 g (graft to body weight ratios of 0.28–0.46). Ligation of the liver remnant portal vein has been done in all patients, without signs of detrimental portal pressure levels in the graft (< 20 mmHg). The patients have undergone two-stage hepatectomy after about 3 weeks without signs of liver failure or small-for-size syndrome. The first patient from the original report in *Annals of Surgery* is now 4 years out, alive and well without evidence of disease. The approach has, understandably, not been without controversy. Concerns have been raised regarding the technical complexity of the procedure and leaving the deportalized liver remnant with intact metastases, while the patient receives immunosuppression [45]. The RAPID concept is still experimental surgery and a "work in progress", but if proven safe and feasible, the prospect of live donation of segment 2–3 grafts could be a promising further development that could mean a paradigm shift in our approach to nonresectable colorectal liver metastasis. Recently, a living donor RAPID procedure has been presented at the 12th Biennial European-African Hepato Pancreato Biliary Association (E-AHPBA) congress in Mainz, May 23–26, 2017 (Nadalin, S et al., Abstract FP2.03).

Living donation offers a range of advantages for the recipient with planned and optimally timed surgery. A limiting factor is however the donor risk. If conventional living donor transplantation with right lobe donation were to be utilized, the issue of significant donor morbidity in 30.35% of the cases and a mortality risk that in the Western experience is 0.2–0.3% has to be considered and evaluated carefully [46–48]. Donation of segment 2–3 grafts, on the contrary, carries a mortality risk on par with that seen for live kidney donors, which is estimated to be about 0.03%. Segment 2–3 grafts can also be harvested safely laparoscopically, thereby further improving the overall strain on donors [49, 50].

The group in Toronto has started a trial to explore the role of neoadjuvant-chemotherapy plus living donor liver transplantation in patients with nonresectable CRLM (https://clinicaltrials.gov/ct2/show/NCT02864485) [42]. An alternative approach to living donation in order to address the scarcity of graft is the utilization of extended criteria donors for patients with malignant disease that fall outside conventional organ allocation criteria [51]. Since patients with colorectal metastasis in the context of this discussion normally do not have portal hypertension or severe liver dysfunction, their requirements with regard to graft function and the tolerability for somewhat inferior graft quality is most likely better than the average liver recipient on the waiting list. Nevertheless, such a policy must always be based on careful assessment of risk, and only be done with fully informed consent in the setting of prospective studies.

Conclusion

Liver transplantation offers a clear survival benefit to patients with nonresectable colorectal liver metastases. Strict selection criteria remain to be defined, but tumor size and CEA levels before transplantation as well as response to chemotherapy and time from resection of the primary tumor to transplantation are predictive factors for survival. Liver transplantation should be restricted to patients with good performance status with no extrahepatic disease. All transplantations for this indication need to be part of prospective trials. Innovative strategies to improve access to liver grafts are needed to further implement transplantation for nonresectable CRLM into clinical practice.

References

1. Masi G, Vasile E, Loupakis F, Cupini S, Fornaro L, Baldi G, et al. Randomized trial of two induction chemotherapy regimens in metastatic colorectal cancer: an updated analysis. J Natl Cancer Inst. 2011;103:21–30.
2. Van Cutsem E, Köhne C-H, Hitre E, Zaluski J, Chang Chien C-R, Makhson A, et al. Cetuximab and chemotherapy as initial treatment for metastatic colorectal cancer. N Engl J Med. 2009;360:1408–17.
3. Bennouna J, Sastre J, Arnold D, Österlund P, Greil R, Van Cutsem E, et al. Continuation of bevacizumab after first progression in metastatic colorectal cancer (ML18147): a randomised phase 3 trial. Lancet Oncol. 2013;14:29–37.

4. Broadbridge VT, Karapetis CS, Price TJ. Cetuximab in metastatic colorectal cancer. Expert Rev Anticancer Ther. 2012;12:555–65.
5. Ekberg H, Tranberg KG, Andersson R, Lundstedt C, Hägerstrand I, Ranstam J, et al. Determinants of survival in liver resection for colorectal secondaries. Br J Surg. 1986;73:727–31.
6. Adam R, Laurent A, Azoulay D, Castaing D, Bismuth H. Two-stage hepatectomy: a planned strategy to treat irresectable liver tumors. Ann Surg. 2000;232:777–85.
7. Hemming A, Reed A, Howard R, Fujita S, Hochwald S, Caridi J, et al. Preoperative portal vein embolization for extended hepatectomy. Ann Surg. 2003;237:686–91; discussion691–3.
8. Jaeck D, Oussoultzoglou E, Rosso E, Greget M, Weber J-C, Bachellier P. A two-stage hepatectomy procedure combined with portal vein embolization to achieve curative resection for initially unresectable multiple and bilobar colorectal liver metastases. Ann Surg. 2004;240:1037–49; discussion 1049–51.
9. Chakedis J, Squires MH, Beal EW, Hughes T, Lewis H, Paredes A, et al. Update on current problems in colorectal liver metastasis. Curr Probl Surg. Elsevier;. 2017;54:554–602.
10. Kanas GP, Taylor A, Primrose JN, Langeberg WJ, Kelsh MA, Mowat FS, et al. Survival after liver resection in metastatic colorectal cancer: review and meta-analysis of prognostic factors. Clin Epidemiol. Dove Press;. 2012;4:283–301.
11. Angelsen JH, Horn A, Sørbye H, Eide GE, Løes IM, Viste A. Population-based study on resection rates and survival in patients with colorectal liver metastasis in Norway. Br J Surg. 2017;104:580–9.
12. Starzl TE. The saga of liver replacement, with particular reference to the reciprocal influence of liver and kidney transplantation (1955–1967). J Am Coll Surg. 2002;195:587–610.
13. Aune S, Schistad G, Skulberg A. Human liver transplantation without azathioprine. Surg Gynecol Obstet. 1972;135:727–8.
14. Mühlbacher F, Huk I, Steininger R, Gnant M, Götzinger P, Wamser P, et al. Is orthotopic liver transplantation a feasible treatment for secondary cancer of the liver? Transplant Proc. 1991;23:1567–8.
15. Hoti E, Adam R. Liver transplantation for primary and metastatic liver cancers. Transpl Int. Blackwell Publishing Ltd;. 2008;21:1107–17.
16. Honoré C, Detry O, De Roover A, Meurisse M, Honoré P. Liver transplantation for metastatic colon adenocarcinoma: report of a case with 10 years of follow-up without recurrence. Transpl Int. 2003;16:692–3.
17. Uskudar O, Raja K, Schiano TD, Fiel MI, del Rio Martin J, Chang C. Liver transplantation is possible in some patients with liver metastasis of colon cancer. Transplant Proc. Elsevier Inc;. 2011;43:2070–4.
18. Kocman B, Mikulić D, Jadrijevic S, Poljak M, Kocman I, Gašparov S, et al. Long-term survival after living-donor liver transplantation for unresectable colorectal metastases to the liver: case report. Transpl Proc. Elsevier Inc;. 2011;43:4013–5.
19. Haug CE, Jenkins RL, Rohrer RJ, Auchincloss H, Delmonico FL, Freeman RB, et al. Liver transplantation for primary hepatic cancer. Transplantation. 1992;53:376–82.
20. Ismail T, Angrisani L, Gunson BK, Hübscher SG, Buckels JA, Neuberger JM, et al. Primary hepatic malignancy: the role of liver transplantation. Br J Surg. 1990;77:983–7.
21. Mazzaferro V, Regalia E, Doci R, Andreola S, Pulvirenti A, Bozzetti F, et al. Liver transplantation for the treatment of small hepatocellular carcinomas in patients with cirrhosis. N Engl J Med. 1996;334:693–9.
22. Hagness M, Foss A, Line P-D, Scholz T, Jörgensen PF, Fosby B, et al. Liver transplantation for nonresectable liver metastases from colorectal cancer. Ann Surg. 2013;257:800–6.
23. Andersen, M. H. et al. Quality of life following liver transplantation in patients with liver metastases from colorectal carcinoma. Scand J Caring Sci. 2012;26:713–9.
24. Dueland S, Hagness M, Line P-D, Guren TK, Tveit KM, Foss A. Is liver transplantation an option in colorectal cancer patients with nonresectable liver metastases and progression on all lines of standard chemotherapy? Ann Surg Oncol. Springer US;. 2015;22(7):2195–200.
25. Hagness M, Foss A, Egge TS, Dueland S. Patterns of recurrence after liver transplantation for nonresectable liver metastases from colorectal cancer. Ann Surg Oncol. 2014;21:1323–9.

26. Chapman JR, Webster AC, Wong G. Cancer in the transplant recipient. Cold Spring Harb Perspect Med. Cold Spring Harbor Laboratory Press;. 2013;3:a015677–7.
27. Burra P, Shalaby S, Zanetto A. Long-term care of transplant recipients: de novo neoplasms after liver transplantation. Curr Opin Organ Transplant. 2018;23:187–95.
28. Grut H, Solberg S, Seierstad T, Revheim ME, Egge TS, Larsen SG, et al. Growth rates of pulmonary metastases after liver transplantation for unresectable colorectal liver metastases. Br J Surg. 2017;105:295–301.
29. Geissler EK, Schlitt HJ. Immunosuppression for liver transplantation. Gut. 2009;58:452–63.
30. Geissler EK, Schnitzbauer AA, Zülke C, Lamby PE, Proneth A, Duvoux C, et al. Sirolimus use in liver transplant recipients with hepatocellular carcinoma: a randomized, multicenter, open-label phase 3 trial. Transplantation. 2016;100:116–25.
31. Rothwell PM, Wilson M, Elwin C-E, Norrving B, Algra A, Warlow CP, et al. Long-term effect of aspirin on colorectal cancer incidence and mortality: 20-year follow-up of five randomised trials. Lancet. 2010;376:1741–50.
32. Rothwell PM, Wilson M, Price JF, Belch JFF, Meade TW, Mehta Z. Effect of daily aspirin on risk of cancer metastasis: a study of incident cancers during randomised controlled trials. Lancet. 2012;379:1591–601.
33. Bains SJ, Mahic M, Myklebust TÅ, Småstuen MC, Yaqub S, Dørum LM, et al. Aspirin as secondary prevention in patients with colorectal cancer: an unselected population-based study. J Clin Oncol. 2016;34:2501–8.
34. Grut H, Revheim ME, Line P-D, Dueland S. Importance of 18F-FDG PET/CT to select patients with nonresectable colorectal liver metastases for liver transplantation. Nucl Med Commun. 2018;39(7):621–7.
35. Hendrik Bläker MD, Elizabeth Alwers M, Alexander Arnold MD, Esther Herpel MD, Katrin E, Tagscherer P, Wilfried Roth MD, et al. The association between mutations in BRAF and colorectal cancer-specific survival depends on microsatellite status and tumor stage. Clin Gastroenterol Hepatol. The American Gastroenterological Association;. 2019;17(3):455–462.e6.
36. Benson AB, Venook AP, Al-Hawary MM, Cederquist L, Chen Y-J, Ciombor KK, et al. NCCN guidelines insights: colon cancer, version 2.2018. J Natl Compr Canc Netw. Harborside Press, LLC;. 2018;16:359–69.
37. Toso C, Pinto Marques H, Andres A, Castro Sousa F, Adam R, Kalil A, et al. Liver transplantation for colorectal liver metastasis: survival without recurrence can be achieved. Liver Transpl. 2017;23:1073–6.
38. Briggs RH, Chowdhury FU, Lodge JPA, Scarsbrook AF. Clinical impact of FDG PET-CT in patients with potentially operable metastatic colorectal cancer. Clin Radiol. 2011;66:1167–74.
39. Lin M, Wong K, Ng WL, Shon IH, Morgan M. Positron emission tomography and colorectal cancer. Crit Rev Oncol Hematol. 2011;77:30–47.
40. Grut H, Dueland S, Line P-D, Revheim ME. The prognostic value of (18)F-FDG PET/CT prior to liver transplantation for nonresectable colorectal liver metastases. Eur J Nucl Med Mol Imaging. 2017;4:283.
41. Dueland S, Foss A, Solheim JM, Hagness M, Line PD. Survival following liver transplantation for liver-only colorectal metastases compared with hepatocellular carcinoma. Br J Surg. 2018;105:736–42.
42. Gorgen A, Muaddi H, Zhang W, McGilvray I, Gallinger S, Sapisochin G. The new era of transplant oncology: liver transplantation for nonresectable colorectal cancer liver metastases. Can J Gastroenterol Hepatol. 2018;2018:1–7.
43. Dutkowski P, Clavien P-A. Solutions to shortage of liver grafts for transplantation. Br J Surg. 2014;101:739–41.
44. Line P-D, Hagness M, Berstad AE, Foss A, Dueland S. A novel concept for partial liver transplantation in nonresectable colorectal liver metastases: the RAPID concept. Ann Surg. 2015;262:e5–9.
45. Hernandez-Alejandro R, Wall WJ. The RAPID concept—novel idea or a bridge too far? Ann Surg. 2015;262:e10–1.

46. Pomfret EA. Early and late complications in the right-lobe adult living donor. Liver Transpl. Wiley-Blackwell;. 2003;9:S45–9.
47. Pomfret EA, Washburn K, Wald C, Nalesnik MA, Douglas D, Russo M, et al. Report of a national conference on liver allocation in patients with hepatocellular carcinoma in the United States. Liver Transpl. 2010;16:262–78.
48. Rössler F, Sapisochin G, Song G, Lin Y-H, Simpson MA, Hasegawa K, et al. Defining benchmarks for major liver surgery. Ann Surg. 2016;264:492–500.
49. Scatton O, Katsanos G, Boillot O, Goumard C, Bernard D, Stenard F, et al. Pure laparoscopic left lateral sectionectomy in living donors: from innovation to development in France. Ann Surg. 2015;261:506–12.
50. Soubrane O, de Rougemont O, Kim K-H, Samstein B, Mamode N, Boillot O, et al. Laparoscopic living donor left lateral sectionectomy: a new standard practice for donor hepatectomy. Ann Surg. 2015;262:757–61. discussion 761–3.
51. Feng S, Lai JC. Expanded criteria donors. Clin Liver Dis. 2014;18:633–49.

External Radiation for Unresectable CRLM

40

Raquel Guimarães Domingos da Silva
and M. Carmen Rubio Rodriguez

Introduction

About 50% of patients diagnosed with colorectal cancer will either present with metastatic liver disease or develop metachronous liver metastases later in their disease course [1]. The term "oligometastasis," introduced by Hellmann and Weichselbaum [2] in 1995, describes an intermediate stage of cancer, between localized and metastatic cancer, that is suitable for local treatment. The benefits of adopting a radical treatment approach in patients with oligometastatic liver disease are now well established.

The introduction of novel treatments, mainly consisting of chemotherapy agents and targeted therapy, has improved the overall survival (OS) of patients with CRLM (colorectal liver metastasis) [3, 4]. Combination of hepatic resection and systemic chemotherapy has improved 5-year survival rates to 50–60% [5]. However, only a minority of patients will be appropriate for surgery (about 25–30%) due to unfavorable disease distribution within the liver, comorbidities precluding surgery, or the presence of extrahepatic disease [6, 7].

Historically, the use of external beam radiation therapy (RT) in treatment of liver tumors has been limited due to the overall low tolerance of liver tissue to radiation [8]. Although radiation can achieve excellent tumor control when delivered to ablative doses [9], dose is limited due to this low tolerance of the surrounding normal liver tissue and adjacent organs. Radiation-induced liver disease (RILD) is a feared complication of treatment, classically manifesting as a triad of anicteric hepatomegaly, ascites, and elevation of alkaline phosphatase. Histopathologically, venous occlusion is the most predominant chance in pathological specimens [10, 11]. Other

R. G. D. da Silva (✉)
Radiation Oncologist, Instituto Nacional de Câncer, Rio de Janeiro, Brazil

M. C. R. Rodriguez
Radiation Oncologist, HM Hospitales, Madrid, Spain
e-mail: crubio@hmhospitales.com

M. M. Correia et al. (eds.), *Colorectal Cancer Liver Metastases*,
https://doi.org/10.1007/978-3-030-25486-5_40

common adverse effects include nausea, vomiting, fever, chills, loss of appetite, and gastritis [12].

With the emergence of more sophisticated treatment planning software and methods of image guidance in the past two decades, more tightly focused treatment fields are now possible, allowing for delivery of higher doses in fewer fractions to discrete individual liver lesions, while minimizing exposure to surrounding normal liver [13–18]. Imaging techniques have also improved, allowing for precise delineation of hepatic tumors [10]. Breathing motion control and image guidance, both before and during treatment delivery, permit tumor-directed treatment with accurate localization, reducing treatment uncertainty, and decreasing the margin of error. Treatment planning techniques and machines have also improved, allowing highly conformal treatment delivery. With increased conformality, comes the potential to deliver higher doses of radiation and thereby increase local control without increasing toxicity [19, 20].

Over the past decade, multiple retrospective and prospective series [10–16] have been published on the use of conformal radiation treatment for hepatic malignancies, and results have been favorable with high rates of local control [9, 21–27]. Though many of these studies were small, and many were retrospective, they have provided ample background data to establish current prospective studies and randomized trials [10].

External beam radiation can be delivered using standard conformal (3D or intensity-modulated RT) or recently developed stereotactic (SBRT) techniques. Stereotactic body radiotherapy (SBRT), alternatively known as stereotactic ablative body radiotherapy (SABR), is a minimally invasive technique for delivering highly focused ionizing radiation with extreme precision. This technique was initially developed in neurosurgical practice and then applied to extracranial lesions. The utility of SBRT as a treatment for unresectable liver tumors was first reported in 1995 by Blomgren and colleagues [28]. Since then, there have been several additional series reporting excellent local control outcomes demonstrating low toxicity, feasibility, and efficacy [29–31].

SBRT delivers large doses of radiation in few fractions, compared with conventional fractionation, where many small doses are generally delivered in a period of weeks. Conformal RT delivers radiation from multiple planar angles, and compared with SBRT, the dose gradient is less steep and the treatment is less conformal, with a greater amount of healthy liver exposed to radiation. In contrast, SBRT can create a rapid radiation dose fall off by using multiple, noncoplanar beams or arcs, and with a coordinate system for localization targets the tumor with millimeter precision, allowing ablative radiation doses to be delivered to gross tumors while sparing adjacent tissue [10].

While SBRT is more costly and requires more intensive planning than conventional RT, this modality combines the local control benefit of dose-escalated fractionated RT with the convenience of short-course RT and an acceptable toxicity profile.

Further advances in radiotherapy technology, such as the development of a magnetic resonance linac for treatment delivery has exciting potential applications for

SBRT. The magnetic resonance image (MRI) linac enables detailed evaluation of target and organ at risk motion and is able to track tumor motion. The ability to acquire real-time high resolution imaging, including functional MRI series, improves the accuracy of both target and organ at risk definition, therefore enabling on-the-fly adaptive therapy, opening up the possibilities for isotoxic dose escalation [7].

As a result, SBRT has emerged as the primary technique of delivering radiation to liver tumors.

Radiobiology of External Beam Radiation

Radiation produces tumor cell kill by depositing energy within atoms, causing transformation into free radicals. This results in direct DNA damage, as well as indirect and cellular damage through generation of reactive oxygen species. Ultimately, generation of DNA double strand breaks leads to tumor cell death [10].

Conventional radiotherapy (i.e., 1.8–2.0 Gy per fraction) results in a tumoricidal effect by means of mitotic death of cancer cells, allowing recovery of late sublethal damage of normal tissues. In contrast, SBRT may provide a novel mechanism of radiation-induced damage: data with higher doses per fraction (i.e., 10–20 Gy per fraction) suggest that, in addition to direct cytotoxicity, a different mechanism involving microvascular damage begins to have a substantial effect on the tumor cell kill [32, 33]. Endothelial apoptosis results in microvascular disruption and death of the tissue supplied by that vasculature [34].

There is a dose–response relationship for radiation and local control outcomes. Nevertheless, as with any other medical procedure, prescription of a course of radiotherapy must represent a balance between risks and benefits. The relative position and shape of the dose–response curves for tumor control and a given radiotherapy complication determine the possibility of delivering a sufficient dose with an acceptable level of side effects.

Major developments in radiotherapy fractionation have taken place during the past three decades and these have grown out of understanding in radiation biology. The relationships between total dose and dose per fraction for late-responding tissues, acutely responding tissues, and tumors provide the basic information required to optimize radiotherapy according to the dose per fraction and number of fractions.

Historically, normal tissue effects are more greatly impacted by fraction sizes than acute effects are, which is why 1.8–2.0 Gy fractionation is considered the standard for conventional radiotherapy, resulting in longer treatment times. In fact, small doses per fraction result in a tumoricidal effect by means of mitotic death of cancer cells, allowing recovery of late sublethal damage of normal tissues at the same time. SBRT may add a novel mechanism of radiation-induced damage: at higher doses per fraction, emerging data suggest that, in addition to direct cytotoxicity, a different mechanism involving microvascular damage begins to have a substantial effect on the tumor cell kill [32, 33]. Endothelial apoptosis results in microvascular disruption and death of the tissue supplied by that vasculature [32].

Thus, even if hypofractionated irradiation may heighten the risks of late toxicity from a radiobiologic point of view, SBRT techniques substantially counteract this concern, reducing the volume of normal tissue exposed to high doses as a result of their precision [35].

As for hepatocellular carcinoma, SBRT is expected to play a role in the treatment of oligometastases from colorectal cancer (CRC). However, negative factors also exist: for example, CRC metastases contain larger proportions of hypoxic cells compared to other tumor types, and hypoxia leads to decrease in radiosensitivity; another is that microscopic extension of oligometastases from CRC may compromise local control. In fact, the local control rates of SBRT in CRC oligometastases are significantly worse than those of oligometastases from other cancers, including NSCLC. Thus, dose escalation should be considered to achieve better local control [36].

It has been proposed that one of the causative mechanisms of local failure are regions of hypoxia, particularly within large regions [37]. In colorectal cancer, tumor hypoxia has been shown to be present heterogeneously throughout resected specimens [38]. Combining SBRT with hypoxia-modifying agents is therefore one potential area of research. Given the propensity for patients to fail at distant sites after SBRT, further work is required to evaluate the optimal sequencing and combination of liver SBRT with systemic therapies [7].

Although the tolerance of the whole liver to radiotherapy is low, as a parallel organ it can tolerate high doses to small volumes as long as the mean dose to the uninvolved liver is low enough no to cause functional compromise [39, 40]. As a result of technical advances in radiation delivery over the past decade, the safe delivery of radiation to the liver has become a realistic prospect, prompting an expansion in its use [9, 41]. Highly conformal dosimetry, together with a steep dose gradient allowing relative sparing of normal liver tissue, makes SBRT a particularly attractive technique for liver irradiation [7].

Patient Selection

Good selection criteria for patients with liver metastases who are candidate for SBRT remain a controversial topic. A multidisciplinary tumor board discussion is recommended before each qualification. For discussion purposes, candidates for SBRT can be divided into three categories: suitable, cautionary, and unsuitable patients [42, 43]. Selection criteria may be based on the lesion number, the lesion diameter, the distance from the organs at risk (OAR), the liver function, and the patient's conditions [44].

In general, indications for SBRT are the same as those for metastasectomy, but without the limits regarding feasibility in patients unfit for surgery. In several reports, the eligibility criteria for SBRT for oligometastatic cancer were defined as follows: a limited number of metastases (one to five), a limited tumor diameter (<4 cm), a locally controlled primary tumor, and no other metastatic sites [45]. Other specific and recently proposed selection criteria to offer SBRT to patients with various oligometastatic tumors include: a controlled primary, favorable histology, limited metastatic disease, the metachronous appearance of metastases, young age, and a good performance status of the patient. In clinical practice, patients eligible for SBRT are essentially those for whom surgery is not feasible because of their age or performance status and because of previous treatment with multiple lines of systemic therapy, when the toxicity of local treatments should be minimized [35].

SBRT Technique

Liver SBRT can be safely and effectively delivered using either a linear accelerator (linac) or a SBRT-specific delivery platform, such as the robotic Cyberknife (Accuray®). These have relative advantages and disadvantages over one another, although broadly the plan quality that can be achieved with either technique is similar. Linac-delivered SBRT enables three-dimensional volumetric imaging acquisition for patient set-up, does not mandate fiducial marker insertion, and generally has shorter treatment times, especially if intensity-modulated arc therapy is used. In contrast, treatment times with Cyberknife are significantly longer, on average being 30–60 min per fraction due to the large number of noncoplanar nonisocentric beams used and respiratory tracking of the mandatory fiducial markers [7].

Fiducial markers are utilized in many institutions to reduce uncertainty from breathing motion and allow tumor tracking [10]. At least two or more gold fiducials should be placed in the vicinity (within 6 cm) of the tumor in a non-colinear fashion by the interventional radiology team, approximately 1 week before treatment planning computer tomography (CT) [36]. Markers are placed percutaneously with image guidance under local anesthesia; it is an outpatient procedure with standard risks from introducing a needle into the liver (bleeding, infection, seeding, pain) and small risk of fiducial migration [10].

Patients are typically simulated with a custom immobilization device (i.e., Alpha Cradle). By delivering the dose in a small number of high-dose fractions, SBRT allows significant dose escalation. Although this will probably be advantageous in improving local control rates, it has the potential to cause late toxicity, particularly if the delivered dose distribution does not accurately reflect that intended at treatment planning. As such, the liver as a target organ for SBRT presents several specific challenges concerning inter and intrafraction motion.

Intrafraction motion occurs due to the effects of respiration. The motion degree can be significant, with intrafraction liver excursion of up to 39.5 mm being reported [46]. Tumor motion is usually predominantly in a craniocaudal direction due to diaphragmatic movement. Strategies to mitigate for intrafraction motion depend on the delivery platform used. A variety of motion management techniques can be used, including abdominal compression [47], gating [48], and breath-hold techniques [49], or alternatively accounted for by the use of four-dimensional computed tomography planning. For respiratory gating or tracking, between three and five fiducial markers are inserted around the tumor to enable intrafraction tracking of tumor motion using kV–kV (kilo Voltage) imaging during treatment [7].

Daily radiotherapy patient set-up is made difficult by the fact that the position of liver tumors relative to bony anatomy has been shown to change between fractions by up to 1 cm [50]. In addition, liver tumors are often of similar density with respect to adjacent normal liver tissue, therefore making daily localization of the tumor with three-dimensional cone beam computed tomography challenging. In view of this, the three-dimensional positions of the whole liver and diaphragm are usually used as surrogates for tumor position [51]. The use of fiducial markers to aid localization is an alternative solution and has been shown to improve confidence in daily tumor visualization before treatment [52].

The liver may also undergo deformation between fractions of radiotherapy. This may be due to temporal alterations in the position of the liver with respect to other abdominal organs, or due to differences in patient positioning at set-up. This has been shown to cause discrepancies >5% in the dose delivered to the tumor and normal tissues compared with that expected from treatment planning, despite using daily cone beam computed tomography for patient set-up [53]. These uncertainties in the delivered dose distribution are particularly relevant when considering dose-escalation strategies for liver tumors, as the normal tissue dose volume histograms calculates at planning may not reflect the delivered dose [7].

After fiducial placement, a pretreatment CT is obtained from radiation planning purposes; this is ideally performed with multiphasic IV contrast in exhale or inhale breath-hold position. A diagnostic MRI or CT is also utilized to define the tumor volume.

The gross volume (GTV) is contoured by the radiation oncologist in each slice of the pretreatment CT. A clinical target volume (CTV) can be added to account for microscopic extension; in many cases, there will be no CTV expansion necessary. Finally, a planning target volume (PTV) expansion is added to the GTV to account for daily setup error and internal organ motion. The size and number of lesions that can be targeted, and dose radiation that can be delivered, is dependent primarily on normal liver reserve and estimated risk of liver complication. Depending on the location, multiple tumors can be treated at the same time. Patients with poor liver function may require dose reduction to reduce the likelihood of complication [24]. Childs Pugh class is one measure of estimating normal liver function; for Childs Pugh category B, reduction in radiation dose may be a consideration. Childs Pugh C is less commonly treated to ablative doses, given poor functional reserve and high risk of toxicity.

The dose prescribed depends on baseline function and normal tissue constraints. In general, the highest allowable dose to the tumor that respects normal tissue constraints is selected.

A useful method of estimating normal liver function is the measurement of the liver effective volume (V_{eff}). In this scheme, the value of V_{eff} for each dose volume histogram is independent of dose units (Gy, %). V_{eff} is utilized as an aid in dose prescription, along with standard metrics such as the mean liver dose. For example, for a five-fraction treatment, the prescribed total dose ranges from 27.5 to 50 Gy depending on the effective liver volume [54]. At least 700 cm^3 of normal liver should receive less than 15 Gy in order to maintain a <5% risk of RILD [10].

For larger volume lesions (>6 cm), achieving ablative doses using a three to five fraction regimen is challenging without exceeding normal liver constraints. For this group of patients, an alternative approach is to use a risk-estratified individualized prescription technique using a normal tissue complication probability model. This effectively allows individualization of tumor dose according to the modeled risk of RILD for each patient, a toxicity of particular concern when treating large lesions. The prescribed dose is dependent on the volume of normal liver exposed to radiation and has been previously described [40, 54]. Outcomes of using this approach in six to ten fraction regimens have reported 1 year local control rates varying from 65% to 71% [40, 55]. Although the use of these more protracted dose fractionation regimens does not meet some definitions of SBRT (e.g., five or fewer fractions), this approach provides a useful option for the safe treatment of larger lesions or when multiple sites are treated [56].

Typically, in smaller lesions, treatment is delivered in three to six fractions, with minimum 1–3 days between each fraction. Depending on location, it is possible to target multiple tumors in a single fraction. The actual radiation treatment is less than 1 h in duration. Because it is a noninvasive and painless, no sedation or anesthesia is required [10].

Prognostic Factors Related to Local Control

Main factors to impact the local control are the target volume and the dose delivered. In most articles, a tumor volume appears as an independent factor predictive of the local control, and smaller volumes are reported to have better outcomes.

Notwithstanding, the dose delivered (and optimal fractionation) is the most important factor affecting local control. Prospective trials with dose escalation demonstrate this dose effect relation. There is a dose–response relationship for radiation and local control outcomes. A variety of dose regimens have been used, varying from single fractions of up to 30 Gy to six fraction regimens where dose is individualized according to the predicted risk of liver toxicity. Several studies have shown a dose–response, with local control improving with higher doses [25, 40, 57]. A meta-analysis concluded that a dose of 46–52 Gy in three fractions or higher is required to achieve 90% of local control at 1 year for the treatment of colorectal liver metastases, equivalent to a biologically equivalent dose (BED$_{10)}$ >117 Gy [58]. Still, more recent studies have persuaded a dose-escalation strategy, using doses of up to 75 Gy in three fractions, reporting local control rates of 94% at 1 year [43]. It should be noted, however, that the mean gross tumor volume in this series was small at 18.7 cm^3 with 60% of lesions being ≤3 cm in size. The feasibility of delivering such high doses to larger lesions is unproven. In general, most series have included lesions up to a maximum size of 6 cm [7].

The size and number of lesions that can be targeted, and dose radiation that can be delivered, are dependent primarily on normal liver reserve and estimated risk of liver complications. For this reason, those with a longer disease-free interval and absence of chemotherapy, adenocarcinoma histology, and metachronous disease presentation seem to have better outcomes.

Clinical Outcomes

A variety of retrospective and prospective studies of SBRT for the treatment of metastatic liver disease have been reported in the literature. The results of these are summarized in Table 40.1. The treatment indications are likely to expand as the evidence base for efficacy continues to grow. Interpretation of the reported survival rates is confounded by the significant variation in primary tumor histology, the volume of metastases treated with radiotherapy dose and fractionation. However, in general, reported local control rates are high, ranging from 70% to 100% at 1 year and 60% to 90% at 2 years [7].

Table 40.1 Summary of reported studies of stereotactic body radiotherapy for liver metastases

Study	Year	Type of study	$N°_{\text{patients}}$	Radiotherapy dose	LC	Toxicity grade ≥3
Blomgren et al. [28]	1995	R	14	8–66 Gy/1–4	80% (24 mos)	14%
Herfarth et al. [62]	2004	Phase I/II	56	14–16 Gy/1	67% (18 mos)	NMT
Schefter et al. [64]	2005	R	18	36–60 Gy/3	NR	NMT
Wulf et al. [63]	2006	R	44	30 Gy/3	61% (24 mos)	NMT
Kavanagh et al. [64]	2006	Phase I/II	36	36–6-Gy/3	93% (18 mos)	NMT
Mendez Romero et al. [24]	2006	Phase I/II	45	37.5 Gy/3	82% (24 mos)	11,8%
Hoyer et al. [39]	2006	Phase II	44	45 Gy/3	86% (24 mos)	6,6%
Katz et al. [64]	2007	R	69	30 Gy/7	57% (20 mos)	NMT
Milano et al. [56]	2008	R	293	50 Gy/5	67% (24 mos)	NMT
Rusthoven et al. [9]	2009	Phase I/II	63	60 Gy/3	92% (24 mos)	2%
Lee et al. [40]	2009	Phase I	68	28–60 Gy/3	71% (12 mos)	NMT
Ambrosino et al. [41]	2009	R	27	25–60 Gy/3	74% (12 mos)	NR
Van de Pool et al. [65]	2010	R	20	37.5–45/3	74% (24 mos)	NMT
Goodman et al. [66]	2010	Phase I	40	18–20 Gy/1	49.4% (24 mos)	NMT
Vautravers Dewas et al. [67]	2011	R	42	40 Gy/3	86% (12 mos)	NMT
Rule et al. [25]	2011	Phase I	37	30–60 Gy/3–5	89% (24 mos)	NMT
Scorsetti et al. [43]	2013	Phase II	61	52.5–75/3	94% (12 mos)	NMT
Yuan et al. [68]	2014	R	57	39–54 Gy/3–7	89.7% (24 mos)	NMT

R retrospective, *LC* local control, *mos* months, *NR* not reported, *OS* overall survival, *NMT* no major toxicity

Higher SBRT doses ($BED_{10} \geq 100$ Gy) and smaller tumor volumes (≤ 40 cm^3) are associated with improved local control and overall survival [18].

Long-term results with SBRT have also shown low toxicity (grade 3 <5%) and long survivals (3 years OS 44%) [71]. Although most of the studies have treated limited number of liver metastases (one to three lesions), patients with multiple liver metastases could be treated safely and benefit from sequential SBRT with high LC (80.6% and 65% at 2 and 4 years) and prolonged survivals (5 year OS of 57.6%) [72].

A further exciting avenue for SBRT research is the discovery that delivering radiation doses within the ablative range seems to enhance antitumor immunity, with activation of the adaptive and innate immune responses. Case reports have described the so-called "abscopal effect" whereby regression of distant metastases outside the radiation field is seen after SBRT [59, 60]. This has stimulated research interest into the potential for combining SBRT with immunotherapy in oligometastatic disease, in order to therapeutically exploit this immune response [7, 61].

Post-treatment Response Evaluation

Serial computed tomography and/or magnetic resonance imaging (MRI) are the most frequent modalities used to assess local response after treatment. Baseline imaging to assess the treatment response is generally carried out at 3 monthly intervals in the first year, the 6 monthly, although computed tomography imaging at earlier time points may be required to confirm a clinical suspicion of RILD. MRI and positron emission tomography (PET) may bring complementary information if the lesion cannot be reliably visualized on computed tomography. However, accurately determining the treatment response using a standard response evaluation criteria in solid tumors (RECIST) alone can be difficult. A phenomenon of pseudoprogression on computed tomography has been described, whereby lesions that have responded to treatment may become necrotic and increase in size, therefore being misclassified as a progression event. Serial imaging may be required to clarify the response, but shrinkage of the hypodense region, vessel displacement, and distinct patterns of contrast enhancement are considered indicative of local control [7].

Toxicity

Respecting individual target volumes and dosing schemes, toxicity rates can be minimized, even for larger volumes. In contrast to primary liver cancer, liver metastases most commonly occur in noncirrhotic livers, and the most predominant toxicity to radiation will be RILD. However, adhering to established dose constraints of normal liver tissue, i.e., keeping below 30 Gy median liver dose in conventional fractionation [62] or application of less than 15 Gy to 700 mL of healthy liver tissue, this may be securely avoided [62].

SBRT in liver metastases is a very well-tolerated treatment, with a low toxicity profile and severe toxicity is exceptional. Most series have reported low rates of treatment-related toxicity, with rates of common terminology criteria for adverse effects (CTCAE) grade 3 or 4 toxicity ranging from 1% to 10%. Historically, the most common toxicity with liver radiotherapy has been RILD. The risk of RILD is known to be proportional to the mean dose delivered to the normal liver and is more common in patients with hepatocellular carcinoma, as underlying liver dysfunction is known to be a risk factor for both the disease and RILD. Most studies of liver metastases treated with SBRT have reported rates of RILD <1% [63].

Conclusions

Historically, conventional radiation therapy has played a limited role in the treatment of liver metastases because of the risk of liver toxicity induced by high doses delivered to normal liver tissue. However, recent technological advances have contributed to the development of SBRT as a precise tightly focused radiation technique that allows the treatment of hepatic metastases with an ablative intent, in few fractions, while significantly limiting dose to the healthy liver and surrounding tissues.

Liver SBRT requires the integration of imaging, in order to properly define the metastases, highly conformed dosimetry to further minimize radiation dose in healthy tissues, and intrafraction control of the liver motion, with image guided systems, to deliver the dose to the metastases with accuracy.

The safety and effectiveness of SBRT has been evaluated with encouraging results in retrospective and prospective clinical studies. Reports of SBRT for primary and metastatic liver disease have been steadily increasing since 2006 and results have been associated with minimal toxicity and high local control rates, most in the range of 70–90% at 1–2 years. As a result of these advances, radiation is being re-explored as a treatment modality for both primary and metastatic liver tumors. SBRT offers an alternative, noninvasive approach, to the treatment of limited hepatic metastases in inoperable patients, or with unresectable metastases with fewest local therapeutic options, and the role of SBRT for the treatment of these patients should therefore be kept in mind in interdisciplinary treatment decisions.

Further clinical evaluation, preferentially in randomized settings comparing to surgery of other locally ablative techniques will further elucidate the full potential of SBRT in patients with liver metastases, especially in the subgroup of oligometastatic patients.

Considering the high propensity for distant progression in these patients, the combination of novel drugs and SBRT needs to be deeply explored with prospective trials in order to improve the overall survival of these patients.

References

1. Abdalla EK. Improving resectability of hepatic colorectal metastases: expert consensus statement. Ann Surg Oncol. 2006;13:1271–80.
2. Hellman S, Weichselbaum RR. Oligometastases. J Clin Oncol. 1995;13(1):8–10.
3. Roberto M, Falcone R, Mazzuca F, et al. The role of stereotactic body radiation therapy in oligomestastatic colorectal cancer. Medicine (Baltimore). 2017;96(48):e9023.
4. Siegel R, Ma J, Zou Z, et al. Cancer statistics,2014. CA Cancer J Clin. 2014;64:9–29.
5. Wei AC, Greig PD, Grant D, et al. Survival after hepatic resection for colorectal metastases: a 10-year experience. Ann Surg Oncol. 2006;13(5):668–76.
6. Hewish M, Cunningham D. First-line treatment of advanced colorectal cancer. Lancet. 2011;377(9783):2060–2.
7. Aitken KL, Hawkins MA. Stereotactic body radiotherapy for liver metastases. Clin Oncol. 2015;27(5):307–15.
8. Marks KB, Yorke ED, Jackson A, et al. Use of normal tissue complication probability models in the clinic. Int J Radiat Oncol Biol Phys. 2010;76:S10–9.
9. Rusthoven KE, Kavanagh BD, Cardenes H, et al. Multi-institutional phase I/II trial of stereotatic body radiation therapy for liver metastases. J Clin Oncol. 2009;27:1572–8.
10. Li D, Kang J, Golas BJ, et al. Minimally invasive local therapies for liver cancer. Cancer Biol Med. 2014;11:217–36.
11. Olsen CC, Welsh J, Kavanagh BD, et al. Microscopic and macroscopic tumor and parenchymal effects of liver stereotactic body radiotherapy. Int J Radiat Oncol Biol Phys. 2009;73(5):1414–24.
12. Zhang S, Zhu G, Li G, et al. Application of stereotactic body radiation therapy to cancer liver metastasis. Cancer Lett. 2015;379(2):225–9.
13. Kini VR, Vedam SS, Keall PJ, et al. Patient training in respiratory-gated radiotherapy. Med Dosim Off J Am Assoc. Med Dosim. 2003;28(1):7–11. 18.
14. Brock KK, McShan DL, Ten Haken RK, Hollister SJ, Dawson LA, Balter JM. Inclusion of organ deformation in dose calculations. Med Phys. 2003;30(3):290–5. 19.
15. Dawson LA, Balter JM. Interventions to reduce organ motion effects in radiation delivery. Semin Radiat Oncol. 2004;14(1):76–80. 20.
16. Dawson LA, Brock KK, Kazanjian S, Fitch D, McGinn CJ, Lawrence TS, et al. The reproducibility of organ position using active breathing control (ABC) during liver radiotherapy. Int J Radiat Oncol Biol Phys. 2001;51(5):1410–21. 21.
17. Hara W, Soltys SG, Gibbs IC. CyberKnife robotic radiosurgery system for tumor treatment. Expert Rev Anticancer Ther. 2007;7(11):1507–15.
18. Mahadevan A, Blanck O, Lanciano R, et al. Stereotactic body radiotherapy (SBRT) for liver metastasis – clinical outcomes from the international multi-institutional RSSearch® patient registry. Radiat Oncol. 2018;13:26.
19. Wagman R, Yorke E, Ford E, Giraud P, Mageras G, Minsky B, et al. Respiratory gating for liver tumors: use in dose escalation. Int J Radiat Oncol Biol Phys. 2003;55:659–668. 81.
20. Wunderink W, Méndez Romero A, de Kruijf W, de Boer H, Levendag P, Heijmen B. Reduction of respiratory liver tumor motion by abdominal compression in stereotactic body frame, analyzed by tracking fiducial markers implanted in liver. Int J Radiat Oncol Biol Phys. 2008;71:907–15.
21. Bujold A, Massey CA, Kim JJ, Brierley J, Cho C, Wong RK, et al. Sequential phase I and II trials of stereotactic body radiotherapy for locally advanced hepatocellular carcinoma. J Clin Oncol. 2013;31:1631–9.
22. Cárdenes HR, Price TR, Perkins SM, Maluccio M, Kwo P, Breen TE, et al. Phase I feasibility trial of stereotactic body radiation therapy for primary hepatocellular carcinoma. Clin Transl Oncol. 2010;12:218–25.

23. Louis C, Dewas S, Mirabel X, Lacornerie T, Adenis A, Bonodeau F, et al. Stereotactic radiotherapy of hepatocellular carcinoma: preliminary results. Technol Cancer Res Treat. 2010;9:479–87.
24. Méndez Romero A, Wunderink W, Hussain SM, De Pooter JA, Heijmen BJ, Nowak PC, et al. Stereotactic body radiation therapy for primary and metastatic liver tumors: a single institution phase I/II study. Acta Oncol. 2006;45:831–7.
25. Rule W, Timmerman R, Tong L, Abdulrahman R, Meyer J, Boike T, et al. Phase I dose- escalation study of stereotactic body radiotherapy in patients with hepatic metastases. Ann Surg Oncol. 2011;18:1081–7.
26. Seo YS, Kim MS, Yoo SY, Cho CK, Choi CW, Kim JH, et al. Preliminary result of stereotactic body radiotherapy as a local salvage treatment for inoperable hepatocellular carcinoma. J Surg Oncol. 2010;102:209–14.
27. Tse RV, Hawkins M, Lockwood G, Kim JJ, Cummings B, Knox J, et al. Phase I study of individualized stereotactic body radiotherapy for hepatocellular carcinoma and intrahepatic cholangiocarcinoma. J Clin Oncol. 2008;26:657–64.
28. Blomgren H, Lax I, Naslund I, Svanstrom R. Stereotactic high dose fraction radiation therapy of extracranial tumors using an accelerator. Clinical experience of the first thirty-one patients. Acta Oncol. 1995;34:861–70.
29. Wulf J, Hadinger U, Oppitz U, Olshausen B, Flentje M. Stereotactic radiotherapy of extracranial targets: CT-simulation and accuracy of treatment in the stereotactic body frame. Radiother Oncol. 2000;57:225–36.
30. Herfarth KK, Debus J, Lohr F, et al. Stereotactic single-dose radiation therapy of liver tumors: results of a phase I/II trial. J Clin Oncol. 2001;19:164–70.
31. Uematsu M, Shioda A, Suda A, et al. Computed tomographyguided frameless stereotactic radiotherapy for stage I non-small cell lung cancer: a 5-year experience. Int J Radiat Oncol Biol Phys. 2001;51:666–70.
32. Fuks Z, Kolesnick R. Engaging the vascular component of the tumor response. Cancer Cell. 2005;8:89–91.
33. Hall EJ, Brenner DJ. The radiobiology of radiosurgery: rationale for different treatment regimens for AVMs and malignancies. Int J Radiat Oncol Biol Phys. 1993;25:381–5.
34. Takeda A, Sanuki N, Kunieda E. Role of stereotactic body radiotherapy for oligometastasis from colorectal cancer. World J Gastroenterol. 2014;20(15):4220–9.
35. Alongi F, Arcangeli S, Filippi AR, et al. Review and uses of stereotactic body radiation therapy for oligometastases. Oncologist. 2012;17:1100–7.
36. Moon DH, Wang AZ, Tepper JE, et al. A prospective study of the safety and efficacy of liver stereotactic body radiotherapy in patients with and without prior liver-directed therapy. Radiother Oncol. 2018;126(3):527–33.
37. Brown JM, Diehn M, Loo BW Jr. Stereotactic ablative radiotherapy should be combined with a hypoxic cell radiosensitizer. Int J Radiat Oncol Biol Phys. 2010;78(2):323e327.
38. Goethals L, Debucquoy A, Perneel C, et al. Hypoxia in human colorectal adenocarcinoma: comparison between extrinsic and potential intrinsic hypoxia markers. Int J Radiat Oncol Biol Phys. 2006;65(1):246e254.
39. Hoyer M, Roed H, Traberg Hansen A, et al. Phase II study on stereotactic body radiotherapy of colorectal metastases. Acta Oncol. 2006;45(7):823e830.
40. Lee MT, Kim JJ, Dinniwell R, et al. Phase I study of individualized stereotactic body radiotherapy of liver metastases. J Clin Oncol. 2009;27(10):1585e1591.
41. Ambrosino G, Polistina F, Costantin G, et al. Image-guided robotic stereotactic radiosurgery for unresectable liver metastases: preliminary results. Anticancer Res. 2009;29(8):3381e3384.
42. Scorsetti M, Clerici E, Comito T. Stereotactic body radiationtherapy for liver metastases. J Gastrointest Oncol. 2014;5(3):190–7.
43. Scorsetti M, Arcangeli S, Tozzi A, et al. Is stereotactic bodyradiation therapy an attractive option for unresectable livermetastases? A preliminary report from a phase 2 trial. Int J Radiat Oncol Biol Phys. 2013;86:336–42.

44. Fundowicz M, Adamczyk M, Kolodziej-Dybas A. Stereotactic body radiation therapy for liver metastasis – the linac-based greater poland cancer centre practice. Rep Pract Oncol Radiother. 2017;22:158–62.
45. Nagata Y, Wulf J, Lax I, et al. Stereotactic radiotherapy of primary lung cancer and other targets: results of consultant meeting of the International Atomic Energy Agency. Int J Radiat Oncol Biol Phys. 2011;79:660–9.
46. Worm ES, Hoyer M, Fledelius W, Poulsen PR. Three-dimensional, time-resolved, intrafraction motion monitoring throughout stereotactic liver radiation therapy on a conventional linear accelerator. Int J Radiat Oncol Biol Phys. 2013;86(1):190e197.
47. Wunderink W, Mendez Romero A, de Kruijf W, de Boer H, Levendag P, Heijmen B. Reduction of respiratory liver tumor motion by abdominal compression in stereotactic body frame, analyzed by tracking fiducial markers implanted in liver. Int J Radiat Oncol Biol Phys. 2008;71(3):907e915.
48. Wagman R, Yorke E, Ford E, et al. Respiratory gating for liver tumors: use in dose escalation. Int J Radiat Oncol Biol Phys. 2003;55(3):659e668.
49. Eccles C, Brock KK, Bissonnette JP, Hawkins M, Dawson LA. Reproducibility of liver position using active breathing coordinator for liver cancer radiotherapy. Int J Radiat Oncol Biol Phys. 2006;64(3):751e759.
50. Case RB, Sonke JJ, Moseley DJ, Kim J, Brock KK, Dawson LA. Inter and intrafraction variability in liver position in nonbreath-hold stereotactic body radiotherapy. Int J Radiat Oncol Biol Phys. 2009;75(1):302e308.
51. Yang J, Cai J, Wang H, et al. Is diaphragm motion a good surrogate for liver tumor motion? Int J Radiat Oncol Biol Phys. 2014;90(4):952e958.
52. Wunderink W, Mendez Romero A, Seppenwoolde Y, de Boer H, Levendag P, Heijmen B. Potentials and limitations of guiding liver stereotactic body radiation therapy set-up on liver- implanted fiducial markers. Int J Radiat Oncol Biol Phys. 2010;77(5):1573e1583.
53. Velec M, Moseley JL, Craig T, Dawson LA, Brock KK. Accumulated dose in liver stereotactic body radiotherapy: positioning, breathing, and deformation effects. Int J Radiat Oncol Biol Phys. 2012;83(4):1132e1140.
54. Dawson LA, Zhu A, Knox J, et al. Radiation Therapy Oncology Group (RTOG) 1112: randomized Phase III study of sorafenib versus stereotactic body radiation therapy followed by sorafenib in hepatocellular carcinoma. Available at: http://www.rtog.org/Portals/0/RTOG%20Broadcasts/Attachments/1112_master_w_update_5.7.13.pdf. (accessed august 2019).
55. Aitken KL, Tait DM, Nutting CM, Khabra K, Hawkins MA. Risk adapted strategy partial liver irradiation for the treatment of large volume metastatic liver disease. Acta Oncol. 2014;53(5):702e706.
56. Milano MT, Katz AW, Zhang H, Okunieff P. Oligometastases treated with stereotactic body radiotherapy: long-term follow-up of prospective study. Int J Radiat Oncol Biol Phys. 2012;83(3):878e886.
57. McCammon R, Schefter TE, Gaspar LE, Zaemisch R, Gravdahl D, Kavanagh B. Observation of a dose-control relationship for lung and liver tumors after stereotactic body radiation therapy. Int J Radiat Oncol Biol Phys. 2009;73(1):112e118.
58. Chang DT, Swaminath A, Kozak M, et al. Stereotactic body radiotherapy for colorectal liver metastases: a pooled analysis. Cancer. 2011;117(17):4060–9.
59. Postow MA, Callahan MK, Barker CA, et al. Immunologic correlates of the abscopal effect in a patient with melanoma. N Engl J Med. 2012;366(10):925e931.
60. Seung SK, Curti BD, Crittenden M, et al. Phase 1 study of stereotactic body radiotherapy and interleukin-2 e tumor and immunological responses. Sci Transl Med. 2012;4(137):137–74.
61. Corbin KS, Hellman S, Weichselbaum RR. Extracranial oligometastases: a subset of metastases curable with stereotactic radiotherapy. J Clin Oncol. 2013;31(11):1384–90.
62. Dawson LA, Normolle B, Balter JM, et al. Analysis of radiation-induced liver disease using the lyman NTCP model. Int J Radiat Oncol Biol Phys. 2002;53(4):810–21.

63. Herfarth KK, Debus J, Lohr F, Bahner ML, Rhein B, Fritz P, Hoss A, Schlegel W, Wannenmacher MF. Stereotactic single-dose radiation therapy of liver tumors: results of a phase I/II trial. J Clin Oncol. 2001;19(1):164–70.
64. Kavanagh BD, Schefter TE, Cardenes HR, Stieber VW, Raben D, Timmerman RD, McCarter MD, Burri S, Nedzi LA, Sawyer TE, et al. Interim analysis of a prospective phase I/II trial of SBRT for liver metastases. Acta Oncol. 2006;45(7):848–55.
65. Wulf J, Hadinger U, Oppitz U, Thiele W, Ness-Dourdoumas R, Flentje M. Stereotactic radiotherapy of targets in the lung and liver. Strahlenther Onkol. 2001;177(12):645–55.
66. Katz AW, Carey-Sampson M, Muhs AG, Milano MT, Schell MC, Okunieff P. Hypofractionated stereotactic body radiation therapy (SBRT) for limited hepatic metastases. Int J Radiat Oncol Biol Phys. 2007;67(3):793–8.
67. Van der Pool AE, Mendez Romero A, Wunderink W, Heijmen BJ, Levendag PC, Verhoef C, Ijzermans JN. Stereotactic body radiation therapy for colorectal liver metastases. Br J Surg. 2010;97(3):377–82.
68. Goodman KA, Wiegner EA, Maturen KE, Zhang Z, Mo Q, Yang G, Gibbs IC, Fisher GA, Koong AC. Dose-escalation study of single-fraction stereotactic body radiotherapy for liver malignancies. Int J Radiat Oncol Biol Phys. 2010;78(2):486–93.
69. Vautravers-Dewas C, Dewas S, Bonodeau F, Adenis A, Lacornerie T, Penel N, Lartigau E, Mirabel X. Image-guided robotic stereotactic body radiation therapy for liver metastases: is there a dose response relationship? Int J Radiat Oncol Biol Phys. 2011;81(3):e39–47.
70. Yuan ZY, Meng MB, Liu CL, et al. Stereotactic body radiation therapy using Cyberknife system for patients with liver metastases. Onco Targets Ther. 2014;7:915–23.
71. Goodman BD, Mannina EM, Althouse SK, Maluccio MA, Cardenes HR. Long-term safety and efficacy of stereotactic body radiation therapy for hepatic oligometastases. Pract Radiat Oncol. 2016;6(2):86–95.
72. Rubio C, Hernando-Requejo O, Zucca Aparicio D, M ALK, Lopez Gonzalez M, Perez JM, et al. Image guided SBRT for multiple liver metastases with ExacTrac((R)) adaptive gating. Rep Pract Oncol Radiother. 2017;22(2):150–7.

41 Lessons from Collaborative Big Data—Insights from *LiverMetSurvey* Registry

Marc-Antoine Allard and René Adam

Background

The management of patients with colorectal liver metastases (CLM) has considerably changed since the first surgical series, showing that resection could cure some selected patients [1]. Since then, surgery has gained wide acceptance and CLM is nowadays the first indication of hepatectomy in western countries [2]. In the era dominated by evidence-based medicine, it is interesting to note that resection of CLM has become a well-established treatment worldwide, on the sole basis of retrospective series.

Although the literature about surgical management of CLM is abundant, there are still numerous pending questions. Among them, we can mention the strategy in synchronous CLM, the definition and objective of resection margins, the role of surgery in presence of extra-hepatic disease, and the place of neoadjuvant chemotherapy. In addition, monocentric studies, even from large volume centers, are limited by the size of study population, precluding definitive conclusions. Moreover, some particular subgroups of patients cannot be studied by using monocentric cohort due to an insufficient number of patients.

M.-A. Allard · R. Adam (✉)
Centre Hépato-Biliaire, AP-HP Hôpital Paul Brousse, Université Paris Sud, INSERM U935, Villejuif, France
e-mail: marcantoine.allard@aphp.fr; rene.adam@aphp.fr

M. M. Correia et al. (eds.), *Colorectal Cancer Liver Metastases*,
https://doi.org/10.1007/978-3-030-25486-5_41

Aims of the Registry

The *LiverMetSurvey* registry aimed:

- To collect on a large scale, the critical information concerning the history of patients surgically treated for colorectal liver metastases
- To prospectively evaluate the outcome after surgery
- To analyze survival data in relation to pertinent prognostic factors
- To provide useful information about pending questions regarding indications, type of surgery, adjuvant treatment, and the role of chemotherapy

This registry includes all patients who underwent surgery for resection of hepatic metastasis of colorectal origin, whether the hepatectomy was performed or canceled during the operation.

Methods

- *Nomination of a scientific committee*

A scientific committee involving 14 expert surgeons coming from different European countries was built to define the critical data needed to explore the different aspects of liver resection for CLM. This meeting led to a questionnaire containing the most clinically relevant information for each patient to be operated on an intention to resect. A particular effort was made to avoid too exhaustive information and to allow the questionnaire to be completed in no more than 15–20 minutes by a young surgeon.

- *Participating centers*

In agreement with the proposal of the scientific board, it was established that all centers managing patients with CLM could participate. Eligibility was not restricted by experience or volume criteria so that the registry might give a true life evaluation of liver resection worldwide. All centers taking part to the *LiverMetSurvey* registry have access to an individualized, auto-administered, confidential and secured database.

The registry is administered by an independent professional data manager. The principal investigator and co-investigators have complete access to data coming from their own centers but no access to data from other registered centers.

- *Managing and Protection of the data*

Data from all contributing centers are collected by a data manager and a control of the quality is made with regular information to the centers concerning incompleteness or incoherence of the specific data for each patient. The registry is secured using SSL protection. Data are therefore encrypted between the user's computer and the *LiverMetSurvey* server, and are only deciphered when they reach the *LiverMetSurvey* server.

- *Services to participating centers*

In order to encourage centers to collaborate and to reward them for including their patients, *LiverMetSurvey* offers different services to the contributing centers. First, the registry can be used as an own web database with descriptive statistical analysis (Fig. 41.2). It also provides a complex statistical analysis of the database for each center available every 6 months (e.g., overall survival, prognostic factors) and makes possible to compare its own practice with the global practice collected in *LiverMetSurvey*. Data can be exported easily. Special statistical analysis can be made on request. Main results are downloadable from the *LiverMetSurvey* website. In addition, every contributing center with updated follow-up of his patients may ask for the global database of LMS to report a paper concerning any topic of interest.

- *Sponsorship*

Sponsorship is crucial to maintain the quality and protection of data included in this registry, which are ensured by dedicated professionals. After being sponsored by Sanofi, *LiverMetSurvey* is now financed by the ARCAD (Aide et Recherche en Cancérologie Digestive) foundation since September 2017.

Results

- *Inclusion*

In December 2016, *LiverMetSurvey* included 27,349 patients, from 346 centers and 71 countries (Fig. 41.1). These patients were collected from all the different continents, but mostly from Europe. Among them 26,707 patients had evaluable data of whom 25,152 were resected (94.2%) and totalized 29,720 hepatectomies (including the repeat resections). A mean of 100 patients are prospectively included every month.

- *Patient outcome*

The survival of resected patients is 42% at 5 years and 25% at 10 years, significantly better than that of operated but unresected patients (9% at 5 years) (Fig. 41.2) with a perioperative mortality of 2.8% within 3 months. Among unresected patients, those who received a treatment during operation such as radiofrequency have still a better survival (22% at 5 years) than that of operated but unresected patients who did not receive any intraoperative treatment (6% at 5 years) (Fig. 41.3). There was no influence of gender in the outcome. Concerning age, the survival of patients

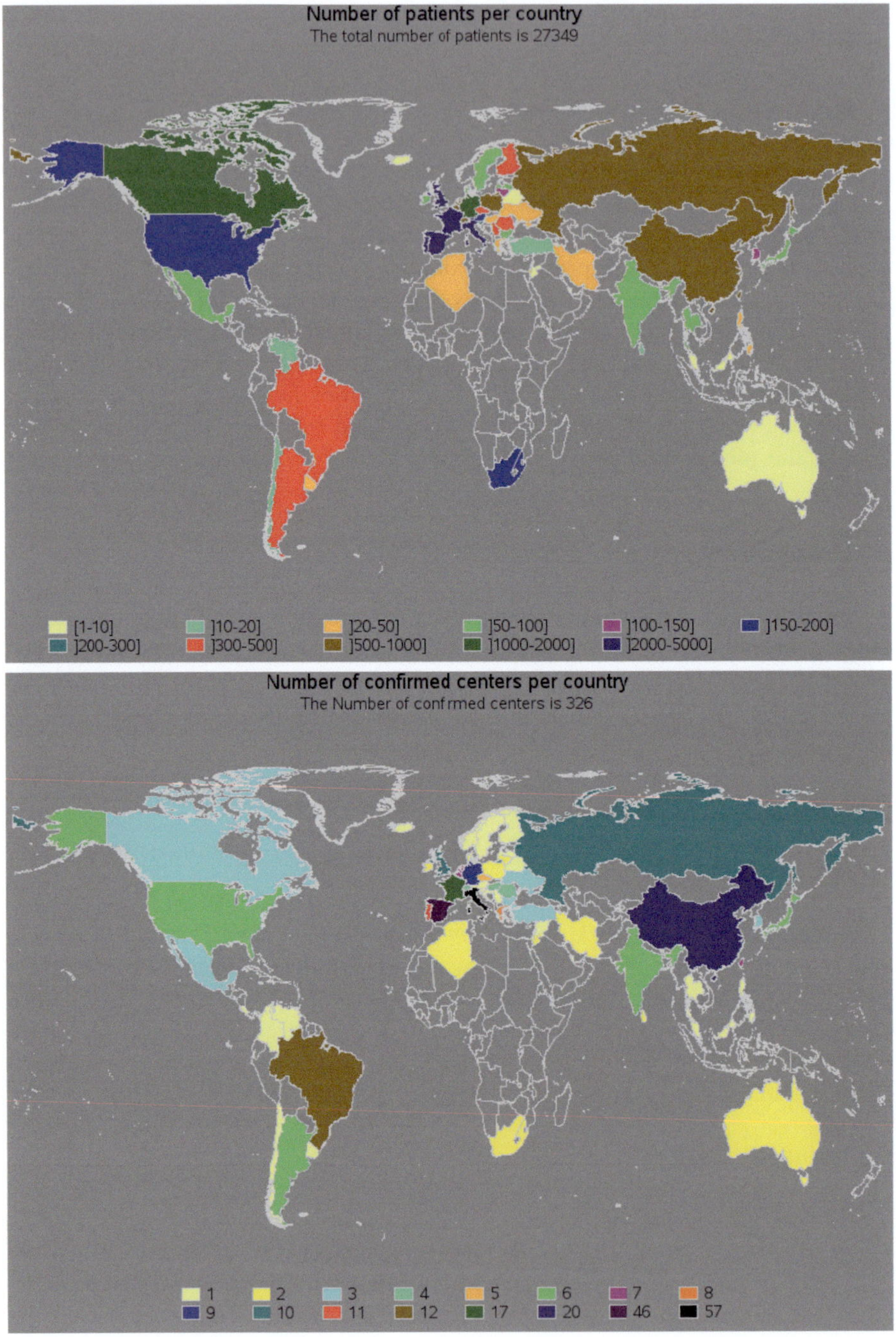

Fig. 41.1 LiverMetSurvey worldwide: number of patients per country and number of confirmed centers per country

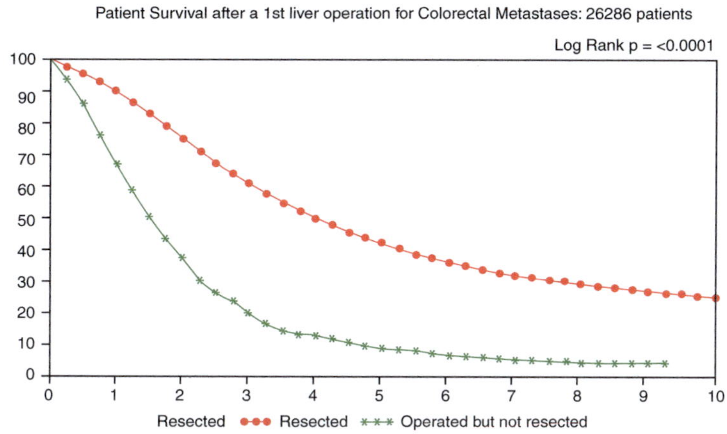

Survival %

Resected	1 yr	2 yrs	3 yrs	4 yrs	5 yrs	6 yrs	7 yrs	8 yrs	9 yrs	10 yrs
Resected	90%	75%	61%	50%	42%	36%	32%	29%	27%	25%
No resected	67%	38%	21%	12%	9%	6%	5%	4%	4%	

Number of exposed patients

	Total	1 yr	2 yrs	3 yrs	4 yrs	5 yrs	6 yrs	7 yrs	8 yrs	9 yrs	10 yrs
Resected	24925	16823	11697	7914	5241	3566	2417	1724	1212	855	608
No resected	1361	648	304	141	67	41	24	12	6	2	0

Fig. 41.2 Survival of resected versus non-resected patients

Details: Log rank p

		proba
Hepat.	Ttwitho	<0.0001
Hepat.	Nointra	<0.0001
Ttwitho	Nointra	<0.0001

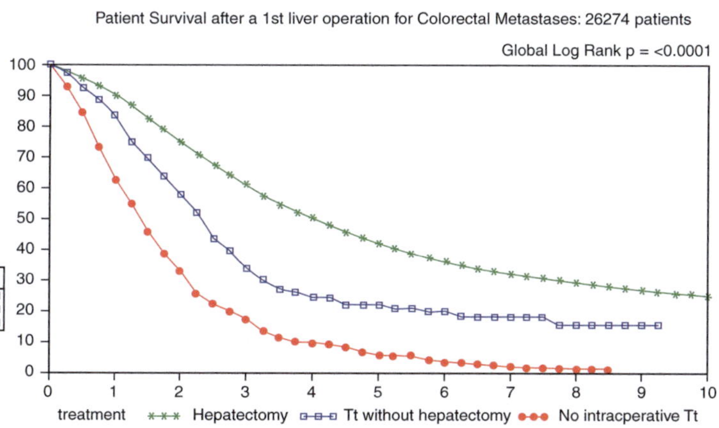

Survival %

treatment	1 yr	2 yrs	3 yrs	4 yrs	5 yrs	6 yrs	7 yrs	8 yrs	9 yrs	10 yrs
Hepatectomy	90%	75%	61%	50%	42%	36%	32%	29%	27%	25%
Tt without hepat	84%	58%	34%	24%	22%	20%	18%	16%	16%	
No intraop. Tt	63%	33%	18%	10%	6%	3%	2%	1%		

Number of exposed patients

	Total	1 yr	2 yrs	3 yrs	4 yrs	5 yrs	6 yrs	7 yrs	8 yrs	9 yrs	10 yrs
Hepatectomy	24925	16823	11697	7914	5241	3566	2417	1724	1212	855	608
Tt without hepat	260	157	93	45	27	19	14	8	5	2	0
No intraop. Tt	1089	486	210	96	40	22	10	4	1	0	0

Fig. 41.3 Survival of resected versus non-resected patients according to the treatment received during operation

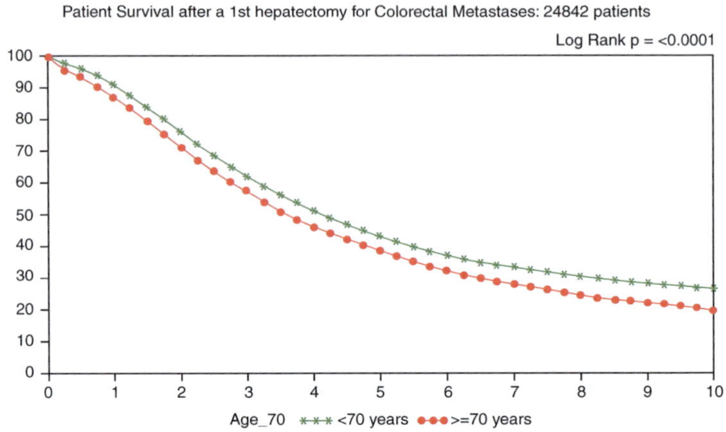

Survival %

Age_70	1 yr	2 yrs	3 yrs	4 yrs	5 yrs	6 yrs	7 yrs	8 yrs	9 yrs	10 yrs
<70 years	91%	76%	62%	51%	43%	37%	33%	30%	28%	26%
>=70 years	87%	71%	58%	46%	39%	32%	28%	25%	22%	19%

Number of exposed patients

	Total	1 yr	2 yrs	3 yrs	4 yrs	5 yrs	6 yrs	7 yrs	8 yrs	9 yrs	10 yrs
<70 years	18410	12687	8964	6087	4084	2798	1928	1400	1000	715	514
>=70 years	6432	4085	2701	1085	1143	758	481	319	209	138	92

Fig. 41.4 Influence of age on the survival after resection of CLM (<70 vs ≥70 years)

younger than 70 years after liver resection was better than that of patients less than 70 (43 vs 39%, $p < 0.0001$) but this difference was not so clinically discriminant (Fig. 41.4).

Also, much other information is obtained concerning the role of primary location, on the size and number of metastases, on the type of hepatectomy, and on the role of preoperative chemotherapy (www.livermetsurvey-arcad.org).

- *Main published studies based on the LiverMetSurvey*

Several studies based on *LiverMetSurvey* data have been published. Here, we briefly present some of the main results.

- Technical considerations

In patients with synchronous CLM, the timing of hepatectomy compared to that of the primary tumor is a matter of debate. The liver first approach (reverse attitude) was compared to the classical approach in the global cohort of *LiverMetSurvey*. Similar survival was observed between the two approaches, provided that the two steps could be completed [3].

The influence of parenchyma-preserving policy for hepatic resection has also been explored within the registry. It was shown that this policy increases the feasibility of repeat hepatectomy in case of hepatic recurrence, thus improving the long-term results of patients with liver only recurrence [4].

More recently, the feasibility, safety, and good long-term results of the strategy of two-stage hepatectomy were assessed with *LiverMetSurvey* [5].

- Role of perioperative chemotherapy

The impact of chemotherapy in the surgical management of patients with CLM is a major topic. An analysis revealed that neoadjuvant chemotherapy has no effect in patients with single, metachronous, small (<5 cm) lesions whereas adjuvant chemotherapy seems to be beneficial, mainly when tumor exceeds 5 cm [6].

Although progression while on chemotherapy is considered a relative contraindication to surgery for multiple hepatic lesions, a *LiverMetSurvey*-based study was designed to explore the potential benefit of resecting patients with progressive disease. This study identified three independents factors of poor outcomes [7]. The authors derived a scoring system giving the survival probabilities after resection in the setting of tumor progression.

Also, the influence on the outcome following liver resection, of the type of preoperative chemotherapy, in patients with unresectable liver metastases has been explored. This study did not evidence any impact of preoperative chemotherapy on survival after resection (ASCO 2018).

The benefit of resection after failure of a second line of chemotherapy has also been evaluated. Although overall survival and disease-free survival was slightly better in patients operated after a first line compared to those resected after a second line, long-term outcomes still remain acceptable [8] and the message addressed to medical oncologists is that surgery should not be denied after the failure of a first line of chemotherapy.

In addition to published studies, analysis based on the registry was used to propose a definition of "synchronous" metastases and international recommendations in the management of patients with synchronous CLM [9].

- Extent of resection

Until which point surgery yields a survival benefit is a permanent question for surgeons and oncologists involved in CLM treatment. It was shown that even in non-resectable lung metastases, resection of CLM might be justified [10]. Another study has proved the usefulness of surgery and identified the main factors associated with acceptable survival after resection of ten or more than ten CLM [11].

- Open versus laparoscopic approach
  A comparison has been made in LiverMetSurvey between 14,484 patients resected by open approach to 915 patients resected by laparoscopy with a further propensity score matching, comparing 1180 open to 590 laparoscopically treated patients. The conclusions were that overall and disease-free survivals were similar with an identical proportion of R1 resections in the two groups, which seemed to validate the laparoscopic approach for selected patients [12].

Conclusions

In hindsight, *LiverMetSurvey* has proved to meet the objectives that were set at the time of its creation, more than a decade ago. By giving a photography of the current practice of liver resection worldwide, the registry has confirmed the curative potential of surgery in CLM. The collection of a large cohort of patients has helped to explore new issues such as the influence of age, of the primary location, of extra-hepatic metastases, the role of chemotherapy, the ways of its optimal association with liver resection, the use of adjuvant techniques to improve resectability, the impact of the center volume on the quality of the results, and the use of laparoscopy.

With regard to the information provided, registries have often been opposed to randomized trials. In fact, both are complementary in providing new information. Clinical trials answer to a single question, in a limited period of time and in a selected group of patients, with the highest scientific value. However, practical feasibility is the main obstacle, because a large number of trials failed, due to recruitment issues. In addition, trials are costly and long-term follow-up is not available.

By contrast, registries make possible to investigate many questions in real time, in an unselected population. The evolution of practices can also be analyzed. The large number of patients in registry allows to make an analysis of specific subgroups of patients, that could not be carried out with prospective randomized studies.

This explains why currently big data through good quality registries such as LiverMetSurvey have increasing support.

References

1. Taylor I. Colorectal liver metastases - to treat or not to treat. Br J Surg. 1985;72:511–6.
2. Dimick JB, Wainess RM, Cowan JA, Upchurch GR, Knol JA, Colletti LM. National trends in the use and outcomes of hepatic resection. J Am Coll Surg. 2004;199:31–8. https://doi.org/10.1016/j.jamcollsurg.2004.03.005.
3. Andres A, Toso C, Adam R, Barroso E, Hubert C, Capussotti L, et al. A survival analysis of the liver-first reversed management of advanced simultaneous colorectal liver metastases. Ann Surg. 2012;256:772–9.
4. Hosokawa I, Allard M-A, Mirza DF, Kaiser G, Barroso E, Eal Lapointe R, et al. Outcomes of parenchyma-preserving hepatectomy and right hepatectomy for solitary small colorectal liver metastasis: a LiverMetSurvey study. Surgery. 2017;162:223.
5. Regimbeau JM, Cosse C, Kaiser G, Hubert C, Laurent C, Lapointe R, et al. Feasibility, safety and efficacy of two-stage hepatectomy for bilobar liver metastases of colorectal cancer: a LiverMetSurvey analysis. HPB. 2017;19:396–405. https://doi.org/10.1016/j.hpb.2017.01.008.
6. Adam R, Bhangui P, Poston G, Mirza D, Nuzzo G, Barroso E, et al. Is perioperative chemotherapy useful for solitary, metachronous, colorectal liver metastases? Ann Surg. 2010;252:774–87.
7. Viganò L, Capussotti L, Barroso E, Nuzzo G, Laurent C, Ijzermans JNM, et al. Progression while receiving preoperative chemotherapy should not be an absolute contraindication to liver resection for colorectal metastases. Ann Surg Oncol. 2012;19:2786–96. https://doi.org/10.1245/s10434-012-2382-7.

8. Adam R, Yi B, Innominato PF, Barroso E, Laurent C, Giuliante F, et al. Resection of colorectal liver metastases after second-line chemotherapy: is it worthwhile? A LiverMetSurvey analysis of 6415 patients. Eur J Cancer. 2017;78:7–15.
9. Adam R, de Gramont A, Figueras J, Kokudo N, Kunstlinger F, Loyer E, et al. Managing synchronous liver metastases from colorectal cancer: a multidisciplinary international consensus. Cancer Treat Rev. 2015;41:729–41.
10. Andres A, Mentha G, Adam R, Gerstel E, Skipenko OG, Barroso E, et al. Surgical management of patients with colorectal cancer and simultaneous liver and lung metastases. Br J Surg. 2015;102:691–9.
11. Allard MA, Adam R, Giuliante F, Lapointe R, Hubert C, Ijzermans JNM, et al. Long-term outcomes of patients with 10 or more colorectal liver metastases. Br J Cancer. 2017;117:604.
12. Eveno C, Cailliez V, Lopezben S, Mirza DF, Kaiser G, Lapointe R, Mentha G, Pardo F, Adam R, Cherqui D. Role of laparoscopic approach in colorectal liver metastasis: an international multi-center data analysis using LiverMetSurvey (Presentation IHPBA meeting Sao Paulo 2016).

Prognosis and Management of Recurrent Metastatic Colorectal Cancer

42

Blaire Anderson and Ryan C. Fields

Introduction

It is predicted that 140,250 new colorectal cancer cases will be diagnosed in the United States in 2018, with an estimated 50,630 cancer-related deaths [1]. Colorectal cancer is the second leading cause of cancer-related death in the Western world [1]. One-half of patients with colorectal cancer will eventually develop metastatic disease. A subset of patients with disease localized to the liver are cured with surgical resection. Unfortunately, approximately 60% of patients will develop disease recurrence with nearly two-thirds having disease within the liver [2–7]. Common extrahepatic sites of metastases include the thorax and peritoneum with metastatic patterns varying based on the site of primary tumor [8].

Techniques including nonanatomic parenchymal-sparing resections, success in induced hypertrophy of the remnant liver by portal vein embolization (PVE), and two-staged hepatectomy as well as associating liver partition and portal vein ligation (ALPPS) have enabled complete extirpation of colorectal liver metastasis (CRLM) at greater rates. Liver-directed therapy, including local and locoregional strategies, has allowed further treatment of liver lesions in distributions unfavorable for resection. Liver-directed therapy is often used in combination with resection with a goal to treat all visible tumors either by resection or tumor destruction with appropriate margins.

B. Anderson
Division of Transplantation Surgery, Department of Surgery at University of Nebraska Medical Center, Omaha, NE, USA
e-mail: blaire.anderson@unmc.edu

R. C. Fields (✉)
Department of Surgery, Barnes-Jewish Hospital, Washington University School of Medicine, St. Louis, MO, USA
e-mail: rcfields@wustl.edu

M. M. Correia et al. (eds.), *Colorectal Cancer Liver Metastases*,
https://doi.org/10.1007/978-3-030-25486-5_42

Tumor recurrence after "curative" resection is a major problem. The majority of patients will die from recurrent disease and liver metastases are the commonest cause of death for patients with colorectal cancer [6]. Of patients who undergo liver resection, 50–75% will develop disease recurrence within 2 years after resection [9, 10]. Many recurrences are extra-hepatic; thus, adjuvant systemic treatment is standard of care after the management of CRLM.

Following liver metastasectomy, 10-year survival rates of 20% have been reported [11]. Of note, this study analyzed patients treated prior to the introduction of modern chemotherapeutic agents. In a contemporary French multi-institutional retrospective cohort study including 2320 patients, Hallet et al. reported 5-year overall survival of 74.3% following hepatectomy in patients who did not have recurrence and 57.5% in patients with recurrent disease. Following hepatic metastasectomy, tumors recurred in 47.4% of patients at a median of 10 months follow-up. About 46.2% had intra-hepatic disease only and 31.8% combined intra- and extra-hepatic metastases. Pre-hepatectomy factors associated with increased rate of recurrence included node positive primary malignancy, more than three liver metastases, and largest metastasis greater than 4 cm. Patients with combined intra- and extra-hepatic recurrence had inferior outcomes with a 5-year overall survival rate of 44.3% compared with 60.8% for intra-hepatic recurrence alone and 64.3% for extra-hepatic recurrence alone. About 89.1% of patients presented within 3 years following initial hepatectomy. Authors emphasized the importance of highlighting to the patient that although extended survival is achievable, survivorship care is paramount, as repeat hepatectomy and further treatment may be needed moving forward [12].

Survivorship Care and Surveillance

There is limited data from which to recommend surveillance in patients with Stage IV colorectal cancer; however, the ability to address recurrent metastatic disease within the liver emphasizes the importance of close surveillance after metastasectomy. A key principle of surveillance is to monitor this high-risk patient cohort for recurrent disease. Timing and duration of follow-up is debatable. According to NCCN guidelines, patients with Stage IV colorectal cancer should be surveyed with a history and physical examination, and carcinoembryonic antigen (CEA) every 3–6 months for 2 years then every 6 months for a total of 5 years. A colonoscopy should be performed 1 year after colon resection, unless pre-operative colonoscopy was not completed due to an obstructing lesion, in which case a colonoscopy is recommended in 3–6 months. Further colonoscopic surveillance is dictated by findings. Computed tomography (CT) scan of the chest, abdomen, and pelvis is recommended at 3–6 month intervals for the first 2 years, then every 6–12 months for a total of 5 years [13].

Interestingly, in a study of post-treatment surveillance of patients with CRLM, frequency of surveillance imaging did not correlate with time to second procedure or median survival. Those who were scanned at 3–4 months intervals had a median survival of 43 months, compared to 54 months in those who were scanned once per year [14]. Positron emission tomography-magnetic resonance imaging (PET-MRI) has recently been investigated for CRLM detection. It was found to be superior to CT ($p = 0.003$) and PET-CT ($p = 0.02$) in detection of CRLM, especially those ≤1 cm in size, but not significantly different from MRI ($p = 0.23$) [15]. Other imaging modalities may be considered for surveillance purposes; however, these are not standard of care.

There is no evidence to recommend routine imaging or CEA beyond 5 years of follow-up. Considering cost and ease, it is not unreasonable to monitor long-term survivors with annual CEA levels. If serial CEAs show elevation, a workup including physical examination, colonoscopy, and CT of the chest, abdomen, and pelvis should be performed. When these investigations do not yield results, a PET-CT should be considered. Alternatively, repeat cross-sectional imaging should be performed in 3 months [13]. Recommendations provided by various organizations are displayed in Table 42.1 [13, 16–20]. Timing and duration should ultimately be determined by individual patient risk profile and performance status. The European Society for Medical Oncology (ESMO) emphasizes social, financial, and emotional aspects as well as functional outcomes to maximize survivors long-term well-being overall [17, 18].

Approach

The strategy in management of patients with liver recurrence after prior hepatectomy is similar to those who initially present with CRLM. Patients should be re-staged to evaluate for other sites of metastatic disease or local recurrence. This should consist of clinical examination, laboratory investigations including liver and renal functional tests, CEA level, as well as a CT or MRI of the abdomen, pelvis, and chest. PET-CT can add additional information on equivocal lesions. In patients with initial occurrence of CRLM, PET-CT should not be done routinely as it rarely changes surgical management [21]. However, PET-CT may detect occult metastatic disease and decrease the number of futile operative procedures; therefore, in the high-risk cohort of patients with recurrent CRLM, PET-CT should be considered [22]. The consensus of a multidisciplinary committee involving surgeons, medical and radiation oncologist, interventional radiologists, and pathologists should drive treatment. Patient co-morbidities, performance status, previous surgical, locoregional, and systemic treatments, residual liver volume and function must be considered and will cumulatively dictate the treatment strategy.

First, one must determine if the patient has potentially resectable disease. If disease is resectable and the patient is an appropriate operative candidate, repeat hepatectomy should be discussed. Residual liver volume and quality must be carefully evaluated, particularly in patients who have had significant exposure to chemotherapy. It is well established that irinotecan and oxaliplatin induce steatohepatitis, sinusoidal obstruction, and periportal inflammation that can affect ability to perform large resections by impairing function of the liver remnant. These hepatic changes

Table 42.1 High-risk/Stage IV colorectal cancer (CRC) surveillance schedule

	History and physical examination	CT (chest/abdomen/pelvis)	CEA	Colonoscopy
NCCN 2018 (stage II, III, IV)	Every 3–6 months for 2 years then every 6 months for the next 3 years	Stage II/III—Every 6–12 months for a total of 5 years Stage IV—Every 3–6 months for a total of 5 years	Every 3–6 months for 2 years then every 6 months for the next 3 years	At years 1 except if no preoperative colonoscopy due to obstructing lesion, colonoscopy in 3–6 months (if advanced adenoma, repeat in 1 year; if no advanced adenoma, repeat in 3 years then every 5 years)
ASCRS 2015 (stage I (increased risk for recurrence), II, III, IV (when isolated metastases are resected for cure))	Every 3–6 months for 2 years then every 6 months for the next 3 years	Annually for 5 years *∗more frequent imaging may be considered for patients at particularly high risk for recurrence including previous liver resection for metastasis. Interval not defined.*	Every 3–6 months for 2 years then every 6 months for the next 3 years	At years 1 except if no preoperative colonoscopy due to obstructing lesion, colonoscopy in 3–6 months *Rectum—colonoscopy as above and proctoscopy (+/– ERUS) every 6–12 months for patients who underwent resection with anastomosis or every 6 months for patients undergoing local excision for 3–5 years*
ESMO 2017 High-risk patients (including patients with metastases)	Every 3–6 months for 3 years	Every 3–6 months for 3 years	Every 3–6 months for 3 years	Completion colonoscopy within the first year if not done at the time of diagnostic workup
JSCCR 2018 After curative resection stage III CRC and after resection of recurrent tumors	Every 3 months for 3 years then every 6 months for the next 2 years	Every 6 months for 5 years *(CT is desirable but plain chest x-ray and abdominal ultrasound is acceptable)*	Every 3 months for 3 years then every 6 months for the next 2 years	At year 1 and 3 for colon cancer At year 1, 2, and 3 for rectal cancer
CCO 2018 Stage II and III resected for cure, (no specific recommendations for stage IV)	Every 6 months for 5 years	Annually for 3 years *(chest x-ray and abdominal ultrasound can be substituted every 6–12 months for 3 years then yearly for years 4 and five)*	Every 6 months for 5 years	At years 1 except if no preoperative colonoscopy due to obstructing lesion, colonoscopy within 6 months with subsequent colonoscopies dictated by findings of the previous one, generally every 5 years if findings are normal *(Sigmoidoscopy may be considered at intervals less than 5 years for high risk rectal cancers)*

NCCN National Comprehensive Cancer Network, *ASCRS* American Society of Colon and Rectal Surgeons, *ESMO* European Society of Medical Oncology, *JSCCR* Japanese Society for Cancer of the Colon and Rectum, *CCO* Cancer Care Ontario, *CEA* carcinoembryonic antigen, *ERUS* endorectal ultrasound

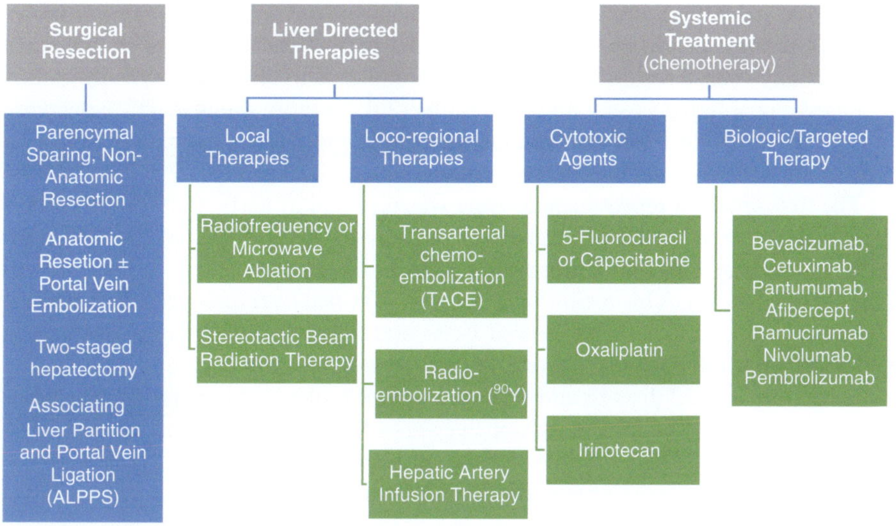

Fig. 42.1 Treatment options for CRLM recurrence

can negatively impact outcomes, with increased risk of liver failure and death [23–26]. When concerned, pre-operative biopsy of normal liver should be performed, and liver volumes should be calculated on imaging.

If disease is unresectable, patient wishes must be reviewed, with prolongation of survival, improved tumor-related symptoms, cessation of tumor progression, and maintained quality of life reasonable goals. The armamentarium of treatment options for palliation has expanded significantly with many systemic, locoregional, and local treatments available. Re-biopsy may be indicated for molecular and genetic analysis to drive newer targeted and immunotherapies (Fig. 42.1).

Surgery

Hepatectomy is the standard of care for those patients with initial presentation of resectable colorectal metastasis and remains the most well studied potentially curative treatment [7]. When disease recurs in the liver after previous resection, re-resection should be considered. In fact, 20–30% of patients will be surgical candidates with disease amendable to surgery [27, 28]. One must consider patient performance status and assess for adequate hepatic reserve. Additionally, surgeons should expect these to be challenging cases with abdominal and perihepatic adhesions, altered liver anatomy with variations in position of vasculature and the biliary system secondary to previous operations and liver regeneration. Longer surgery times, greater risk of operative bleeding, increased risk of organ damage, and post-operative complications have been reported [3].

The SEPTRA-C2T Phase II randomized control trial supports the use of bioresorbable membranes to reduce abdominal and perihepatic adhesions in two-stage hepatectomy. These results can likely be extrapolated to re-resection, as this study included repeat hepatectomy up to 6 months [29]. Authors showed a 33% decrease in time to complete liver mobilization and the proportion of patients with one or more complications was half that observed in the control group [29].

The first series of repeat hepatectomy was reported as early as 1989 [30]. Since then, many centers have published their results, with survival rates of 29–70%, mortality of less than 3%, and perioperative complications comparable to initial resection [27, 28, 31–34]. A bi-institutional analysis of repeat liver resections for recurrent CRLM including 126 patients showed 1-, 3-, and 5-year survival rates of 86%, 51%, and 34%, respectively [35]. Favorable outcomes likely reflect careful selection of patients with limited disease and favorable tumor biology, the majority of patients in this study (71%) underwent minor liver-resections. Nanji et al. in a population-based study of 1310 patients who underwent hepatic resection for CRLM with 6% ($n = 78$) undergoing repeat resection, showed comparable short-term postoperative outcomes with trends towards higher rates of postoperative mortality and readmission rates although these were not statistically significant. Median overall-survival was 86 months and cancer-specific survival 74 months from time of initial liver resection. 5-year overall survival from time of first resection was 60% [36]. A systematic review of repeat hepatectomy for CRLM, included 22 observational studies with a total of 1610 patients reporting a recurrence rate of 64% at median follow-up of 32 months. Median overall survival was 35 months, with 3- and 5-year survival rates of 55% and 42%, respectively [37]. As mentioned, parenchymal-preserving strategies with initial hepatectomy, afford further options for subsequent operation in the case of liver recurrence.

Resection may be of benefit in the setting of concurrent extrahepatic disease. Leung et al. in their retrospective review of 219 patients who underwent hepatectomy for CRLM and resection of synchronous extrahepatic disease showed that long-term survival was possible but that true cure was rare [38]. Pulmonary colorectal metastases are amendable to resection when the primary tumor has been resected for cure (R0) and complete resection of lung disease with maintenance of adequate lung function is attainable. Additionally, re-resection of pulmonary lesions may be considered in select patients [13]. Five-year overall survival of 49% has been reported for re-resection of hepatic and pulmonary metastasis [39]. Other modalities for management of pulmonary metastases include ablative techniques and stereotactic beam radiation therapy (SBRT) both of which are potential treatment options for liver disease and will be discussed further.

There are scenarios where even when disease is resectable, this may not be the best option for the patient. Passot et al. looked at outcomes comparing *RAS* mutation status, with mutated *RAS* representing 15–35% of colorectal cancer patients. They defined three high-risk factors associated with poor prognosis: largest liver metastasis >3 cm, more than seven cycles of pre-operative chemotherapy, and node positive primary tumor. Those patients with all three factors were found to have a median survival of only 22 months with no 4-year survivors. Their survival outcomes are comparable to patients treated with modern chemotherapy alone leading authors to conclude that hepatectomy may be ill advised in patients with this mutational status [40]. Additionally, *RAS* mutations have been associated with a higher incidence of extra-hepatic brain, bone and lung relapse, reflective of poor tumor biology [41, 42].

Similarly, *BRAF* mutations, reported in 2–4% of CRLM, are poor prognostic biomarkers associated with worse survival outcomes after liver resection [42–44]. The low frequency of this mutation in resected CRLM is likely attributable to the fact that *BRAF* mutant colorectal cancer patients more commonly develop peritoneal metastases and less frequency liver-limited disease and are therefore often are not amenable to surgical metastasectomy [44]. In a multicenter trial from Italy, patients who underwent liver resection for CRLM with available mutational status data were analyzed. *BRAF* mutants had the worst recurrence free and overall survival, 5.7 and 22.6 months, respectively [42]. As we begin to better understand tumor genomics, mutational status should be considered in clinical decision making of CRLM management.

Systemic Treatment

Systemic chemotherapy plays an important role in the multimodal treatment of CRLM. With disease recurrence that is unresectable the realistic goal of systemic treatment is palliative. Modern chemotherapeutic and biologics have resulted in prolonged median overall survival in patients with CRLM between 29 and 37 months [45, 46]. Standard first-line combinations include cytotoxics 5-fluorouracil or capecitabine in combination with oxaliplatin (FOLFOX or CAPOX) or irinotecan (FOLFIRI). A 3-drug combination (FOLOXIRI) can be considered in younger patients with good performance status, but it is associated with significant toxicity. Targeted agents including bevacizumab for *RAS* mutants and bevacizumab, cetuximab, or panitumumab for *RAS* wild-type tumors are now standard of care.

Generally intensive first line strategies are used for a period followed by less intensive, maintenance therapy, until progression. The CAIRO3 study, a Phase III multicenter randomized controlled trial, assessed capecitabine plus bevacizumab maintenance therapy following six cycles of intensive first line treatment, CAPOX-bevacizumab. This regimen was found to be effective without compromising quality of life [47].

Testing for mismatch-repair (MMR) status is indicated, as immunotherapy is an option in a subset of patients based on genetic status. Le et al. evaluated pembrolizumab, an antiprogrammed death 1 immune checkpoint inhibitor, in patients with treatment refractory metastatic colorectal cancer. MMR-deficient colorectal cancer was compared to MMR-proficient colorectal cancer and MMR-deficient other primary cancers. Immune-related objective response rate and immune-related progression-free survival rates were reported as 40% and 78%, respectively, for

MMR-deficient colorectal cancer patients, superior to MMR-proficient patients, 0% and 11%, respectively. Similar results were observed for MMR-deficient non-colorectal cancer [48]. Newer targeted therapies and clinical trials of such may be options for patients and should be explored for treatment refractory patients.

Once tumors become chemo-refractory, survival estimates are poor, 4–5 months [49–51]. Palliative chemotherapy was once the only option; however, locoregional strategies have been investigated in patients with chemo-refractory disease with reasonable results. Options include ablation, hepatic artery infusion (HAI) chemotherapy, radioembolization (^{90}Y), transarterial embolization (bland or chemo), and SBRT (Fig. 42.2).

Locoregional Therapy

Ablation

Ablation includes radiofrequency, microwave, cryoablation, and irreversible electroporation. It is a locoregional alternative to resection that can be used with curative or palliative intent. If complete ablation can be performed, which may be more parenchymal sparing for certain tumors, especially in patients who have previously undergone liver resection, this treatment option can be potentially curative. Under image guidance, ablation can be performed percutaneously, laparoscopically, or by open surgery destroying liver tumors without removing them. Ideal candidates are patients with inadequate liver function, anatomic distribution incompatible with resection, or significant comorbid conditions making resection less desirable. Complications range from low-grade fevers, transient elevations of liver function tests and abdominal pain to hemorrhage, abscess, biloma, biliary fistula, hepatic insufficiency, arteriovenous fistulas, portal vein thromboses, diaphragmatic hernia, tumor implantation, and thermal injury to surrounding structures [52]. A standardized post ablation protocol has not been defined. Both laboratory (CEA) and imaging (contrast enhanced ultrasound, CT, MRI, or PET-CT) surveillance at 1 and 3 months is recommended to ensure complete treatment, followed by return to previous surveillance protocol.

No randomized data is available comparing ablation to resection for CRLM or CRLM recurrence. A meta-analysis including 13 studies published between 2003 and 2011 compared radiofrequency ablation to surgical resection finding inferior overall survival and disease-free survival with ablation [53]. Otto et al., in a prospective nonrandomized trial of radiofrequency ablation compared to resection in early CRLM amenable to surgery found that survival did not depend on the treatment modality, but that local recurrence was significantly higher after ablation (32% vs. 4%, $p < 0.001$) [54]. Similarly, when compared to surgical re-resection, ablation results in shorter progression free survival (10.2 vs. 4.3 months, $p = 0.002$); however, median overall survival was reported as the same,

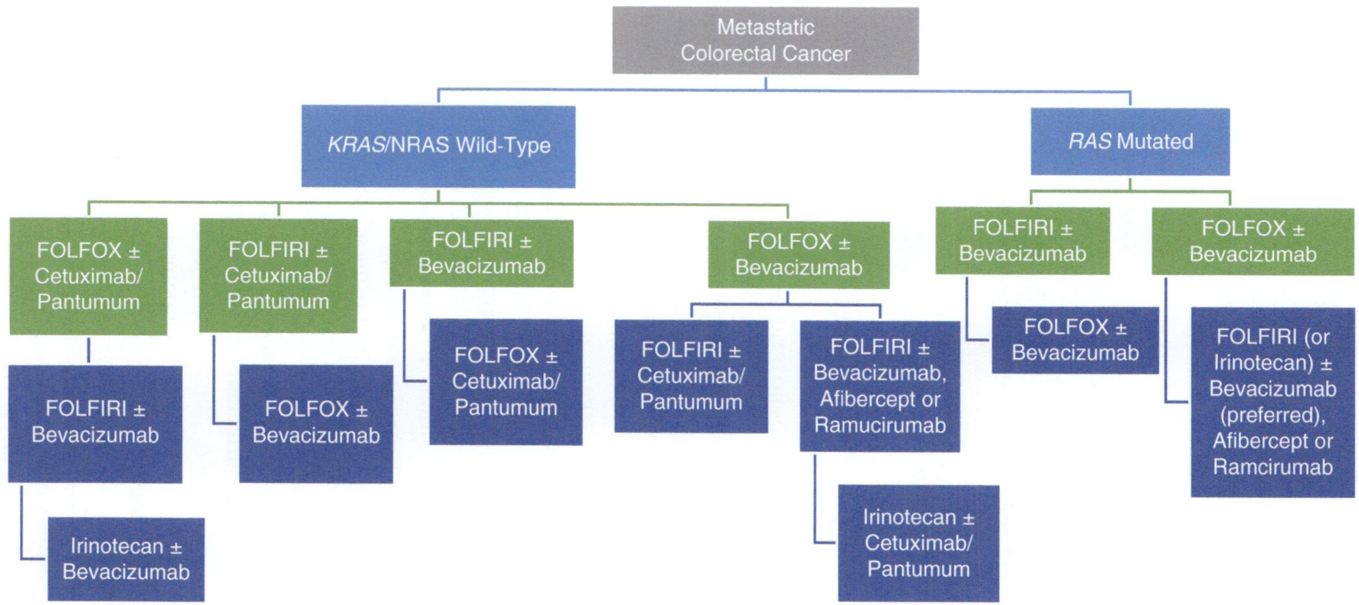

Fig. 42.2 Systemic treatment options. 5-fluorouracil (5-FU) can be substituted with capecitabine. FOLFIRI, 5-FU and irinotecan; FOLFOX, 5-FU and oxaliplatin. Cytotoxic triplet therapy of FOLFOXIRI (5-FU, oxaliplatin and irinotecan) can be considered in carefully selected, fit patients

33.3 months. Ablation is associated with shorter hospital stay (1 vs. 5 days, $p = 2 \times 10^{-10}$) and post-procedure morbidity has been reported as significantly lower (12.1% vs. 38.7%, $p = 0.021$) [55]. So long as a complete ablation can be performed, the results would be expected to be similar to an adequately performed resection.

Synergy of ablative techniques with other treatment modalities has been demonstrated. Combining intra-operative ablation with resection in cases that would otherwise be unresectable has shown favorable results [56]. The CLOCC trial, a prospective randomized trial comparing systemic therapy alone to systemic therapy in combination with ablation with or without surgical resection for unresectable CRLM, demonstrated both improved progression free survival and overall survival with combination therapy ($p = 0.01$) [57]. The therapeutic debate continues for CRLM amenable to resection; however, ablation has established a role and is particularly appealing in cases of CRLM recurrence when resection may be particularly challenging if not impossible.

Hepatic Arterial Infusion (HAI) Chemotherapy

HAI of chemotherapy, specifically floxuridine (FUDR), is possible through a surgically implantable subcutaneous pump connected to a catheter placed in the gastroduodenal artery. Hepatic lesions derive the majority of their blood supply from hepatic arterial inflow in comparison to normal liver parenchyma, receiving majority of blood from the portal vein, thus maximizing treatment effects. HAI treatment is complex and requires multidisciplinary skills in placement and management. The chemotherapeutic agent of choice, FUDR, is ideal because of its high first pass extraction in the liver. This enables high doses of treatment with minimal systemic exposure [58]. Biliary toxicities can be significant. The administration of dexamethasone through the pump has been found to decrease rates; however, it is important to closely monitor liver function tests while receiving treatment [59]. Other complications include thrombosis, dislodgement, extrahepatic perfusion, incomplete perfusion, pump malfunction, pocket infection, hematoma, pump migration, catheter occlusion, dislodgement, erosion, arterial hemorrhage [60].

Ammori et al. reported a decade of experience with HAI in combination with systemic therapy for conversion of unresectable CRLM. Despite extensive disease, 25% of patients responded sufficiently to undergo resection or ablation of their CRLM. During the study period, 14 patients underwent repeat resection or ablation for recurrence. Median 5-year survival from pump placement was 59 months in the conversion group compared to 16 months in the nonconversion group ($p < 0.001$) [61]. With combination HAI and systemic chemotherapy for unresectable CRLM, conversion rates as high as 47% have been reported [62].

Randomized controlled trials are needed in the assessment of HAI treatments to better define their role in the current era of systemic chemotherapeutics. In patients with unresectable CRLM HAI given in conjunction with systemic chemotherapy can improve response rates and increase the number of patients who go onto liver resection. Currently, HAI chemotherapy should be considered in patient with disease confined to the liver who have progressed on first line chemotherapy.

Selective Internal Radiation Therapy (SIRT)

Selective internal radiation therapy (SIRT) or radioembolization with yttrium-90 (^{90}Y), a high-radiation beta-emitter bonded to resin or glass microspheres, has been used in tumors refractory to chemotherapy. Colorectal cancer cells are highly radiosensitive and tumors have increased microvascular density; therefore, delivery of intra-arterial brachytherapy results in high tumoral concentrations based on the principle that the blood supply of hepatic tumors is different than normal liver parenchyma. Segmental or lobar delivery can be utilized.

SIRT for liver tumors was first reported in 1965 [63]. It utilization for salvage therapy has shown consistent results with median overall survival of 10.5 months reported in several studies [64–67]. Common side effects include fatigue, abdominal pain, and nausea. Importantly, low rates of biochemical toxicity have been reported. Providers should be aware of uncommon, but serious side effects including radiation induced gastric ulcers, lymphocytopenia, jaundice, cholecystitis, lung toxicity, hepatic abscess, radiation hepatitis, and liver failure [68].

The Metastatic colorectal cancer liver metastases Outcomes after RadioEmbolization (MORE) study included 606 patients reporting a median overall survival from the first treatment with ^{90}Y of 9.6 months. Performance status, tumor burden, number of previous chemotherapeutics, liver function, and no extra-hepatic disease predicted better survival. The collection period predated utilization of biologic chemotherapy agents and included a large proportion (35%) of patients with extra-hepatic disease who benefit less from liver-directed therapy (7.4 vs. 12.1 month survival; $p < 0.001$) [69]. Hickey et al. in a multi-institutional review of 531 patients reported median overall survival from diagnosis of primary colorectal tumor of 48.7 months, from diagnosis of CRLM of 37.7 months, and from ^{90}Y treatment of 10.6 months. Again, outcomes were significantly better without extra-hepatic disease 14.4 months vs. 6.6 months ($p < 0.001$). Of note, 18% of patients had prior hepatic resection, 14% of patients had prior ablation, and 4% prior transarterial chemoembolization (TACE) [64]. Combined analysis of three multicenter randomized phase 3 trials, FOXFIRE, SIRFLOX, and FOXFIRE-Global showed that addition of SIRT to first-line chemotherapy for patient with liver-only or liver-dominant CRLM resulted in equivalent survival [70]. Given the results of these studies SIRT, and in particular ^{90}Y microspheres, should be considered in highly selected patients with chemotherapy-refractory disease and predominant hepatic metastases.

The use of SIRT in down-staging for resection has been reported with favorable results [71, 72]. Conversion to resection has been reported at rates of 9–85%; however, most series include population with mixed primary pathologies and are biased by patient selection [72–74]. With the combined benefits of selective tumor treatment and induction of hypertrophy of untreated liver segments, the role of SIRT in down-staging should be further explored. Of note, traditional perfusion of hepatic segments cannot be assumed following previous liver resection; therefore, SIRT treatment and subsequent resection in the case of CRLM recurrence must be carefully planned.

TACE

Another transarterial treatment modality, TACE, targets tumor ischemia by embolization with delivery of intraarterial chemotherapy. TACE is most commonly used for unresectable hepatocellular carcinoma, but both bland hepatic artery embolization and TACE have been used for local control after CRLM progression during systemic chemotherapy. A randomized controlled trial of 70 patients compared drug-eluting beads with irinotecan (DEBIRI) in combination with FOLFOX to systemic chemotherapy alone showing improved overall response rate (76% vs. 60% at 6 months, $p = 0.05$) and median progression-free survival (15.3 vs. 7.6 months) with the addition of TACE [75]. Subsequent systematic review, including this study as well as 5 observational studies, of TACE with the use DEBIRI for unresectable CRLM reported improvement in median survival from 15 to 25 months [76]. This treatment is indicated after failure of other modalities, and more recently in conjunction with other locoregional treatments.

Stereotactic Bean Radiation Therapy (SBRT)

SBRT has enabled delivery of greater combined doses of radiation over the course of fewer treatments with local-control results comparable to resection with far fewer risks. Outcomes of SBRT for CRLM in a 60 patient cohort reported local control of 50% at 1-year and 26% at 4-years [77]. The results of the international multi-institutional RSSearch® Patient Registry, which included 427 patients with liver metastasis, CRLM being the most common (44%), showed a median overall survival of 27 months with 76% 1-year survival [78]. Risk of recurrence correlates with increased tumor size as well as dose regimen with documented tumor control of greater than 80% when optimized [79]. Radiation has also been used as salvage therapy for bilateral CRLM not amenable to second-stage hepatectomy [80].

Systematic prospective studies are required to further endorse this treatment option in the setting of CRLM. Currently SBRT can be considered in carefully selected patients or in the setting of a clinical trial. The benefits of this treatment modality include the short treatment time course with delivery over only a few fractions, the lack of need for recovery, as well as a favorable toxicity profile.

Conclusion

In summary, approximately 60% of patients with treated CRLM will develop disease recurrence. Of these, two-thirds will have recurrent liver metastases. Overall survival of 74.3% following hepatectomy in patients without recurrence and 57.5% in patients with recurrent disease have been reported by Hallet et al. in the era of contemporary chemotherapy [12]. The ability to address recurrent metastatic disease within the liver justifies close surveillance after metastasectomy with frequent clinical encounters, tumor markers, and imaging based on local guidelines. Intra-hepatic recurrence should be approached similarly to the initial presentation of CRLM. Re-staging must be performed to assess both intra- and extra-hepatic disease burden. In the case of liver recurrence amenable to resection hepatectomy should be considered, taking into account patient performance status and volume of the future liver remnant. Systemic therapy will play a role for all patients, with new targeted therapies and clinical trials providing options for chemorefractory disease. Liver-directed therapies including ablation, HAI chemotherapy, SIRT, TACE, and SBRT provide a large armamentarium of options for palliation. With continuously evolving treatment options, multidisciplinary care is critical in CRLM recurrence.

References

1. Siegel RL, Miller KD, Jemal A. Cancer statistics, 2018. CA Cancer J Clin. 2018;68:7–30.
2. Wei AC, Greig PD, Grant D, et al. Survival after hepatic resection for colorectal metastases: a 10-year experience. Ann Surg Oncol. 2006;13:668–76.
3. Wicherts DA, Miller R, de Haas RJ, et al. Long-term results of two stage hepatectomy for irresectable colorectal cancer liver metastases. Ann Surg. 2008;248:994–1005.
4. Choti MA, Sitzmann JV, Tiburi MF, et al. Trends in long-term survival following liver resection for hepatic colorectal metastases. Ann Surg. 2002;235:759–66.
5. Nanji S, Cleary S, Ryan P, et al. Up-front hepatic resection for metastatic colorectal cancer results in favorable long-term survival. Ann Surg Oncol. 2013;20:295–304.
6. House MG, Ito H, Gonen M, et al. Survival after hepatic resection for metastatic colorectal cancer: trends in outcomes for 1,600 patients during two decades at a single institution. J Am Coll Surgeons. 2010;210:744–52. 752–745.
7. Abdalla EK, Vauthey JN, Ellis LM, et al. Recurrence and outcomes following hepatic resection, radiofrequency ablation, and combined resection/ablation for colorectal liver metastases. Ann Surg. 2004;239:818–25.
8. Riihimaki M, Hemminki A, Sundquist J, et al. Patterns of metastasis in colon and rectal cancer. Sci Rep. 2016;6:29765.
9. Kun-Ming C, Tsung-Han W, Chih-Hsien C, Wei-Chen L, Jy-Ming C, Jinn-Shiun C, Jeng-Yi W. Prognostic significance of the number of tumors and aggressive surgical approach in colorectal cancer hepatic metastasis. World J Surg Oncol. 2014;12:155.
10. Min-Su P, Nam-Joon Y, Sang-Yong S, Tae Y, Suk-Won S, Young Rok C, Ki H, Geun H, Kyoung Bun L, et al. Histopathologic factors affecting tumor recurrence after hepatic resection in colorectal liver metastases. Ann Surg Treat Res. 2014;87(1):14–21.
11. Tomlinson JS, Jarnagin WR, DeMatteo RP, et al. Actual 10-year survival after resection of colorectal liver metastases defines cure. J Clin Oncol. 2007;25:4575–80.

12. Hallet J, Sa Cunha A, Adams R, et al. Factors influencing recurrence following initial hepatectomy for colorectal liver metastases. BJS. 2016;103:1366–76.
13. NCCN Clinical Practice Guidelines in Oncology (NCCN Guidelines): Colon Cancer. Version 2.2018, March 14, 2018. Available at: https://www.nccn.org/professionals/physician_gls/pdf/colon.pdf.
14. Hyder O, Dodson RM, Mayo SC, et al. Post-treatment surveillance of patients with colorectal cancer with surgically treated liver metastases. Surgery. 2013;154:256–65.
15. Lee DH, Lee JM, Hur BY, et al. Colorectal cancer liver metastases: diagnostic performance and prognostic value of PET/MR imaging. Radiology. 2016;280:782–92.
16. Steele S, Chang G, Hendren S, et al. Practice guideline for the surveillance of patients after curative treatment of colon and rectal cancer. Dis Colon Rectum. 2015;58:713–25.
17. Glynne-Jones R, Wyrwicz L, Tiret E, et al. Rectal cancer: ESMO clinical practice guidelines for diagnosis, treatment and follow-up. Ann Oncol. 2017;28:iv22–40.
18. Van Cutsem E, Cervantes A, Nordlinger B, et al. Metastatic colorectal cancer: ESMO clinical practice guidelines for diagnosis, treatment and follow-up. Ann Oncol. 2014;25:ii1–9.
19. Watanabe T, Muro K, Ajioka Y, et al. Japanese Society for Cancer of the Colon and Rectum (JSCCR) guidelines 2016 for the treatment of colorectal cancer. Int J Clin Oncol. 2018;23:1–34.
20. Cancer Care Ontario: Colorectal Cancer Follow-up Care Pathway Map. Version 2018.03, March 14, 2018. Available at: https://www.cancercareontario.ca/sites/ccocancercare/files/assets/DPMColorectalFollowUp.pdf.
21. Moulton CA, Gu CS, Law CH, et al. Effect of PET before liver resection on surgical management for colorectal adenocarcinoma metastases: a randomized clinical trial. JAMA. 2014;311:1863–9.
22. Fernandez FG, Drebin JA, Linehan DC, et al. Five-year survival after resection of hepatic metastases from colorectal cancer in patients screened by positron emission tomography with F-18 fluorodeoxyglucose (FGG-PET). Ann Surg. 2004;240:438–47.
23. Fernandez FG, Ritter J, Goodwin JW, Linehan DC, Hawkins WG, Strasberg SM. Effect of steatohepatitis associated with irinotecan or oxaliplatin pretreatment on resectability of hepatic colorectal metastases. J Am Coll Surg. 2005;200:845–53.
24. Vauthey JN, Pawlik TM, Ribero D, et al. Chemotherapy regimen predicts steatohepatitis and an increase in 90-day mortality after surgery for hepatic colorectal metastases. J Clin Oncol. 2006;24:2065–72.
25. Zorzi D, Laurent A, Pawlik TM, Lauwers GY, Vauthey JN, Abdalla EK. Chemotherapy-associated hepatotoxicity and surgery for colorectal liver metastases. Br J Surg. 2007;94:274–86.
26. Morris-Stiff G, Tan YM, Vauthey JN. Hepatic complications following preoperative chemotherapy with oxaliplatin or irinotecan for hepatic colorectal metastases. Eur J Surg Oncol. 2008;34:609–14.
27. De Jong MC, Pulitano C, Ribero D, et al. Rates and patterns of recurrence following curative intent surgery for colorectal liver metastasis: an international multi-institutional analysis of 1669 patients. Ann Surg. 2009;250:440–8.
28. Butte JM, Gonen M, Allen PJ, et al. Recurrence after partial hepatectomy for metastatic colorectal cancer: the potentially curative role of salvage re-resection. Ann Surg Oncol. 2015;22:2761–71.
29. Dupre A, Lefranc A, Buc E, et al. Use of bioresorbable membranes to reduce abdominal and perihepatic adhesions in 2-stage hepatectomy of liver metastases form colorectal cancer: results of a prospective, randomized controlled phase II trial. Ann Surg. 2013;258:30–6.
30. Lange JF, Leese T, Casting D, Bismuth H. Repeat hepatectomy for recurrent malignant tumors of the liver. Surg Gynecol Obstet. 1989;169:119–26.
31. Adair RA, Young AL, Cockbain AJ, et al. Repeat hepatic resection for colorectal liver metastases. Br J Surg. 2012;99:1278–83.
32. Pinson CW, Wright JK, Chapman WC, et al. Repeat hepatic surgery for colorectal cancer metastasis to the liver. Ann Surg. 1996;223:765–73. discussion 773–6
33. Lee H, Choi SH, Cho YB, et al. Repeat hepatic resection in patients with colorectal liver metastases. World J Gastroenterol. 2015;21:2124–30.

34. Saiura A, Yamamoto J, Koga R, et al. Favorable outcome after repeat resection for colorectal liver metastases. Ann Surg Oncol. 2014;21:4293–9.
35. Petrowsky H, Gonen M, Jarnagin W, et al. Second liver resections are safe and effective treatment for recurrent hepatic metastases from colorectal cancer: a bi-institutional analysis. Ann Surg. 2002;235:863–71.
36. Nanji S, Tsang ME, Wei X, et al. Outcomes after repeat hepatic resection for recurrent metastatic colorectal cancer: a population-based study. Am J Surg. 2017;213:1053–9.
37. Lam VWT, Pang T, Laurence JM, et al. A systematic review of repeat hepatectomy for recurrent colorectal liver metastases. J Gastrointest Surg. 2013;17:1312–21.
38. Leung U, Gonen M, Allen P, et al. Colorectal cancer liver metastases and concurrent extrahepatic disease treated with resection. Ann Surg. 2017;265:158–65.
39. Bellier J, De Wolf J, Hebbar M, et al. Repeated resections of hepatic and pulmonary metastasis from colorectal cancer provide long-term survival. World J Surg. 2018;42(4):1171–9.
40. Passot G, Denbo JW, Yamashita S, et al. Is hepatectomy justified for patients with *RAS* mutant colorectal liver metastases? An analysis of 524 patients undergoing curative liver resection. Surgery. 2017;161:332–40.
41. Kemeny N, Chou J, Capanu M, et al. KRAS mutation influences recurrence patterns in patients undergoing hepatic resection of colorectal metastases. Cancer. 2014;120:3965–71.
42. Schirripa M, Bergamo F, Cremolini C, et al. BRAF and RAS mutations as prognostic factors in metastatic colorectal cancer patients undergoing liver resection. Br J Cancer. 2015;9:1921–8.
43. Teng HW, Huang YC, Lin JK, et al. BRAF mutation is a prognostic biomarker for colorectal liver metastectomy. J Surg Oncol. 2012;106:123–9.
44. Yaeger R, Cereck A, Chou JF, et al. BRAF mutation predicts for poor outcomes after metastectomy in patients with metastatic colorectal cancer. Cancer. 2014;120:2316–24.
45. Heinemann V, von Weikersthal LF, Decker T, et al. FOLFIRI plus cetuximab versus FOLFIRI plus bevacizumab as first-line treatment for patients with metastatic colorectal cancer (FIRE-3): a randomised, open-label, phase 3 trial. Lancet Oncol. 2014;15:1065–75.
46. Cremolini C, Loupakis F, Antoniotti C, et al. FOLFOXIRI plus bevacizumab versus FOLFIRI plus bevacizumab as first-line treatment of patients with metastatic colorectal cancer: updated overall survival and molecular subgroup analysis of the open-label, phase 3 TRIBE study. Lancet Oncol. 2015;16:1306–15.
47. Simkens LH, van Tinteren H, ten Tije AJ, et al. Maintenance treatment with capecitabine and bevacizumab in metastatic colorectal cancer (CAIRO3): a phase 3 randomised controlled trial of the Dutch colorectal cancer group. Lancet. 2015;9:1843–52.
48. Le CT, Uram JN, Wang H, et al. PD-1 blockade in tumors with mismatch-repair deficiency. N Engl J Med. 2015;372:2509–20.
49. Grothey A, Van Cutsem E, Sobrero A, et al. Regorafenib monotherapy for previously treated metastatic colorectal cancer (CORRECT): an international, multicentre, randomised, placebo-controlled, phase 3 trial. Lancet. 2013;381:303–12.
50. Karapetis CS, Khambata-Ford S, Jonker DJ, et al. K-ras mutations and benefit from cetuximab in advanced colorectal cancer. N Engl J Med. 2008;359:1757–65.
51. Jonker DJ, O'Callaghan CJ, Karapetis CS, et al. Cetuximab for the treatment of colorectal cancer. N Engl J Med. 2007;357:2040–8.
52. Gervais DA, Goldberg SN, Brown DB, et al. Society of interventional radiology position statement on percutaneous radiofrequency ablation for the treatment of liver tumors. J Vasc Interv Radiol. 2009;20:S42–7.
53. Weng M, Zhang Y, Zhou D, et al. Radiofrequency ablation versus resection for colorectal liver metastases: a meta-analysis. PLoS One. 2012;7:e45493.
54. Otto G, Duber C, Hoppe-Lotichius M, et al. Radiofrequency ablation as first-line treatment in patients with early colorectal liver metastases amenable to surgery. Ann Surg. 2010;251:796–803.
55. Dupre A, Jones RP, Diaz-Nieto R, et al. Curative-intent treatment of recurrent colorectal liver metastases: a comparison between ablation and resection. Eur J Surg Oncol. 2017;43:1901–7.

56. Van Amerongen MJ, van der Stok EP, Futterer JJ, et al. Short term and long term results of patients with colorectal liver metastases undergoing surgery with or without radiofrequency ablation. Eur J Surg Oncol. 2016;42:523–30.
57. Ruers T, Van Coevorden F, Punt CJ, et al. Local treatment of unresectable colorectal liver metastases: results of a randomized phase II trial. J Natl Cancer Inst. 2017;109:djx015.
58. Ensminger WD, Gyves JW. Clinical pharmacology of hepatic arterial chemotherapy. Semin Oncol. 1983;10:176–82.
59. Kemeny N, Conti JA, Cohen A, et al. Phase II study of hepatic arterial floxuridine, leucovorin, and dexamethasone for unresectable liver metastases from colorectal carcinoma. J Clin Oncol. 1994;12:2288–95.
60. Allen PJ, Nissan A, Picon AI, et al. Technical complications oand durability of hepatic artery infusion pumps for unresectable colorectal liver metastases: an institutional experience of 544 consecutive cases. J Am Coll Surg. 2005;201:57–65.
61. Ammori JB, Kemeny NE, Fong Y, et al. Conversion to complete resection and/or ablation using hepatic artery infusional chemotherapy in patients with unresectable liver metastases from colorectal cancer: a decade of experience at a single institution. Ann Surg Oncol. 2013;20:2901–7.
62. D'Angelica MI, Correa-Gallego C, Paty PB, et al. Phase II trial of hepatic artery infusional and systemic chemotherapy for patients with unresectable hepatic metastases from colorectal cancer: conversion to resection and long-term outcomes. Ann Surg. 2015;261:353–60.
63. Ariel IM. Treatment of inoperable primary pancreatic and liver cancer by the intra-arterial administration of radioactive isotopes (y90 radiating microspheres). Ann Surg. 1965;162:267–78.
64. Hickey R, Lewandowski RJ, Prudhomme T, et al. ^{90}Y radioembolization of colorectal hepatic metastases using glass microspheres: safety and survival outcomes from a 531-patient multicenter study. J Nucl Med. 2016;57:665–71.
65. Saxena A, Meteling B, Kapoor J, Golani S, Morris DL, Bester L. Is yttrium-90 radioembolization a viable treatment option for unresectable, chemorefractory colorectal cancer liver metastases? A large single-center experience of 302 patients. Ann Surg Oncol. 2015;22:794–802.
66. Lewandowski RJ, Memon K, Mulcahy MF, et al. Twelve-year experience of radioembolization for colorectal hepatic metastases in 214 patients: survival by era and chemotherapy. Eur J Nucl Med Mol Imaging. 2014;41:1861–9.
67. Kennedy AS, Coldwell D, Nutting C, et al. Resin 90Y-microsphere brachytherapy for unresectable colorectal liver metastases: modern USA experience. Int J Radiat Oncol Biol Phys. 2006;65:412–25.
68. Riaz A, Awais R, Salem R. Side effects of yttrium-90 radioembolization. Front Oncol. 2014;4:198.
69. Kennedy AS, Ball D, Cohen SJ, et al. Multicenter evaluation of the safety and efficacy of radioembolization in patients with unresectable colorectal liver metastases selected as candidates for (90)Y resin microspheres. J Gastrointest Oncol. 2015;6:134–42.
70. Wasan HS, Gibbs P, Sharma NK, et al. First-line selective internal radiotherapy plus chemotherapy versus chemotherapy alone in patients with liver metastases from colorectal cancer (FOLFIRE, SIRFLOX, and FOXFIRE-Global): a combined analysis of three multicentre, randomised, phase 3 trials. Lancet Oncol. 2017;18:1159–71.
71. Braat MNGJA, Samim M, van den Bosch MAAJ, et al. The role of ^{90}Y-radioembolization in downstaging primary and secondary hepatic malignancies: a systematic review. Clin Transl Imaging. 2016;4:283–95.
72. Justinger C, Kouladouros K, Gartner D, et al. Liver resection after selective internal radiotherapy (SIRT): proof of concept, intial survival, and safety. J Surg Oncol. 2015;112:436–42.
73. Whitney R, Tatum C, Hahl M, et al. Safety of hepatic resection in metastatic disease to the liver after yttrium-90 therapy. J Surg Res. 2011;166:236–40.
74. Moir JA, Burns J, Barnes J, et al. Selective internal radiation therapy for liver malignancies. Br J Surg. 2015;102:1533–40.

75. Martin RC 2nd, Scoggins CR, Schreeder M, et al. Randomized controlled trial of irinotecan drug-eluting beads with simultaneous FOLFOX and bevacizumab for patients with unresectable colorectal liver-limited metastases. Cancer. 2015;121:3649–58.
76. Richardson AJ, Laurence JM, Lam VW. Transarterial chemoembolization with irinotecan beads in the treatment of colorectal liver metastases: as ystematic revie. J Vasc Interv Radiol. 2013;24:1209–17.
77. McPartlin A, Swaminath A, Wang R, et al. Long-term outcomes of phase 1 and 2 studies of SPBRT for hepatic colorectal metastases. Int J Radiat Oncol Biol Phys. 2017;99:388–95.
78. Mahadevan A, Blanck O, Lanciano R, et al. Stereotactic body radiotherapy (SBRT) for liver metastasis – clinical outcomes from the international multi-institutional RSSearch® patient registry. Radiat Oncol. 2018;13:26.
79. Rule W, Timmerman R, Tong L, et al. Phase I dose-escalation study of stereotactic body radiotherapy in patients with hepatic metastases. Ann Surg Oncol. 2011;18:1081–7.
80. Colbert LE, Cloyd JM, Koay EJ, et al. Proton beam radiation as salvage therapy for bilateral colorectal liver metastases not amenable to second-stage hepatectomy. Surgery. 2017;161:1543–8.

Index

M. M. Correia et al. (eds.), *Colorectal Cancer Liver Metastases*,
https://doi.org/10.1007/978-3-030-25486-5

M

R

T

MIX
Papier aus verantwortungsvollen Quellen
Paper from responsible sources
FSC® C105338

If you have any concerns about our products,
you can contact us on
ProductSafety@springernature.com

In case Publisher is established outside the EU,
the EU authorized representative is:
Springer Nature Customer Service Center GmbH
Europaplatz 3, 69115 Heidelberg, Germany

Printed by Libri Plureos GmbH
in Hamburg, Germany